Victory over Fat

Victory over Fat

6 Steps to Permanent Fat Loss and Super Health

Dr. Ric Alexander

Galahad Publishing   North Hollywood, California

Victory over Fat
6 Steps to Permanent Fat Loss and Super Health

Galahad Publishing
P.O. Box 5451
North Hollywood, CA 91606-5451

GalahadPublishing.com

Book design by Galahad Publishing design staff & Casa Graphics, Inc.

First Edition: 2005

Publisher's Cataloging-in-Publication
Alexander, Ric, 1950-
    Victory over fat : 6 steps to permanent fat loss and super health / Ric Alexander. – 1st ed.
    p. cm.
    Includes bibliographical references and index.
    LCCN 2005923529
    ISBN 0-918483-10-7

    1. Weight loss. 2. Nutrition. 3. Mind and body.
I. Title.

RM222.2.A3795 2005   613.2'5
                                 QBI05-200083

Printed in the United States of America
Printed on acid-free paper

10 9 8 7 6 5 4 3 2 1

*This book is dedicated to everyone who makes the choice
to trust in the wisdom of Nature to help them find the truth
of healthful and joyful living.*

*A special dedication goes to D.J.
for her encouragement, love and support.*

SPECIAL NOTICE TO THE READER

The information contained in this book is not intended as medical advice or to replace the professional services of a qualified physician. All information is true to the best of the author's knowledge. Sources used were deemed to be accurate and the author's opinions are based on almost forty years of nutritional and psychological study, personal experience and the observation of others.

The information contained herein is not intended to diagnose or recommend treatment for any disease. It is meant solely to entertain, educate and to stimulate the desire for balanced health and further study. Readers should always use their own good sense and seek the advice of a qualified professional in any area that they may have questions. The consequences of any actions recommended in this book are the sole responsibility of the person taking those actions.

CONTENTS

three

Meet Your New Friends

four

five

six

For Your Body Only

seven

Making the Change

eleven

Lean for Life—Physical Causes of Excess Fat

twelve

Lean for Life—Emotional Causes of Excess Fat

thirteen

Being Lean   399

PREFACE

I have always been fascinated by the incredible vehicle we call the human body as well as extremely curious about the workings of the human mind and spirit. Most of my life has been spent learning about these three aspects of our being. My goal has been to learn how to supply each one with what it needs for optimal health and how to achieve and maintain balance among them. I felt that doing this would lead to the healthiest, happiest and most productive life possible.

I am not sure what motivated me to study these things, but I remember observing older people when I was a young boy. Some were fat and plagued with diseases such as diabetes or heart disease. They looked tired and old. Many of these people's actions did not make sense to me. I also saw other people of the same age, who were lean, active and healthy. It seemed obvious that they had to be living a different lifestyle than the others were. I wanted to be like the healthy ones and hoped to someday be able to inspire others to be lean and healthy. I set out to learn all I could about being healthy in body, mind and spirit. I wanted to embody the best qualities of all those who inspired me.

As I observed people and their behaviors, I noticed that those who had high blood pressure were put on low salt diets. It seemed that eating less salt would be helpful at preventing that problem and perhaps many others. I saw people who got fat and developed diabetes put on low sugar diets so it seemed wise to eat as little sugar as possible. This is how I have continued for more than thirty-seven years—constantly striving to learn more about the function of the human body, mind and spirit and how to supply their needs so optimal health and happiness can be enjoyed. I felt that many of the answers I was seeking could be found by comparing the habits of healthy people to those of unhealthy people. I also believed that studying Nature (our Creator) would supply vital answers to my questions. Of course, I read everything I could get my hands on about physical, emotional and spiritual health and used what I was learning to improve myself and my life.

This book could have been expanded with useless facts, figures, recipes and other fillers. It would have ended up being a thousand pages or more with the truth of healthful eating hidden under tons of trivia. This may have kept you from reading it, and if you did read it, you would have had a much harder time finding and learning the vital concepts. On the contrary, how to eat well could be written in approximately twenty-five pages. Few people, however, would follow the guidelines without first having the knowledge contained in the rest of this book.

You will learn not only what to eat, but also how, why and when. You will discover that eating and exercise are only part of the fat-loss process and you will be surprised by the many emotional and spiritual components. After you have read this book you should have all the pieces needed to complete the permanent fat-loss puzzle and see the big picture. You will have a practical understanding of how your body works and what it needs to be healthy and free of excess fat.

Repetition is the key to successful learning and why the most important ideas in this book are repeated a few times. Sometimes the principle applies in different circumstances but it was often done on purpose because before most of us truly understand something we usually have to see it a number of times. For the information in this book to improve your life, it must be thoroughly understood and then become a permanent part of your lifestyle.

I feel that I have discovered the answers to most of my questions and incorporated these truths into my life, but learning about these subjects is never-ending and always fascinating. I have done my best to share some of these answers in a way that can be easily understood and applied in your life so you can start enjoying the incredible benefits as soon as possible.

Dr. Ric Alexander

ACKNOWLEDGMENTS

I want to give recognition and thanks to all the nutrition and health researchers and pioneers who taught me most of what I know about being lean and healthy. Some wrote books or articles and others taught seminars. I also want to thank the authors of the thousands of magazine and newspaper articles who wrote about better health and improving one's life. I am in debt to all of them not only for my own health but also for providing most of the facts and many of the insights into healthful eating and joyful living found within the pages of this book.

Thanks go out to all of the patients who shared with me their nutritional experiences and insights or who offered encouragement and motivation for me to finish this book. I also want to give thanks to those who instilled in me the desire to be healthy and strong—my parents, numerous spiritual teachers, philosophers, psychologists, visionaries, and health pioneers. Men like Paul Bragg, Jack LaLanne, Ralph Waldo Emerson, Paavo Airola, Peary Radar and Ralph Waldo Trine to name just a few.

I want to recognize some of the role models who motivated me to work with consistent dedication toward the accomplishment of some of my physical goals. Some of these men include Charles Atlas, Steve Reeves, Larry Scott, Mike Mentzer and Bruce Lee.

I also want to thank David Pinion, D.J., Lois Carruth and Donna Maas for their help in editing this book, Jesse Farless and Peter Stiefel for their work on the cover, and Patty Weckbaugh for her formatting efforts.

An extra special thank you goes to Gerda, who gave her love, support and suggestions during many of the years that this book was being written.

I especially want to thank Nature for helping me to understand the principles of healthful living and for giving me the desire to be healthy and to share what I have learned with others.

You cannot teach a man anything;
You can only help him find it for himself.

Galileo

one

Why Another Book on Nutrition and What Can It Do For Me?

Congratulations, you now hold in your hands the information that explains how you can attain permanent fat loss and live a longer, healthier life. *If you choose*, you can finally end your struggle with excess fat and eliminate the frustration, wasted time and wasted money that go with it.

This book is different from other books about nutrition or weight loss because you will learn about providing healthful nutrition not just to your body but to your mind and spirit as well. To enjoy balanced health you must nourish all three because you are a total being—a triad of body, mind, and spirit. If your mind is unhealthy, even the most nutritious foods can be turned into harmful substances in your body. And, if your spirit (soul) is starving, your nutritional program will almost surely fail.

You will learn what to do *and* why you are doing it. If you do not have a good reason for eating well or do not understand the "why" of what you are doing, maintaining motivation and control is difficult. You will learn truths about yourself and about how Nature intends you to nourish your body. These truths will give you the power to change your thinking, which in turn will create the behaviors necessary to make and keep your body lean. This knowledge is vital, because if you do not thoroughly understand why you are following each step of the program your efforts will fall short of what could be achieved. Worse yet, you might give up, and this will ensure failure. Nevertheless, even if you follow just a few of my recommendations you will have less excess fat and be far healthier than you would have been.

Whenever you see the word *Nature* capitalized throughout this book, you may want to replace it with God, the Creator, Infinite Intelligence or whatever Higher Power you may believe exists. It is implied that Nature has intelligence because when I refer to Nature I am referring to the Creator of our bodies and the foods and other nutrients that will keep them healthy and lean.

The information in this book comes from more than thirty-seven years of nutritional study and personal experience, and almost twenty years of counseling others in proper eating and exercise. It is based on good sense, logic, scientific knowledge, discoveries of past researchers and aware individuals, human behavior, practical experience, and the observation of Nature's laws in an attempt to learn the truth about how to supply the human body, mind and spirit with what they need for optimal health. My comprehensive program consists of simplified and practical ways to apply everything I have learned. This information is meant to furnish you with what you need to accomplish your health goals and save you many years of wasted time and effort. Nature supplies the foods; I simply share with you the knowledge of how to enjoy optimal health from those foods. I have no "miracle" meals or diet drinks to sell you. These would need processing and would therefore not be healthful products. I have only one special interest to promote—your good health!

Not a "Diet" Book

This is not a "diet" book. It is a book about lasting change—changing you and your body from the inside out. This is the only way you can succeed, because the source of all permanent change is from within. You will learn how to get and stay lean the way Nature intended—by supplying your body with the nutrients it needs to be healthy—not by dieting. As you have most likely already experienced, diets do not work. Many do create temporary weight loss, but most are unbalanced and unhealthy. Some cause a loss of lean, healthy tissue, making it easier to gain fat after the diet ends.

One definition of insanity is repeating a behavior over and over but expecting a different outcome each time. Many people follow a diet, gain the weight back and then follow the same or a new diet hoping for different results each time. The yo-yo effect experienced is unhealthy—physically, mentally and emotionally.

After reading this book you will know more about the truth of healthful eating than most nutritionists. They have gone to school and studied nutrition but have seldom learned to eat healthfully or in a truly balanced way. That is why many of them have fat and unhealthy bodies. Some college nutrition teachers I had were grossly obese. They can quote the recommended dietary (daily) allowance (RDA) of every vitamin and give you the side effects of inadequate amounts, but with the balanced nutrition you will be getting, a vitamin deficiency is the last thing you need to be concerned about.

People often joke about how bad the food is in hospitals, not just for patients but for the staff as well. Unfortunately, this is no joke. These meals are some of the worst dietary atrocities you will ever see, yet are designed by people with college degrees in nutrition.

In 2002 I read an article in a "health" magazine that gave the fat loss suggestions of a university professor who teaches nutrition. She suggested drinking two cups of coffee and eating a bagel prior to exercising. Does using a stimulant like caffeine and eating a worthless processed flour product sound like a good way to supply energy for exercising to build strength or lose fat? You could take amphetamines to get energy and lose weight but I do not recommend it.

The same article suggested eating a processed cold cereal, milk, flavored yogurt, sponge cake, chocolate, and unripe bananas for workout energy. A few healthful foods were also listed but not many. It then suggested cornflakes, honey, pretzels, rice cakes and white bread after exercise to build muscle or increase endurance. I guarantee you that none of those foods will do either. Suggestions for the rest of the day included cheese pizza, ice cream, soft drinks, and table sugar. Keep in mind that this advice comes from someone who is teaching our future nutritionists.

Not long ago a patient gave me a list of foods her nutritionist said she could eat at any time, with or without meals. They were called "free foods." Out of twenty-one items there were only five I consider healthful. Most nutritional seminars taught by "experts" have coffee, soft drinks and unhealthful foods available for those who attend. Many people have fat bodies because of a lack of knowledge or misinformation. It is easy to understand why this is such a common problem when you look at the advice being given by dieticians, nutrition "experts" and through various "health" magazines, books, and other means.

Long before you finish this book you will know far more about nutrition and healthful eating than most doctors. You may already, because few medical schools even teach nutrition, and what is taught is about the equivalent of a high school health class. The students memorize trivial information about various vitamins and minerals instead of learning how to supply good nutrition to the body. Did you ever notice that many doctors are not lean or healthy? Studies have shown that the diets of doctors and their families are worse than the diets of average Americans. The life expectancy of doctors is fewer than sixty years—far below the national average. No, it is not the stress of their work that is killing them early because many of the rest of us have just as much stress. Most doctors spend many years studying disease but little time, if any, learning how to achieve or maintain good health. I was lucky because I had studied health for more than twenty-five years prior to becoming a doctor.

This book is not about losing "weight." It is about losing internal waste and excess body fat, enjoying optimal health, and *gaining* many other valuable benefits. In upcoming pages you will learn how to discover the physical and emotional causes of why you have excess fat. Prior to that you will learn what to eat that is right for your unique body, and also when, how and why. You will finally understand what "balanced nutrition" means and be taught how to harness the powers that made your body fat to make it lean. You will learn how to *be* a lean person instead of a fat person. You will learn that being lean and healthy is not difficult, time consuming or expensive. It is no harder than being fat and unhealthy. In fact, being fat is often more difficult, expensive and time consuming.

Look at what you are about to embark on as a grand adventure that will change you and your life forever in many wonderful ways. Do not fear the changes; embrace and enjoy them. You deserve them whether you believe you do or not.

Why Are So Many People Fat?

Every day you see magazines, newspapers, tabloids, fitness magazines, and numerous other media with headlines promising "Instant weight loss with no effort," "Lose 10 to 30 pounds in one week," "Lose weight without changing what you eat," and so forth. Supermarket shelves overflow with products labeled "Lite," "No fat," and "Natural" along with instant meal replacements and weight-loss shakes. News programs entice you to watch the entire broadcast with an upcoming story about the latest diet drug, diet book, celebrity weight-loss program, miracle cream or magic soap that promises to melt or wash your fat away. Weight-loss clinics make millions as their members lose weight and then usually gain it right back again. Bookstores often devote large sections to all the new "diet" crazes and celebrity cookbooks, and rarely does a day go by that you do not get a sales letter, e-mail, or flier on your windshield announcing some miraculous new weight-loss product.

With all these low-calorie foods, drugs, meal replacements and fat-burning supplements, along with hundreds of books, clinics, computer programs, articles, consultants and even hypnosis centers and tapes, you would expect to see a nation of lean, healthy people. Instead, we are seeing a rapidly increasing number of fat people in all age groups. The number of overweight children has more than doubled since 1980. This is an especially sad statistic.

In a July-September 2000 article in *Sports Medicine Bulletin*, Jeffrey P. Koplan, M.D., M.P.H., the director of the U.S. Centers for Disease Control and Prevention, indicated that the United States is in the midst of an alarming epidemic of increasing obesity and physical inactivity, especially among young people. He went on to say that these two trends now contribute to more than 300,000 deaths a year from cancer, heart disease and diabetes. In the four years since that article was written, the number has increased to 400,000 deaths a year. Only tobacco, which kills 418,000 each year, contributes to more deaths. He believes that flawed urban design that makes walking unpleasant and unsafe, aggressive marketing of fast foods and snack foods, and modern conveniences are the three main forces contributing to the epidemic. You will learn of more throughout this book. His article also stated how poor diets and ineffective weight control compound the adverse health effects of inactivity.

The United States government has declared obesity a disease. The cost of fat loss (even this book) can now be included on your income tax return along with other deductions for health care. I believe we need someone to develop a program to educate U.S. citizens, especially the youth, about the truth of proper eating and exercise—a campaign to counteract the misinformation and constant advertising that is causing the problem. I do not believe that the government's current efforts will ever do much to help the problem.

Surveys indicate that people are eating more of everything and you will soon learn why. Currently, almost 31 percent of the American population are considered obese. Another 35 percent are labeled overweight. Just look around and you'll see. In 1961, the obesity rate was only 13 percent but had grown to 23 percent by 1990. It has increased by five percent in the last two years. The obesity rate among children has doubled in the last fifteen years. Be aware that even some people who look thin have abnormally high body fat percentages. The strange thing is that with all the eating going on almost everyone is undernourished. It is ironic that with our greater understanding of nutritional needs and numerous advances in technology that the health of most people is deteriorating faster than ever. Americans are eating more despite the fact that at any time almost half of the women in America are on a diet. Another sad statistic is that more than 40 percent of overweight Americans believe they are underweight or normal weight.

Another factor influencing the ever-growing number of obese Americans is that there are more single, working parents leaving older children to care for themselves. The children prepare processed foods at home or are given money to eat at fast-food restaurants. Fewer families sit down together at mealtime. I believe that there are other factors involved: the amount of processed foods, junk foods and fast foods being eaten is increasing with each generation, people are less physically active and nutritional ignorance is being passed on to many children. I also believe that fewer children are being taught healthy ways to deal with some of the most common causes of overeating—stress, depression and boredom.

So, almost one out of every three Americans is obese. Your lifetime risk of getting cancer is also about one out of three. Coincidence? I don't think so. Research has already shown that being fat increases your chances of getting cancer and most other diseases.

How do you know if you are obese? One general definition is weighing more than 20 percent of the weight shown in height and weight charts. This is inaccurate for muscular people and may also show an obese person with low lean body mass to be normal weight. Another definition of obesity is having a body mass index (BMI) greater than 30. You are considered overweight with a BMI of 25 to 29.9. Someone with a BMI of 40 or more is morbidly obese.

The BMI is determined by dividing weight in kilograms (2.2046 pounds) by the square of your height in meters (39.37 inches). Another method is to divide your weight in pounds by the square of your height in inches and multiply the result by 703. For example, a 5'-2" (62 inch) woman weighing 140 pounds would have a BMI of 25.6 (140 divided by 62^2 (62 x 62) = .0364 x 703 = 25.6). The BMI is inaccurate for unusually tall or muscular people. I do not like using either of these two methods because they can be deceptive and were based on populations of people who were not in good physical condition. I prefer measuring body fat percentage using the bioelectrical impedance method. It is fast, easy, and inexpensive. You will learn more about it later.

We are always hearing about new discoveries like adding fiber to your diet to reduce cholesterol and improve bowel function, or eating a particular vegetable to help protect you from a certain type of cancer. Books written more than a hundred years ago talked about most of these so-called "new" discoveries. Why are so many people just hearing about them now? The authors of these old books observed and learned from Nature. You will soon learn that most of these "discoveries" are simply good sense (I do not call it common sense because I think it is uncommon) or just one piece of a puzzle that is useless without the others.

The primary problem seems to be that too many people now trust man's science more than Nature's wisdom. Scientists often believe that they are smarter than Nature when it comes to keeping the human body healthy and lean. Because our health is rapidly declining, and more people are obese than ever before, we are clearly moving in the wrong direction under the guidance and "wisdom" of science. My belief is that Nature has the answers and if you want a lean and healthy body with a sound, active mind, you must return to a simpler and more natural diet. You will also be able to handle the stresses of our fast-paced society better. Nature will teach you if you just listen.

Have you ever noticed that you do not see many wild animals (excluding those that need excess fat) or primitive peoples with excess fat? This is because they are guided by their instincts to eat what is right for them. A polar bear eats completely different foods than a black bear and most primitive peoples stay lean and healthy by eating the whole, natural foods of their environments. They are not influenced by constant advertising telling them to eat distorted, unbalanced foods sadly lacking in nutritional value. When it comes to health and nutrition, it is easy to see who the real "primitives" are.

Please do not let some "expert" convince you that alcohol, processed sugar and chocolate are good for you and talk you out of the good health and lean body that is rightfully yours. The attitude of many nutritionists seems to be that adding expensive supplements can easily fill in the gaps created by eating and drinking worthless or even harmful products. Scientists have even begun to make what they call engineered foods. These processed products claim to be "foods" you can survive on and be healthy. They are healthy for the manufacturer's pocketbook but I would not trust my body's health to them.

Even with all the information available, it is obvious that a great deal is still missing in the understanding of how to get and stay lean and healthy. Most books and programs give you just a few pieces of the permanent fat-loss puzzle. Conflicting information abounds and simply adds to your confusion and frustration. I have talked to hundreds of people who are extremely confused about how to eat healthfully.

Stop waiting for a magic pill that will instantly melt your fat away. This worked in the 1996 movie *The Nutty Professor* but, like most diets, the results were short-lived. No pill will ever take the place of the fresh, wholesome and balanced foods supplied by Nature. This book gives you most of the pieces needed to complete the puzzle and understand the mystery of permanently losing excess body fat. It also teaches you how to discover the few pieces unique to your body. You will find out that being lean is the natural state of your body, not a complicated process of counting calories or points, food substitutions, weighing portions, incessant exercising or constant deprivation. You will learn why your body either stores fat, stays the same or burns excess fat. The goal of this book is to supply the pieces you have been missing so you can finish the puzzle and see the big picture. Then (I hope), the proverbial light will go on and you will say "Aha, now I see why my past efforts failed." Your new knowledge should renew your hope and show you that structural, chemical, mental, emotional and spiritual balance is the key. Throughout this book you will be taught how to attain these balances for yourself.

I am always actively searching to learn more about correct eating, as you should be also. I do not claim to have all the answers, but enough to help you succeed if you truly want to, and your true self does want you to be successful. The principles you will learn in this book have been proven to work. Use your own good sense and experiment with what you read here to determine what is best for your unique body. These principles worked hundreds of years ago, they work now and they will work hundreds of years from now because they are based on how Nature intended us to keep our bodies lean and functioning at their best. You do not have to wait for some new discovery. You just have to learn and apply the truths that have always been.

If you have made the choice to get and stay lean—chosen to accept responsibility for your health and appearance—you will learn how to achieve your goal. If you are not yet ready to choose, I hope that you will find within these pages what you need to make that healthy choice. Understand that until you have changed emotionally no permanent physical changes will occur.

Why Diets and Fat-Losing Gimmicks Do Not Work

In chapter thirteen a number of diets are discussed and reasons are given for why almost all of them are stressful and unhealthful and why some even promote fat gain. Almost everyone who follows them fails to achieve lasting fat loss because the underlying causes of why the person is fat are still there.

You can not be lean for life without first eliminating the physical and emotional causes of your excess fat. I use the word *causes* because if someone's primary cause is emotional the excess fat and internal waste that accumulates will create a physical problem. Similarly, if the primary cause is physical, the stress and frustration created will cause an emotional problem. No program will work for long if the underlying causes are still there.

The greatest nutritional program in the world will fail if you do not follow it because of an emotional reason. Even the power of hypnosis usually fails to create a subconscious suggestion strong enough to overcome the one that made you fat and is keeping you that way. When hypnosis does succeed, constant reinforcement is usually necessary and the right nutritional plan for the person is rarely determined. Diets and gimmicks just treat the symptoms, giving you temporary relief (weight loss) at best. Only about five percent of those who lose excess fat keep it off for three years. Most people quickly gain all or more of it back. You will learn why this happens and why those five percent are successful.

The bottom line is that many people are in an ongoing war with fat. They are always looking for new ammunition in the form of pills, diets, exercise, herbs and more. They may win a battle occasionally but lose even more, so the war continues. You will soon learn how to end your war by making your enemies your allies.

The Six Steps to Permanent Fat Loss and Super Health

There are six steps you must take if you want to be lean and healthy and enjoy life more fully. By the time you have finished this book, you will know how to complete each step. These steps should be within the ability of almost anyone. You will be taught how to find motivation to begin and be given alternatives to use if certain steps cannot be accomplished. These steps can be expressed as faculties we all possess. Listed here are brief descriptions of the six steps.

1. Find Your Reason to Be Lean
   [Desire]
Why do you want to be lean? Answering this question is the first and most important step you must take because until you find *your* reason you will do nothing else. If your reason is strong enough it may be able to overpower an emotional cause that you are unable to eliminate.

2. Discover and Eliminate Your Causes for Excess Body Fat
   [Non-resistance]
This is a vital step if you want to stay lean without any struggle. Even if this step cannot be achieved, you should still be able to accomplish your goals. There may be some effort involved now and then, but if you follow the other steps you can often overcome the causes or gradually eliminate them.

3. Learn What, Why, How and When to Eat and Drink
   [Knowledge]

It has been said that "Ignorance is bliss," but when it comes to eating, ignorance is excess body fat and poor health. It has also been said that "Knowledge is power." For healthful eating, knowledge is the ultimate power, because without it you will be unaware of your other faculties and powers or not know how to use them effectively. Applying the knowledge found in this book can make and keep you lean and healthy.

Many natural laws exist and some of them apply to eating. If you break a nutritional law you will experience negative consequences just as surely as if you were to jump off a cliff and break the law of gravity. You cannot fool Mother Nature, nor should you try. Once you know and understand Nature's nutritional laws—whether you choose to follow them or not—you will know what reaction you will get from each action. You will be given reasons to follow the laws of Nature and learn how to stop sabotaging your goals.

Eating well is far more than just knowing what to eat. How to eat and when to eat is vital. You must learn what foods are right for your unique body, what foods to eat at certain times of the day, what foods to eat together and what foods to eat during different seasons of the year. Another vital concept is when to drink water and when not to drink it. Learning the why of what you are doing helps motivate you and helps you to know how to eat in different situations. You will learn how to eat healthfully at a party or restaurant and how to develop your own favorite meals.

4. Harness the Six Powers that Make People Fat to Make You Lean
   [Creation or Control]

Extremely strong powers are working to make you fat and they are difficult to overcome using will power. For most people they are impossible to overcome, but it does not have to be that way. Like other powers, they can be used for destructive or constructive purposes. You will be taught how to use these powers to help make and keep you lean. You will learn that when you make your enemies your allies the war ends. You can then spend your time and money in worthwhile pursuits instead of constantly fighting the "battle of the bulge." With these powerful forces available at your command, the only way to fail is not to use them.

The six powers you will learn to harness are:

The power of Nature – Nature supplies nutritious, balanced foods full of vitamins, minerals, phytonutrients, enzymes and other nutrients your body needs to be lean and healthy. Satisfying your body's needs with natural foods eliminates abnormal cravings and makes it difficult to overeat. You will also learn how to let your body's true nature guide you and keep you lean as it is designed to do.

The power of habit – All success is based on repetition. Once people find what works for them to make money, stimulate happiness or anything else, all they have to do is keep repeating it to continue being successful. If you exercise regularly and eat well most of the time, you will experience success at being lean and staying healthy. After a behavior is repeated enough times it becomes a habit. Once habits are established, they tend to perpetuate themselves. By repeating healthy behaviors, you will soon replace the habits that made you fat and unhealthy with habits that will make and keep you lean and healthy.

The power of inertia – This law of physics essentially states that a body at rest tends to stay at rest and a body in motion tends to stay in motion unless acted upon by an outside force. You will learn how to use this power to get and keep yourself moving toward your goals.

The power of momentum – This power creates the "snowball effect" that often causes problems to progress faster and faster. For example, after people gain some excess internal waste and body fat, their systems become less efficient. This makes it easier to gain body fat because they must now eat more in an attempt to supply the nutrition their bodies need. Decreased muscle mass slows the metabolism, which also makes it easier to gain excess body fat. You will learn how to replace the numerous negative cycles now working against you with positive cycles that will work for you. Learning to make momentum work for you will reverse the snowball effect and make losing fat easier and easier as you progress. After you have achieved your goal, the power of momentum will help keep you lean.

The power of the subconscious mind – I believe this is our greatest creative power. You will learn how to use this awesome power to create the leanest and healthiest body genetically possible for you.

The power of love – This is the ultimate power we can experience and harness. Once this is done, the other powers are simple to learn and use. If we do not love ourselves, we may feel unworthy of having a lean and healthy body. Without love, no amount of effort will accomplish much of anything. Even if you do not love yourself, you may still be able to achieve your goal if you love someone else enough to do what is necessary to keep your body healthy. For example, a man may not eat himself into an early grave if he loves his wife and children enough to be there for them.

5. Shape and Strengthen Your Body
   [Work, Use or Action]
Having strong and well-developed muscles has numerous benefits. They shape your body, making it more attractive, and help make you more resistant to injury, stress and other physical problems. A stronger body also keeps you feeling younger and gives you the ability to get more enjoyment from and

perform better at physical activities. More muscle mass also increases your metabolism, which makes it easier to get and stay lean.

6. Be a Lean Person
[Being]
Being fat usually comes from thinking and behavioral patterns you have developed. So does being lean. Luckily, it is rarely too late to change the patterns that create your appearance and your life. You will learn how in chapter thirteen.

What Your New Nutritional Program Can Do For You

The benefits of eating nutritiously and in harmony with Nature are numerous. Read through the following benefits carefully so you will fully understand what your new nutritional program can do for you. You will experience more energy, lose fat, feel less depressed, and enjoy many other benefits. These changes should inspire you to continue, making the program easier to follow and feel more natural as you progress. In the beginning you might need a great deal of motivation just to make that first small change. Each step gets easier, but nothing will happen until you take that crucial first step. Use these benefits to help you develop your personal reason or reasons to begin.

Normal Body Weight

Being too fat or too thin each presents different health problems. Following this program allows your body to achieve the best body weight for you naturally. If you are underweight and exercise intensely enough to stimulate muscular growth, you will gain muscle. You may also gain some fat if you are below healthy levels. If you have excess body fat, it will start to burn off naturally as your whole system normalizes and moves toward balance. This will happen without starving yourself or "dieting."

Reducing to a more normal body weight can lessen or eliminate many aches and pains. Misalignments of your knees, hips, back, feet, ankles, shoulders, and even neck will cause more stress and pain if your body has excess fat. Conditions such as arthritis, bursitis, neuritis and tendinitis worsen faster if you are carrying excess weight. Achieving and maintaining your normal body weight in conjunction with having a healthy fat-to-lean body mass ratio is a major key to good health. Many serious health problems and even premature death can be prevented. Attaining normal body weight is the foundation for most of the other benefits you can enjoy.

Increased Vitality

The most frequent complaint I have heard from patients, people I have met, and those I have counseled in nutrition, is that their get-up-and-go got up and went. Often they are simply not providing their bodies with good energy-producing foods. Many people expect their bodies to perform well with no fuel or with a fuel that produces hardly any power. This is like expecting your car to run great with no gasoline or with a cup of gasoline diluted with a gallon of water. Some people eat good foods but at the wrong time. This has a similar effect and often causes the good energy foods to be stored as fat. Good nutrition also produces the energy to do the exercise that helps the nutritional program impart even better results.

Poor eating habits create an accumulation of internal waste that causes obstructions and friction throughout the body. This reduces the efficiency of most functions. Energy that could be used for exercise, pleasure, work, and positive accomplishments is used up internally. Following the program in this book gives your body the chance to cleanse itself of these obstructions and then stay clean and energy efficient.

Another common cause of fatigue is a lack of trace minerals in the diet. Much is still unknown about most of these vital elements, but a lack of them can greatly reduce one's energy level. Many of the recent "miracle" energy supplements contain primarily trace minerals. Unfortunately, most of them are extremely overpriced and people soon stop buying them. They then go without these vital nutrients and their fatigue returns. Kelp and other products from the sea supply these vital nutrients inexpensively and in the perfect balance our bodies need.

A number of things can drain someone's energy or cause insufficient energy production. These include lack of exercise, certain spinal misalignments, internal imbalances, overeating, nutritional deficiencies, low thyroid function, chronic illness, anemia, hypoglycemia, depression, boredom, carrying around excess body fat, negative emotions and a lack of "soul" food. You will learn more about these throughout this book. Some negative emotions, internal imbalances, illnesses, depression and other emotional problems will be eliminated or improved as your body becomes better nourished and more balanced. A positive cycle, where each improved area helps the others to improve, will be created. The power of momentum will start working *for* you instead of against you. Because your energy level, nutritional status, and emotional balance affect sexual desire and function, your sex life should also benefit greatly.

Improved Self-Image

Your self-image has perhaps the greatest influence on your success and happiness. It may be the most valuable benefit you will get from normalizing your body weight, supplying good nutrition to your brain and having more energy. When you look better, you feel better, and your brain can do more of what you ask of it if you supply it the nutrients it needs. And, more energy increases your motivation to accomplish your goals and do the other things you desire. This leads to greater self-confidence and an even better self-image. Improving your health usually leads to progress in all other areas of your life. Your enhanced self-image will help you to love yourself enough to not return to unhealthy behaviors during times of excessive stress or depression. An improved self-image makes it easier to get through the challenges of life we all sometimes experience.

Following the program in this book will also make you feel more in control of your body and your life. You will no longer feel powerless to change things you previously felt you had no control over. Your entire life will improve dramatically.

A Longer and Healthier Life

I have never heard anyone say, "I want to live to be old but I don't care if I'm healthy." Naturally, everyone would prefer to live as long as possible and be healthy. Sadly, few people plan for a healthy future and if you do not plan to be healthy when you are old, you will probably not be. Always remember that *what you do today* has a tremendous influence on whether you will be healthy or even alive tomorrow.

Some people do financial planning and investing for many years so they will have enough money to live comfortably, travel and enjoy life when they are older. Unfortunately, many of them die prematurely or are in poor health and unable to enjoy their later years. A number of people have said to me jokingly, "If I had known I was going to live so long, I would have taken better care of myself." For most of them, however, it is not a joke. Health planning is even more important than financial planning because if you have your health you can still enjoy life tremendously even if you do not have much money. On the other hand, millions of dollars cannot buy back lost health. Planning and investing in both areas should be started as early in life as possible. A mere $7 a month invested at 15 percent interest will grow to one million dollars by age sixty-five if you start at age fifteen. A goal within easy reach of most people if they start soon enough. An investment of only $14 a month will create two million dollars by age sixty-five. Makes you wish you had started that program at age fifteen, doesn't it? The program will have to be different, but it is never too late to start. Similarly, the sooner you start investing in your health and the more you invest, the more benefits you will enjoy.

Start your children off investing $10 each month in a good no-load mutual fund and they will probably have between one and three million dollars by the time they reach age sixty-five. Start them off with good nutritional habits and they will have a good chance at living long enough and being healthy enough to enjoy it. Be aware that they will fight and rebel while growing up— especially during their teenage years—but most of them will eat just like you have taught them, once they are out on their own.

You may feel that you have little to live for but this feeling could change at any moment, especially after your brain starts getting adequate nutrition. There must be at least a spark of hope deep down inside or you would not be reading this right now. I know what despair and hopelessness is like because I have been there. For years during my twenties, I suffered with intense lower back and sciatic nerve pain along with severe hypoglycemia (low blood sugar). I also had a very low income. Fortunately, things did change for me and improved nutrition had a great deal to do with it. Your current state of affairs may improve dramatically, especially after you start following the guidelines in this book.

Being fat ages you. It stresses your heart, lungs and all other glands and organs. It overloads your joints, especially your lower back, pelvis, hips, knees and ankles. It also creates emotional stress because of the negative impact it has on your self-image. If you get fat when you are ten years old, you could have the body of the average fifty-year-old by the time you are thirty. Your life will be limited in numerous ways and shortened by a number of years. Many people who believe suicide is a sin essentially commit it by ending their lives years prematurely. They dig their own graves with their forks and spoons. Overeating and not supplying the body with adequate nutrition also speed the aging process.

Studies indicate that if you are overweight by age forty your life will be shortened by approximately three years. If you are obese you will lose six to seven years. Can you imagine how many years could be lost if someone was obese by age fifteen or twenty? Smoking cigarettes will shorten your life by another seven years. A grossly obese person who smokes could die twenty-five years earlier than necessary. And remember that the years you do have will be less vital and enjoyable if you have excess fat.

Eating properly allows your body to eliminate internal waste and toxins and this provides many benefits. Your body will function better and produce more energy. Combine this with exercise and you will feel more alive and motivated to accomplish good works in the world. You will almost surely live longer and greatly reduce your risk of heart disease, cancer, stroke, diabetes and many of the lesser problems and deterioration normally associated with aging. As your body gets cleaner inside, your chronic skin problem, asthma or nagging allergy could soon be history.

Being clean inside also decreases your chances of contracting common viral and bacterial diseases. You should rarely, if ever, experience a common cold because it is simply your body's way of cleansing itself of excess waste. By following the right nutritional program for you, there will never be enough build-up of waste to create the need for your body to cleanse itself. If you do experience a cold (cleanse), you should determine and eliminate what you are eating that is causing excess waste to accumulate.

Another common benefit of less internal waste is having cleaner and fresher breath. The lungs act as organs of elimination, so if your body is constantly working to excrete excess waste, your breath will always have a bad odor. The skin is a major organ of elimination so another benefit should be reduced body odor. Cuts and other injuries will heal faster and your sexual and other bodily functions should improve. Your bowel movements will probably be much more regular.

Normal body weight with a good fat-to-lean ratio, structural balance, proper nutrition, regular (and correct) exercise, internal cleanliness, and uplifting thoughts, feelings and deeds are the primary keys to a longer and healthier life. These and many others will be explained in a unique book I have planned about natural longevity. Get in touch with the publisher of this book for more information.

A More Attractive Appearance

In his book *Psycho-Cybernetics*, Maxwell Maltz, M.D., F.I.C.S., gives many examples of dramatic improvements in the lives of his patients after *minor* cosmetic surgeries. This demonstrates how a small change in your appearance can make a big difference in how you feel about yourself.

The saying "Clothes make the man" refers to how dressing well and looking sharp makes you feel better about yourself and your life. Because your body is the clothes of your soul—the true person that you are—improving your appearance can be an important step in knowing the wonderful being that you are. The more your true self shines forth, the faster and easier bad habits and other things you do not like about yourself will be eliminated.

There will be far more to your improved appearance than just a more shapely body. Your hair will shine, your skin will be clear and healthy, your eyes will sparkle and you will stand taller and walk with a spring in your step. You will look younger and be more attractive because you will smile more. We all do when we are feeling good. You will be more confident with the opposite sex, on your job, and in your other personal relationships. How you feel about yourself will probably improve dramatically. Looking better also makes you feel more like improving yourself and your life in other ways. All of these changes will not happen overnight and there may be some emotional and mental work necessary, but improving your appearance is a giant first step—one that makes all the others easier.

Everyone (including you) will act differently toward you. Most people will respect and congratulate you. Use this to feel even better about yourself and to create new opportunities and friendships. Take pride in your leaner body and give it more of the respect, care and love that it deserves.

Millions of people spend billions of dollars every year in an attempt to look younger and more attractive. Much of that money is spent on skin care products that do little to give them healthier skin. Eating well, exercising, limiting sun exposure and losing excess fat will keep your skin and you looking and feeling younger. Put your time and money into these effective activities instead of wasting it on products that rarely deliver on the promises they make.

The act of taking charge and developing a large degree of control over how you look will prove to you that you have far greater power than you ever imagined. You can then choose to use that power to improve other areas of your life. Many new opportunities will open up for you and your increased confidence will allow you to take advantage of them.

Improved Emotional Health

What does nutrition have to do with emotional health? A better question is, what *doesn't* nutrition have to do with it? Unfortunately, little consideration is usually given to the influence poor nutrition has on emotional health and behavior. As the quality of nutrition has declined, the incidence of murders, rapes, alcohol and drug abuse have increased. Suicides, spousal and child abuse and other violent, senseless acts are also on the rise. Why? I believe it is because an increasing number of people are failing to supply their bodies and minds with the nutrients needed to cope with the stresses of their lives. Our brains need good nutrition if we are to function calmly and rationally in this busy, competitive and stressful world. If the brain does not get what it needs, the end results are depression, laziness, negative and confused thinking and greater susceptibility to negative influences. A large drop in blood sugar level can turn a calm, loving person into a stark raving lunatic. I know because I have experienced it. Many alcoholics, mentally disturbed people, murderers and other violent criminals suffer from hypoglycemia.

A *minor* nutritional deficiency can make teenagers feel like life has no meaning and turn to drugs for the answer. To them, it is the logical thing to do. After all, most children are given drugs of some kind by their parents whenever anything is wrong with them. Many of them were exposed to drugs even before they were born. Our youth see drugstores on many street corners, drugs in the supermarket, ads for drugs in magazines and numerous television commercials pushing drugs. Drugs are being sold everywhere they look and more and more are being designed especially for children. Drug ads usually shout "extra strength" or "fast relief" for your problems. It should not be a mystery why so many young people turn to drugs in an attempt to solve their emotional problems. That's what everyone else does, isn't it? Even mom and dad are probably using alcohol or another drug of some kind to relax, sleep, feel better or cope with the stresses of their lives. The vast majority of people (even children) in the United States use a drug of some kind *every* day. Sadly, if the first drug does not work, our youth often look for something stronger that promises faster or longer-lasting relief.

If you want to keep your children off drugs, teaching and providing good nutrition and natural health care is the best way to start. Being exposed to natural methods builds a strong foundation because it shows them that almost all problems can be solved in a healthy and positive way. Adequate nutrition will prevent many potential problems from even happening and could help them to feel good enough about themselves to solve the others without drugs. Of course, you must practice what you preach and be a good example or nothing you say will have meaning or value to your children.

People can experience low self-esteem because of a simple nutritional imbalance. This feeling could turn them to crime, make them associate with the wrong crowd or rebel against everything. Some may even take their own lives or someone else's because they just don't care. A minor nutritional imbalance can make people feel so worthless and depressed that they sit and cry or eat junk food all day. Empty, lifeless foods just make things worse and cause their bodies to ask continually for nutrition to meet their needs. The constant input of lifeless food creates poor physical and emotional health and excess body fat. This lowers their feelings of self-worth and further reduces the desire to improve anything.

The mental and emotional stresses we all experience daily cannot be dealt with rationally unless our brains get the nutrients necessary to function normally. Small stresses can seem overwhelming if someone is deficient in even one vital nutrient. It is sad to think that the most likely cause of a teenage suicide or a mother killing her crying infant is an easily resolved nutritional deficiency.

Emotional health alone should be motivation enough for us to improve our own diets and the diets of our children. Think about what a fantastic world it would be if we all got the nutrients our bodies and minds need to function as Nature intended. World hunger, unemployment, crime, war, drug abuse, many birth defects and numerous social problems would be greatly reduced or completely eliminated. Few prisons or mental institutions would be needed and the productivity and progress achievable is almost unimaginable.

How to Get the Most from This Book

Read this entire book thoroughly. Some of the information you need the most will be found in chapters or sections you may think do not apply to you. For example, it is especially important for those with excess fat to learn about gaining muscular body weight, because a lack of lean body mass (LBM) is a common reason why people—especially inactive or older ones—have excess body fat. It is also an important part of staying healthy. Most people who are overweight with fat are underweight with muscle. This is why the term overweight is extremely inaccurate. The term *overfat* best describes what is really happening because someone could be considered "normal" weight yet be obese and another could be labeled overweight but have a low body fat percentage.

If you are thin, you still need to learn the health secrets found in the fat-losing sections. Just because you are lean does not necessarily mean you are healthy. You may have to cleanse your body thoroughly and restore its efficiency before you can start gaining muscle and improve your appearance. The causes that make other people fat may be making you sabotage your life with drugs or in some other way. Throughout the book you will also learn how to help your children keep from getting fat or to lose excess fat they already have.

Look at this book as a true friend who will be brutally honest with you—a friend who cares about you, accepts you as you are and wants you to learn to help yourself but gives you support and encouragement when you need it. See it as the kind of friend who will give you a swift kick in the rear to help you wake up and see the truth. Some of what you read may initially offend you because the truth often hurts. Please do not let this be a problem for you. People usually fail in their quests to be lean because they are afraid to face the truth of why they have excess body fat. This is a common cause of failure in other areas of life but seems especially powerful when it comes to being lean. Most people are always searching for a magic pill to melt their fat away instead of looking for and facing the truth—the only thing that can free them from their bondage to fat, poor health and constant dieting.

One cornerstone truth is that your body is programmed to be lean. We all have different potentials but, barring some rare genetic defect, no "body" wants excess fat, because it is unhealthy and impedes normal function. We do not have brown fat cells like bears do that were designed to release energy slowly during months of hibernation. Do not keep looking for some drug, gimmick or person to assume responsibility for your health and physical appearance. Take an honest look at yourself and realize that the responsibility is yours and that once you accept it you should be able to achieve your goal by applying the knowledge found within this book. I want you to succeed. I do not want this book to be read once and stuck on a shelf while you wait for the next book about some new miracle diet.

Another truth is that there will never be a magic pill developed, but it will certainly not be from mankind's lack of effort. Scientists will keep trying, because the market for a product like this is so enormous it could generate billions of dollars in profit, and because of an ever-increasing number of fat people, the market is constantly growing.

The information contained here can help you no matter what your age, gender, or physical condition. It does not matter if you are a thin person wanting to gain muscular body weight or extremely obese and desperate to lose excess body fat. Even though all normal human bodies function essentially the same, many variables need to be considered. They include differences in age, frame size, speed of metabolism, ancestry, digestive efficiency, gender, hormone levels, muscle mass, nerve flow, internal cleanliness, type, amount and intensity of activity, and others. Some of these are genetic variations but others come from past and present habits and lifestyle. These variables make it imperative that you customize your nutritional program to meet the specific needs of your unique body. You will learn how to do this in chapter six.

This book contains practical, usable information to help you reach your goals. The purpose is to give you the knowledge of how to plan and develop meals that will supply your body's needs based on your specific requirements and the varying circumstances of your life. I will not attempt to impress you with a bunch of technical mumbo jumbo that would take a biochemist to understand.

This book does not contain fancy recipes that most people will never look at or charts and food tables listing calories, protein grams, carbohydrate grams, fat grams, and various vitamin and mineral amounts. You will learn later why calorie counting is negative and a waste of time. It is not necessary, but you may want a small, inexpensive book to learn about fat, carbohydrate and protein contents of certain foods. These can often be found near supermarket checkout counters.

I have purposely used two different styles of writing throughout this book. Part of the time I will be talking about how the human body functions and about people's behavior in general. At other times I will be talking to you. This was done because I want this book to be like your personal nutritionist. It would have been difficult to be direct and personal all the time but I did want to "talk" to YOU much of the time instead of to a generic person. It is important that you relate personally to what I am saying and vital that you assume responsibility for your own health and appearance.

As you read, highlight or underline key points and ideas of particular importance to you. This way you can review these ideas quickly and easily. This is vital because you will not remember most of the information until you review it several times. Once learned, these ideas will never be forgotten, but you must keep studying until you learn them. A summary of the most important principles is included at the end of the book.

Now, settle back and get ready to digest the material presented here (pun intended). Read on and learn how to fill the remaining years of your life with more vitality, accomplishments, happiness and superior health. Always remember that what you hear, see, read, feel, think, eat or drink becomes a part of you and influences your health and happiness in one way or another. Be selective and make healthy choices.

If we keep well and cheerful we are always young, and at last die in youth,
even when years would count us old.

Tyron Edwards

Every man is his own ancestor, and every man his own heir.
He devises his own future, and he inherits his own past.

Frederick Henry Hedge

The beginning is the most important part of the work.

Plato

There are two ways to live your life.
One is as though nothing is a miracle.
The other is as though everything is a miracle.

Albert Einstein

People need loving the most when
they deserve it the least.

John Harrigan

All I have seen teaches me to
Trust the Creator for all
I have not seen.

Ralph Waldo Emerson

two

The *Victory Over Fat* Program

This chapter gives you basic insights into eating well and explains how my *Victory Over Fat* program works. Each part of the program is explained more thoroughly later so you will fully understand how to do everything correctly.

If you asked a hundred people the question, "What is a balanced nutritional program?" you would probably get a hundred different answers. Unfortunately, for many people it means eating a balance of sugar, salt, saturated fat, and processed grain products. You will learn what a *healthful* balanced program is and how to customize it to supply the needs of your unique body. You will also learn about the inefficiency spiral that causes most people to gain fat and internal waste at an ever-increasing rate. You will learn how to reverse this spiral and lose unwanted weight at an increasingly faster rate.

Nature's Plan—What a Concept

The more I observe Nature's handiwork and see the incredible balance in natural environments, the more I am convinced that Nature has the answer to how we should eat. After all, our bodies and minds were created by and are a part of Nature. Sadly, few of us know how to listen to and learn from the wisdom of Nature. Our diets and lifestyles are becoming less natural and this moving away from balance correlates with the increase in the number of fat and sick people.

Mankind has disrupted many of Nature's delicate balances. Our instincts are clouded and our actions distorted by misinformation and advertising. The planet we live on is sick and unbalanced for the same reasons we are. The imbalances in our diets, lifestyles and environments often originate from the love of money being greater than the love of our planet, its creatures, our fellow human beings and ourselves. The wealthy businessman who is polluting the air or raping the land will probably live a life of sub-optimal health and die prematurely because he has been convinced to eat the nutritionally void foods produced by others.

Nature puts the foods we should eat right under our noses and essentially tells us if we just eat a variety of the whole, natural foods it supplies, we will be lean *and* healthy. Wow, what a concept! These foods not only supply our bodies with the nutrients necessary to function efficiently but also contain substances that help protect us from the negative effects of an unhealthy environment. Nature's foods contain substances that help our bodies detoxify the thousands of toxic chemicals found in our water, air, food, home and the products we use. These same foods also help keep us comfortable in our environment.

Eating for good health and a lean body should be easy. Unfortunately, most of us are no longer in touch with our natural instincts because of the abundance of misinformation and advertising we are exposed to on a daily basis. It should not be difficult to understand that if you put unbalanced, distorted foods into your body, its function will be unbalanced and its shape distorted. To make matters worse, we usually eat these foods at the wrong times and with little variety. Ironically, the processing, packaging and advertising make these processed foods cost more than natural foods. People who eat processed foods pay a premium for their poor health and excess body fat. Then they pay for expensive supplements, drugs, medical care, and for other programs and products in an attempt to regain lost health and to lose their excess fat.

Eating Nature's way and wisely investing the money you save will improve your financial status. Amazing! Nature also wants you to be prosperous. Last, but not least, think about the extra time that you will have to do the things you love, and enjoy the wonders and beauty Nature has created. Great bonus benefits just for eating wholesome natural foods, wouldn't you say?

Just What Should We Eat?

The controversy over what we should eat has been raging for hundreds, if not thousands, of years. Some say to consume dairy products and others say absolutely not. Some say not to eat red meat and others say you must if you want good health. Some say we should just eat fruit and others recommend eating mostly brown rice. What is confusing about these varying opinions is that they all give fairly convincing reasons for doing what they recommend. With all the foods Nature has created for us, I doubt if many people would want to eat fruit or brown rice all day, nor does it make sense to do so. Let's take a look at the primary controversy of eating meat (fish, fowl or red meat) versus being a vegetarian.

Human beings have been eating the flesh of other creatures for thousands of years, just as many other animals have. Perhaps this was not the original intent of Nature but it is how things are now. Some animals instinctively eat little else but meat. Coyotes eat rabbits, rabbits eat the grass and other vegetation supplied by Nature, and they both fertilize the grass with their wastes. This is an example of the cyclic nature of the food chain. Nature tells the coyote to have only two or three young in the spring because that is all the food chain can support. Rabbits multiply more often and have numerous offspring each time because they are here primarily as food for coyotes and other carnivorous animals. Nature's food chain is incredible and precisely balanced with humans at the top.

Native Americans and others who lived off the land were in tune with Nature and most of them respected life in all forms. They ate fish, fowl and red meat, especially in the winter when many other foods were unavailable. They were a balanced part of the environment and ate animals only for survival.

If you compare the human body with those of other animals, you will see that some of our teeth are like the teeth of meat-eating animals and some are like those of plant-eating animals. The length of our intestinal tract is approximately somewhere in between the two and we have digestive enzymes capable of digesting both meat and vegetarian foods. It appears that our bodies were designed, or have adapted, to eat meat and the other foods Nature supplies.

Meat is about the only adequate source of certain amino acids, vitamin B_{12}, and the mineral cobalt. A deficiency of these nutrients can lead to some extremely serious health problems. Therefore, I believe that Nature designed humans to eat some meat, but I do not believe it intended animals to live in cruel, overcrowded environments, be fed unnatural diets or injected with antibiotics, growth drugs and other toxic chemicals. All animals, especially those used for food, should be treated with love and respect. They are a part of Nature, just as we are. Being at the top of the food chain makes us responsible to help Nature maintain its delicate balance. We should respect all creatures and do our best to preserve their homes and prevent their extinction. The animals we raise for food should be fed their natural foods and raised in clean, uncrowded environments where they can be healthy. It is foolish to believe we can get health-building nutrients from sick and tortured animals that have been fed improperly and polluted with drugs and other chemicals.

Red meat is high in iron, phosphorus and B-complex vitamins. It also contains vitamin A and varying amounts of calcium. Meat is almost completely digested and is used well by the body. Carnivorous animals eat organ meats along with muscle meat and I feel that we were also meant to do this. Organ meats are richer in nutrients than muscle meats and I believe may contain substances not yet discovered that help keep our organs functioning properly. They are generally less expensive. I do not recommend eating them more than occasionally, however, because of environmental toxins, possible heavy metals and infectious organisms that may be found in organ meats now. The most dangerous organ meats to eat are brains. Please avoid them. Poultry is similar in nutritive value to red meat but is generally lower in fat, except duck and goose. Seafood is also similar in nutritive value to red meat except for lower amounts of iron. Shellfish and saltwater fish are rich in iodine, fluorine, and cobalt. They also contain high amounts of omega-3 fatty acids unless they are farm-raised and fed improperly. Herring and oysters are high in zinc. Shellfish are low in fat but contain considerable amounts of cholesterol, which, as you will learn, is not normally harmful. Unfortunately, they may contain contaminants if they live in waters polluted with toxic chemicals. Many fish contain unsafe levels of mercury. You will learn more about mercury and the safest seafood to eat in chapter eight.

The problems associated with eating meat—especially red meat—do not come from the meat itself if it comes from healthy animals that eat their natural diets and are raised in healthful environments. The main problem is that many people eat far more meats (and grains) than they need and not enough fruits, vegetables and legumes to maintain a normal pH balance in their bodies. You will soon learn about this vital balance and how to maintain it.

The main problem is that much of our meat comes from animals (cows, sheep, pigs and fowl) that are fat, diseased, tortured, fed unnatural diets, and full of antibiotics and growth-enhancing hormones. Even farm-raised fish are given antibiotics when they are confined in crowded ponds, which makes them more susceptible to diseases. The residues of these drugs can increase the risk of certain cancers and other diseases. The insecticides sprayed on animals are usually absorbed into their bodies and end up in the meat that people eat. This is not the kind of meat Nature intended us to eat. Meat may also be contaminated with dangerous bacteria and fecal matter if proper sanitation methods are not followed during processing. Buying and eating hormone-free organic meats is well worth the money spent.

Feeding cows the waste products of sheep is completely unnatural, yet mankind did it and caused a serious problem. Cows are not carnivorous so obviously something negative was going to happen eventually. Some of the sheep were diseased and this led to the development of bovine spongiform encephalopathy or "mad cow disease." A number of people have already died from eating the meat of infected cows and tens of thousands of animals have had to be destroyed.

Another part of the meat-eating problem comes from the way people cook it, process it and what they eat with it. Overcooked meat contains carcinogens, and the nitrite and nitrate additives in cured and processed meats are converted into carcinogenic (cancer-causing) nitrosamines. Meat that is eaten with oils or alkaline foods (you will learn about these soon) or that is overcooked is not digested efficiently and may not be broken down into a usable form. As any undigested meat travels through the intestinal tract it can putrefy and release harmful toxins. The deficiency of fiber in the average person's diet extends the time from ingestion to elimination and this increases the amount of toxins that are absorbed. This lack of fiber comes from not eating enough fruits, vegetables, legumes and whole grains.

Eliminate as much fat as possible from the meat you eat. You do not need the saturated fat and most of the drugs or environmental toxins explained earlier are stored in the fat.

I believe most of us need *some* meat to enjoy optimal health. Some people have the capability to do well as vegetarians but many others do not. While following a vegetarian diet for two years, I created numerous imbalances and health problems in my body. After adding fish and fowl to my diet, most of my problems were resolved, but I began having joint pains throughout my body after I resumed heavy exercise. None of the herbs or other supplements that were claimed to relieve joint pain gave me any relief. Eating some red meat once a week was what resolved this problem. I have also done nutritional counseling for fat and sickly vegetarians who needed some animal protein in their diets to achieve proper balance and health. Because we all have different needs and digestive capabilities we must each determine and eat what is right for us. You will learn later how to figure out what foods your body does best on and how much meat it needs, if any.

In the Season Thereof

Many years ago I read the recommendation to eat foods "in the season thereof." This is healthful advice and makes perfect sense, because the foods available in each season have different effects on our bodies. Nature supplies foods to meet our specific needs during different times of the year. This occurred naturally in the thousands of years before refrigeration. We should still eat this way, however, because it's in harmony with the way Nature intended. It is most important to eat this way if you live where the winters are cold and snowy and the summers hot and sunny. If you live in a temperate climate, such as Southern California, your diet will vary less from season to season.

Changing your diet to match the season should be as natural as wearing seasonal clothes. You would probably not go out in a snowstorm in shorts and a tee shirt or wear your heavy winter coat outside on the hottest day of summer. The same principle applies to matching the foods you eat with the temperature of your environment.

In the winter your body needs more animal protein, fats, lentils, corn and whole grains. These foods are acid forming and generate more internal heat to help keep you warm. Some people say they thicken your blood and act something like anti-freeze. Eating these foods makes sense because dried legumes, whole grains and foods high in protein—such as eggs, meats, nuts and seeds—can be stored without refrigeration or obtained fresh in the winter. Other good winter foods are the hard vegetables that can be stored for a few months without refrigeration. These include potatoes, rutabagas, parsnips, onion, yams, turnips and many kinds of squash. Apples, pears, oranges and avocados are the fruits in season during the winter. You can also eat dates, figs, prunes, raisins and other dried fruits.

After winter come the warmer days of spring. This is when your body does its spring-cleaning and when Nature supplies the fruits and other foods that stimulate this cleansing process. Grapes, cherries, and berries are especially cleansing. This is why they have a laxative effect on some people, especially those with the most internal waste. Cleansing out the residue of the heavier winter foods gets your body ready for the upcoming heat of summer. I believe that this is why so many people get colds in the spring.

At last summer arrives, and the green leafy vegetables and wide variety of other lighter vegetables come in season—foods like zucchini, summer squash, string beans, peas, lettuce, spinach and numerous others. Summer is the time for a variety of melons and a large selection of other fruits. These lighter vegetables and fruits help keep your body cool in the summer heat. You have probably noticed that you do not feel as much like eating heavier meals of grains and complete protein foods in the summer. Your appetite is lighter and different than it is in the winter. Do you think your body is trying to tell you something? Because of this conditioning effect, if you were to eat watermelon, bananas, berries and other fruits during the winter, you would probably feel cold most of the time. Likewise, eating excessive amounts of grains, meats and other winter foods makes you uncomfortable in hot weather. This is why many people seek out air-conditioned environments all summer.

Think about the Eskimo. Eskimos eat a great deal of meat and fat, primarily because that is what's available to them. It is impossible to grow bananas in northern Alaska. Eating as they do would kill an average person, but for them it is a necessity to condition their bodies for the harsh environment in which they live. Their bodies are also short and round, helping them to conserve internal heat.

Now think about African tribesmen. Their diets of fruits and complex-carbohydrate foods keep their bodies conditioned to live comfortably in an extremely hot environment. The majority of them do not eat much meat. Their bodies are often tall and lean to better dissipate the heat. As you can well imagine, if an Eskimo and African tribesman traded diets, they would each have serious problems. The Eskimo would freeze and the tribesman would die from the heat. It would be as if they wore each other's clothes.

In general, if a food can be freshly grown in the climate where you live, or stored without refrigeration through the next season, it will probably be good for you at those times. You will learn more about this later.

What is a Healthful Nutritional Program?

Contrary to what you may have read or been taught, eating in a healthful and nutritious way is not complicated. It is not always easy to do, but it is not complex and time-consuming as some people might lead you to believe. It is not something only hardcore "health nuts" will do. You just have to learn the truth about how your body is best nourished and then follow those guidelines.

The human ego always looks for ways to complicate everything in an attempt to feel important and get attention. To find the truth in any aspect of life you must simplify it. You must clear away the superfluous and trivial so you can see the truth shining forth. This is as true for healthful eating as it is for everything else.

In a nutshell, a good nutritional program has the following four aspects.

1. The Right Food at the Right Time

Good nutrition is not simply what you eat, but also when you eat it. In all areas of life, timing can make all the difference between success and failure. When you are ready for something to happen, it will happen. When the student is ready, the teacher will appear and vice versa. Likewise, when your body needs a particular food or nutrient, if you supply it, all will go well and health will be enjoyed. If you do not, there will be negative health consequences. Even good nutrition *at the wrong time* will rob you of energy or be stored as excess fat or internal waste.

2. Simple and Positive

A healthful nutritional program must be simple and relatively easy to follow. If it requires spending hours and hours counting calories, looking up protein and fat grams in charts, weighing food down to the ounce and other trivial pursuits, it is not a good program. These time-consuming activities are negative because the constant focus is on what you cannot have. No one is going to follow a regimen like that for long; therefore, it is doomed to failure. Your program should take a minimal amount of time and effort.

A good nutritional program must be positive and create a healthy state of mind that gradually improves. It should focus on what you *can* eat and the *benefits* you are enjoying from eating well. If you concentrate on the positives, you will not have time to think about (or miss) what you are not eating.

3. Inexpensive

Eating well is not costly. Good health is available to anyone with even a moderate budget for food. A healthful nutritional plan should not be based on expensive or exotic foods. In times past, peasants often ate simple, homegrown, whole foods and the aristocracy and wealthy people ate expensive and exotic foods. Healthwise, the peasants were far better off because of the greater nutritional value they got from their simple meals. They also usually did not overeat, but many of the rich did. You will learn later why overeating is almost impossible if you eat wholesome natural foods. Your meals should consist of very few costly processed foods.

4. Balance

Balance is listed last but is certainly not least. You were probably taught in school about the four basic food groups (bread and cereal, meat, fruits and vegetables, and milk) and told you would be healthy if you ate a certain number of servings from each group every day. Unfortunately, this is a frequent cause of excess fat, poor nutrition and ill health. I believe this four-food group concept has conditioned the minds of many people and created a great deal of illness, death and tragedy.

Complete nutrition comes from a number of different forms of balance. A large part comes from eating a variety of whole foods that give your body many different nutrients from which to choose. Balance also comes from the ratio of "live" (raw) foods to "dead" (cooked) foods. Perhaps the most important balance you should pay attention to is between acid-forming and alkaline-forming foods that maintain the proper pH in your system. A balanced amount of carbohydrate, protein and fat in your diet is also important. If nutritional supplements are taken, it is important to have proper ratios among various minerals and other nutrients. Imbalance can be created from any of these aspects and because health is balance, any imbalance creates some form of ill health. You will learn how to easily maintain all of these balances.

Acid/Alkaline Balance

Would you like to know the simple secret of losing fat and staying lean even without exercise? And here's the best part. You get to eat *more* food, not less. In fact, the more of the right foods you eat, the faster your body will burn stored fat. It's simple chemistry. Isn't Nature's plan great? Both Nature and I do recommend exercise along with correct nutrition but we will get to that subject later. If you are raising an eyebrow in skepticism at this point, read on and you will learn why these statements are true.

Your body is constantly striving for homeostasis (balance) in many different ways, like maintaining a pH (acid/alkaline balance) of 7.41 in your blood. It does not want your blood pH higher or lower. Your body has a few ways of maintaining this balance but I am going to explain only those important to our goals of optimal health and permanent fat loss. First, I will explain what happens when the blood is acidic.

When the pH is acidic (lower than normal), your body often steals calcium from your bones. Because calcium is alkaline it neutralizes some of the excess acid. If the pH is still too low, your body will store the remainder of the acidic food as fat because this gets it out of your bloodstream and increases the pH back to normal. Neither of these reactions is healthful. One contributes to osteoporosis and the other to excess body fat. Many people's bodies are almost always acidic. This increases inflammation, making all your aches and pains worse and creating an ideal environment for cellular mutation and disease-causing organisms. Now, let's examine what happens when the blood is alkaline.

When the pH is alkaline (higher than normal), your body burns stored fat because this creates acid and lowers the pH back to normal. This reaction is good for you. The more alkaline your blood is the more stored fat your body will usually burn. Correct exercise is extremely good for you but is not necessary for this fat burning to occur. Don't worry that you will lose too much fat by eating alkaline foods. Your body has ways of preventing that. You will learn about this later. After you reach your goal, eating a balance of alkaline- and acid-forming foods will maintain your body weight and fat-to-lean ratio.

What foods create an acid residue (ash) and lead to fat gain when excessive amounts are eaten? Complete protein foods (mainly meats, fish, fowl and eggs), most grains and grain products, milk and fats are the main ones. Lentils, peanuts, walnuts and Brazil nuts also leave an acid ash after being digested. What makes these foods acidic is a high phosphorus, iron and sulfur content. Complete protein foods, processed wheat products and fats (usually unhealthful ones) are the primary components of most people's meals. Another part of the problem is that these foods are highly concentrated (many calories in a small portion) compared to most of the alkaline foods needed to maintain a balanced pH. That means you have to eat a much larger quantity of alkaline foods than acid foods if you do not want to gain fat. Look at the typical meals most people eat and it is easy to see why so many of them have excess fat.

What are the alkaline foods that stimulate fat burning? Fruits, vegetables and all legumes except lentils are the main ones. Other alkaline foods are lima beans, soybeans, baked beans, navy beans, carob, coconut, chestnuts, almonds, mushrooms, molasses and amaranth. Millet, buckwheat and quinoa are the only grains I know that are alkaline. These foods are alkaline because they contain high amounts of potassium, calcium and magnesium. Even pineapples, oranges and tomatoes are alkaline because the alkalinity I am referring to is what enters the bloodstream after the food is digested, not what the food is like when you eat it.

There you have it. Losing stored fat is normally just a matter of eating more alkaline-forming foods and fewer acid-forming foods. Eat more alkaline foods to restore the balance lost from eating an excess of acidic foods. It is that simple and simplicity is the way of truth and Nature. After a normal body fat percentage is achieved, people can then eat more acidic foods and fewer alkaline foods. If they maintain a normal acid/alkaline balance they should not gain body fat unless they eat excessive quantities of food. This should rarely be a problem because overeating is difficult to do if you eat a balance of whole, natural foods. On the other hand, gaining fat is *extremely* easy when processed and other highly concentrated acid-forming foods are eaten.

The fat burning generated by an alkaline pH can be slowed down in different ways. Eating salt can do it, as can having a slow metabolism. For some people, a slower metabolism is natural for their bodies, but for most, it has been created by vertebral misalignments at the base of the neck, excessive dieting or the loss of lean body mass due to a lack of correct exercise. It may be a combination of two or more. These and other reasons are explained in upcoming chapters.

Losing excess fat as just explained is extremely healthy for two primary reasons. The alkaline-forming foods are full of the enzymes, vitamins, minerals and phytonutrients needed to burn the stored fat for energy. This is one of the reasons why you can lose more fat by eating this way than by fasting. The second reason is because your pH stays relatively balanced during and after the losing period. A balanced pH has many health benefits besides keeping you lean. You will have more resistance to disease. I have seen serious conditions (cancer and others) cured simply by restoring the pH of the body back to normal. Other health benefits you will experience from losing fat this way—Nature's way—are a normal metabolism and improved bodily function including better digestion, assimilation and elimination. You will soon learn how important these functions are to good health and a lean, attractive body.

Many of the "diets" people follow are acidic or pH balanced. Most of them force the body to burn fat and this causes an acidic condition to develop. Because this is a stressful and unwanted condition, the body slows its metabolism so it can function on fewer calories. For example, say a person's body needs 2,000 calories a day to function normally. What would happen if a diet program created a balanced pH, but contained only 1,200 calories a day? Remember that if the pH is balanced, the body does not want to store or lose fat. The body would get perhaps 1,500 calories a day: the ingested 1,200 and 300 from *forced* fat burning and the catabolism (burning) of muscle. Because the body does not like the acidic condition this creates, it will slow its metabolism down as soon as it can. Some weight will be lost (water, fat and muscle) until the metabolism slows down so the body can survive on the 1,200 calories. This is why most dieters' progress stops after they lose 15 to 20 pounds. Most people then get discouraged and return to their old eating habits. When dieters start eating 2,000 calories again, first they would gain weight from retaining normal or excess amounts of water. Then, the slower metabolism they developed because of the diet and the loss of muscle mass, which slows the metabolism even more, would cause them to gain excess fat back quickly. Most people end up with more fat than when they started. Many reducing programs just reduce your metabolism, lean body mass, energy level, eating enjoyment, health and your pocketbook. People on low-calorie diets usually feel deprived psychologically because the quantity of food is less than normal. This often causes them to overeat after the diet ends.

If you were to get 1,200 calories primarily from alkaline-forming foods, you would not feel deprived because you could eat large quantities of these low-calorie foods. Your body will get an abundance of the nutrients it needs to burn the stored fat and maintain your muscle mass, good health and vitality. Will your metabolism slow down? Hardly any or not at all, because your body will be getting the 2,000 calories of energy it needs to function normally. The other 800 calories will come from stored fat being burned naturally (not forced) to balance the pH. Will your fat loss plateau? No, because the fat burning creates the pH your body wants. Your progress should continue until you lose as much unhealthful weight as you want to lose. Then you can eat a pH balanced diet of 2,000 calories without gaining back any fat.

The Inefficiency Spiral

The majority of people I have known and most of the fat ones I have counseled nutritionally were caught in an inefficiency spiral. I am referring to the inefficient digestion, assimilation and utilization of the foods they eat. It starts with people eating foods low in nutritional value or eating in such a way that their bodies are unable to digest efficiently, process properly, or use the nutritious foods they are eating. Either of these scenarios requires them to eat larger than normal quantities of food to supply the nutritional needs of their bodies. This is why people can eat junk food all day long and still be hungry. Their bodies are literally starving and craving the nutrients needed to function properly. Until someone's body gets what it needs, it will keep asking for more. Even healthful nutrition, if supplied at the wrong time, will be stored as fat or accumulate as internal waste. Either way the person's body gets less efficient at processing and utilizing the next meal.

This inefficiency spiral worsens as more fat and waste accumulate in the body. As the body becomes less efficient, it requires even more food to get the nutrition it needs. As people eat more in an attempt to supply the nutrition their bodies are craving, more excess accumulates and their bodies become increasingly less efficient. This negative cycle is why it is easier for people to gain more after they gain 10 or 15 pounds of fat and waste. Like a snowball rolling down a hill it gains more momentum and greater power.

A build-up of fat and internal waste decreases energy production and creates the need for more energy to perform internal bodily functions. It is like having dirty, sticky oil in your car's engine causing excessive friction that robs the engine of power. More stress is also placed on all parts of the engine. Similarly, internal friction creates more stress and work for the body and takes energy away from vital processes and physical and mental activities. Energy is also used up carrying the excess weight around.

My *Victory Over Fat* program stops and then reverses the inefficiency spiral by creating an efficiency spiral that improves bodily function and moves someone toward better health. The body gets more and more efficient as it gets internally cleaner and eliminates excess body fat. Now, less food is required to supply the nutrients the body needs. Eating less helps to further reduce fat and internal waste, making the whole process even easier. Positive results are experienced as the power of momentum works *for* you instead of *against* you. Eating less also saves money. As your weight normalizes and internal friction decreases, more energy becomes available for physical and mental activities, because less is needed for vital internal functions and less is used carrying the excess weight around.

The Four Steps for Reversing the Inefficiency Spiral

You have probably heard the saying "You are what you eat," but it is not true. People can be fat and unhealthy even though they eat good wholesome foods. What you eat is just the first of four steps necessary to reverse the inefficiency spiral and deliver health-building nutrition to your body. Let's go over these steps and you will see what I mean.

Step 1: Eat Nutritious Foods

The first step, of course, is to eat nutritious foods. You cannot expect to get good nutrition and enjoy optimal health unless the foods you eat contain nutritional value. Unfortunately, most people do not even take this step. Health-conscious people do, but usually leave the other three steps purely to chance. Many of them wonder why they do not get the results they expect and some stop eating well for that reason.

You will soon understand that much more is involved than just eating nutritious foods. Even the best foods can create fat gain, discomfort or harmful toxins if cooked improperly, eaten in poor combinations or when emotionally upset, eaten at the wrong time or with fluids, or if an excess of acid-forming foods is eaten. Nonetheless, eating nutritious whole foods is the key first step you must take if you want to enjoy normal body weight, boundless energy and optimal health.

Step 2: Obtain Efficient Digestion

The right nutritious foods can do your body little good if they are not digested well and broken down into their usable forms. This step is rarely considered but is as important as the foods you eat. What good is nutritious food if it is eaten in such a way that it simply generates internal waste, carcinogenic toxins, or supplies little nutritional value? People may have the illusion of eating well when in reality their bodies are starving for good nutrition. This is why you must have a practical understanding of how your body digests food and know how to optimize your digestive function. You will learn that even your thoughts are important to attaining this goal.

Step 3: Assimilation

After nutritious foods are broken down into usable forms, they must be assimilated into the bloodstream to be available for use. Most nutrients are absorbed in the small intestine, so the key to optimal assimilation is to make sure the small intestine is functioning at peak efficiency. Size of meals, when you eat, combinations of foods eaten, physical condition and mental state are also important.

Step 4: Utilization—The Bottom Line

This final step is vital because even if highly nutritious foods are eaten, digested well and efficiently assimilated, without utilization the prior three steps will have been wasted. The primary key to utilization is when food is eaten. For example, if someone were to eat the same amount of the same foods between eight in the morning and noon, or from five in the afternoon until nine at night, you would see extremely different results. Eating in the morning would allow for relatively normal function throughout the day and maintain someone's body weight or cause some fat loss. I do not recommend doing this because it requires eating so much in a short time that it would overload your digestive system. I am explaining this simply to make a point. In contrast, a person eating at night would probably be tired during the day, muscle tissue would be cannibalized for energy, and much of the food would be stored as body fat because it is not needed at night. You must eat foods that supply what your body needs, *when* it needs it. Do this and the powerful principle of timing will work for you.

The saying "You are what you eat" should be "You are what your body utilizes." If your body is fat, you might say, "You are what your body *hasn't* utilized." You now know the three additional steps beyond eating nutritious foods. This does not make eating healthfully more complicated, it just means a few more simple steps need to be taken. The bottom line is the nutrition your unique body utilizes.

Throughout this book, most of the things you learn will improve one or more of the preceding four steps. This allows you to supply the nutrients your body needs from a minimum amount of food so you can live longer and enjoy a more attractive body, a healthy fat-to-lean ratio and improved health.

What we hope ever to do with ease we must first learn to do with diligence.
Samuel Johnson

We should believe only in deeds; words go for nothing everywhere.
Fernando Rojas

Faith is the substance of things hoped for, and
proof of things invisible to mortal sight.
Dante

The only happy man is he who thinks he is.
French Proverb

Nothing is worth more than this day.
Goethe

Do good, and don't look back.
Dutch Proverb

three

Meet Your New Friends

This book was written to teach you, among other things, how to eat for optimal health, not just fill your head with hundreds of nutritional facts and add to your confusion. But, to understand healthful eating you must first have a basic knowledge of the types of foods and nutrients your body needs to be lean and function at its best.

You probably already know something about the three macronutrients: carbohydrates, proteins and fats. I will briefly explain each of these and five more that are vital to good health—water, oxygen, carbon dioxide (surprise), sunlight and sleep. Before we discuss different kinds of foods, you need to understand the form in which they should be eaten.

Whole Foods for Balanced Health

It is best to eat foods in their most whole and natural states. Instead of drinking apple juice or orange juice, eat the whole apple or orange. Eating part of a food creates imbalance, but when a whole food is eaten each part supplies something complementary to the others. A synergistic action occurs between them. In other words, the whole is greater than the sum of the parts. Some exceptions to this now exist because of pesticides and other chemicals certain foods may absorb or have on the outside. Sometimes using part of a food can help restore lost balance more quickly, but once balance has been regained, eating the whole food helps prevent imbalance.

Whole grains consist of three parts: endosperm, bran and germ. Almost all bread is nutritionally incomplete and causes imbalance in our bodies because it is made from only the endosperm. The bran and germ are removed during processing because the bran makes the flour too coarse and the germ causes the bread to need refrigeration to prevent it from going bad quickly. This creates the need to supplement our diets with bran to get the fiber necessary for normal bowel movements and with germ oils to supply healthful fats to our bodies.

When separated and sold individually, parts of foods make larger profits. For example, many years ago it was discovered that wheat germ oil greatly increased energy and endurance. To capitalize on this discovery it was advertised and sold as an energy tonic. It had positive effects because it contained something missing from people's diets. But, it is unbalanced because it is only one part of the whole. Later, the part of the germ oil that increased endurance was isolated and named octacosanol. It is now sold as a more expensive food supplement but is even more incomplete. Nature intended the octacosanol to be ingested with the rest of the germ and all of the bran and endosperm, not taken separately. A whole grain gives you all three parts at one time and in the perfect ratio your body needs for good health. The balance and completeness of whole foods is a vital key to good nutrition and is missing from many foods eaten today in modern societies.

Many of my nutritional clients believed they ate relatively healthful diets, but after telling me they frequently drank orange juice and ate "whole-wheat" bread we found that our definitions of a healthful diet were extremely different. When I told them that drinking orange juice was not healthful, they often replied, "But it's a natural food." I then asked if they had ever seen a carton of orange juice growing on a tree. The reply was no, of course, and then I explained that the orange that grows on the tree is the whole, natural food they should eat. Drinking just the juice creates imbalance because some of the orange's complementary and synergistic nutrients are missing. For example, the white pulpy part of an orange contains the bioflavonoids important for capillary strength. Bioflavonoids (now often just called flavonoids) are necessary for the proper absorption and use of the vitamin C in the juice. These two nutrients work together to keep our collagen healthy. The indigestible fiber of the orange cleans your intestinal tract and supplies bulk for normal bowel function. Fruits contain a healthful sugar called fructose, but fruit juices contain excessively high concentrations that stress your body's blood sugar balancing system. Nature seals the juice inside the orange for a good reason. It reduces the fructose concentration and prevents exposure to light and air that quickly destroys the vitamin C.

Another comment I frequently heard was, "But, it's from a natural source." If you think about it, everything in our world originates from natural sources, whether it is a poison, a nutritious food, a plastic grocery bag, or anything else. Scientists can modify natural substances to create extremely unbalanced and toxic products. Just because something is derived from natural sources does not mean it is good for us. When it comes to food, wholeness and natural form are extremely important.

Eating whole foods creates a positive cycle of health and efficiency. When you supply your body the health-building nutrients found in these foods, it can function optimally and because it is satisfied, it will not stimulate you to overeat.

Carbohydrates

The two basic forms of carbohydrates are simple and complex. Fruits are simple-carbohydrate foods that help you to be lean and healthy. They undergo little digestion and supply relatively quick energy. Fruits are great as snacks or as an entire meal during the warmer months. Refined sugar is also a simple carbohydrate, but is detrimental to the goal of permanent fat loss.

Complex carbohydrates are found primarily in vegetables, grains, legumes and milk. They contain some incomplete protein, but are mostly carbohydrate. Complex carbohydrates generally supply longer lasting energy than simple-carbohydrate foods because the energy is released as the food is gradually broken down into simple carbohydrates by your digestive enzymes. Some carbohydrates have been rated with what is called the glycemic index. This rating tells you how fast the foods energy is released and can sometimes be helpful in determining the best time to eat a certain food. This is explained in greater detail in chapter five.

The primary function of carbohydrate foods is to supply energy. They are broken down into glucose, the main energy source for your body. Energy can also be derived from fats and proteins, but is most easily obtained from carbohydrates. Most people get the largest percentage of their calories from carbohydrate sources.

Your body needs energy for your muscles to work, your internal organs to function, to build new tissues, to dispose of worn out cells and for your brain to function. In fact, your brain uses about 25 percent of your energy and uses glucose as its sole source. To carry out internal and external functions your body needs energy. It prefers carbohydrates as an energy source over both fat and protein and a daily input is needed. This is why Nature provides such a large variety of carbohydrate foods and why you should eat more carbohydrates than proteins or fats.

If your body needs energy but does not have enough carbohydrates or fats, it will convert protein into glucose. Because this requires much more energy than the conversion process for carbohydrates or fats, it reduces the energy available for work, play or internal functions. Toxic byproducts are also created. Eating carbohydrates allows the body to use protein for its primary functions and not for energy. Also, protein utilization is improved when carbohydrates are eaten in the same meal.

Carbohydrates are required for normal fat metabolism. If insufficient carbohydrates are available, the body burns more fat than it can handle. This results in an acidosis condition that can lead to dehydration and sodium imbalance. Some people say fat burns in a fire kindled by carbohydrates because fats require carbohydrates in order to be broken down in the liver. This is another reason why fruits, vegetables and most legumes are considered fat-burning foods. You have already learned how these foods stimulate fat burning to balance the pH of the blood and why even most whole grains are not considered fat-burning foods even though they are complex carbohydrates.

Carbohydrates supply significant amounts of incomplete protein, enzymes, vitamins, minerals and phytonutrients. They contribute bulk to the intestinal contents and improve the peristalsis (progressive wave of contraction and relaxation) of the gastrointestinal tract. This helps maintain a normal transit time for food through the system and improves elimination. Carbohydrates also help the body eliminate toxins, reduce cholesterol levels in the blood, supply the framework for making nonessential amino acids, and are precursors to nucleic acids, connective tissue matrix and a certain part of nerve tissue.

Many people have been led to believe that carbohydrates make you fat. Nothing could be further from the truth. In fact, eating the *right* carbohydrates is the key to stimulating your body to burn stored fat naturally and healthfully. What few "experts" explain are the differences in the various carbohydrate foods and the effects they have in our bodies. Here is the simple truth. Carbohydrates from *processed* grains (wheat, primarily) make people fat. You will learn why later.

Please read the next sentence carefully and memorize it. **Any carbohydrates eaten but not used are stored as body fat.** This is why utilization is such an important step and why even good foods can make you fat if eaten to excess or at the wrong time.

Protein

Protein foods are classified as either complete or incomplete. Complete protein foods contain the ten amino acids essential for normal growth and function. These amino acids must be obtained from foods because they cannot be made in the body at all or in sufficient amounts. Complete protein foods are meats, poultry, fish, eggs and milk. Milk is usually classified as a carbohydrate but does contain the complete protein casein.

There are a total of twenty different amino acids. They are used for repairing damaged tissues and for building new tissue. Infants and children need far more essential amino acids than adults because of the greater growth they are experiencing. Adults require only about 20 percent of their amino acids to be the essential ones. Most foods contain amino acids but any not supplied can be made from the essential ones. Remember that carbohydrates furnish the framework for this. The protein in grains, vegetables and legumes is considered incomplete because it lacks one or more of the essential amino acids. If you do not get the missing amino acid from another source, you will become deficient and experience health difficulties.

Protein can be used as a source of heat and energy, but is extremely inefficient because the conversion process uses up to 30 percent of the energy produced. In contrast, fats and carbohydrates use only about five percent of their calories for the conversion process. Therefore, protein should be used for its primary functions and not for energy. High-protein diets are expensive, stress the body and can cause harmful physical and emotional imbalances.

Most body fluids such as enzymes, hormones, mucus, milk and sperm are made from protein. Bile and urine are the only ones without protein. Immunoglobulins (antibodies) are also made from protein. Blood proteins, particularly albumin, are important for maintaining a normal osmotic relationship among body fluids. Not enough blood protein can lead to edema. Blood proteins also transport other substances to where they are needed. Proteins help maintain pH balance in the body and are needed for a variety of other metabolic functions.

The best time to eat protein foods is in the evening so the amino acids are available for building and repair at night. The nutrients eaten within a few hours after exercise are also used for growth and repair, so some complete protein should be eaten soon after intense strength and bodybuilding workouts. Carbohydrates should also be eaten soon after strength training to replenish the glycogen (stored glucose) in the muscles. Walking or other aerobic exercise rarely breaks down any muscle, so complete protein is unnecessary after this type of exercise.

I believe that the majority of people in the United States eat far more protein than they need. Excessive amounts of complete protein overwork the digestive system making it less efficient. You now know what that can cause. Excess protein also contributes to the development of a variety of problems, such as osteoporosis and hypoglycemia. You will learn how this occurs in chapter ten.

The recommended dietary allowance for protein is 0.8 gram per kilogram of ideal body weight. A kilogram is 2.2 pounds so the RDA is 0.36 gram per pound. Therefore, a man whose ideal weight is 150 pounds would need 54 grams (150 x 0.36) of protein a day and a woman whose ideal weight is 100 pounds would need 36 grams. The minimum protein requirement is about 0.2 gram per pound if the person is getting adequate energy from fats and carbohydrates. This equals 30 grams for a 150-pound man and 20 grams for a 100-pound woman. These recommendations are based on eating complete and incomplete protein foods. These amounts must be adjusted somewhat based on the quality and utilization rate of the proteins being eaten. For example, vegetarians need more because of the lower biological value of the proteins they eat.

I believe that most people would be healthier if they ate one gram of protein for every two to four pounds of lean body weight. For instance, if a woman's lean body mass is 100 pounds, she should eat between 25 and 50 grams of protein a day. Keep in mind that if she had 20 percent body fat her total weight would be 125 pounds. If a man's lean body mass is 200 pounds, he should eat between 50 and 100 grams of protein a day. Even this estimate may be excessively high for some people because certain variables must be taken into account, like amount, intensity and type of exercise, occupation, age, speed of metabolism, and others. Remember that only about 20 percent of the total protein needed has to come from complete protein foods like meats and eggs. Even a lean, hard-training 200-pound bodybuilder (not a growth-enhancing drug user) should not need more than 90 total grams a day and only about 18 grams from complete protein. That's far less than most smaller, inactive people eat.

Those who market protein powders and drinks often recommend 300 or more grams of complete protein a day. This is absurd but sells more of their products. What most of us need are more good fats and carbohydrates for the energy, vitamins, minerals and other nutrients they supply. People who exercise intensely and eat excess protein usually also gain body fat because muscular growth is not a fast process. Ingesting excess complete protein in an attempt to force muscles to grow does not work unless you are using growth-enhancing anabolic steroids or similar drugs. It is harmful to your body, expensive, uses a large amount of energy and is unnecessary. Chapter fifteen has more guidelines for determining your personal protein needs.

Eating excess complete protein also leads to excess body fat because most of the foods (mainly meats and cheese) contain saturated fat. These fats increase cholesterol and triglyceride levels in the blood and lead to other negative health effects for those who do not burn the fat as energy. This fat used to be necessary for keeping the body warm in cold weather and during times of famine or poor harvests, back when most people did hard physical work that burned the fat for energy. Because nowadays most of us are not out in the cold much, do not have to worry about famine and do little hard physical work, we need to reduce our consumption of saturated fats.

Like carbohydrates, **any complete protein eaten but not used is stored as body fat.** Once again, the bottom line is proper timing to ensure nutrient utilization.

Fats

Because of advertising, various books about dieting, numerous articles and fad diets, many people believe fat is bad for them. The fear of eating fat often causes them to eat a worthless processed food just because the label says "low fat" or "no fat." Most of these products are made from foods that contain no fat to begin with or are loaded with sugar and other unhealthful ingredients. Many people see "no fat" on the label and assume it is good for them. It is usually labeled this way to sell more of the product.

Some people believe all they need to do to lose body fat is eat less fat. This often creates nutrient imbalances, because they eliminate the good fats along with the bad ones and most people replace the fat with *processed* complex carbohydrates. Eating excess fat can cause someone to gain body fat, but the majority of people I have counseled got fat by eating processed grain products and dairy foods. Getting caught up in some low-fat diet craze may create serious imbalances and starve your body for the vital nutrients found in fats.

This could lead to some puzzling health problems and probably to an increase in body fat.

Fats are vital nutrients with many important functions that contribute to good health and even to being lean. They act as carriers for the fat-soluble vitamins: A, D, E, and K. Fats are important for the conversion of the provitamin carotene (alpha, beta and gamma) to vitamin A. If you get less than 10 percent of your total calories from fat, you may develop a deficiency in carotene and vitamins A, D, E and K. This could lead to many serious deficiencies and subsequent health problems. Because vitamin D is important for making calcium available to the body, fats help us get adequate calcium. For this reason, a low-fat diet may contribute to the development of osteoporosis. Fats supply long-lasting energy, because one gram contains about nine calories—more than twice the amount found in one gram of carbohydrate or protein. I believe most of us should supply more of our energy needs from healthful fats. Fats also create a satisfied feeling after eating and contribute to the pleasing taste of many foods. Rather important, wouldn't you say? We do not need a low-fat, low-taste diet—we need a right-fat, great-taste diet.

Most glands and organs in your body are protected and held in place by internal deposits of fat. About 45 percent of your total fat is used for this purpose. A layer of fat also insulates your body against changes in temperature and helps preserve body heat. Some fats are a part of your cell walls and help other fats to pass into and out of the cells. Other fats improve your bowel function and help keep your joints well lubricated and your skin moist and supple. I recently read a magazine article in which a dermatologist said that if you are well hydrated and still have dry skin the best thing to do is apply lotion. Based on this statement it does not seem like this skin specialist knows much about keeping the skin healthy.

Instead of applying creams and lotions to your skin to keep it soft, feed your skin with nutritious fats. The best way to have healthy skin is to nourish the live skin cells, not just soften the dead cells on the outside. Some skin creams and lotions contain healthful nutrients that can be absorbed into the skin but many also contain unhealthful ingredients. Nature wants us to eat more fat in the winter not only to keep us warm but also to protect our skin from the elements and prevent it from drying out.

Understand that not all fats are created equal and that some are much better for us than others. For instance, some fats contain saturated fatty acids. These saturated fats are usually hard at room temperature and come from animal fat, butterfat, coconut oil, palm oil and palm kernel oil. All of these, with the exception of coconut oil, should be kept to a minimum in your diet. Fats with unsaturated fatty acids are usually liquid at room temperature and come from vegetable, nut and seed sources. Monounsaturated fatty acids are found in avocado, olive, peanut, and canola oils. Polyunsaturated fatty acids are found in corn, sesame, sunflower seed, flaxseed, soybean, walnut, grapeseed, cottonseed, safflower and fish oils.

Three unsaturated fatty acids—linoleic, linolenic and arachidonic—have what is called essential fatty acid (EFA) activity. Fatty acids with EFA activity are precursors to compounds important in the regulation of blood pressure, heart rate, vascular dilation, lipolysis (breakdown of fat), blood clotting and the proper function of the central nervous system. Essential fatty acids help reduce inflammation, water retention and blood platelet stickiness. They have sometimes completely eliminated the symptoms of premenstrual syndrome. Cholesterol levels of the blood are also lowered by EFA activity.

These fatty acids are called "essential" because they must be supplied in the diet. The two most important essential fatty acids are omega-6 (linoleic acid) and omega-3 (linolenic acid). A recommended ratio I have seen is 3.5 parts omega-6 to 1 part omega-3. A one-to-one ratio may be healthier but no one knows for sure. Primary sources of omega-6 are evening primrose, safflower, sunflower seed, sesame, cottonseed, grapeseed, peanut and corn oils, as well as meat and poultry. Omega-3 EFAs are found in flaxseed and its oil, borage oil, salmon, sardines, mackerel, herring, fish oils, walnuts and its oil, pumpkinseeds and green leafy vegetables. Soybeans, soybean oil and hemp oil are sources of both types of EFAs.

If farm-raised fish are not fed dietary sources of omega-3s they will not contain this vital nutrient. The same holds true for the eggs of chickens that are denied a natural diet. If animals do not eat as Nature intended they are unhealthy and their meats or eggs will not supply us with the nutrients we need.

Eggs high in omega-3 fatty acids are now available from chickens that are fed plants that are rich in omega-3s. The meat from chickens, pigs, cows and sheep used to contain omega-3 fatty acids because the animals ate their natural diets. Unfortunately, many of them, and some fish, are now fattened up with grains like corn that contain only omega-6 fatty acids. The beef and lamb raised in New Zealand contain omega-3 fatty acids, as does the beef you can buy from grasslandbeef.com. And, these meats taste much better than the meat lacking in this essential nutrient.

It is estimated that the average diet supplies 20 to 40 times more omega-6 fatty acids than omega-3s. An excess of omega-6s may limit the amount of omega-3s your body can use and create other unhealthful imbalances. Most people should probably increase their consumption of omega-3 fatty acids and decrease intake of omega-6 sources. The only omega-6 oils I recommend using occasionally are cold-pressed sesame, grapeseed and sunflower seed. I believe that many people suffer from health problems caused by a deficiency of EFAs, primarily omega-3. Most saturated fats interfere with the metabolism of omega-3 and omega-6 fatty acids. This is another good reason to limit your intake of saturated fats.

I once attended a nutritional seminar during which the instructor said that if you have enough fatty acids in your body, the herpes virus cannot cause blisters. Herpes simplex viruses cause what are commonly called cold sores or fever blisters in the mouth or on the lips and face. Genital herpes and herpes zoster (shingles) are also caused by this virus. The instructor said that all of these conditions could be prevented or helped by essential fatty acids. Based on personal experimentation and reports from a few patients, EFAs seem helpful for preventing cold sores.

Cholesterol has gotten a bad reputation that is completely undeserved. Some food companies have taken advantage of this false information to sell more of their products, many that never even contained cholesterol. But if people think cholesterol is bad for them, a product label that reads "No Cholesterol" will increase sales. Let me give you a few facts.

Cholesterol is a type of fat known as a sterol and has many vital functions. It is a major part of brain and nerve cells and is found in many glands. Without cholesterol, your body could not make male and female sex hormones and adrenal hormones. These hormones are important for your sex drive and performance, muscle development, other normal functions and some help your body burn fat. Important functions, wouldn't you say? Instead of looking for an aphrodisiac, supply your body with the precursor nutrients and then stimulate more sex hormone production with strength-building exercise. The bile that emulsifies fat so it can be further broken down and used by your body is made from cholesterol and vitamin D is produced from it when your skin is exposed to sunlight. Cholesterol is a part of the secretions of the oil glands that keep our skin well hydrated and protected from the environment. This vital fat also helps maintain normal flexibility of our cell walls.

A normal human body produces far more cholesterol than most people get from what they eat and only about 40 percent of ingested cholesterol is absorbed. Eating large amounts of foods that contain cholesterol barely raises your blood cholesterol level because your body simply makes less if you eat more. There is one exception—eating processed sugar with cholesterol increases your blood cholesterol levels significantly. Do not stop eating eggs and other healthful foods that contain cholesterol—stop eating sugar. Remember that commercial salad dressings, sauces and similar products are often loaded with sugar. Eating more foods that contain cholesterol may be healthful, because your liver will not have to produce as much cholesterol.

Polyunsaturated fats lower your blood cholesterol level but most saturated fats (butterfat, palm and palm kernel oil, and meat fat) increase it dramatically. Therefore, these saturated fats are the real enemy and you should avoid them whenever possible. Cheese is probably the main contributor to excessive saturated fat in the average American's diet and is widely known as being constipating. I especially recommend avoiding it.

Coconut oil is a saturated fat that has gotten a bad reputation but in reality is one of the healthiest fats you can eat. Other saturated fats are made up of long-chain fatty acids (LCFAs) that digest slowly and once absorbed combine with protein to form lipoproteins. They often end up inside fat cells. Coconut oil is completely different because it is composed of medium-chain fatty acids (MCFAs) like the healthful fat found in human breast milk. Medium-chain fatty acids are much smaller molecules that do not need pancreatic enzymes for digestion. They are absorbed quickly and go directly to the liver where they are used to produce long-lasting energy. They create a cumulative increase in endurance in those who use them for a while. Because of their energy production, MCFAs stimulate the metabolism enough to burn up the calories in the oil and some from other foods. Therefore, coconut oil is not only an excellent energy source but also stimulates fat loss.

You can buy energy supplements made from MCFAs but it is better and less expensive to use coconut oil or coconut butter. Medium-chain fatty acids have been shown to improve digestion, strengthen the immune system and protect against bacterial, viral and fungal infections. An effective natural treatment for overgrowth of the yeast *Candida albicans* is caprylic acid, a fatty acid found in coconut oil. MCFAs reduce the risk of heart disease by protecting the heart and arteries from harmful conditions. Polynesian and Asian people who use coconut and its oil have the lowest rates of heart disease in the world. Medium-chain fatty acids improve the absorption of B vitamins, fat-soluble vitamins, amino acids, and minerals, especially calcium and magnesium. Coconut oil is the best oil to use for high heat cooking. As the health benefits of coconut oil become more widely known, its availability will probably increase. If you want to use it but cannot find any at your local health-food store it can be ordered online at celtic-seasalt.com. Two products are available. The oil has a pleasant flavor and the coconut butter is tasteless.

Nature clearly did not intend everyone to use coconut oil because coconuts grow only in certain climates. You could use it to help you lose fat but it is not necessary to accomplish your goals. Remember that you should be able to be lean and healthy by eating the foods that can be grown in the environment where you live.

Fatty acids are usually found in the body as combinations called triglycerides. This is the form of most of the fats we eat and also the form found in our fat cells. Eating *refined* carbohydrates is unhealthful because it increases the triglycerides in our blood.

Cholesterol and triglycerides are carried in the bloodstream by lipoproteins. High-density lipoproteins (HDL, or "good" cholesterol) carry them to the liver. The liver can use them or send them to other parts of the body using low-density lipoproteins (LDL, or "bad" cholesterol). Our cells get the fatty acids they need from the LDL but when needs have been met, the excess fats and cholesterol are either transferred to HDL and carried back to the liver or transported to fat cells for storage. A direct correlation has been determined between the amount of saturated fats eaten and the level of LDL cholesterol in the blood.

Most of the fat you eat should come from foods containing healthful fat. Nature seals many vital nutrients inside foods to prevent them from being destroyed by exposure to heat or oxygen. This is true of oils and juices. Mother's milk is sealed inside for the same reasons. If you eat whole grains, seeds, nuts, eggs, fish, avocados and a variety of different vegetables, you should get most of the fats you need. Eating the whole food is the preferred way to get them but you can also use coconut oil and some unsaturated oil from seed sources or olives. The oils I prefer are coconut, olive, sunflower seed, grapeseed and sesame. Walnut and pumpkinseed oils are also good because they are sources of omega-3 fatty acids. I do not recommend using vegetable oils, animal fats, butterfat, palm oil or any hydrogenated or partially hydrogenated oils. Fats are hydrogenated to harden them and extend the shelf life. Hydrogenated fats disturb your normal cholesterol metabolism. Most commercial baked goods contain hydrogenated fat. This is just one of many reasons to avoid those products.

High heat changes the molecular structure of unsaturated fats and creates unhealthful trans-fatty acids. They start to form at 320°F and the higher the heat, the more of them that will form. Because trans-fatty acids fit only partially into the receptor sites of enzymes and membranes, they cannot do the job of a normal fatty acid and they block normal fatty acids from binding and doing their jobs. This impairs the protective barrier around the cells that keeps out invading allergens, bacteria and viruses. Some molecules that would normally be kept out of our cells can get in and those that should stay in our cells can now get out. Heart function may also be abnormally affected because it is fueled by fatty acids. Butterfat is a natural source of trans-fatty acids and should definitely be avoided. Trans-fatty acids are more destructive to our health than saturated fats. This is just one good reason to completely avoid deep-fat fried foods.

Most commercial oil producers use high heat and chemicals to extract the oil from seeds, vegetables and grains. They usually first press the oil-containing foods. Then they soak them in chemical solvents so more oil can be extracted. The oil is then degummed, refined, bleached and finally deodorized using steam distillation under pressure. The oils are usually heated to 464° to 518°F for 30 to 60 minutes to remove the chemicals and peroxides used during refining and bleaching. At this point, essentially all the nutritional value has been destroyed. When heated to more than 302°F, unsaturated fatty acids become mutagenic, meaning they can damage the genes of those who eat them and the genes of their future offspring.

Canola oil is considered healthful by many but I do not recommend it. It contains about 10 percent omega-3 fatty acids but they are destroyed if it is heated higher than 120°F. Few manufacturers process this oil at temperatures low enough to maintain any health benefits, and canola oil also contains erucic acid, a toxic fatty acid.

You should only use oils obtained by cold-pressing techniques that are stored in dark, light-blocking containers. Except for olive and coconut oils, it is best to store oils in your refrigerator after they are opened. Raw nuts and seeds are also best kept refrigerated to protect them from heat and light.

Extra virgin olive oil does not contain many essential fatty acids but is beneficial to health because it contains chlorophyll, vitamin E and beta-carotene. Being monounsaturated makes it more stable than polyunsaturated oils. It can be heated up to 325°F without destroying nutrients. It is best used raw but can be used for medium-heat cooking. It is a great-tasting salad dressing when eating vegetables.

Monounsaturated fats reduce the amount of LDL cholesterol in our blood but do not affect the HDL amount. These fats can be used frequently. Besides olive oil, avocados and almost all nuts contain monounsaturated fat. Polyunsaturated fats lower both the LDL and HDL cholesterol. They do have important uses in the body, but do not use them often. Avoid peanuts and peanut products, because they are legumes containing omega-6 fatty acids.

Even if you are eating foods containing healthful fat it is still a good idea to use cold-pressed oil as a salad dressing for your lunch or on whole grains at breakfast. Fats and oils are best ingested early in the day so the calories are used as energy and do not accumulate as body fat. Unsaturated fats are absorbed more rapidly than saturated fats and are made available to the body for energy faster. Ingesting healthful fats reduces your craving for unhealthful fatty foods, such as cheese, meat fats or greasy fried foods. They also help satisfy your hunger throughout the day.

Almost all tissues can use fatty acids for energy. The body prefers saturated and monounsaturated sources for this purpose. Muscular tissue derives much of its energy from fat even when glucose is available. This explains why exercise is helpful for losing body fat and staying lean.

Like carbohydrates and proteins, **any fat eaten but not used is stored as body fat**. Once again, the key to ensure utilization is proper timing.

Water

Water is the most important nutrient you can ingest but many people do not get enough. Approximately 60 percent of your body weight is water. Even your bones are about 22 percent water. It is needed for almost all bodily functions such as digestion, absorption and elimination. Water transports nutrients into cells and transports waste out. It helps maintain a normal body temperature. It is needed to manufacture digestive enzymes, hormones and many other substances. Water is also needed to cleanse out toxins and keep your body clean and functioning at peak efficiency.

Your muscles are approximately 70 percent water, and if they dehydrate even a small amount your muscular efficiency is greatly reduced. They act like emergency storehouses for water. Because your internal organs are vital to sustaining life, if you do not drink enough water they will get what they need from your muscles and your muscles will dehydrate. This causes fatigue and muscular weakness. Many people frequently suffer from fatigue that they could eliminate simply by drinking more water and restoring normal muscle function.

The body of a sedentary adult male weighing 150 pounds contains approximately 45 quarts of water and loses about three quarts a day. In the desert he would lose about 10 quarts or more. A sedentary 120-pound female has about 36 quarts of water and loses about two and a half quarts each day. If you are outdoors, exercising or perspiring excessively, you need more water to replace what you are losing. Drink some before and during your activities not just after. A rule of thumb when active is to drink 16 ounces of water for every 500 calories you burn. For example, if you ride an exercise bike and it indicates that you burned 500 calories, you should drink 16 ounces of water. Because most people eat excess protein and not enough fruits and vegetables, this amount will be best for them. When you are eating a more balanced diet, you should not need as much, but I still recommend drinking about this amount because of the body's need for water to flush out the numerous toxins we are exposed to in our modern environments. Normally, drinking a bit more water than you need won't hurt you but not drinking enough could.

If you are taking antidiuretic hormone (ADH) for diabetes or another condition, you must be more aware of your water intake. Because this hormone prevents the normal loss of water, you could become water intoxicated if you drink more than you need. The symptoms of this condition range from a mild headache to confusion, coma, seizures and even death. Consult with your doctor if you take ADH.

You get water from drinks like coffee and tea but your body does best on pure water. Some people I have counseled were not drinking any water. After I explained the importance of it, they began drinking water and reported dramatic improvements in how they felt; increased energy was always one of the benefits. Drink more water and less junk liquids like soft drinks that can create nutritional imbalances and fat gain. As you will learn, even diet sodas contribute to making you fat. If you do not like water, add a little lemon or lime juice or drink various caffeine-free herbal teas.

You get water from most of the whole foods you eat, especially fruits and vegetables, but you should still drink extra. The thirst mechanism of your body usually works well, but extreme heat or sweating may make it lag behind your need. You may not get the message to drink until you are almost two percent dehydrated. Sickness, age or abnormal function of certain parts of the body can make the thirst mechanism inaccurate, as can drinking junk liquids. For these reasons, the majority of older people probably do not drink enough water. Many of them take drugs for symptoms caused by not getting enough. Some people drink carbonated water, but because of the carbon dioxide gas released in their stomachs they feel full before they get enough.

Even the "experts" disagree on how much water we should drink. Understanding why is easy if you consider such variables as the different foods and drinks people ingest, varying body sizes, activity levels, gender, age, internal organ function and overall health status. One person may need two glasses of water a day but another may require seven or eight. Even the amount you need varies from day to day. Therefore, it is impossible for me to tell you how much water to drink but I am going to give you a rule of thumb to help you determine the right amount for you.

Normally your urine should be clear. If it is yellow, you probably need more water. It's that simple. You may already know that if you take supplemental B vitamins your urine is more yellow than normal because any of the water-soluble vitamins not used are flushed out of your system. You will learn later how wasteful this is and even if you are taking them, it is still easy to figure out how yellow your urine will be when getting an adequate amount of water. Simply determine how much water you generally need when not taking the vitamins and then drink the same amount with the vitamins and check the color. After you determine approximately how much water you need, it is simple to fill up a bottle with that amount each morning. Drink from it throughout the day and when the day is half over, half of the water should be gone and it should all be gone when the day is done. This is a simple method to use if you feel that you are not drinking enough water.

Some of the most common symptoms experienced when not getting enough water are headaches, dizziness, fatigue, irritability, cramps, nausea, constipation, itchy skin, incoherent speech, acute mental confusion, loss of coordination, blurred vision, elevated pulse and rapid breathing. Severe dehydration can even result in death.

Some doctors believe that water will cure many of the ailments that plague people today. I agree it is vital to good health but believe that many other variables are usually involved in causing these problems. As with losing excess fat, the true cause or causes must be discovered and eliminated for any condition to be resolved healthfully and permanently.

Obesity decreases the amount of water in the body to as low as 45 percent. This explains why obese people frequently have many of the symptoms of dehydration, and why it is more important for an obese person to drink adequate amounts of water and to avoid products that cause water loss. The importance of drinking adequate amounts of water cannot be overemphasized.

Chlorine and fluorine are harmful

Chlorine and fluorine are two toxic chemicals you do not want in your water. Many city water systems add numerous chemicals to the water to kill bacteria, inhibit algae growth and for various other reasons. Your water supply may have as many as fifty different chemicals added. They are considered "safe" by the agencies adding them, but no one knows the detrimental long-term health effects. I believe that these chemicals cause cumulative damage and are the primary causes of certain health problems often seen in older humans and animals. The elderly have ingested small amounts of these toxins over a long period of time. It is like being slowly poisoned. Many people drink bottled spring water partly because tap water tastes bad. This may seem like a healthy alternative but pollution in the air and soil finds its way into our mountain lakes and springs. Also, according to Hulda Clark, Ph.D., N.D., author of *The Cure for All Cancers*, bottled water is a major source of isopropyl (propyl) alcohol, the chemical she believes is the primary cause of cancer. Because her research and ideas make sense to me, I avoid untested bottled water.

Chlorine is an essential mineral but is found throughout the body in the form of chloride. Many scientists, doctors and health researchers believe the chlorine added to water is extremely harmful. Chlorine is a highly reactive chemical with the potential to join with other chemicals and minerals to form harmful substances. Chlorine in drinking water destroys vitamin E and many of the good intestinal bacteria important for optimal health. These friendly bacteria make vitamin K and keep the intestinal yeast *Candida albicans* in check. I believe that the excessive growth of this yeast is the cause of numerous health problems that have medical science baffled.

Ten to twenty years after chlorination of water became more common, the incidence of heart attacks and arteriosclerosis (hardening of the arteries) began increasing significantly. I believe that this is because chlorine damages the inner lining of the arteries. The damage is then repaired with a patch made of cholesterol and other substances. This patch decreases the inside diameter of the artery and if enough damage occurs, could completely plug the artery. A study I read many years ago indicated that the people living in a city with a chlorinated water supply had a much higher incidence of arteriosclerosis than those in a nearby city where the water was not chlorinated. Those who moved from the city without chlorinated water to the city with it began to develop the problem.

Because your skin can absorb chlorine from water, I recommend using a chlorine filter on your shower. These can be purchased for about $50. Methods are available that can eliminate the need for or reduce the amount of chlorine used in swimming pools. This would be a worthwhile investment if you have a pool you use frequently. Inhaling chlorine fumes is another way it can get into your system. Many older people may have fallen when showering because the chlorine fumes overcame them. I believe these fumes and the chlorine in water used for washing the face could contribute to the development of cataracts.

Fluorine is an essential trace mineral found in the body in the form of fluorides. The form in natural foods is calcium fluoride but the form added to drinking water is sodium fluoride. Sodium fluoride is poisonous; it is used in insecticides and rat poison. Numerous scientific reports show it to be a selective and *cumulative* poison. Excess amounts of fluorine (from sodium fluoride) destroy the enzyme phosphotase, which is important for many processes in the body including the metabolism of vitamins. Fluorine inhibits the activities of other important enzymes and seems especially harmful to brain tissue.

Sodium fluoride is a toxic byproduct of aluminum manufacturing, and aluminum toxicity is suspected as a possible cause of the brain damage that causes Alzheimer's disease. I believe that fluorine is also a part of that cause. I recommend avoiding all products containing sodium fluoride (toothpaste, fluoridated water and others) or aluminum. I also recommend wearing gloves when washing dishes so your hands are not exposed to water that contains fluoride and chlorine.

High levels of fluorine can depress growth, cause calcification of ligaments and tendons and create degenerative changes in the kidneys, liver, adrenal glands, heart, central nervous system and reproductive organs. It also makes bones brittle and more susceptible to breaking. Some doctors believe sodium fluoride contributes to young people growing excessively tall and women having abnormally wide bottoms. Because it interferes with all the enzymes in the body and with the function of the thyroid gland, it contributes to obesity. Certain research suggests a direct relationship between fluoridated water and the incidence of Down's syndrome. During World War II, the Russians and Germans added fluoride to the water to make concentration camp prisoners docile and apathetic. It is sometimes added to the drinking water of animals to make them more manageable.

Most countries in the world have forbidden the fluoridation of water. Their lawmakers must believe the scientists, doctors, dentists, biochemists and enzymologists who say it is harmful. It is illegal in all European countries except Ireland, where it is added to the water. It is also illegal in all European countries to import fruits and vegetables sprayed with fluoride-based pesticides.

Many people believe fluoride is necessary to prevent tooth decay. I believe that scientists working for industries that produce sodium fluoride helped to spread this belief. It may help during the formation of the teeth, but is unnecessary after age eighteen. An excess of fluoride can cause a mottling (uneven discoloration) of the teeth. Because most fruits, vegetables, whole grains, eggs, meats and fish contain calcium fluoride, no one should have a problem getting plenty of fluoride if a few whole foods are eaten. Some of these foods contain even more calcium fluoride if grown with fluoridated water. These whole foods are where I recommend getting fluoride throughout life. I believe the healthful form of fluoride found in these foods has health benefits scientists have yet to learn.

Because so many foods contain calcium fluoride, you might think you would get an excess of fluorine but you do not because your body simply uses what it needs and the rest stays harmlessly bound to the calcium. The antidote for fluorine poisoning is calcium. I believe this is because calcium fluoride is formed, thereby preventing the excess fluorine from causing problems.

A young person wanting healthy teeth should eat whole, natural foods and limit or completely avoid foods that cause cavities. Older people should do the same, because the natural foods keep them lean and healthy and the cavity-causing foods have many other harmful effects. In chapter four you will learn about these harmful foods and about groups of people that never had any cavities until they began eating certain processed foods.

The best water to use

The type of water you drink is extremely important. Controversy has raged for many years over drinking distilled water that is mineral free or drinking well or spring water containing inorganic minerals. If you observe Nature and look at history you will see that most of the water ingested by humans and animals contains minerals; therefore, I believe that this water is healthful. Rainwater is distilled but most people and animals do not use it as their main source and these days even rainwater is often full of pollution.

Thousands of pesticides, herbicides, chemical fertilizers, detergents, dyes and other harmful chemicals pollute our environment. This makes many natural water sources unhealthful for us. The Environmental Protection Agency (EPA) sets standards for about ninety different contaminants in our drinking water. Therefore, we need to find a healthful source. Distilled water can be beneficial for people with certain health problems and imbalances but should probably be discontinued after balance has been reestablished. I drank distilled water for a few years and my body developed symptoms of chronic mineral deficiencies even though I was eating well and taking supplemental minerals. This problem may be specific to the individual, because some people have stayed healthy drinking distilled water for a period of many years. If you do want to drink distilled water, I suggest adding two or three tablespoons of purified seawater to every gallon to replace the minerals removed during distillation.

Most water filters do not filter out many of the harmful substances found in our water supplies. Some can become breeding grounds for bacteria, especially if the filter's inner cartridge is not changed often enough. Because even distilled water can contain certain chemical toxins, I believe that the best water to drink is produced from a process known as reverse osmosis. Water treated by reverse osmosis goes through pre-filters and then the water is forced through a membrane that only the water can go through. The toxins are washed away and eliminated. The water then goes through another filter. Water purified this way is like the *pure* spring water Nature probably intended us to use. Once you taste it, you will not want to drink the chemical-filled "dishwater" coming out of most taps.

I recommend drinking water that is room temperature. People who would never put their hands or feet in ice water think nothing of pouring it into their stomachs, which are far more sensitive. Drinking ice water actually makes you hotter because your body has to heat the water to body temperature. I also recommend avoiding hot drinks and soups. Wait until they cool to a moderate temperature. Many Japanese people eat foods heated to extremely high temperatures. I believe that this is one of the reasons why Japan has such a high incidence of stomach cancer.

You should now have a good idea of why the type of water you drink and use for personal hygiene is so important. Because water is vital for normal bodily function and considerable volume is ingested each day, it is essential to have the purest available. The timing of when you drink it also has extreme significance. You will learn about this in chapter five.

Oxygen and Carbon Dioxide

You can live more than a month without food, more than a week without water, but only a few minutes without oxygen. It is vital, of course, to keeping us alive, but you must learn how to supply the oxygen your cells need. When your body oxidizes (burns) fat, it must use oxygen. If your brain and body get adequate oxygen, they can function optimally and better protect you from disease and degenerative processes. As you will soon learn, carbon dioxide (CO_2) is also a vital nutrient and not just a metabolic waste product.

People often use sugar or caffeine to give them energy when what they need is more water or more oxygen. Develop the habit of taking breathing breaks instead of coffee breaks. Do this on arising, during breakfast, midmorning, at lunch, midafternoon, after you get off work, during dinner, whenever you feel stressed and before retiring at night. Breathing properly could become one of your most important and beneficial health habits. Generally, you should breathe in through your nose and out through your nose or mouth. Having some extra oxygen for dessert will certainly make you feel better than eating a pastry made from sugar, fat and flour. Oxygen decreases emotional stress, which is a major cause of overeating. Because more oxygen to your brain improves your self-image and your thinking, it will be easier to make better choices in all areas of life.

Contrary to popular belief, I am not going to recommend taking deep breaths to get more oxygen. You learned in the last chapter that utilization of nutrients is what counts. This is also true for the nutrient oxygen. This may seem contradictory but to get more oxygen to your bodily tissues you have to breathe shallow and slowly. I know most of you are probably raising an eyebrow in disbelief so let me explain.

Our breathing is controlled primarily by the amount of carbon dioxide in our blood. Carbon dioxide levels also affect how much oxygen our blood picks up in our lungs and how much is released in our bodily tissues. A higher level of carbon dioxide delivers more oxygen to our tissues and a lower level leads to less oxygen to the tissues. This occurs because of what is known as the Bohr effect. Therefore, deep breathing, which causes us to exhale excess carbon dioxide, decreases the amount of oxygen our cells get.

Think about what happens during hyperventilation. Breathing faster and deeper does not increase the amount of oxygen that goes to your cells, as most people would assume. Deeper breathing *decreases* the amount of oxygen your cells get. You may already know what it feels like to hyperventilate. It does not take long before you start to feel the effects—dizziness, increased pulse rate, nausea, tetany (muscle cramp), numb or blue lips, tingling in your arms and hands. You may feel like you are not getting enough air and may even faint. These are the symptoms of hypoxia, or an inadequate amount of oxygen going to the cells, and breathing excessively can create it. Some people believe that excess oxygen causes the symptoms felt during hyperventilation but they come from not getting enough oxygen. If you suffer from angina, anxiety, allergies, migraines, asthma, epilepsy or similar health conditions, hyperventilating could bring on the symptoms of your condition. Breathing into a paper bag helps people who are hyperventilating because they breathe back in the carbon dioxide they are eliminating and restore more normal CO_2 levels.

Carbon dioxide has many more important functions. It is a smooth muscle dilator. Not enough of it could cause spasms of the blood vessels in the brain, triggering migraine headaches, strokes or epileptic seizures, and if the blood vessels in the heart spasm, it could cause angina or a myocardial infarction (heart attack). Chronic contraction or spasm of the bronchial muscles can lead to asthma. Carbon dioxide also acts as a catalyst for numerous bodily functions. It assists the normal function of proteins, fats, carbohydrates, enzymes, vitamins, minerals, antibodies and hormones, primarily by changing the pH of the blood. People who over-breathe have hormone deficiencies, particularly the female sex hormone. Deep breathing may not be the entire cause but is usually a part of it. Carbon dioxide seems to work something like a hormone that is produced by every tissue and probably acts on every organ. It is as vital as oxygen because without it you will not get adequate oxygen and will have numerous other imbalances and dysfunctions.

Almost all of us over-breathe because we do not know how to breathe correctly or have been taught incorrectly. Most of us do not usually do it to the degree that we experience extreme hypoxic symptoms, but few of us get adequate oxygen to our cells. We experience mild hypoxic symptoms but assume they are normal or look for other causes. Over-breathing creates imbalances in our body that must be corrected if optimal health is to be enjoyed. Why does meditation help people feel better, decrease stress, and reduce sleep needs? Because during meditation we breathe slowly and more shallow. This is also how biofeedback and other relaxation techniques produce most of their results. Thousands of years ago, Buddha taught his followers breath awareness as a vital step to reaching enlightenment. Even today, yogis of India perform what seem to be superhuman feats. Everything is done with breath control, because breathing is the only thing they can consciously regulate. For example, they can slow their heart rates dramatically. This cannot be done except by increasing the amount of carbon dioxide in their blood by breathing less. It is easy to understand how this works. Over-breathing increases the heart rate because the cells get less oxygen, and breathing less slows it because the cells get more oxygen.

Our atmosphere used to be well over 10 percent carbon dioxide. The alveoli of our lungs contain about 6.5 percent carbon dioxide, and while developing in the womb our bodies get about 7 to 8 percent carbon dioxide. The problem of over-breathing exists because the amount of carbon dioxide in the air is much less. It was only .035 percent in 1996. How do we compensate for such low levels of carbon dioxide in the air? We need to learn to breathe slower and shallower so we always maintain higher carbon dioxide levels in our blood, which leads to more oxygen going to our cells. Although it varies for everyone, the average amount of air we should breathe is 3 to 4 liters per minute.

Many of us have a habit of over-breathing because we have been taught that it is good for us by people who did not know or understand the Bohr effect. It is nothing to feel badly about. Most of us have not been taught how to breathe, eat, exercise, have good posture or take care of our health in other ways, or we have been instructed incorrectly.

We can improve our retention of carbon dioxide if we know and reduce the things that stimulate over-breathing. Overeating greatly increases breathing as does lack of physical work or activity, so this gives you another good reason to eat well and exercise. Other causes of deeper breathing are intense emotions (positive or negative), stress, heat, stuffy environments, bed rest, prolonged horizontal lying and excess sleep. Eating animal products increases breathing more than plant products and cooked foods increase it more than raw foods. Anything that stimulates your sympathetic nervous system leads to over-breathing. This is the body's way of eliminating carbon dioxide in preparation for the physical action that will create more. Often we are sitting in traffic or in other situations where we are unable to do anything physical. Knowing how to breathe properly is especially important at these times. It should be obvious how to prevent over-breathing. Just do the opposite of what causes it. I believe that an insufficient amount of natural balanced light also stimulates over-breathing. You will learn about this vital nutrient in the next section.

K. P. Buteyko, Ph.D., a Russian scientist, has been researching breathing for more than forty years and has helped thousands of people resolve their severe and chronic health conditions by teaching them how to breathe correctly. His research has linked deep breathing to being the entire or partial cause of over 150 diseases. Professor Buteyko's goal has been to help people recondition their breathing patterns by using his deliberate volitional breathing method (DVBM). It is now known as the Buteyko Method and is best learned from a qualified instructor. It teaches people to relax their respiratory muscles until they feel a slight shortage of air. With practice, I believe it will reset your respiratory mechanism so you will be less sensitive to carbon dioxide levels and naturally breathe a lesser and healthier amount of air.

Professor Buteyko developed a test he calls the "Control Pause." To get an accurate reading you need to be relaxed and must not have eaten for at least an hour. Just inhale and exhale normally (do not exaggerate) and then hold your breath while pinching your nose. Look at a clock with a second hand and time from the start of holding your breath until you get the first urge to breathe. Do not make an effort to hold your breath as long as you can. This test is designed to measure your respiratory sensitivity, not your will power. A control pause of 60 seconds indicates that you are breathing the medically recommended amount. For more than forty years, all the people tested with a control pause close to 60 seconds were extremely healthy. A time of 30 seconds means you breathe an average of twice the recommended amount, 20 seconds indicates three times the amount and 10 seconds or less means six times more than normal. The lower the control pause is the more you are over-breathing.

People who learn correct breathing report feeling a new inner calm, having fewer struggles in their lives and responding to situations logically and calmly instead of emotionally. All of their symptoms of stress are greatly reduced. I highly recommend that you read more about Professor Buteyko's research and the success of his method. Learning to breathe as he suggests will probably influence your health and well-being more than any other change you make. Search the Internet to find more information and a listing of instructors. I have met and talked with Christopher Drake, a knowledgeable and qualified instructor of the Buteyko Method.

Unfortunately, many of us breathe polluted air. This makes it even more important to get the nutrients our bodies need to protect us from these pollutants. Breathing less is also helpful because it decreases the amount of toxins we inhale. I highly recommend doing as much as you can to breathe clean air whenever possible. To clean *all* the air in your home and office, get an air purifier (not an air filter) that produces ozone and negative ions. This is how Nature purifies the air. If you cannot find one, get in touch with the publisher of this book and they will help you locate one. A less expensive alternative is a negative ion generator (about $30) and a good air filter. Some filters also have negative ionizers. Filters are limited because the air is not cleaned until it passes through the filter, but using a filter is far better than breathing unclean air.

Sunlight

This nutrient is vital to all life—plant or animal. Without sunlight, there would be no food for anyone or anything. But sunlight is vital for good health in other ways. Have you ever felt less energetic and ambitious when the sky is gray and overcast? People in certain parts of the world get extremely depressed and develop a condition called seasonal affective disorder (SAD). It is caused by a deficiency of sunlight, but is easily resolved if the person spends a few hours a day exposed to full-spectrum lights that duplicate sunlight. A similar but milder condition called the winter blues affects millions.

I believe that sunlight, like love, is an essential nutrient that is sadly lacking in many people's lives. Getting ultraviolet (UV) light through the pupils of our eyes seems to feed and balance the pineal and pituitary glands. This in turn has a balancing effect on all other glands of our endocrine system. Normal function of these glands is critical to good health and maintaining normal weight. Some people have excess body fat simply because their thyroid glands are functioning below normal due to an insufficient amount of UV light getting to their pineal glands. I believe that balanced light is extremely important for maintaining a normal appetite. Many pets that are indoors most of the time are fat and have more health problems because of an inadequate amount of natural light.

You do not need to nor should you ever stare directly at the sun. To get the UV light you need, all you have to do is sit in the shade outside or indoors by an open window. You can also work or play outdoors. Whenever possible, you should avoid wearing eyeglasses and contact lenses outside, or have them made from plastic that lets UV light pass through. I especially recommend not wearing sunglasses. Whenever possible, I work near an open window so I can get Nature's balanced light. Numerous health problems, including cancer, have improved when the afflicted person got more natural light. Many of the health benefits obtained at the health retreats of the past were probably due to the natural light exposure. Years ago, I was working in an office doing drafting and design work under regular fluorescent lights. My eyes began to get strained easily when working or reading. I learned about natural light and found that I could read for hours without eyestrain if I was outside or under full-spectrum lights. My office and home both have full-spectrum lighting throughout.

Many of us do not get enough UV light because we are stuck indoors or behind glass or certain clear plastics that block the passage of UV light. If the window near you in your home, office or car is closed or you wear UV-blocking eyeglasses, contact lenses or sunglasses, you are not going to get this vital nutrient. Air pollution also reduces the amount of UV light we get.

I began wearing eyeglasses when I was five years old and got my first pair of bifocals at age twelve. I enlisted in the Army at age eighteen and was issued glasses for distance vision. While serving in Vietnam I didn't wear them for reading and the close up work I was doing. About ten months later I noticed that when I wore them my eyes hurt, so I stopped wearing them altogether. When I returned home almost a year after that, my eyesight was perfect and had been for many months. About ten years later I learned that the constant exposure to the natural light of the sun (we did not have glass windows) is what had restored my vision back to normal. Now, after more than thirty years, my distance vision has weakened a little because I am usually in my office treating patients or looking at a computer screen, but I can still read fine print without glasses. I plan to have an office someday where I can replace the windows with UV-transmitting clear plastic; I expect to see rapid improvement in my distance vision soon after. You may experience improved vision after you get more balanced light through the pupils of your eyes.

Sunlight has other health benefits, because it contains a balance of colors. Even the light Nature supplies is balanced. Unfortunately, most man-made lights are not. For example, a regular incandescent light bulb has more of the red color spectrum or wavelength. This creates imbalance and problems. The cells of animals subjected to red light weakened and then ruptured. Could the red color spectrum of incandescent lights be damaging to our cells? I think it is highly possible. The reaction of cells exposed to blue light was like that of cells being attacked by viruses. Could this make cells more susceptible to viral disease? Again, I believe it is a possibility. During certain studies, adult male rats under regular fluorescent lights were irritable and tried to bite, but those under natural light were docile and helped care for their young. Mink exposed to sunlight through pink glass became aggressive and sometimes vicious. People wearing pink-tinted lenses have gone from being extremely aggressive and disturbed to relaxed and confident after changing to gray tinted lenses. Color therapy helps people by reestablishing the balance of vibrations we should be getting from balanced light and different colored food. You can read many fascinating and thought-provoking stories about natural light in *Health and Light* by John N. Ott. I highly recommend it.

It is important to reduce your exposure to unbalanced light sources like incandescent light bulbs, regular fluorescent lights, halogen lights, computer monitors and televisions. The more exposure you have to these man-made light sources, the more important it is to counteract their negative effects with as much balanced light as possible.

Some regular-shaped light bulbs are labeled "full spectrum" and are sold as plant lights. These are healthier for plants and animals because they have a balance of colors but they do not contain UV light. Ultraviolet light can be produced only from a fluorescent light. Thanks to John Ott, these are now available in different lengths of straight tubes and even small curved fluorescent tubes that can be used in a regular light socket. These lights are initially more expensive, but save you money by using less energy and lasting for many years. The ones currently in my office have been there for more than ten years.

Sunlight is an essential nutrient for good health, vitality and normal metabolism and body weight. Do your best to get as much each day as you can. If you are often indoors, use full-spectrum "Ott-Lites™" at home and work. These have a balance of colors *and* ultraviolet light, just like the sun. Do not wear sunglasses. Instead, wear a hat or visor to shade your eyes. When our eyes get UV light, the pupils dilate more than if the UV is blocked. If you block the UV with sunglasses, regular glasses, contact lenses or windows in your home, office or automobile, your eyes will get excess visible light. I believe this could possibly damage them and contribute to the development of cataracts or other eye problems. If nothing else, this excess of visible light causes eyestrain, squinting and wrinkles.

You can get contact lenses and eyeglasses made from plastics that let UV light through. I highly recommend them if you wear corrective lenses. You may also want to replace some glass windows with UV transmitting clear plastic in the area of your home or office where you frequently spend time. This way, you get the balanced light without having the window open, as this is difficult during certain weather.

I believe that most adults taking mood-altering and anti-depressant drugs could feel great and throw their pills away if they got more sunlight, better nutrition and regular exercise. The same goes for hyperactive children taking various drugs. Hyperactivity in children is reduced after exposure to natural light during recess and is almost nonexistent in classrooms with full-spectrum lighting. Instead of spending money on drugs for your children, stop feeding them foods loaded with sugar and caffeine and donate some full-spectrum lights to the schools they attend. Full-spectrum lighting has also been shown to reduce the number and severity of dental caries (cavities) in animals and schoolchildren.

I do not recommend exposing your skin a great deal to sunlight or UV tanning lights. Your body needs some sunlight exposure to produce vitamin D but because this vitamin can be stored in the body, exposure to the face and arms for a few minutes a day during the summer produces enough for the entire year. Most of us get more than that even when we attempt to avoid sun exposure. Because the ozone layer of the earth has been depleted, the sun's rays seem more harmful to the skin than they were in the past. Therefore, it is probably better to keep sunlight exposure on your skin to a minimum (especially if you are fair skinned) and supplement your diet with vitamin D. This could prevent age spots and reduce the risk of various forms of skin cancer, including one that can be fatal. Use natural sunscreen lotions and special clothing to protect yourself, find out from your doctor what skin cancers look like and make a habit of checking your skin regularly. Have any suspicious changes checked by a competent physician as soon as possible. Sun exposure causes wrinkling by creating free radicals that damage the collagen connective tissue under the skin. I believe free radicals also contribute to the development of skin cancer. Antioxidant supplements help protect us from free radicals. You will learn more about free radicals and antioxidants in chapter eight.

If you feel you need some sunlight exposure to your skin, I recommend alternately exposing different parts of your skin like the thighs, back or stomach. Cover up other areas, especially the face, arms and hands.

Some people say sunlight is bad for our eyes. True, we get more UV light now because of man-made chemicals destroying some of the ozone layer, but this should not be a problem for the majority of us, because we spend most of our time behind glass that blocks the UV rays. Billions of people in the world spend most of every day with their eyes getting natural sunlight and I have not heard of an epidemic of eye problems because of it. They probably have far fewer eye and other health problems than people who rarely go outside or the ones who wear special wraparound sunglasses to prevent any UV light from getting to their eyes.

I believe that incomplete, unbalanced nutrition and exposure to chemical toxins or other environmental influences that create imbalances in our bodies cause the eye problems blamed on UV light. Exposure to unbalanced light sources could be a major cause of many problems. Numerous imbalances are actually caused by a lack of UV light through the pupils of the eyes. Also, remember that the pupils do not dilate as much if glasses or windows block the UV light. This lets in more visible light that may cause eye damage. Studies mentioned in the book *Health and Light* indicated that numerous animals developed retinal damage after exposure to green light, the color of light your eyes are exposed to while wearing most sunglasses.

If you are afraid of the UV light from the sun, illuminate your home and office with full-spectrum lights having a balance of colors and some UV. I believe that the Ott-Lites™ that John Ott helped develop are the best. You and your children, plants and animals will all be healthier.

Sleep

Sleep is another nutrient vital to good health and the normal function of our bodies and minds. A major purpose of sleep is to restore balance and normal sensitivity to the central nervous system. Because this system controls all other parts of the body, it should be obvious that adequate sleep will improve all bodily functions. During sleep, our bodies also repair cellular damage and create new cells, and our brains sort, organize and file what we have learned during the day.

We sleep in 90-minute cycles, gradually going into a deeper sleep during the first 45 minutes and coming back into a lighter sleep the next 45 minutes. This pattern repeats throughout the night. If you awaken at night, it will usually be at or near the end of one of these 90-minute cycles. It is best to sleep in increments of these cycles because it is easier to wake up at the end of one. This means that six hours, seven and one-half hours or nine hours are the best amounts of sleep for most of us.

We all need our own unique amount of sleep, depending on mental and physical activities, genetic predisposition, age, individual metabolism, overall health and nutritional status. Because most of these variables change frequently, we sometimes need more sleep and when we lose sleep, we need to catch up to restore balance. I recommend that children get a minimum of ten and one-half hours, teenagers a minimum of nine hours and most adults a minimum of seven and one-half hours each day. Teenagers need more sleep than adults because they are learning more and still growing physically. Children need the most because they are growing rapidly and learning a tremendous number of things every day.

Experiment to determine the best amount of sleep for you and realize that you will sometimes need more. I suggest that you arrange one day each week when you can sleep as long as your body needs so it can catch up on sleep that you may have missed during the week.

Most Americans do not get enough sleep and this contributes to the obesity epidemic as well as to a number of other problems. This topic will be discussed more in the fatigue section of chapter eleven.

Along with sleep and the other nutrients just explained, we all need other "vital nutrients" for good health and permanent fat loss. These nutrients feed your mind and your soul, which in turn *dramatically* affects the health of your body. You will learn about them in upcoming chapters.

Variety

It is often said that variety is the spice of life and this especially applies to eating well. Why do you think Nature produces such a large assortment of foods with different shapes, tastes, textures, smells and colors? Nature knows we need a variety of foods to get the wide spectrum of nutrients necessary for good health. It also produces many foods to satisfy our personal tastes and because we live in different environments and have unique digestive capabilities and nutritional needs.

Natural foods stimulate all five of our senses. The shape of foods has a visual effect on us like the shapes of other things in our environment. Because the same taste quickly gets boring, the tastes of different foods get us to eat more variety so we supply the balance of nutrients our bodies need. The texture of a food stimulates our touch receptors when we prepare it and chew it. And, the right touch sensations are important to our health, happiness and feeling satisfied. The sound made when chewing foods also has significant influence on our health and well-being. A variety of whole, natural foods is necessary to get a balance of these effects.

The color of foods has a specific purpose. Each color has a unique wavelength or vibration that affects us differently. For instance, yellow (lemon) is cleansing, red (chili peppers) is hot and stimulating and green (lettuce) and brown (nuts) are neutral. You see an abundance of green and brown in natural environments because they are neutral or balanced colors. The color of a food is often determined by the nutrients it contains. If you have a variety of colors in yours meals, you will probably get a good balance of nutrients.

The different smells of foods have significance by inputting their special vibrations into our olfactory sensors. The goal of aromatherapy is to restore lost balance. Eating a variety of foods should keep you balanced so you do not need aromatherapy. Nature has created thousands of different plants and flowers to supply us with even more colors and smells. Stop and smell the roses—literally. This is one of the ways Nature offers us the "soul" food we all need. You will learn about this special "food" in chapter nine. Throughout this book the term *soul food* will refer to food for the soul, not the ethnic food with the same name.

Most processed foods no longer have their natural and varied textures. They are usually soft and gooey or dry and crunchy. Most of them have also had their natural colors processed out and artificial colors added. Their shapes have been changed, their smells lost or altered, and most would be completely tasteless if not cooked in oil or coated with sugar or salt. This dramatically limits the variety of tastes. Often, all five of the healthful stimuli intended by Nature have been distorted or eliminated.

Many people believe that eating healthfully requires eating limited, drab and boring meals but this is opposite of the truth. With a little imagination, simple and nutritious meals can be some of the tastiest you will ever eat. A wide variety of natural foods keeps your meals fresh, new and exciting, and supply an abundance of the nutrients your body needs to be healthy. You may need only a small amount of a particular nutrient, but if you are in a rut with your eating, you may not get enough of it. An adequate variety of foods increases your chance of getting a nutrient that could prevent you from developing a serious illness or experiencing puzzling and annoying deficiency symptoms. Most people assume that the dry skin, brittle hair, fatigue, nervousness, bad moods or other health problems they suffer with are normal, when in reality they are symptoms of minor nutritional deficiencies. I believe you will be pleasantly surprised at the health improvements you will enjoy after following a balanced nutritional program for a while.

If you want to see drab, boring and limited, just take a look at the average person's diet. You will probably be shocked by the lack of variety. Being bored with their meals is why people often have such a hard time deciding what to eat. It is a source of stress, wasted time and poor food choices. Some people's main choices are between hamburgers, pizza and fried chicken. This is the "Standard American Diet" that is appropriately called SAD. Boredom is a common reason why people overeat.

Think about what people often eat. Hamburgers or cheeseburgers on processed white buns, pizza with cheese or meat on a processed white crust, processed white spaghetti with meatballs and cheese, meat or cheese sandwiches on processed white bread, meat with processed white rolls. Starting to see a trend? Many meals are primarily meat, cheese and processed wheat—foods that leave an acidic ash that leaches calcium from your bones and is often stored as fat. Processed wheat has negative effects on your health, and because it is almost tasteless, salt and other harmful condiments are usually added. These further undermine your health and add to the fat gain. Large amounts of meat and cheese supply excess protein and saturated fat that add to the fat gain and harmful effects. Besides these foods, a large number of many people's calories come from processed sugar and processed corn. Because the body is physically unsatisfied, it stimulates more eating in an attempt to supply its needs. And, because many of these meals taste the same, there is limited emotional satisfaction—another common cause of overeating.

Because every food has its own unique blend of nutrients, getting into an eating rut by frequently having the same foods for breakfast and eating similar lunches and dinners can create imbalances that lead to poor health. I have known people who ate the same exact breakfast every day. This probably sounds ridiculous and it is. Variety in your diet supplies the many different nutrients your body needs and decreases the chance of developing a deficiency.

Look for New Taste Treats

When you go to the supermarket, keep an eye out for natural foods you have never eaten before. Buy something new and try it. I think you will be surprised by the many taste treats and new healthful foods you will find. Look at the large variety of fruits and vegetables. Think of the different species of fish to choose from and do not forget about all the whole grains, legumes, nuts and seeds. A few of these foods must be purchased at health-food stores or by mail, but it is not difficult to find sources in the yellow pages or on the Internet.

How long has it been since you had trout, halibut or mahi mahi? When was the last time you ate some okra, Brussels sprouts, leeks, Jerusalem artichoke, yucca root, lotus root, eggplant, rutabaga, pumpkin, parsnip, sweet potato or hominy? Pumpkin is good for you if it is not in a pie, and yams and sweet potatoes are not just for Thanksgiving. What about pecans, pine nuts, sunflower seeds, almonds, pumpkinseeds, figs, dates, raisins or even prunes? Prunes are not just good for you when you're constipated. How about kidney beans, pink beans, lima beans, lentils and other legumes, or quinoa, kamut, spelt, millet or buckwheat to name a few grains? You have probably rarely eaten, never eaten or even heard of some of these nutritious foods. Most of my nutritional clients absolutely loved the majority of new foods I introduced them to once they tried them. Have some lamb, buffalo or turkey instead of beef and chicken, and eat meats whole or ground. With a bit of experimentation, many foods you have never even tried before could be added to your list of favorites as the number of foods in your diet increases.

Another way to create variety in your diet is by alternately using similar foods. For example, do not always eat romaine lettuce. Sometimes use green leaf, red leaf, or butter lettuce. Use different varieties of cabbage as the primary ingredient of your salad or along with lettuce. Use radish sprouts or daikon radish in place of regular radishes. A few varieties of potatoes are purple, white, red and russet. A few different onions are white, red, yellow and green.

The most health-building foods to eat in the summer are fruits, yet many people probably do not even eat one or two servings a week. Fruits condition your body for the heat and supply clean-burning energy. This is why Nature supplies so many different kinds of fruit when the weather is hot. Apples and certain other fruits are available in quite a few varieties. If you are lacking in this area, start eating more and different fruits. They are delicious and nutritious as snacks or as breakfast or lunch.

Squashes are some of the most nutritious foods you can eat and Nature supplies a large variety. The lighter ones are great for summer and the hard, heavier ones are ideal for winter. Here are just a few of the most common squashes: acorn, banana, butternut, crookneck, hubbard, spaghetti, straightneck, and zucchini. How many have you even heard of? How many have you ever eaten? How often do you eat them? If you want to be lean and healthy, instead of eating spaghetti (an incomplete processed grain product) and meatballs for dinner, eat some spaghetti squash and meatballs instead. Most people who have tried it say they love it.

What if you have never liked vegetables? If you try the hundreds of different varieties available, you are bound to find some whose taste you enjoy. Because your taste buds will normalize as your body gets cleaner and more balanced, make sure to always try something again that you may not have liked before. A food you disliked could easily end up on your list of favorites. It may help you to discover and enjoy the taste of certain vegetables if you mash them. Everyone has eaten mashed potatoes but what about mashed banana squash, parsnip, turnip or rutabaga. Mash certain vegetables and see if you like them better that way. Add some olive oil and see how good they can be. Try mixing the new ones with a vegetable that tastes good to you. Mix some mashed banana squash, parsnip or rutabaga with some mashed potatoes or try different combinations of steamed vegetables cooked in an omelet. You may discover a unique taste treat. On the other hand, you may not have liked poi (made from taro root) when you tried it in Hawaii, but you may like sliced and steamed taro root.

Another alternative until your taste buds normalize is to *drink* your vegetables. Fresh vegetable juice supplies concentrated amounts of enzymes and other vital nutrients that help your body return to balance faster. The whole vegetable is preferred but the juice can be used in the beginning of your program and even later if you eat large amounts of cooked foods or just want more of these vital nutrients. Vegetable juices are available in many health-food stores or you can buy a juicer and make your own. Green vegetable juices are what I recommend using most often. Carrot juice contains a large amount of concentrated sugar so is not good for fat loss. The sugar causes it to go bad fast, so make sure you always drink it soon after making or opening a bottle of it. If you use carrot juice, I suggest buying it separately and combining it with green vegetable juice. Avoid the unnatural combination of vegetable and fruit juices.

Two other ways to create variety in your meals is to prepare your foods differently and vary what you eat in the same meal. Have fun developing numerous taste combinations you enjoy. Exercise your mind and express your creativity, but follow the food combining and other guidelines you learn from this book. If eating nutritious foods ever seems drab and boring, you can easily change it.

Foods to Eat

Such a large number of whole, natural foods are available that even after you customize your list just for you, it will still be a long one. Nature seals inside whole foods the perfect balance of nutrients that work together to create good health. The first thing often removed during processing is the most vital part— the life force. This is why most processed foods are lifeless and incapable of building or sustaining good health. They are unbalanced products that create chemical imbalances in your body that can cause abnormal function, disease and excess fat storage.

Scientists are genetically engineering corn and creating many other unnatural foods that I recommend avoiding. No one knows the long-term effects of eating these foods or the meat of animals fed these foods. Chapter four covers a few items I believe should rarely, if ever, be ingested but remember that a healthful program should be positive. Your primary focus should always be on the hundreds of delicious and nutritious whole foods you *can* eat to be lean and healthy. Let's now briefly discuss some of the different food groups.

Vegetables

Any vegetable can be included in your nutritional program and once you start discovering what is available, you will probably be amazed at how many you are unfamiliar with or have never eaten. Remember that the heavier vegetables are best eaten during cold weather and the lighter vegetables during warmer weather. Vegetables are best eaten raw, steamed, baked, or quick stir-fried. Experiment by steaming up different combinations of three or four vegetables for lunch along with a salad and some olive oil for dressing. Find some combinations that appeal strongly to your personal tastes.

Not all methods of processing ruin a food. Frozen and canned vegetables can be used, but are usually not as nutritious as the same foods eaten fresh. Whenever possible, go with a recently harvested food. Frozen should be your second choice and canned your last. Because frozen foods are often frozen soon after harvest, they may be more nutritious than "fresh" foods in the supermarket that may have been harvested days before. Organic produce is more readily available either fresh or frozen. Many canned foods are essentially whole but generally lose some nutritional value during processing. This lack can be partially made up for with a good multivitamin and mineral supplement. I say partially because whole foods contain many other nutrients besides vitamins and minerals. Use canned vegtables when your time is extremely limited, but avoid those with added salt or sugar.

Grains

Many people have never eaten more than one or two of the foods in this far more limited group. Some people live their entire lives without ever eating a whole grain. Here is a list of the most common grains: wheat, barley, corn, brown rice, buckwheat, rye, quinoa, brown Basmati rice, millet, spelt, kamut, oat groats and wild rice. Sorghum, teff and other grains are staple foods for millions of people but are not commonly seen in the United States. Amaranth is a seed but because it is often used more like a grain it will be discussed with grains.

Whole grains are inexpensive and buying them in bulk (loose or in five-pound bags) is the most economical way to get them. You can buy them in health-food stores, wholesale outlets or by mail order.

I like to combine three different grains and eat them for breakfast, as a lunch entree or as part of a lunch containing vegetables, legumes or avocado. Use a large grain (wheat, kamut, barley, rye, oat groats or brown rice) for about 70 percent of the total. Then add a lesser amount (20 percent of the total) of millet, spelt or wild rice. Next add a bit (10 percent) of quinoa, buckwheat or amaranth. Try different variations to learn the taste combinations you prefer. Because they cook at different rates just start one cooking and set a timer for when to add each of the other two. This makes it simple to cook up three at a time. Most grains take less than an hour to cook and buckwheat takes only five minutes. I suggest eating each grain separately to experience its unique flavor and to test how your body reacts to it. The flavor of some grains may not appeal to you alone but will taste great in combination with others. Some combinations will be less acidic if one or two of the grains used are alkaline but I do not recommend grains when fat loss is your primary goal.

Here is a simple way to prepare a whole grain that normally takes 30 to 45 minutes to cook. At night put some of the grain in a thermos bottle (perhaps half full) and then fill it with boiling water and secure the lid. In the morning you will have a nutritious ready-to-eat breakfast. How's that for fast food?

Because some grains have been a major part of the diet of some races or cultures for only a short time relative to other foods, your body may not digest or utilize some of them efficiently. This is why it is important to experiment with each kind to see how they affect you. Even if you handle them well, they should be used sparingly, because most are acidic and concentrated sources of calories. It is best to cycle the use of grains by not eating the same kind more than every two to four days. I recommend eating wheat less often than the others, because many people have been overloaded with processed wheat products. Wheat is a common allergen and should be avoided if your body cannot handle it.

For energy during cold weather, eat more whole grains, good fats, legumes and winter vegetables. During warmer weather, get most of your energy from healthful oils, some legumes and whole grains, and a large variety of fruits and summer vegetables. A good way to get the nutrition from grains during the summer is by sprouting them for use in your lunch salads. They are especially nutritious when sprouted so you may want to read a book about how to do this.

When eating grains for lunch, I usually put a little sesame, grapeseed or sunflower seed oil on them. It may sound unusual but is a good combination and tastes great. Give it a try. For breakfast, I often put coconut oil and amazake (a cultured brown rice drink) or rice milk on the whole grains. Sometimes I warm them all up and sometimes I eat them cold. Amazake is often combined with nut milks and is sold in some health-food stores. Soymilk or other "milks" made from various grains or nuts, could also be used. Adding pine nuts to grains adds a unique taste. You may like your grains plain or with seed oils *or* a bit of pure maple syrup on them. Try adding some raisins, dates or figs. Use what you prefer, or better yet, vary what you put on your grains.

A whole grain contains the germ, bran and endosperm in perfect balance. Processing removes the germ and the bran. The flour produced from endosperm is then made into bread, crackers, cookies, pasta and other baked goods that affect your body much the same way refined sugar does. Processed-grain products are a *major* contributor to people being fat and unhealthy. Processed grains are tremendously unbalanced and often stored as fat, not just because they are acidic but because the endosperm cannot be used properly without the other two parts. Also, the endosperm is broken down so fast that it causes a rapid increase in blood sugar. The body then releases insulin, which stimulates the food to be removed from the blood and stored as fat. This lowers the blood sugar level back to normal.

When you eat a *whole* grain, it releases its energy at a slow, gradual rate. This is like burning a log in your fireplace. It gives off a certain amount of heat for a long time as the fire slowly consumes the log. When a grain is processed into flour, it is digested fast and gives the body a large amount of energy quickly. This is like grinding up the log into sawdust and burning it. It will give off a tremendous amount of heat quickly and be used up in a short time.

Processed-grain products also create nutritional imbalances and excess waste that lead to frequent colds (body cleanses) and increased susceptibility to many other diseases. Eating processed grains often leads to overeating because people crave them. Unfortunately, eating more just makes the imbalance worse and the people fatter. Most people do not know that their bodies are craving them because of a blood sugar imbalance or as a futile attempt to get the two missing parts. Think about it, have you ever heard of someone craving healthful, *whole* carbohydrates like fruits and vegetables or even whole grains? Now you know why.

Your body cannot build health without all three parts of a grain in perfect proportion. Similarly, without the proper amounts of water, cement and sand you cannot make concrete and build a strong foundation. Like the grains, concrete must contain all three ingredients in correct proportions. Take away the water (germ) and cement (bran) and all you have left is sand (endosperm) that cannot be used to build a solid foundation (good health). As you add more you just get a larger and larger pile of sand (unused endosperm stored as fat).

Because the endosperm is essentially worthless and creates imbalance, we are sold the bran separately to lower our cholesterol levels, reduce our risk of certain cancers, and normalize our bowel function. We are also sold the germ oil to give us essential nutrients and vitality. Germ oils are often called "super foods." You could eat a piece of processed bread, a spoonful of bran and a bit of germ oil in an attempt to get a whole food. This would be expensive and unless you knew the perfect proportions would be either unbalanced or wasteful. Like making concrete with excess water, cement or sand, an improper ratio of ingredients will not turn out right. It is much easier to let Nature supply all three parts in perfect balance and the germ oil unaffected by light or air.

A large variety of breads are labeled "whole wheat" but if they do not need refrigeration they are not whole. A few contain the bran along with the endosperm but they do not have the germ. Numerous other products (pasta, crackers, and so on) are also falsely labeled. It is extremely misleading to consumers.

There are some nutritious breads that are whole and still have their life force. They are frozen when you buy them and must be kept in the refrigerator. These breads are unleavened and are made only from sprouted grains and water. The one I buy is called Manna® Bread. There are a few varieties and some also contain sprouted seeds. They are dense, moist and must be sliced prior to eating. They are naturally sweet because the sprouting process breaks down the complex carbohydrates of the grain into simple carbohydrates. The germ oil adds to the taste, making these breads taste great even plain.

Legumes

Here is another group of nutritious foods sadly neglected by many people. Legumes consist of various dried beans and peas. Peanuts are a legume also known as goobers or goober peas. Legumes are best eaten primarily in the winter, because they are dried and can be stored without refrigeration. Most of them (except lentils) leave an alkaline ash that helps balance the acid ash of the meats and grains eaten in the winter. Some people's bodies can efficiently break down and get the nutrition from legumes but others cannot. My body does not digest most legumes well. This is probably the main reason why it developed severe protein deficiency symptoms when I was a vegetarian for a few years. It was unable to get certain essential amino acids from the legumes. Theoretically, my diet should have been perfectly balanced, but it was not because of my body's digestive limitation. Think about the four steps to good nutrition—eating nutritious foods, efficient digestion, assimilation, and utilization. Just because someone else's body thrives on a particular food does not mean your body will. I eat legumes now but not in the quantity necessary to be healthy on a vegetarian diet. In chapter six you will learn how to customize your diet to your unique needs and digestive capabilities.

There are products available that can eliminate some of the bloating and gas that legumes are famous for producing. These may help your body get more nutritional value from legumes, but first you should experiment with the many different types of legumes to see how they react in your body. You may be able to find a few that your body digests well. Soaking legumes in water overnight before cooking them improves their digestibility. This probably helps because it starts the sprouting process. As with grains, sprouting is a good way to get the nutritional value of legumes during the summer. Legume sprouts are also digested easier. You could try the digestive aid products, but if you cannot find any legumes your body digests effectively, you may be better off eating more of the foods that it does digest well.

Nuts and Seeds

Nuts and seeds should be eaten primarily during cold weather because they are storable foods containing mostly protein and fat. Raw (sometimes dry roasted) nuts can be used as a nutritious meal when you are out and about and healthful foods are unavailable. If you are prepared, you will not have to eat unhealthful foods or go without eating, because neither is a good choice. You can eat one particular type of nut or a combination of two or more. Try some roasted unsalted pistachios sometime. Nuts taste great and are nutritious snacks, especially when combined with raisins, dates or figs. Avoid pre-made trail mix combinations containing peanuts (legumes), salt, sugar, oils and other unhealthful ingredients. Almond, cashew and other nut butters are excellent foods but use only the raw, natural ones that do not contain salt or other added ingredients. Your body will probably digest and use nut butters better than peanut butter, which I do not recommend.

Seeds are highly nutritious foods that can be used in a variety of ways. They can be eaten for breakfast either in combination with each other or added to grains. Just soak a few different kinds in water overnight in the refrigerator and on arising eat them as a breakfast treat either alone or with grains. Add a grain drink, soymilk or dried fruit if desired. Raw seeds can be eaten separately or in combination with nuts or other seeds. They supply nutritious oils that you already know are important for good health, and eating the whole seed is the most natural and balanced way to get these oils. Just like whole grains, you get the oil and the other parts in perfect proportion. The most commonly used seeds are sunflower, sesame, poppy, hemp, pumpkin, and flax. Try these and others to determine the ones that taste good to you. Seeds, especially the smaller ones such as poppy, hemp and flax, can be ground up to release more of their nutritional value. Use them soon after grinding, because they get rancid quickly once their oils are exposed to oxygen. Tahini (sesame seed butter) tastes great and is nutritious, containing a substantial amount of calcium. Raw tahini is better than the kind made from roasted seeds. In some countries, pumpkinseeds are used to maintain male potency, because they supply zinc and other nutrients necessary for a healthy prostate gland and to produce the sex hormone testosterone.

Sprouting seeds greatly increases their nutritional value. Using seed sprouts in your salads is a great way to get nutrition from them in warmer weather. Some of the most commonly used seed sprouts are alfalfa, radish, broccoli, clover, and sunflower. A book about sprouting will teach you how to grow these wonderfully nutritious foods.

It is best to eat nuts and seeds raw, and buying them in bulk is the most economical way to get them. Find a source near your home or buy them mail order. Avoid any that have been roasted in oil and covered with salt. They are expensive and unhealthful because the salt stimulates you to eat excessive amounts and the oil adds excess calories.

Fruits

Fruits are the food of choice in the summer for snacks or even as a great breakfast or lunch. Many fruits can be taken with you to supply the nutrition you need when you are out, thereby preventing you from going hungry or eating something that is not good for you. During the winter, apples, pears, avocados and citrus fruits are the best ones to use. Fruits are best eaten raw so you get their nutritious stores of enzymes, vitamins, minerals and phytonutrients.

Fruits contain the natural sugar fructose along with other forms of sugar. Fructose is a healthful energy source that needs no digestion. It is absorbed less than half as fast as glucose or galactose (a type of sugar) and needs no energy for transport into the body. It is also by far the sweetest of all natural sugars.

Fresh fruits are usually the best, but frozen fruits are close behind and sometimes more nutritious because they are fresher or allowed to fully ripen before freezing. Canned fruits can be used occasionally if they do not contain added sugar, corn syrup or other unhealthful ingredients.

Meats

Some kind of meat will generally be the main ingredient of your evening meal. Because meats need more energy to digest than most other foods, the best time to eat them is in the evening when you are usually inactive. They also supply the essential amino acids your body needs for repair and rebuilding during the night. Foods classified as meat are red meats, fowl and fish. When eating meats, eliminate as much of the fat as you can. I do not recommend eating pork and suggest limiting your consumption of shellfish and fish without scales. Pork is difficult to digest, shellfish are scavengers and could be polluted. One research study found that people's vitality was reduced after eating the varieties of fish without scales and increased after eating the varieties of fish that have scales. Many fish without scales, like sharks and swordfish, are near the top of the food chain and therefore often contain concentrated amounts of mercury and other environmental toxins.

Eggs

Eggs are extremely nutritious but because they contain cholesterol many people are afraid to eat them. You have learned how important cholesterol is to good health and that ingesting it normally has a negligible effect on your blood cholesterol level. I say "normally" because if you eat processed sugar at the same time, your blood cholesterol does go up. I eat two dozen eggs a week often with pure maple syrup or natural (no sugar added) jelly at the same meal and my blood cholesterol level is only 133 and my triglycerides are 44. I am not sure how the ridiculous idea that eggs (yolks especially) are unhealthful got started, but I heard it was from an experiment years ago that used artificial, processed eggs not real ones.

Here are a few facts about eggs that you probably do not know. Eggs are easily digested and used almost entirely. They contain a complete, high-quality protein that is ranked equal in distribution of essential amino acids to that of human milk. Eggs and human milk are the standard that all other proteins are rated against. The yolk contains half of the protein and almost all of the vitamins and minerals. It is an excellent source of iron, copper, phosphorus, sulfur, vitamin A, riboflavin, vitamin B_{12}, vitamin D, pantothenic acid and thiamin. Egg yolks are also rich in choline, an essential nutrient that acts similar to a vitamin. It helps prevent development of a fatty liver and is good for the brain and nerves. It has been used to treat numerous mental disorders. The yolk contains all the fat, but the fat is *unsaturated* and finely emulsified which makes it easily assimilated. I believe it is the healthiest fat you can eat. It is also what gives eggs most of their taste. Egg yolks contain numerous phospholipids having important functions in the body. For example, lecithin aids in the transport and use of fatty acids that help protect against hardening of the arteries and heart disease. It also helps keep the brain, liver and kidneys healthy. In contrast, the egg white contains only the other half of the protein, some sulfur and some riboflavin. People who eat only egg whites lose out on almost all of the nutritional value of an egg and most of the taste. Remember that it is always best to eat the whole food, not just part of it.

I prefer fertile eggs because they are more complete and come from chickens that roam free and eat natural foods. These eggs are higher in the omega-3 fatty acids that are lacking in many people's diets. Because many chickens are not allowed to eat a natural diet, the amount of this important fatty acid in their eggs is low. You can now buy omega-3 eggs from farms where the chicken feed is fortified with algae that contain these essential fatty acids. There is no difference in nutritional value between eggs with brown shells and eggs with white shells. They just come from a different breed of chickens. I believe that eggs, nuts and seeds are some of the most nutritious foods you can eat because they are all origins of new life.

Many animals and some humans eat raw eggs. This is probably the best way to ingest them but you may have heard that a substance called avidin, found in raw egg whites, depletes the vitamin biotin. What you have probably not heard is that the egg yolk is a good source of biotin and that you would have to eat more than twenty-four egg whites a day to produce a deficiency. Eating the whole egg raw would not cause a deficiency. Another concern is that eggs may be contaminated with *Salmonella* bacteria. Author and health researcher Dr. Hulda Clark has found it on the shell of some eggs but never in the egg itself. I have eaten at least six raw eggs every week for many years without a problem, but remember that the eggs I eat come from healthy chickens. If someone did want to eat a raw egg, a good precaution to take is to put the egg in boiling water for about 30 seconds. Doing this should sterilize the shell and will denature the avidin, thereby preventing it from binding with and making the biotin unavailable for use. Nevertheless, eat raw eggs at your own risk.

Continue to Learn

The previous sections just briefly described the different types of foods. To learn more, you can purchase a book listing the various nutritive components of different foods, such as calories, vitamin and mineral content, and grams of fat, protein and carbohydrate. This is not necessary, but will help you learn more about different foods. These books are inexpensive and can usually be found at bookstores, magazine stands and near supermarket checkout counters.

The primary purpose is for you to discover and eat more of the wide variety of foods available, and secondarily to learn their nutritive value. For example, if you believe a particular food has little value, you may avoid it even though it is highly nutritious. Do not focus on or worry about calories. This creates negative feelings that make being lean and healthy an unnatural struggle. You will learn later why calorie counting is actually detrimental to losing fat. Use the information in these books to help you find more foods you like and the foods that work best for you. As time passes, you will get more in tune with your inner self and be naturally guided to the best foods for your unique body.

How Much of Each Type of Food?

Now that you are getting an idea of what foods to eat, it is important to determine the healthiest amounts of each. Numerous opinions exist on this subject and now you are going to get mine, along with my reasoning for why I think this way. I strongly believe in it because it is Nature's way and because it works—plain and simple. The common amounts and ratios taught in schools and found in "health" pamphlets are a major reason so many people are fat today. They make no distinction between whole nutritious foods in a group and processed products with hardly any nutritional value. They also fail to mention any difference in winter, spring, summer or fall diets. These dietary guidelines are often shown in pyramid form. First, let's take a look at the recommendations of the United States Department of Agriculture (USDA) and the United States Department of Health and Human Services. Then we will look at my recommendations.

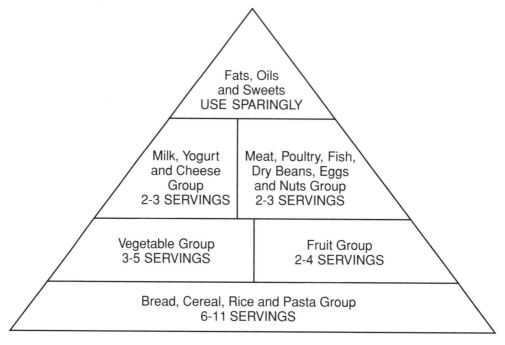

Source: United States Department of Agriculture and the
United States Department of Health and Human Services

Following those guidelines will give you far more concentrated acidic foods than unconcentrated alkaline foods. You will be uncomfortable in the heat of summer and be fat and unhealthy. You will probably be deficient in good fats. This food pyramid contains the milk, yogurt and cheese group you will not find in any of mine. You will get large amounts of bad fat from that one. It also recommends refined grain products (breads and pasta) that you will not find in any of my pyramids. Can you imagine how much body fat people would gain if they ate eleven servings of processed bread and pasta every day?

My pyramids give you basic guidelines of what to eat more or less of during different seasons, but I do not list specific numbers of servings. This is unnecessary because when you eat whole, natural foods your body gets the nutrients it needs and is satisfied. It is difficult to overeat. You naturally eat when you are hungry and do not eat when you are not. These guidelines will vary to some degree depending on if your body will do best with mostly vegetarian foods or if your body needs more meat than average. You will learn how to determine your unique needs in chapter six. Now let's take a look at my food pyramids.

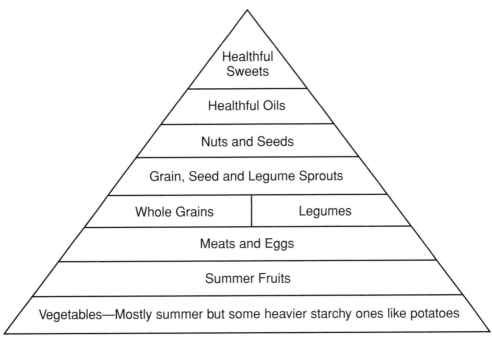

Summer Pyramid

I especially enjoy summer because of all the clean, cooling and delicious fruits available. As you can see, the bulk of your diet should consist of alkaline foods that will maintain a normal blood pH and keep you comfortable in the summer heat.

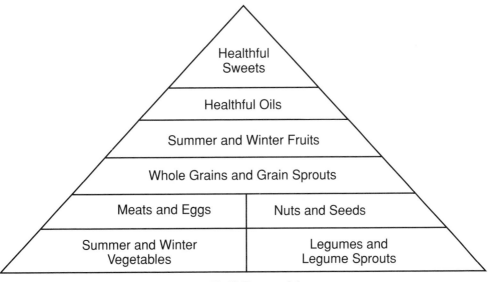

Fall Pyramid

My fall food pyramid includes some fall foods and more of the acidic foods that prepare your body for colder weather.

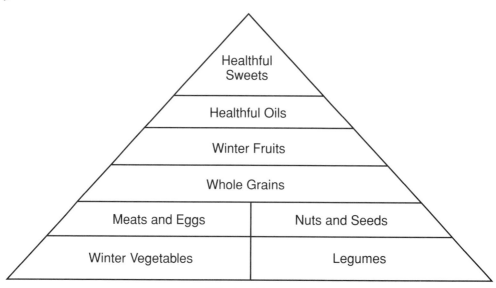

Winter Pyramid

This pyramid contains quite a few acidic foods like meats, eggs, grains, nuts and seeds. These foods (and avocados) all contain the healthful fats your body needs more of during cold weather. To maintain a normal blood pH it also contains legumes and winter fruits and vegetables, all of which are alkaline. Eating more of the acidic foods does not cause an imbalance, because many of these foods produce energy for our activities and to keep us warm during the winter. If you live where the winters are mild (like Florida or Southern California) you should follow the fall pyramid guidelines during the winter.

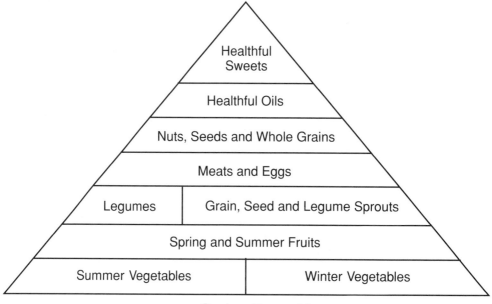

Spring Pyramid

During springtime, the foods (primarily spring fruits) come into season that stimulate our bodies to cleanse the heavier winter food residues. Nature supplies them to get our bodies ready for the warmer temperatures of summer. You will also start to eat summer vegetables and fewer winter vegetables.

You now have an overview of some of the foods you should eat and what time of year to eat them. In chapter five you will learn more about why the time of day that you eat a particular food is so vital to the results you get.

Super Foods?

Some books on nutrition include information about miracle foods for good health. Most of these "super foods," such as wheat germ oil, are not foods at all. They are parts of foods that create health improvements by filling in some of the gaps created by the lifeless processed foods many people eat. Wheat germ oil and wheat bran supply what is missing from the processed grain products people eat by supplying the nutrients you would get in perfect balance if you ate some whole wheat. As you have learned, getting these nutrients separately is an improvement, but they are not supplied together or in the perfect ratios Nature intended.

Yogurt is often called a super food. It is a fermented milk product containing various bacteria. They are considered friendly bacteria because they help keep your intestines healthy. Some of them can synthesize certain B-complex vitamins (especially biotin and folic acid) and vitamin K. About one hundred different species of bacteria can be found in a normal intestinal tract. If you eat in a well-balanced way and do not kill them, there will be no need to replenish these bacteria. Unfortunately, many of us do not supply the nutrients our friendly bacteria need to multiply and be strong. Also, pesticides, the chlorine in our water and the antibiotics contained in some meats or that we take to fight infections kill off these naturally occurring bacteria.

I do not recommend eating yogurt, but taking a supplement that contains a variety of these beneficial bacteria is helpful to compensate for our diets being less than perfect and for the various chemicals we cannot avoid. These supplements can be found in capsule form in most health-food stores. One or two capsules a month should be adequate for most people. Eating garlic has been shown to increase the growth of these good bacteria and reduce the amounts of harmful bacteria in our systems. Many people consider it a natural antibiotic. With pure water, balanced light, good nutrition and regular exercise, you should rarely, if ever, need antibiotic drugs. They are helpful for certain severe conditions but the excessive use of antibiotics weakens the immune system just like relying on a wheelchair for a month would weaken the legs. If you ever take antibiotic drugs, I suggest using two or three capsules daily to replenish the friendly bacteria being killed by the drugs. Take them during the course of treatment and for at least a week after. Eating some garlic every day during this same period would also be helpful.

You now have some of the basics about the foods you will be eating. As you read on, you will learn when to eat these foods, what to eat them with, how to cook them, how to determine the right ones for you, and how to develop many nutritious *and* delicious meals.

One's destination is never a place but rather a new way of looking at things.
Henry Miller

Life will bring you pain all by itself. Your responsibility is to create joy.
Milton Erickson, M.D.

You are a child of the universe, no less than the trees and the stars;
you have a right to be here.
Desiderata

Your future depends on many things, but mostly on you.
Frank Tyger

It is the wisest who grieve most at loss of time.
Dante

Celebrate what you want to see more of.
Tom Peters

four

Banish Your Enemies

This is perhaps the most important chapter in this book, because the following items cause most of the excess body fat people have and increase the risk of getting almost every disease. If you cut your intake of each of these items by just one half, your problems with excess fat could be gone and your health greatly improved.

Never look at your nutritional program in a negative way or feel your diet is restricted. Your goal is to expand your horizons and find more good foods to eat and more ways to get balanced nutrition. Nevertheless, a few things are *extremely* harmful to your health and can ruin an otherwise good program.

This chapter contains a brief explanation of these items and their negative effects. Most of them are nutritional vampires. Besides not supplying nutritional value, they suck some of the nutrients you have obtained elsewhere right out of your bloodstream. This causes deficiencies of many vital nutrients. For each item I recommend avoiding, you should find five to ten new health-building foods. Very few people will stop using all of these "things" (they cannot be called foods) but I hope the following information will inspire you to eliminate some and reduce your consumption of the others. Because they are *all* detrimental to getting and staying lean and healthy, the more you avoid them the better off you will be.

Alcohol

As you should know, alcohol is extremely detrimental to your physical and emotional health. It is also tremendously destructive to society and people's lives. It can kill you instantly if you drink and drive or slowly if you just drink it. Alcohol abuse is the third leading cause of preventable death. Alcohol can kill or injure you even if you do not drink it. Here are a few statistics that will probably shock you. Alcohol use is seen in 75 percent of domestic assaults, 70 percent of all child abuse, 50 percent of all emergency room visits, 52 percent of all rapes, and a staggering 86 percent of all homicides. Forty percent of all traffic deaths (16,000 people every year) are linked to alcohol consumption. The traffic fatalities alone amount to more American lives lost in four years than during the Vietnam War, which lasted more than ten years. One out of every four hospital beds is filled because of alcohol and 100,000 deaths are linked to it every year. It costs more and kills more than all illegal drugs combined.

Alcohol interferes with the activation of vitamins in the liver, and because it is a toxic chemical it places a great deal of stress on the liver and other parts of the body. You may feel that you drink only in moderation and that this is not excessively stressful to your liver. But what if your liver is the weakest link in your health chain? Moderate consumption, along with the many other liver stressors of our modern environment, could easily break it. Even minor damage gradually accumulates over the years into major damage. Many alcoholics started out by drinking socially and "moderately."

Let's say for now that moderate alcohol consumption will cause only minor liver damage. Still, every drink you take destroys brain cells that can never be replaced. You have probably heard that most of us use only about five percent of our brain. You may feel like you have plenty of cells to spare but that five percent refers to what we consciously use. We would not have all those brain cells if we did not need them. Millions of subconscious functions are occurring all the time—breathing, smell, sight, memory, hearing, digestion, elimination, immune functions, blood flow, lymph flow and many more. These automatic functions are controlled by the other 95 percent of your brain cells.

To maintain mental and physical health you need to retain as many brain cells as possible. Keep in mind that most of us are frequently exposed to other chemicals that destroy brain cells. It is difficult to avoid everything that kills brain cells and damages the liver but you can easily avoid one of the worst— alcohol. When they are older, many people are going to wish they had the brain cells they are currently destroying with alcohol.

The B vitamins are the most vital to the health and normal function of your brain and nervous system. Drinking causes a deficiency of these nutrients because your body uses them to burn the sugar in the alcohol. Alcohol either inhibits proper absorption or causes a loss of vitamin A, magnesium, zinc and calcium. Taking B-complex vitamins, those three minerals and vitamin A can reduce the short-term effects of alcohol quite a bit, and some—but far from all—of the long-term negative effects.

Alcohol is a depressant and because so many people already suffer from depression they do not need to add to the problem. If you are depressed, drinking alcohol is like pouring gasoline on a fire; it makes things worse. And, when you are feeling good, why do something to depress you? Drinking, especially to excess, also makes you feel weak-willed and unable to control yourself and your life. This often leads to more drinking, overeating and other problems.

People often suffer from depression because of imbalances that can usually be corrected. It is frequently caused by a lack of proper nutrition to the body, mind and spirit. When these aspects are well nourished, people do not need alcohol to relax, forget their problems or attempt to cover up how depressed they already are. Most people, however, look to alcohol as a quick fix. Unfortunately, the alcohol they turn to further depletes the specific nutrients they need to feel better. Many people take a drug to treat the depression caused by drinking alcohol. This often leads to an expensive and destructive cycle. Because depression is a major reason why people overeat or make poor food choices, it is clearly best to never drink alcohol if being lean and healthy is your goal. Learn to relax, increase your self-confidence or get whatever else you feel you need in positive, healthy ways instead of from alcohol, which amplifies current problems and usually creates new ones.

Alcohol often reduces a person's inhibitions and self-control. This frequently leads to physical violence, dangerous activities, eating to excess, drinking more, unwanted pregnancies, making poor food choices, and numerous other problems. Alcohol also impairs your judgment and reaction time possibly leading to injury or death.

Alcohol contributes to gaining excess body fat by supplying empty calories. Because most people do not reduce their food consumption to compensate for the calories in the alcohol, they end up getting excess calories. To make matters worse, their bodies usually stimulate them to eat more to replace the vitamins and minerals used up by the alcohol. This leads to more fat gain. Some people drink large quantities of alcohol and do not eat much. They may gain less fat but are usually malnourished and suffer from numerous nutrient deficiency symptoms.

Alcohol causes inflammation of the stomach, pancreas and small intestine and this interferes with normal digestion and absorption of foods. The inflammation can affect the ability of the pancreas to secrete insulin to maintain a normal blood sugar level. The alcohol causes ingested carbohydrates to trigger a rapid rise in blood sugar followed by a drop below normal. Alcohol blocks gluconeogenesis (the conversion of protein to glucose) and this can also cause low blood sugar. The resultant hypoglycemia makes people feel so terrible that they often drink more alcohol or eat sugar and other unhealthful foods in an attempt to feel better. The results are temporary at best and a destructive cycle is created. For more information, refer to the sections on hypoglycemia and alcoholism in chapter ten.

Forget about drinking wine to improve your digestion, because you can easily get the beneficial effects without any of the harmful ones. If you follow the guidelines in this book, your digestion will be optimized, and the positive effects of drinking wine come from the phytonutrients, not the alcohol. You can get the same phytonutrients from drinking grape juice or better yet by eating grapes or other fruits and vegetables containing these health-building nutrients. Alcohol is dehydrating and this can lead to numerous negative health consequences, including poor digestion.

Alcohol consumption increases the risk of developing cancer. Mouth, throat and laryngeal cancer risk is significantly increased with alcohol use, especially if the drinker also smokes. Alcohol has also been shown to increase the risk of colorectal and breast cancer. Beer is low in alcohol but contains carcinogenic nitrosamines. Some studies indicate that alcohol may damage DNA. This could lead to birth defects in the children of parents who drink.

I do not recommend drinking alcohol in any form or amount. You may choose to drink some alcohol occasionally. If you do, please do what you can to minimize some of its negative effects. Take supplemental forms of calcium, zinc, magnesium, vitamin A and the B-complex vitamins and eat a healthful diet containing other nutrients that help reduce the damage caused by alcohol.

Caffeine

Caffeine is a stimulant. It will wake you up when you are tired, but if you are eating well, you will not need a stimulant to get or keep you going. You will have plenty of natural get-up-and-go. If you do not, it is because you have an imbalance that is either reducing energy production or causing an abnormal energy drain.

If your body is balanced and functioning normally and your diet is good, when you feel tired it is because you are. Listen to your body and give it the rest it needs. Remember that sleep is a vital nutrient. If you feel tired without a good reason, using a stimulant is like whipping a horse that is weak from overwork and lack of food. It may keep going for a while, but will get weaker and finally collapse. Many people use drugs to stimulate their bodies to keep going when what is needed is proper nutrition, regular exercise or adequate rest.

Using a stimulant can easily become habit forming. Think about how many coffee addicts you know. Are you one? Using stimulants prevents people from learning how to have energy and vitality naturally or keeps them from finding and eliminating the cause of their low energy. If the cause is the beginning of a serious health problem, if detected early, much grief, expense and even premature death may be prevented. If you find yourself dragging in the morning or at other times of the day, instead of reaching for a cup of coffee, look at your diet and the amount of rest you are getting. Our bodies dehydrate some during the night and that causes fatigue. The best thing to get you going in the morning is water. Start your day with a glass or two of water and then eat nutritious foods to keep you energized all day long. If you feel tired between meals, drink some water. If that doesn't perk you up within 10 to 15 minutes, eat a nutritious snack.

Stimulants put excessive stress on your heart and nervous system and have negative effects on other parts of your body as well. Most of us have excess stress in our lives already, so we do not need something to increase it. Some people believe that caffeine improves the performance of physical skills but studies have shown that it does the opposite. Also, after stimulation by any source, the body must later get additional rest. Stimulants such as nicotine, tea and coffee often cause symptoms like those of hyperthyroidism (overactive thyroid gland). Some of these symptoms are progressive weakness, increased pulse rate, shaking, insomnia, sweating, heart palpitations, and weight loss even though the appetite is good. All of your mental and physical functions are affected by the thyroid hormone, so it is extremely important to have normal thyroid function. Excessive stimulation to the thyroid gland over a period of years can weaken it and make it underactive. Hypothyroidism (underactive thyroid gland) slows the metabolism and is a common physical cause of people gaining and having difficulty losing excess fat.

One survey indicated that pregnant women who ingested more than 600 milligrams (mg) of caffeine daily experienced more complications and more of them lost babies through miscarriage or stillborn births. That's about the amount of caffeine found in four cups of coffee, but keep in mind that many other products contain caffeine. More than one cup of coffee a day during pregnancy has been linked to low birth weights. Coffee may also adversely affect a woman's fertility. In ancient times, women drank strong coffee to prevent conception. Mothers can pass caffeine to their babies through their breast milk. This may cause the baby to become addicted and to cry frequently and have difficulty sleeping.

Caffeine is a powerful poison that acts like arsenic and lead. It is especially harmful to brain and nerve tissue. One expert believes caffeine can damage the pancreas of a fetus. I believe that the nervous system of a growing fetus is also adversely affected. It takes women longer than men to detoxify from caffeine and it is more harmful to women because it causes damage at lower doses. If you are a woman wanting to bear healthy children, I highly recommend avoiding caffeine before, during and after pregnancy. The developing fetus may suffer extensive damage during the critical first few weeks.

When caffeine contacts the lining of the stomach, it increases the flow of digestive juices including hydrochloric acid. This is especially detrimental to anyone with an ulcer. Look at all the products designed to absorb or inhibit excess stomach acid. Many of those suffering from this condition could resolve it by not using caffeine products. Caffeine stimulates excess acid and then another drug is taken to reduce the excess. Does this make any sense? Do you think it is good for your body? Caffeine also produces the same changes in the blood vessels of animals that prolonged resentment, hostility and anxiety does.

Dr. Hahnemann, the founder of homeopathic medicine, says coffee drinking can cause the following diseases: headaches, toothaches, shooting pains, spasms in the chest and stomach, constipation, diseases of the liver, uterus and bones, difficult breathing, inflammation of the eyes, erysipelas (inflammation of the skin and mucous membranes) and bowel diseases. It also gives you bad breath and has been shown to sometimes cause diarrhea.

A study I read many years ago indicated that drinking even two to three cups of coffee a day doubles your chance of having a heart attack. One cup a day may be too much for someone with an existing heart condition. Coffee often raises the blood pressure, placing stress on the heart and vascular system. Coffee may also inhibit the absorption of calcium, iron and other essential vitamins and minerals.

Caffeine stimulates your adrenal glands to produce epinephrine (adrenaline) that converts stored glycogen into glucose. This increase in blood sugar is why you get a fast energy boost. The result, however, is short-lived, because insulin is released and your blood sugar falls quickly. You then look for another quick pick-me-up. This often creates a hypoglycemic condition that makes you feel terrible and leads to storage of excess body fat. Repeated stress to the body's blood sugar balancing system may lead to chronic hypoglycemia or diabetes. You will learn more about these conditions in chapter ten.

Caffeine dehydrates you, causing fatigue and numerous other negative symptoms. Many people get caught in the negative cycle of ingesting more caffeine in an attempt to fight the fatigue it causes. It also raises your blood sugar level and stresses your entire body. What you wanted to give you energy makes you tired and stresses you instead. Do those sound like healthy effects? Time is wasted, the body is stressed and permanent damage is done.

There is a wide range of amounts of caffeine contained in some common drinks, because caffeine is water-soluble. The longer hot water is exposed to ground coffee beans, the more caffeine it will extract. Eight ounces of coffee contain anywhere from 78 to 178 mg of caffeine. The drip or vacuum method of brewing coffee produces less caffeine than percolating. A cup of decaffeinated coffee has only 2 to 7 mg, but eight ounces of tea contain from 83 to 178 mg. If you drink tea instead of coffee, you may be getting more caffeine than coffee drinkers are. A cup of cocoa can contain as much as 409 mg of caffeine. Wow! Have you ever wondered why those "nice" hot cups of cocoa you gave your children had them bouncing off the walls and you pulling your hair out? Now you know. You may have made it worse by adding sugar and marshmallows made from sugar. One large marshmallow contains one and one-half teaspoons of sugar. If that's not bad enough, you will soon learn that cocoa contains another chemical with the same adverse effects as caffeine. Cola and many other soft drinks have approximately 36 to 68 mg of caffeine in a 12-ounce can and are made almost entirely of sugar. They are not a good alternative for you or your children. Be aware that children are affected much more by caffeine than adults are.

Coffee plants used to grow naturally in the shade of large trees, but one plant produces only about one pound of coffee beans. Because coffee is the second largest crop in the world, unnatural things were done to meet the demand. Many large trees were cut down and a hybridized coffee plant was developed that could grow in the sun. This caused destruction of the natural habitat of insects, birds, monkeys and other animals. Many plants were also eliminated. It seems a shame to destroy the natural environment to grow coffee that is harmful to all who drink it. Because this land is being farmed, wouldn't it be far better if it was producing nutritious foods to help feed the starving people of the world?

Coffee trees that can grow in the sun are more susceptible to insects and need heavier spraying with pesticides. Coffee is the third most heavily sprayed crop and three-quarters of the coffee grown in the world is sprayed with DDT, chlordane, paraquat and zineb. These are some of the most toxic chemicals in existence. This is why they were banned in the United States many decades ago. If you drink organic, shade-grown coffee, you will avoid these toxic pesticides but it is still far better just to drink something that is good for you.

If you have been ingesting caffeine, when you stop using it be prepared for withdrawal symptoms such as headaches, irritability, restlessness, nervousness and the inability to work productively. All of these are usually made worse by lethargy. If you experience these symptoms between hits of caffeine, chances are caffeine is the cause. Many people use other drugs to treat the symptoms caused by caffeine. These drugs lead to other imbalances, unpleasant side effects and even more damage to your body. Drugs containing caffeine give relief because they stop the caffeine withdrawal symptoms. Stopping and starting is difficult, so it is usually best to quit cold turkey instead of tapering off gradually. Give your body a chance to purge itself of this addictive toxin. If you do not, the unpleasant symptoms and damage to your body will continue. I highly recommend that you avoid coffee, tea, soft drinks, cocoa, chocolate and other products containing caffeine. Be aware that many pain remedies and some weight-loss products contain caffeine. The other harmful ingredients in these drinks and products are even more reasons to avoid them.

A new problem with drinking coffee has developed and it is making people fat. "Designer" coffeehouses are springing up all over the country. Like fast-food outlets, aggressive marketing is used to sell unhealthful products at high prices. Many people drink these products thinking it is the trendy thing to do. They order a cappuccino or latte and usually get a large number of calories. People are also making them at home. Many of these drinks have 300-plus calories and some contain more than 500. Can you imagine getting more than one-quarter of your daily caloric needs in one drink containing nothing but unhealthful ingredients? Certainly not something you should ingest if your goal is to be lean and healthy. These drinks give you the negative health effects of coffee, milk, whipped cream, sugar and chocolate. You will soon learn how bad these other ingredients are for your body.

Some people say they do not have time to eat breakfast, but spend more time waiting in line to buy a designer coffee and donut (doughnut) than they would preparing and eating a healthful breakfast. Others say that healthful foods cost too much, but spend more money every month for expensive coffee drinks and junk-food lunches five days a week than I spend for *all* of my healthful meals.

Do not let advertisers convince you that tea is good for you just because some teas contain phytonutrients that produce positive effects. Scientists are currently working hard to create a form of coffee containing antioxidants. This will be a powerful marketing tool because you can then be told that drinking coffee is good for you, for the same reason you have been told that wine is good for you. Just because a future man-made coffee hybrid may contain one healthful ingredient does not mean it will be good for your health. It will still contain numerous harmful ingredients and the positive will not outweigh the negative. We may soon be told that smoking some new "designer" cigarette is good for our health because it contains one healthful ingredient along with all of the unhealthful ones. Keep in mind that you can get the good without the bad by eating whole, natural foods.

Caffeine is tasteless, so if you feel you must drink coffee use decaffeinated but be aware that coffee contains many other harmful substances such as coal tar, a known carcinogen, and oils and acids that irritate your stomach lining. Decaffeinated coffee may also contain unhealthful chemicals used to remove the caffeine. It is much easier just to drink something that is healthful. Like pure water. Why put a sharp stick in your eye when you can enjoy a beautiful sunset instead?

Dairy Products

Many people have been led to believe that dairy products are good for them but nothing could be further from the truth. Do you think Nature intended humans to be the only animals that drink milk after being weaned *and* to drink the milk of an extremely different species? This is an abnormal behavior instilled in humans by billions of dollars of advertising designed to convince us that cow's milk is good for us. Here are some reasons why you must avoid dairy products if you want to be lean and healthy.

Dairy cows are mutant animals developed by mankind. Nature did not create these creatures. The cow Nature created would have a calf and then develop enough milk to supply the nourishment needs of its offspring. Milk production would stop after the calf was weaned. This is how it is with all other mammals and how I believe it should be with humans. A few hundred years ago some people saw a way to make money by selling the milk of a cow to humans. No, I do not know if one of them was named Frankenstein. Selective breeding was done over a period of years and now we have animals producing about *seventy-five* times more milk than Nature intended. These milk-producing "machines" would die if not milked regularly by humans. It is obvious they are abnormal because they would have never survived naturally. Here are just a few of the results of this distortion.

The milk of today's cows is diluted because of the overproduction that has been bred into them. Because their calves do not get the nourishment Nature intended, they grow more slowly and get sick easier. To reduce the incidence of disease, many of them are given antibiotics. These drugs find their way into the milk that humans drink and cause weakened immune systems and destruction of the friendly intestinal flora. It also makes the next generation of cows weaker and sicklier. The antibiotic residue in milk also plays a major role in the development of antibiotic-resistant bacteria.

Why did people think the milk of a cow was suitable for human consumption? Cow's milk was given to a human infant and the infant grew faster than one fed with human milk. It was then falsely assumed that the cow's milk was as good, if not better, than the human milk. A great new moneymaking industry was envisioned. Most certainly, cow's milk makes a human infant grow faster than mother's milk, but this is not a good thing. A calf is supposed to grow four times faster than a human infant does and stimulating rapid growth in an infant is a risky thing to do. If growth occurs too fast, certain parts of the body may develop abnormally. A tumor producing excess growth hormone will turn a child into a giant who will probably not reach his fortieth birthday. Clearly, this is not something parents would choose for any of their children. Giving anabolic steroids to babies will also make them grow faster but do you think this would be healthful?

Numerous abnormal developments are probably created in infants fed cow's milk. These abnormalities may haunt many of them with mysterious health problems for their entire lives. If you wanted your baby to grow fast and become huge, you could use the milk of certain other animals, but the side effects of doing this would be even worse than those caused by cow's milk. Because certain nutrients found in mother's milk are not found in cow's milk, other developmental problems are likely to occur. Forcing rapid growth on infants could also lead to the development of an excess number of fat cells, making it easier for them to be fat for their entire lives.

What is the real purpose of milk? We have to examine infant development to answer that question. Before a mammal is born, it is attached to the bloodstream of its mother and gets everything (good or bad) from her blood. After a baby is born, it is meant to suckle at its mother's breast and ingest milk unaffected by light or oxygen. The mother and infant are still closely connected frequently but not continuously. Can you see the gradual transition Nature intended? The baby is getting everything in the milk except for what the lungs are now doing. The milk of an animal is similar to the blood of the animal. About the only thing missing is the red blood cells that carry oxygen to the cells and carbon dioxide away from the cells. If your baby needed a blood transfusion would you want the doctors to use cow's blood? Your baby's body would reject it. Giving cow's milk to a human baby is almost the same thing.

The milk of each species of animal is different because the needs of each infant animal are different. For example, human milk contains almost five times the amount of protein-digesting enzymes that cow's milk does. Human milk is six to seven percent protein, consisting mostly of lactalbumin (whey) that forms soft, easy-to-digest curds in a human infant's stomach. Cow's milk is 20 percent protein, consisting mostly of casein that forms tough curds that are hard for a human stomach to digest. This is why infants given cow's milk frequently suffer with colic (stomach cramping). Cow's milk contains three times as much calcium, sodium and potassium and six times as much phosphorus as human milk. Just right for a calf but too much for a human infant. The high level of phosphorus can lead to a loss of calcium and a resultant deficiency that is often made up for by calcium from the bones.

The composition of human milk changes to meet the needs of a growing infant. Human milk and colostrum (the milk secreted for a few days after giving birth) contain antibodies and other protective ingredients not found in cow's milk. One important immunoglobulin helps protect the infant's immature digestive tract from infection. All infectious diseases are less frequent in breast-fed infants. Certain amino acids needed for proper development are found in much higher concentrations in human milk. Growth of the friendly intestinal bacteria *Lactobacillus bifidus* is enhanced by the beta-lactose of human milk. This ingredient also produces organic acids that improve the absorption of phosphorous, calcium and magnesium, and it produces many of the B vitamins. Cow's milk contains alpha-lactose that has none of these beneficial effects. Cow's milk leaves three times more ash or residue than human milk and this increases the workload on the kidneys. Human milk contains more cholesterol than cow's milk. It is believed this is important for the normal development of the brain and nervous system. It is also thought to stimulate the production of certain enzymes that, later in life, lead to normal cholesterol levels.

Numerous contaminants have been found in cow's milk throughout the years but many of these have been eliminated. Some health researchers today state that milk must be boiled before use but one allergy expert says that if milk is boiled or heated, it becomes highly allergenic.

Galactose, a sugar produced from the lactose found in milk and dairy products, seems toxic to human egg cells. This is probably why women who live where milk consumption is high experience the largest decrease in fertility as they age.

Some people can handle milk products better than most of us. This is probably because their ancestors have been drinking it for hundreds of years and their bodies have retained the lactase enzyme that digests lactose (milk sugar). They are usually Northern European Caucasians and certain Caucasian American ethnic groups. The vast majority of adult humans in the world are lactose intolerant because their ancestors did not drink cow's milk. Humans are usually born with the lactase enzyme but lose it after a few years because it is no longer needed. If your body does not produce it, do not think something is wrong with you. You are normal. If you drink milk but are missing the lactase enzyme, the lactose inhibits the absorption of calcium. You may not get much calcium from the milk and it could even reduce the amount you absorb from other sources. Symptoms of lactose intolerance are bloating, flatulence, cramps and diarrhea. The diarrhea can lead to a loss of vital nutrients (or medications being used) because of the rapid transit time through the intestines. It has often been pointed out to me that cats will drink milk, but cats are also lactose intolerant and usually get diarrhea when they drink milk. I do not have any facts on the subject, but I believe that other adult mammals are lactose intolerant just like cats and almost all of us.

Cow's milk can cause chronic gastrointestinal blood loss that leads to anemia. Perhaps this is why the American Academy of Pediatrics (AAP) does not recommend using whole cow's milk in the first year of life. Why they think it is healthful to use after that is a mystery to me.

Researchers have determined that ancient and modern peoples who drank cow's milk developed numerous dental caries even though it contains twice as much fluoride as human milk. The bacteria *Lactobacillus acidophilus* was always found in the cavities. It was also learned that those who did not drink milk (other than human milk) did not have cavities. And, they did not floss, brush or see a dentist. Do not worry about getting more fluoride to protect you from cavities; just stop using milk products and processed sugar.

Mammals go through a natural transition while growing to adulthood. They drink milk when young, but not after being weaned and eating as an adult. The bodies of human beings (mammals) do the same. We are born with the enzyme to digest and use milk but lose it a few years after gaining the ability to digest and use our natural adult foods.

After a woman has a baby, she naturally starts producing milk. This continues for as long as the baby is nourished in this way. As the baby starts eating foods, it is gradually weaned (generally between six months and two years of age) and the milk production stops. It does not make sense that it stops because the baby is now supposed to drink the milk of a cow. It also does not make any more sense for a human baby to drink cow's milk than it does for an adult human to eat hay and grass.

People who consume milk and other dairy products commonly experience at least one of two major side effects—excess body fat or frequent illness, especially colds. The cold is caused by a constant build-up of mucus in their systems. The mucus is formed to carry the unusable products out of the body. Because cow's milk is extremely mucus forming, the body works hard to reject it. The slogan of the dairy producers should be "Got mucus?" and the answer would be a resounding yes.

The cleansing reaction most people call the common cold has been created in many of my clients just by improving their diets. It is nothing more than their bodies cleansing out excess internal waste. The next time you have a "cold," be happy. Your body has simply accumulated an excessive level of internal waste and is cleansing itself to prevent a worse disease or prevent you from polluting yourself to death. Blocking a cold with drugs, large amounts of vitamin C or anything else just prolongs the inevitable and is extremely unhealthful. Remember that Nature made your body to be self-healing and self-cleansing. The cleansing is a part of the healing.

Some of my patients have stopped consuming dairy products. After just a few months, they have reported things like less nasal congestion, losing weight, feeling cleaner inside and not getting sick even though everyone around them is. I grew up about a block away from a dairy farm and would walk there to get milk for my family. Prior to that I used to go across the street and milk the neighbor's cow with their son and bring some of it home. I used to drink large quantities of milk. I also used to get sick frequently and always had sinus problems. Every night before bed I had to use nose drops to clear my sinuses so I could breathe. I stopped drinking milk approximately thirty years ago and have not been "sick" since, except for a few self-induced cleanses you will learn about later.

Naturally, those who make money selling dairy products will tell you their "foods" are wonderful for your body. Some even label cow's milk as the "perfect" food. Perfect for a calf, but not for a human. They also tell you about the vitamins, calcium and other nutrients in milk, but they do not tell you that the calcium and many of the other nutrients are poorly absorbed. They also fail to mention any of the negative effects like tooth decay, frequent colds and excess fat. You now know that the majority of us are intolerant to milk and dairy products because, like other mammals, we are not supposed to drink milk after we are weaned. Mankind, however, in a never-ending quest for profit, has developed artificial enzymes to help you digest the milk sugar and eliminate some of the negative reactions. Calciferol (synthetic vitamin D) is artificially added to cow's milk in an attempt to increase calcium absorption. Unfortunately, it binds with magnesium and carries this vital nutrient out of the body. Some researchers believe pasteurization changes the calcium in cow's milk so it cannot be assimilated into the body. The sizes of the butterfat particles in milk are changed by homogenization and this may make them a contributor to the development of arteriosclerosis. Mankind also removes the fat from milk to reduce its fat-gaining side effect. These changes help to some degree, but as you will learn, 38 percent of the calories in 2-percent milk come from fat. Good sense will tell anyone that something should be avoided if it needs so many modifications to escape just a few of its negative effects.

Even with all the changes made to cow's milk, it still causes problems for many people because of the inability to digest and use the milk protein casein. Remember that casein is different from the protein in human milk and much harder to digest. Like lactose intolerance, casein allergy causes diarrhea and abdominal pain. My faith and belief is in the natural way we were intended to nourish our bodies. I do not believe cow's milk is a part of this. Cow's milk (the way it used to be) is a wonderful food for calves but even they are smart enough (and they are not very smart) not to drink it after they are weaned and able to eat carbohydrate foods. Their bones continue to grow and stay strong even though milk is never ingested again. This occurs with other animals as well. It makes no sense that the animals known as humans should be any different. Eating a variety of whole, natural foods will supply our calcium needs just like the natural foods of other animals do for them.

Some researchers believe that drinking milk as an adult causes cancer cells to multiply much faster than normal. This rapid growth makes it harder for the body to eliminate the mutant cells. This may be partly because of the high sodium levels of milk. Nutritional biochemist T. Colin Campbell has found that rats briefly exposed to aflatoxin (a carcinogen produced by food molds) often developed liver cancer when given casein. He was able to "turn on" the cancer growth by giving them more casein (about 10 percent of the diet) and "turn it off" by decreasing the casein in their diets.

Epidemiological research suggests a correlation between milk consumption and breast and prostate cancer. Breast cancer is rare in Asia where people do not drink milk. Two large studies in the United States linked dairy consumption to prostate cancer and another found that men who frequently consumed dairy products had a 70 percent higher risk for this disease. Those who were also taking calcium supplements dramatically increased the risk.

Do not worry about where you will get your calcium from if you stop using milk products. You will learn how to get all the calcium you need from the healthful sources Nature intended.

Some nutritionists believe a deficiency of riboflavin (vitamin B2) may develop if someone does not consume dairy products. Because riboflavin is found in green leafy vegetables, whole grains, eggs and meats, especially organ meats, this is highly unlikely and would be a problem only for someone eating a diet containing few of these healthful foods. This nutrient is in all good multivitamin and mineral supplements so even someone eating poorly could get enough from this source.

You may be thinking, "What about yogurt?" Many people say it is good for you, including brainwashed nutritionists and anyone making money selling it. You will learn the secret of the long-living Hunza people later and it is not because they eat yogurt. Besides, the yogurt they eat and the sugar-laden yogurt you buy in the supermarket are as different as night and day.

If you still feel the need to use milk, especially during your nutritional transition period, you will probably do best drinking raw unprocessed goat's milk. Most people's bodies can digest and use raw goat's milk and raw goat milk cheese and yogurt fairly well. Goat's milk is naturally homogenized, it contains the enzyme that helps your body digest it, and the ingredient balance is closer to that of mother's milk. Even still, I recommend using raw goat's milk products in moderation and soon "weaning" yourself off of them entirely.

Sugar, Honey and Artificial Sweeteners

Sucrose (processed sugar) is extremely harmful to your body. If good health is your goal, you must reduce or eliminate it from your diet. It cannot be called food because it is devoid of nutritional value and is therefore nothing like a real food. It creates negative side effects and addiction, just like many drugs.

Mankind had another "brilliant" idea when it was decided to take a healthful food and strip it of everything except its sweet taste. All the nutrients necessary to burn it for energy are removed and the concentrated sweetness is much higher than our bodies were designed to handle. This unbalanced product places a great deal of stress on our bodies because they were intended to get the natural sugar concentration found in whole foods, along with the vitamins, minerals and other nutrients necessary to use those sugars. Eating incomplete and unbalanced foods creates imbalance—imbalance of bodily functions, imbalance of our internal chemistry and imbalance in our appearance because of excess body fat, poor skin tone, vascular damage, and wrinkles from frowning and depression.

Nature gave us the ability to taste sweetness because foods that taste sweet are loaded with vitamins, minerals, enzymes and phytonutrients. The sweet taste was intended to attract us to eat foods containing many of the nutrients we need for good health. Nature never intended us to process away the life-giving parts and use only the sweet-tasting part of healthful foods to make lifeless, tasteless foods palatable. Refining everything but the sweet taste out of certain foods is about the same as processing a poppy seedpod into the drug opium. Our taste capabilities (sweet, sour, salty and bitter) were given to us to attract us to the variety of foods needed to keep us lean and healthy or to prevent us from eating something toxic to us. Many of the deadly toxins found in poisonous plants are alkaloids, which have an intensely bitter taste. Nature gave us the bitter taste to prevent us from eating something harmful.

For the rest of this section, the word *sugar* will refer to processed sugar. Many processed foods are loaded with sugar because food producers know it acts like a drug to keep people eating their products. Eating an excess of concentrated sugar-containing foods distorts a person's sweet taste mechanism. These food producers also know that if their products are not loaded with sugar, all the people with desensitized taste buds will not buy them. Many of the products would taste like cardboard if they were not covered with sugar. A popular soft drink has more than nine teaspoons of sugar in 12 ounces. Most soft drinks are just carbonated water, sugar and a small amount of flavoring. Just one-sixth of a medium cherry pie has 14 teaspoons of sugar, and you will find four teaspoons of sugar in just one-quarter cup of a certain children's breakfast cereal. Many people will tell you fruit yogurt is good for you, but it contains seven and one half teaspoons of sugar in just eight ounces. Unless it is sugarless, one half cup of applesauce has more than four teaspoons of sugar. The same amount of ice cream usually has less than that but how many people eat applesauce instead of ice cream and think they are eating for good health?

Check the labels of a few processed foods for the sugar content. You will be amazed not only by the amount but also by where you find added sugar. Once you decide you want to, it is not difficult to stop using sugar. Avoiding it has numerous health benefits and helps restore your taste sensitivity for natural sugars. Fructose (fruit sugar) is rated at 173 on the sweetness scale compared to the baseline of 100 for sucrose, but because it is found in healthy amounts in fruit it may not seem as sweet as foods containing extremely high concentrations of sugar.

The negative effects of eating sugar would fill many pages, so remember that the following are just a few of them. I hope they will give you ample reasons to greatly reduce the amount of sugar in your diet. It is close to impossible to eliminate sugar completely unless you make all of your own meals and never eat in restaurants or at other people's homes where there is almost always sugar in some of the foods.

Sugar contains "empty" calories that cannot produce energy unless B vitamins are available. Because it has no nutritional value, your body is robbed of nutrients just to use it. Sugar works essentially the same way alcohol does to rob your body of B vitamins, magnesium and other nutrients. This usually creates a deficiency of the nutrients vital to keeping the brain, nervous system and other parts of your body healthy. If your brain and nervous system are not functioning normally, it is difficult to think straight, feel good and follow a healthy lifestyle.

The natural foods sugar is processed from contain the B vitamins necessary to use it. As always, Nature puts nutrients that work together in the same food. Then mankind comes along and separates the parts creating imbalance in the food and the health of those ingesting it. Do you want to reduce your stress? Do you want to feel better, experience less depression and have more energy and ambition? If so, cut out the sugar in your diet and start enjoying the benefits of the B vitamins the sugar was previously depleting. You will learn more later about the vital functions of the B vitamins.

Sugar distorts your appetite for good foods and takes the place of the nutritious foods you should be eating. The more sugar you eat, the fewer good foods you will eat and the more depleted your body will become in the nutrients necessary to use the sugar and the nutrients you would have gotten from the good foods. And, any sugar not burned for energy is stored as fat.

Everyone knows sugar is bad for the teeth and is a major cause of cavities. Numerous studies have shown that primitive peoples (with no floss, brushes, toothpaste or dentists) who had never eaten sugar did not have cavities until after being introduced to and eating refined sugar. Even in populations with poor nutrition, if the sugar consumption was low, so was the incidence of cavities.

Sugar seems to be a primary cause of tartar formation that can lead to periodontal problems and loss of teeth. Conversely, the teeth of many people with periodontal problems have tightened in the bone after sugar and white flour products were eliminated from their diets.

Eating sugar stresses the blood sugar balancing system of the body. The main stress falls on the pancreas, whose job it is to secrete insulin to maintain a normal blood sugar level. Insulin reduces the blood sugar level by stimulating the body to store the excess sugar as fat. If the pancreas is stressed enough it could malfunction, with diabetes as the result. The high blood sugar condition *diabetes mellitus* is discussed in chapter ten. High sugar levels in the blood are extremely harmful, especially to the blood vessels carrying it.

When your body is subjected to abnormally high blood sugar concentrations, it often overreacts causing your blood sugar level to drop below normal. This makes you feel terrible so you look for another "fix" of sugar to feel better. This frequently leads to overeating, especially of the foods most lacking in nutritional value and the ones that rob us of health and add excess fat at a rapid pace. Chronic hypoglycemia may then develop.

Eating sugar creates a negative cycle that undermines your health and stimulates body fat gain. Here is how it works. Sugar depletes the B vitamins and other nutrients essential for normal brain and nerve function. This leads to nervousness and the inability to think and act rationally. Excessive amounts of sugar can also create a low blood sugar condition, causing symptoms such as fatigue, nervousness, inability to concentrate, anxiety, depression, erratic behavior, low self-esteem and apathy. When this occurs, most people reach for a quick pick-me-up to relieve them of these uncomfortable feelings. The most common choices are alcohol, caffeine, nicotine, processed grains or products loaded with sugar. These produce a quick energy boost, but it is short-lived so they soon experience the same uncomfortable symptoms. This perpetuates the negative cycle and leads to overeating worthless foods that cause rapid fat gain and a decreased ability to resist disease and function normally. Excess body fat and the depletion of vital nutrients make the body more susceptible to the hypoglycemic condition and further lowers the self-image. This is the same negative cycle created by alcohol, caffeine and nicotine. You will soon learn how to reverse this cycle and replace it with a positive cycle that makes it easy to stay feeling and looking your best.

Because B vitamins are important to muscles, a lack of them affects our most important muscle, the heart. Pigs fed a diet deficient in thiamin (vitamin B_1) showed scarring on the right side of their hearts. Beriberi, a disease caused by thiamin deficiency, causes heart damage, increased pulse rate and palpitations, high blood pressure and a number of other undesirable symptoms. Eating refined sugar and a diet relatively low in B vitamins could easily lead to these problems. Many of the chronic conditions that modern people suffer from are caused by minor nutrient deficiencies that could easily be prevented. A major shortcoming of modern medicine is the failure to diagnose health problems until they are extreme and causing severe and easily recognized symptoms. By then, unfortunately, permanent damage has often already occurred or it is too late to prevent or successfully treat the problem.

The damage a high blood sugar level does to the inner wall of the arteries is widely known. When a concentrated form of sugar is ingested, the blood sugar level will be excessively high until the body has a chance to lower it.

Damage to the arterial walls can occur during the times when the blood sugar level is high. This could contribute to the development of atherosclerosis (arterial plaque formation).

Sugar has a dramatic effect on increasing the cholesterol level of the blood, and a diet without sugar has been shown to reduce cholesterol levels. A research study found that when rats were fed corn oil and starch their cholesterol levels were low, but when they were given corn oil and sugar their cholesterol levels more than doubled. Even rats fed lard or hydrogenated oil along with starch had lower cholesterol levels than the rats given the healthier oil and sugar. Remember that a cholesterol-containing food has almost no effect on raising your blood cholesterol level unless sugar is eaten at the same time. Sugar seems as much, if not more, of a cause of high cholesterol as bad fat. Also, when sugar was included with fat, the rats stored more of the food as body fat. This is another way that sugar causes excessive stress to the body.

Eating refined sugar stimulates cancerous tumors to grow rapidly. Sugar does not contain any nutrients to nourish your normal cells and it depletes your body of the protective nutrients you may be getting from other sources. Cancer and diabetes have been increasing proportionately with the rise in sugar consumption. Some people have had certain cancers go away in a few months after sugar was eliminated from their diets. Primitive groups of people with no history of cancer soon began developing it after "civilized" men introduced them to refined sugar. One doctor stated that cancer sufferers in the final stages could be pain-free if they lived on natural foods and eliminated all sugar.

A book was once written about the fact that sharks do not get cancer. I would like to see an experiment where sugar is fed to sharks and see if they still do not get cancer.

Strong solutions of sugar are an irritant to our tissues, especially the stomach and intestines. Sugar also irritates the nerves and causes symptoms expressed most dramatically in children and women. It can cause hyperactivity in children and menstrual pain in women. Evidence indicates that an excess of sugar has a negative effect on the liver and can cause numerous symptoms of poor liver function.

An acid intoxication is produced when sugar and meat are combined. Neither meats nor sugar contain oxalic acid but when eaten at the same time, oxalic acid is produced. A soft drink, which is mostly sugar, consumed with meat will produce a large amount of oxalic acid. Be aware that sugar is often contained in sauces people eat with meat. Oxalic acid can cause conditions such as rheumatism, inflammation of the respiratory tract with excess secretions, adenoid nasal growth and inflamed tonsils. Is sugar the cause of the tonsil problems seen in our children? I believe tonsils have an important purpose and am happy I still have mine. I have resolved snoring for many people by realigning a particular vertebra in their necks, but sugar may be the cause of snoring for some people. Oxalic acid combines with calcium in the digestive tract to form calcium oxalate, which cannot be absorbed. Because calcium oxalate is the primary composition of almost 75 percent of all kidney stones, I believe an excess of calcium oxalate increases the risk of developing them.

People who eat sugar often have chronic dyspepsia (indigestion), bad body odor, poor complexions, constipation, and are often bad-tempered. Those who like sweets often dislike fresh fruits, vegetables and meats. Their natural tastes have obviously been distorted by excess sugar consumption.

Sugar disrupts the important balance between calcium and phosphorus. Initially it increases the calcium but after the effect has worn off, the phosphorus is increased. This leads to a decrease in calcium and could be part of the cause of osteoporosis. As you now know, health is balance and anything creating imbalance causes health problems.

When large amounts of refined sugar are eaten, the sugar concentration in the blood gets so high the body does everything it can to eliminate the excess as fast as possible. First, the pancreas is stimulated to secrete insulin, a hormone that inhibits fat utilization and increases fat synthesis. This causes the body to use some of the excess sugar for energy instead of using fat. The liver and muscles store some of the excess sugar as glycogen, but any unused sugar is stored as body fat. Because the glycogen storage locations are full, even glucose (sugar) from good foods at the next meal is stored as body fat if it is not used for energy. All of this is done in an attempt to protect the body from the harmful effects of unnaturally high concentrations of sugar in the blood. As you can imagine, the end result is more body fat.

Many "sugar-holics" can be found where sugar consumption is high. These people have a condition much like alcoholics because the input of empty calories robs the body of B vitamins and often leads to hypoglycemia. Some people can eat a small amount of sugar or drink a little alcohol, but others find it difficult to stop once they get started. Like the alcoholic who cannot have a single drink, some people need to completely avoid sugar or they will go on a destructive binge. Alcoholics or sugar-holics often indulge in alcohol or sugar when nervous, upset or emotionally fatigued. A negative cycle occurs because both of these substances deplete the B vitamins essential for proper function of the brain. The hypoglycemia usually created also negatively affects brain function. Some people ingest alcohol and sugar to celebrate and then have to deal with the negative effects. These products also stress the endocrine glands and this may be the cause of the excessive alcohol or sugar consumption in the first place. It is obvious why both of these conditions often continue to worsen.

How much sugar do Americans eat? In 1940 it was 106.5 pounds per person annually. That is about one pound every three days. If you eliminate infants, people who are nutritionally aware, and many elderly, it was probably close to one-half to one pound a day for many. In 1999 sugar consumption was about 156 pounds per person annually—almost a 50 percent increase.

That's three-quarters of a pound to one-and-a-half pounds a day for many. For some people, it may be two or three times higher. The strange thing is that more and more artificial sweeteners are being used, but sugar consumption is still increasing.

Conditions that have been helped (or eliminated) by eating less sugar are chronic fatigue, high blood pressure, migraine headaches, food allergies, asthma, alcoholism, sinus troubles, neuroses, ulcers, epilepsy, depression, rheumatic fever and various degenerative conditions such as arthritis. Sugar contributes to the development of urinary tract infections, intestinal cancer, indigestion, diverticulosis (pouchlike herniations of the colon), hormone disorders, mental illness and kidney stones. I believe that sugar contributes to the development of every disease.

Not eating sugar may help prevent insects from biting you. Vitamin B1 works well as an insect repellent but is depleted when you eat sugar. Therefore, if you want to decrease your chances of being bitten by a tick, mosquito or any other insect, eat less sugar.

Here is another good reason to avoid sugar. Because your body needs three ounces of water to store one ounce of sugar, it takes barely more than five ounces of stored sugar to add one pound of excess weight.

Eating sugar is an acquired bad habit that does not have to control you, and it does not take long to develop the good habit of avoiding it. Following the eating guidelines and other advice in this book makes it an almost effortless task. It will be easy because you will be providing the minerals (primarily chromium) your body needs to eliminate your physical craving. And, as your brain starts functioning better and your energy stabilizes, your improved self-image and sense of well being will make it easy to eliminate your psychological craving. After you eliminate sugar from your diet, get ready to enjoy the tastes of foods you have disliked in the past. This is a common reaction to a sugarless diet. Get rid of the sugar in your children's diets and watch their hyperactivity decrease, their attention spans improve, and their taste for nutritious foods increase.

Processed honey causes about the same effects in the body as sugar. It contains a few vitamins and minerals, but in insignificant amounts. Eating honey as it was eaten in ancient times is healthful and nutritious because it is raw and contains the comb and the bee pollen. This reduces the sugar content, supplies more nutrients and maintains the balance Nature intended. Unfortunately, it is not readily available in this form unless you are a beekeeper or have a friend who is.

Most honey is unhealthful because it is processed into a concentrated and unbalanced product. Just like grain processing, the healthiest parts (bee pollen and royal jelly) are taken out and sold separately as "superfoods." These are the parts that gave ancient people the positive results they got from eating honey. They did not have our modern methods of processing and separating the parts. It was also used sparingly because they thought of it more as a medicine than a food.

Do not be tempted to replace sugar with artificial sweeteners. These products are bad for your health and do nothing to help you get or stay lean. Saccharin is a product of coal tar and my belief is that anything made from coal tar is harmful to the body. One report in a medical journal stated that children in a particular town who used saccharin exclusively all suffered from goiter (enlarged thyroid gland). In large doses it can cause headaches, gastrointestinal disturbances and depression. Some people have experienced severe allergic reactions that included skipped heartbeats, a rash and cold sweats. As far back as 1935 there were doctors who believed saccharin might cause cancer. It has since been proved to be carcinogenic. Amazingly it is still on the market as a non-prescription drug.

One researcher soaked peas in various solutions and then recorded how many sprouted. Of those soaked in water, 94 percent sprouted. Eighty-seven percent of those soaked in sugar water did. Even when soaked in salt water, 44 percent still sprouted, but not a single pea soaked in the saccharin solution sprouted. The life force that causes the peas to sprout was destroyed. This researcher concluded that saccharin is a protoplasmic poison and, if you did not already know, our bodies are made of protoplasm—the living substance of a cell regarded as the physical basis of life. Sounds pretty important to good health, if you ask me. Saccharin appears to be far worse for us than sugar.

Cyclamate was another sweetener that was popular for a while. It was banned in 1971 because it caused cancer in laboratory animals.

Forget about drinking diet sodas and foods sweetened with aspartame, because it causes you to crave carbohydrates and overeat; not exactly helpful if you want to be lean and healthy. Aspartame is the technical name for the registered brand names NutraSweet, Equal, Spoonful and Equal-Measure. It has reportedly caused ninety-two different symptoms including headaches, dizziness, seizures, nausea, numbness, rashes, depression, fatigue, irritability, muscle spasms, tachycardia (abnormal heart rate greater than 100 bpm) and insomnia. A few other symptoms are hearing loss, heart palpitations, difficult breathing, vision problems, slurred speech, tinnitus (ringing in the ears), loss of taste, anxiety attacks, joint pain, vertigo, and memory loss. It is also believed by some researchers and physicians to trigger or worsen the following chronic illnesses: brain tumors, epilepsy, Parkinson's disease, Alzheimer's disease, lymphoma, birth defects, multiple sclerosis, chronic fatigue syndrome, diabetes, fibromyalgia (tendon and muscle pain) and mental retardation.

Aspartame is made of aspartic acid, phenylalanine and methanol. The first two are amino acids but methanol (wood alcohol) is a deadly poison that breaks down in the body to the toxic chemicals formic acid and formaldehyde. Dr. Hulda Clark believes that methanol is the root cause of diabetes. Is the widespread use of aspartame why the incidence of diabetes is increasing rapidly, especially among young people? I hope I have presented enough information to convince you to avoid the toxin aspartame. It is now found in more than five hundred products and in Uganda it is even added to the sugar they produce. Read labels or ask for ingredients to avoid unknowingly ingesting this harmful product.

Another sweetener is sucralose. It is sold commercially as Splenda® and can be found in many low-carb snack products. Sucralose is made by processing sugar with the toxic chemical chlorine. Not exactly healthful sounding, is it? It can have unpleasant side effects like stomach pain and gas and is not recommended.

Corn syrup is often used to sweeten foods that have had their natural tastes removed. This product is about 42 percent sugar, mostly glucose. I do not recommend using it although it is probably far better than ingesting high-fructose corn syrup, which is sweeter and mostly fructose. It is now used in large quantity in hundreds of products. Fructose is the natural sugar used by Nature to attract us to the nutritious foods containing it, but our bodies do not do well with abnormally high amounts. Evidence also indicates that high levels of fructose increase the triglycerides circulating in our blood to excessively high levels. Our bodies were not designed to use the high levels of fructose contained in high-fructose corn syrup or even in fruit juices. This is why I recommend avoiding both of them. You should not use pure, granulated fructose for the same reason. I recommend avoiding all current man-made sweeteners and any that are developed in the future—even the ones like stevia and xylitol that are claimed to be healthful. They are not whole foods. Eat whole natural foods that are sweet, do not use sweeteners to make processed foods taste better.

People have often asked me why a land of milk and honey is considered a healthy place if we are not supposed to eat milk products or honey. The answer is simple. A land of milk and honey simply describes a fertile land containing plants for the bees and food for animals (including humans) to multiply and thrive.

Do not worry about missing sugar, honey and artificial sweeteners. They are all unnatural, unbalanced and unhealthful. Nature supplies a multitude of sweet and nutritious foods for our health and enjoyment and other *whole* foods have their own unique tastes and should not need to be sweetened.

Salt

Some natural sodium and chloride is contained in almost every food we eat. Our bodies need 0.5 to 3 grams (500 to 3,000 mg) of sodium each day, yet many teenagers get about 25 grams a day. That is more than ten times the RDA of 2.4 grams. The average American gets 10 to 12 grams a day. Approximately three grams are found in natural foods, three to five grams come from processed foods and about four grams are added during cooking or just prior to eating. As you can see, even the highest requirement is met just from natural foods. Milk (which you should not be ingesting) contains almost 250 mg in two cups. Five ounces of meat, fish or fowl contains slightly more than 100 mg. Most other natural foods are low in sodium. Following my program will probably give you less than three grams a day but this should be plenty.

Unless otherwise indicated, the salt referred to in this section is refined salt that has been ruined by the high heat and other processing steps used to refine it. Salt originally contains eighty-four minerals, but when the refining process is over only two remain—sodium and chloride. Over 90 percent of this salt is used in industrial manufacturing. It works fine for these applications, but creates tremendous imbalance in a human or animal body. What about the sea salt you see sold in health-food stores? Unfortunately, it has also usually been processed until it is almost entirely sodium chloride.

Excess salt intake causes hyperacidity because the chlorine of the sodium chloride causes increased hydrochloric acid production. This is a common problem that plagues millions of people. Alcohol, refined sugar, caffeine and even decaffeinated coffee also increase acid production. Most people usually reach for a drug to reduce the excess acid. Instead of introducing another unbalanced product (the drug) into your system, stop using salt (and the other acid stimulators) and chances are you will end your suffering.

Most sodium is held in the tissues and tends to reduce the effect of calcium, which has many important functions. Salt also increases the body's loss of potassium, another mineral with numerous vital functions. Potassium was an essential part of a once-famous cancer treatment. Instead of worrying about getting more calcium and potassium, reduce your salt intake so the calcium you have is not limited in its crucial functions and you do not lose what potassium you already have. I believe that excess salt is the main reason why so many people have an imbalance of minerals in their bodies.

Some primitive nations still have groups of people who have never tasted salt and many others will not eat salted food. Some of these people were given salt by civilized man and they then developed a craving for it. This does not mean they need salt any more than craving chocolate means you need it for good health. Ranchers often give salt to their animals thinking they also need it. These are animals that have survived for thousands of years without excess salt. Animals need some unprocessed salt if their foods do not contain it or if they are confined to small enclosures and unable to eat their natural diets that contain the sodium and many other minerals their bodies need.

Salt has a stimulating effect on the adrenal glands. This can lead to increased stress and adrenal exhaustion. In this way it is almost like a drug. Some people believe it acts as an emotional stimulant that is pleasurable on some level. But, like other drugs, this pleasure is unnatural and brings with it many negative effects, including overeating. Some researchers believe that salt stimulants cancer cells to grow faster than normal. A much lower incidence of cancer exists among people who use small amounts of salt and a higher incidence is seen among people who ingest larger amounts.

Excess salt irritates the delicate membranes of the body. You would not want salt in your eyes or an open wound, so why would you ingest it so it can come in contact with sensitive internal bodily tissues? This affects normal function. For example, salt over-stimulates the digestive tract and interferes with proper absorption, especially of protein.

Because every gram of salt is held in suspension with 70 grams of water, excess salt causes an abnormal accumulation of fluid. This extra fluid affects the normal function of the body and plays a part in the cause of many diseases. In heart and kidney ailments, the body often develops edema. The cause is not excess water, but excess sodium. Reducing sodium intake and drinking more water helps these conditions immensely. Lowering their salt intake has helped many people with heart conditions.

People generally lose about 10 pounds shortly after starting a diet. Because most diets restrict the intake of salt and sugar, the body quickly eliminates 10 pounds of water. This lost "weight" is regained almost overnight when people stop the diet and start eating more salt and sugar again.

Ingesting excess salt is most likely a major cause of kidney problems, because the kidneys excrete 90 to 95 percent of the sodium we lose. Ingesting four to twenty-four times (if you get 12 grams but need only 0.5 grams) more than the body needs will put a great deal of stress on the kidneys and could cause a breakdown.

Fluid retention can cause a waterlogged condition in the ears and sinuses. One woman who had been deaf for years had her hearing come back after just three weeks on a salt-free diet. Millions of people suffer from sinus conditions. Many of them could be helped, or perhaps completely cured, just by eliminating the excess salt in their diets. A few other conditions that have been helped by using less salt are hives, insomnia, epilepsy, nervous tension, rheumatic joint swelling and cirrhosis of the liver.

Because salt creates havoc with the body's delicate water balance, it is extremely difficult to lose fat or stay lean if you are ingesting excess salt. Because water is formed when fat is oxidized in the body, normal water balance is imperative. If it is not balanced, stored fat will probably not be burned, because your body does not want to create more water if it is already drowning in excess. In the beginning of a good fat-burning program, your weight may stay the same or even increase because fat is becoming water. In fact, 100 ounces of fat yields more than 107 ounces of water. You get more water because oxygen from your blood combines with the hydrogen from the fat. In a day or two your water metabolism will adjust and the water weight will be eliminated. If you are not eating salt, that is. Most fat people are waterlogged, which is partly why their flesh is excessively flabby. Excess salt and sugar are the main reasons why. I believe that many fat people have excess water stored where it is not supposed to be and not enough water where it is supposed to be. By eating properly, your distorted fat and sugar metabolisms move closer to balance, but more importantly, normal water balance is restored. Some diet programs create weight loss through dehydration. This is harmful and produces only temporary results.

In the past, athletes and other people exercising in the heat were told to take salt tablets to replace the salt believed lost from excessive sweating. This could actually be harmful. First of all, the body does not lose much sodium through perspiration. Second, the body adapts to working or exercising in hot climates. Third, those exercising or working in the heat will probably eat more and therefore get more natural sodium. Finally, if they truly needed more, their bodies would create a craving for foods naturally high in sodium. Think of the primitive peoples who get only small amounts of sodium from the foods they eat but usually do hard physical work in high temperatures. They have fewer health problems because of it, not more. Luckily, most athletic trainers and coaches now know better than to give their athletes salt tablets.

Excess salt consumption can cause hypertension (high blood pressure) in some people. They are placed on low-salt diets after the problem develops. Stop using excess salt before health problems develop and you will save yourself many difficulties. It will also be much easier to stay lean. This is an additional benefit for the heart because being fat puts stress on the heart and can also cause hypertension.

Salt stimulates you to eat by increasing the flow of saliva. Now you know why you can't eat just one potato chip, pretzel, salted nut or other salted food. If you want to get and stay lean, you cannot ingest something that stimulates you to keep eating.

Pregnant women placed on a salt-free diet in the last weeks of pregnancy experienced shorter labor and reported less pain. Death from eclampsia (a severe form of toxemia of pregnancy) was much lower during the Second World War when food was rationed. Less salt was being ingested during that period. In countries where salt is rationed, eclampsia is almost unknown and the number of miscarriages is small.

Another research study found that people could reduce their hair loss substantially (50 to 60 percent) by having less salt in their tissues. Perhaps you can keep your big bushy head of hair far longer if you cut back on the salt.

Many common preservatives contain sodium. Sodium alginate, sodium pectinate, disodium phosphate and monosodium glutamate are a few examples. Avoiding everything with the word "sodium" in it will help keep your sodium levels normal.

What about getting enough iodine? Potassium iodide is added to table salt after iodine and eighty-one other minerals have been removed during processing. This does not make sense to me. Why add back only one of eighty-two? Some foods (especially seafood) naturally contain a healthful form of iodine and vegetables contain it if iodine is in the soil where they are grown.

These foods are healthful sources of this vital mineral. Some multivitamin and mineral supplements also contain it. Many people in the United States and other developed countries get excess iodine because of the high amounts of salt consumed and from the iodate used as a conditioner in making bread. Even if you made an effort to get as little salt as possible, it is unlikely you would ever develop an iodine deficiency. Some people are sensitive to iodine and could have severe reactions to the iodine added to salt. Iodine excreted through the skin can make acne worse. If you have this problem, reducing your salt intake could help dramatically.

Refined salt often contains other unhealthful chemical additives like yellow prussiate of soda, corn sugar and alumino-silicate of sodium. You will learn later why this last additive containing aluminum should be avoided. Salt is also often contaminated with bacteria and mold that can cause health problems.

I believe Nature intended some people to eat fish and vegetables from the sea to get the trace minerals they need. Those who lived far from the sea were to get them from meats and from foods and herbs grown in the soil. Powdered kelp (seaweed) is a good source of many minerals, including numerous trace minerals. It is only about 18 percent sodium chloride. Unfortunately, kelp and other types of seaweed may now be contaminated with toxic chemicals so are no longer healthful.

The eighty-four minerals found in seawater are similar in kind and ratio to the minerals found in our blood. Numerous physical problems could probably be eliminated if people got these important minerals. Especially many of the trace minerals scientists have not even determined the function of yet. Nature knows they are important. That is why they are included in whole, natural foods. Numerous "miracle" health products are currently available that primarily contain trace minerals. It is not a mystery why so many people feel much better when using these products if you realize that most people are deficient in these vital trace minerals. These products are usually extremely overpriced and are unnecessary if you eat naturally and balanced.

An inexpensive source of trace minerals is available. Believe it or not, it is salt—unrefined salt with nothing taken away or added. Celtic Sea Salt® contains nothing but the eighty-four minerals found in seawater and would be a healthful additive if you are deficient in trace minerals. It could be used in moderation by almost anyone. Your health-food store may sell it. If not, you can order it online at celtic-seasalt.com. If you feel you need more unrefined salt you should be tested to see if you do and if so, how much. You will learn later about various testing methods.

Refined salt deadens the taste buds on your tongue making great-tasting, natural foods seem bland and unappetizing. Many people cannot taste anything except salt, so everything tastes about the same. You will be amazed at how flavorful natural foods are as your taste buds come back to life in the coming weeks. You will soon start to enjoy the great variety of tastes Nature provides. Avoid most condiments because they are usually loaded with salt and sugar. If you need something for the transition period use products such as allspice, curry, kelp, ginger, lemon or lime juice, peppermint, saffron, caraway, tarragon and other herbs and spices. It is fine to use some of these products in moderation, but I suggest you strive to develop a refined palate so you will be able to savor the different natural tastes of the foods you will be eating.

Chocolate and Cocoa

Chocolate and cocoa are not conducive to good health or being lean. Both are made from processing the cocoa bean. The cocoa beans are roasted and then ground and compressed to extract most of the fat, which is sold as cocoa butter. What's left is still 20 to 30 percent fat and is called bitter chocolate. When finely ground, it becomes cocoa. Sugar is added to make sweet chocolate and sugar and milk are added to make milk chocolate. So far we have a large amount of fat and usually some sugar and milk. Doesn't sound especially healthful, does it? And do not forget about the caffeine.

Chocolate and cocoa are extremely high in calories. For example, a pound of plain processed chocolate has about 2,500 calories that come mostly from fat. A pound of fat contains 3,500 calories. Now you can see why it does not take many chocolate bars to produce a one pound gain of body fat.

Anyone with acne is normally told to avoid chocolate products so it must be part of the cause. Another condition often caused by chocolate is pruritus ani (itching anus). This problem has frequently been resolved when the affected person stopped eating chocolate. Citrus fruits and juices and some cola drinks can also cause this condition.

As you have learned, cocoa and chocolate contain caffeine. What you probably do not know is that they also contain theobromine, a chemical that has effects like caffeine. It is a poisonous powder used chiefly as a diuretic, myocardial (heart) stimulant and vasodilator (blood vessel relaxant). An average-sized chocolate bar has about 75 to 80 mg of caffeine. Parents who would never dream of letting their children drink coffee think nothing of giving them cocoa, chocolate and soft drinks that contain as much, if not more, caffeine than coffee. These two stimulants are what give people the fast energy boost that they get from eating chocolate. You already know some of the negative effects of caffeine. Now you know that you will get the negative effects of caffeine, theobromine, numerous calories from fat, sugar and milk if you eat milk chocolate. These all contribute to the addiction many people have to chocolate.

Chocolate and cocoa also contain oxalic acid that prevents calcium absorption and may cause kidney stones. Instead of worrying about getting enough calcium, avoid these two products that rob your body of this vital mineral.

Processed Foods

The Aborigines of Australia, the Eskimos of North America and other people who still live as their ancestors did are usually healthy. A behavior they all share is *not* eating processed foods. Also, their water does not contain chlorine, fluoride and numerous other chemicals. They enjoy good health and vitality even though their diets are extremely different. The key is that their foods and drinks are whole, natural and free of harmful chemicals.

I believe that the consumption of processed foods is the greatest health hazard (physical, emotional and social) of modern society. It is also the primary cause for being fat. To make them convenient and storable, these "foods" are pre-cooked, pre-mixed, pre-sweetened, pre-shaped, pre-packaged and essentially pre-pare you to have excess fat, live a depressing life with low energy and poor health, and to die young. Most, if not all, of the vital health-building nutrients originally contained in the foods have been eliminated. This is why they can sit in your cupboard and still be the same years later—still as worthless as ever. There may be some protein, carbohydrate, fat and a few vitamins and minerals that survived the processing or were added later but most of the nutrients and the life force are gone—the nutrients and life force we need to live a long and healthy life. To add insult to injury, the food processors usually add salt, sugar, hydrogenated oils, artificial colors, artificial flavors and chemical additives and preservatives. Many processed foods have added milk or lactose. Most of these additions create more imbalance, weakness and disease in our bodies. Keep in mind that most processed foods and drinks are not made with pure water and that many of them may be contaminated with toxic chemicals used during processing.

Salt, sugar and artificial flavors often added to processed foods inhibit our natural ability to taste if a food is bad. This could cause people to eat something that will make them ill. On the other hand, if a natural food is spoiled or contaminated in some way, you will usually smell or taste it and avoid eating it.

I recommend that you avoid eating processed meats. Many of them contain carcinogenic chemicals like nitrite, and during processing the chance of bacterial contamination increases. The four most common bacteria found in processed meats and certain other foods are *Campylobacter*, *E. coli*, *Salmonella* and *Listeria monocytogenes*. Incidences of the first three have been decreasing but the rate for *Listeria* infection has changed very little. *Listeria* is often found in processed lunchmeats, hot dogs and certain cheeses. Any of these bacteria can cause illness or death.

More than 90 percent of processed foods contain hydrogenated or partially hydrogenated oils. These oils contribute to heart disease, elevated cholesterol and triglycerides, non-insulin dependent diabetes, cancer and obesity. Research also indicates a connection between hydrogenated oils and attention deficit disorder (ADD).

Dr. Hulda Clark says that most processed foods are contaminated with isopropyl alcohol. Eat real foods, not artificial ones, if you want to be lean and healthy. Mankind may think it knows better than Nature, but it should be obvious to you by now that the more that humans mess with things, the more we mess up our own health and the health of our planet.

You have already learned about some of the worst processed items like sugar, alcohol, coffee, cocoa and salt. Another extremely harmful one is processed flour. It is almost as common as salt and sugar. Practically all processed foods contain flour, salt or sugar and many contain at least two of them. It is amazing how far away from natural balance most processed foods are.

To make flour, food processors start with a whole grain (usually wheat) that naturally contains essential oil, fiber, vitamins, minerals and other healthful nutrients, all in perfect balance. Then they strip away the germ and the bran and grind the endosperm into flour. This destroys most, if not all, of the remaining vitamins, minerals and other vital nutrients. The end result is something completely unbalanced and lifeless. The processor then adds a few artificial vitamins and minerals and has the nerve to label it "enriched." A worthless product with some artificial nutrients added is still worthless, because vitamins usually act as coenzymes and can do nothing unless certain other nutrients are present.

Processed white rice is poorly utilized and becomes mucus forming because the B vitamins needed to use the carbohydrate in the rice are removed from the original brown rice. Food processors seem to think that if a food is processed until it is white that it will sell better because it can be labeled "pure." This is just another example of that belief.

We do not yet understand the function of many nutrients found in whole, natural foods but scientists are discovering more of them and why they are vital to maintaining good health. A few nutrients known as phytonutrients have been discovered and researchers believe that many more exist. If you eat a variety of whole, natural foods you can get all the health-building nutrients Nature created now. Do not wait for scientists to find more and put them in a pill. It will not be the same, it will be much more expensive and you will probably be long gone before they even come close.

Eating processed foods creates a negative cycle that leads to sub-optimal health of body and mind, life-threatening diseases and excess body fat. The cycle goes something like this. Unbalanced and lifeless foods contain almost no nutritional value. In an attempt to get the nutrients it needs, your body stimulates your appetite and often creates abnormal cravings. This leads to overeating and eating more processed foods. Overeating leads to increased body fat storage and more internal waste. As more fat and internal waste accumulates, the efficiency of your body decreases, thereby creating the need to eat even more to get the nutrients your body requires. The excess fat and waste also decrease your vitality and contribute to the development of numerous diseases. On the other hand, whole, natural foods create a positive cycle that has the opposite effects.

Foods are often processed so they can sit on a shelf for many years. To accomplish this they are literally processed to death. All the nutritional value is eliminated. Many whole foods (dried beans, grains, nuts and seeds) can be stored for years, but Nature has sealed the life force and nutrition inside, not removed it.

If your body does not get the nutrients needed for good health, you will suffer from various physical ailments you probably think are normal simply because they are common. A frequent complaint is fatigue. Fatigue reduces your enjoyment of the good things in life, keeps you from being as active as you want to be and reduces the desire to exercise. Less physical activity and exercise lead to poor health, more fat gain and perpetuation of the negative cycle.

When your brain does not get the nutrients it needs to function well, your self-image and work performance suffer. Even your favorite recreational activities will be less enjoyable if you are functioning below par mentally. Your libido and sexual performance will also decline dramatically. Depression is a common result and usually leads to overeating that leads to more fat and internal waste, and these then lead to less efficiency and energy along with more depression and feelings of hopelessness. Are you starting to get the picture?

Now, combine this negative cycle with the one created by low blood sugar and others caused by a lack of exercise and various emotional reasons. With these negative cycles working against them, it is easy to see why so many people have excess fat and can never get rid of it no matter what they do. You can replace these negative cycles with positive ones that make being lean and healthy easy and natural.

Processed foods do not just rob you of optimal health, a more enjoyable life and an attractive appearance, they also rob you of money. They are much more expensive than natural foods because of what I call the three Ps—processing, packaging, and propaganda (advertising). These three Ps cost billions of dollars a year and the consumers of processed foods pay for it. *Processing* usually involves substantial cost for machinery and manpower. *Packaging* designed to stimulate the consumer to buy a product is where much time and money are spent. Package designers know all the right buzzwords, colors and other psychological tricks to influence you to buy foods that will make you fat and unhealthy. *Propaganda* (advertising) expenses are astronomical and ads use proven sales techniques to convince you that an unbalanced product with little, if any, nutritional value is good for you. Just check out the production and airtime costs of a 30-second television commercial. You must realize that most food processors are in business to make money, not improve your health. Sometimes cheap ingredients are used and the money this saves is spent on advertising or kept as profit. It is sad that millions are spent figuring out how to make more profit, and small amounts, if any, are spent trying to offer a healthful product.

Here is just one example of how costly processed foods are. I recently went to a supermarket and did some price comparisons. A two-pound bag of brown rice cost $1.59 or five cents an ounce. This makes about six to seven pounds of food after it is cooked. This means that this nutritious food costs one-and-a-half cents per ounce. The price of a one-pound box of a popular breakfast cereal was $4.49 or 28.1 cents an ounce. If you spent that money on brown rice you could make 17 to 20 pounds of food for the same cost as one pound of breakfast cereal. The price range among the cold cereals was 23 to 39 cents per ounce. Therefore, the cost of these unbalanced, processed cereals with limited nutritional value is between fifteen and twenty-six times more than the nutritious whole grain. And, if the grain was purchased in bulk, its cost would be about one half as much and the cost of the processed cereals would be between thirty and fifty-two times more than the whole grain. You can now buy processed breakfast cereals in the form of a candy bar so you do not even have to sit down for a few minutes to eat breakfast. This unhealthful product costs even more than the processed cereal and prevents families from spending time together. Compare the cost of instant mashed potatoes to real potatoes or any of thousands of examples and you will see how outrageously expensive unhealthful processed foods are compared to healthful natural foods.

Now let's compare a bag of processed candy to an apple. The bag of candy contains about 10 pieces and costs the same as a large organic apple. The candy has no nutritional value except for some sodium and is made of corn syrup, sugar and artificial colors and flavors. Three pieces of the candy contain as many calories as the apple. The apple contains a number of vital nutrients like potassium, calcium and vitamin A, and has real colors and flavors. The candy will stimulate you to eat more to get the nutrition your body needs but the apple supplies some of that nutrition so you will eat less.

Fast-food restaurants also spend billions on advertising and little or nothing attempting to offer anything healthful to eat. Many believe that this aggressive marketing is the cause of the epidemic of obesity in America. Fast-food outlets are even spreading to schools, hospitals and mass-merchandising stores. Fast foods are undermining the health of the people in hundreds of foreign countries as thousands of new fast-food restaurants open each year. Many people in these countries—especially the younger ones—will soon follow in our fat and unhealthy footsteps. It has already happened to many Polynesian people, Native Americans, Mexican Americans, and African Americans who have replaced their traditional foods with the typical American diet. If the Hunza and other long-living, healthy people ate pizza, hamburgers, fries, soft drinks and other processed foods they would also get fat and die young. Put them in automobiles and behind desks all day and their health would deteriorate even faster.

Another extremely detrimental side to fast foods is the serving sizes. Have you noticed that they have increased dramatically as fast-food outlets compete for your business? What used to be a large soft drink is now called a mini. Everything seems to have names like super, big, giant, colossal, jumbo, extra-large, gigantic, and king-size. At the movies you can buy a bucket of popcorn that contains almost an entire day's worth of calories. This competition was getting so out of hand there would have been soon gallon cups for soft drinks. Because that would have looked ridiculous and been difficult to handle, they just let you pay more and get as many refills as you want. This same portion size competition can be seen in many junk-food products. Have you also noticed that as the portion sizes have increased so has the size of the people consuming them? It is not difficult to understand why.

Fast-food outlets are adding additional drive-up windows as they compete to see who can be the fastest. They are making it possible to get fat even faster. Many of these fast-food outlets are now open 24 hours a day so people can get fat day or night. Because most fast foods are high in calories but low in nutritional value, your body stimulates overeating in its attempt to get what it needs. Fast foods can be eaten fast and this also leads to overeating.

Have you ever noticed that a large percentage of television commercials are for processed foods, fast foods or drugs? It is quite ironic. You are being sold drugs to treat the health problems most likely caused by eating the processed and fast foods.

Do not worry about missing fast foods. Eating well does not take much time and effort. Because we lead busy lives, many people fall into the trap of eating at fast-food outlets frequently and using TV dinners and other processed products. My life has been—and still is—extremely busy, but I have been able to eat well for more than thirty-three years. Being busy is not an excuse—it is all the more reason to eat well. You will learn that eating healthfully just takes knowledge and a bit of planning. You will not be spending hours in the kitchen preparing your nutritious meals. In fact, many meals will need no preparation at all. You will also learn how to make relatively healthy choices when dining out.

The effects that whole, natural foods have on our five senses are vital to the balance and health of our bodies and minds. These effects, and our health, are lost or distorted when most foods are processed. When the five healthful stimuli intended by Nature are changed or eliminated, it creates numerous imbalances and distortions in the body. You will learn about this in chapter fourteen.

I occasionally eat a few minimally processed foods, such as frozen or canned fruits and vegetables, raw nut and seed butters, grain drinks, tofu, and unleavened breads made from only sprouted grains and water. Many of these foods are close to their natural states and are therefore quite nutritious. Most of them are still balanced. The body uses them well as they are or because of the other whole raw foods usually eaten at the same time. If your body normally gets an abundance of life force from healthful, balanced, live foods, when dining out or occasionally at home, you can eat some minimally processed foods. But it is always best to choose foods as close to their natural states as possible. Read the labels carefully. If some of the foods you eat are derived from healthful sources, only slightly processed and used in moderation, they should not have any detrimental effects on your health.

Chemicals

Even if your diet contains absolutely no processed foods, you will still be ingesting a large number of chemicals. Chemicals found in fertilizers and pesticides, in the air you breathe, and in the water you drink and use for washing your body. Many of these chemicals are transmitted into the soil and absorbed by the foods grown there. You also breath in or absorb chemicals when you use soaps, deodorants, perfumes and colognes, face creams, nail polish, shampoos and many other products.

More than three thousand different chemicals are added to foods. The vast majority of them are detrimental to the normal function of your body. They poison you in some way and create imbalances that cause a myriad of perplexing health problems. Some safety tests are done on many of these chemicals before their use is approved, but most of the time the chemical or food producer wanting to use it does the tests. Wouldn't you feel more secure if an independent company was doing the testing? Because of political pressures, the Food and Drug Administration (FDA) even allows food processors to add known cancer-causing substances. Also, safety tests are done only on individual additives, not combinations of them. Who knows what health problems certain combinations could cause. Another problem arises because many of these chemicals accumulate in your tissues or cause cumulative damage. The long-term effects of most of them are still unknown.

I believe that many of the diseases common to older people affect them because they have been exposed to certain chemicals longer. I also believe that a correlation will eventually be found between particular physical complaints and the chemicals a person ingested or was exposed to throughout the years, as has happened to industrial workers who developed cancer and other diseases after being exposed to chemicals on the job. Problems just take longer to manifest because the exposure level is lower.

Because of the abundance of chemicals in our modern environment, it is impossible to eliminate exposure to all of them. But, if you avoid processed and radiated foods, buy organically grown produce and eat meats that do not come from tortured and drug-filled animals, you can greatly reduce your exposure. Some of these foods cost a bit more but are well worth it, and because eliminating processed and prepared foods reduces your food costs tremendously, you will most likely save a substantial amount of money. I spend far less on food every month than most of the people I know who do not eat healthfully. Chances are you will also spend much less on medical expenses. Also, remember that the nutrients found in natural foods help protect you from some of the harmful effects of chemical exposure you cannot avoid.

Just because a label reads "no preservatives" or "natural ingredients" does not mean the product is free of harmful additives. You cannot rely on the labels of processed foods to tell you the whole story. For one thing, you probably do not know what most of the chemicals are or what short- or long-term harm they may cause. Also, manufacturers often put harmful chemicals such as monosodium glutamate (MSG) into a mixture of some kind and give it an innocent-sounding name. Is this done to conceal that the product contains MSG? I do not know, but it happens, so be aware. A few hidden sources of MSG are malt extract, autolyzed yeast, bouillon, hydrolyzed vegetable protein, natural flavors, seasonings, lunch meats, sausages, soups, condiments, chips, fast foods and maltodextrin. According to specialists in this field, most processed foods contain it. MSG can cause a variety of symptoms such as migraines, numbness and tingling, seizures, diarrhea, panic attacks, asthma and heart problems. Unfortunately, you may have no idea that MSG or other harmful additives are in a product until after you have a bad reaction. This is another good reason to avoid as many processed foods as possible.

Sodium nitrate and sodium nitrite are often found in processed meats. They combine with other chemicals in the meats or in your body to form carcinogenic nitrosamines. I have been hearing about the cancer risk of eating nitrates and nitrites for almost 40 years.

I do not recommend using most of the butter, sugar and salt substitutes available because the chemicals used to make them are probably more detrimental to your health than what they are replacing. Think about the saccharin example.

I highly recommend using natural cleansers, cosmetics, deodorants, shampoo, toothpaste, and other personal or environmental care products. Many of these products are much better for you and the environment. Sadly, even many natural products are contaminated with toxic chemicals. Dr. Hulda Clark gives many suggestions and substitutes in her book *The Cure for All Diseases*. Store food and water in glass or ceramic containers. Hard plastic containers can be used if they are clear and imprinted with the number one. Toxic chemicals may leach into the food or water that is stored in plastic containers labeled with a two or higher number. Do your best to reduce your exposure to harmful chemicals. If a certain chemical causes cancer or Alzheimer's disease after 60 years of exposure at a particular level, if you limit your exposure to half of that amount it will take 120 years. You probably won't be here long enough to see the problem develop.

Nicotine

Nicotine is a toxic poison that causes cells to mutate and after a few mutations become cancerous. It is also extremely addictive. Cigarette smoking reduces your life expectancy by many years and increases your chances of getting almost every known disease. It doubles the risk of a woman having a miscarriage. Smoking is the leading cause of preventable death, not just because of the nicotine but because of the tar, carbon monoxide, benzene, hydrogencyanide, arsenic, formaldehyde and more than 4,000 other toxic poisons also contained in cigarettes. All of these chemicals are extremely harmful and you must stop smoking if you want to be healthy. Here now are only a few of the detrimental effects of nicotine.

Nicotine is extremely detrimental to good nutrition. It interferes with vitamin C absorption and destroys vitamin C you already have in your blood. It also restricts your blood vessels, reducing the amount of vital nutrients going to all parts of your body. Nicotine decreases the amount of oxygen your cells receive and causes a release of adrenal hormones that raise blood glucose levels. High amounts of sugar cause vascular damage and could lead to the development of hypoglycemia. Smokers drink more coffee, eat more sugar and drink more alcohol. All of which can stimulate a hypoglycemic reaction along with having other detrimental health effects. Smoking makes the pH of the blood more acidic and also decreases the sense of taste.

Some people use smoking to stay lean. Because nicotine causes a release of glucose, they get a temporary pick-me-up from a cigarette. This is like ingesting alcohol, sugar and other processed carbohydrate products. Holding the cigarette and putting it in the mouth replaces holding and putting food in the mouth. People often get fat after they stop smoking, because they replace the smoking habit with excess eating.

Improving your nutrition, exercising regularly, being more aware, and feeding your mind and spirit all make eliminating the destructive use of nicotine easier. You may need special assistance to quit but these healthy habits are extremely helpful and of great value in preventing you from smoking again. Following most of the same steps used to get and stay lean can help you to permanently stop smoking.

Banish Them Forever

You already knew most of the products discussed in this chapter were harmful to your body and mind but did you ever imagine how bad? And the sad thing is that they have far more negative effects. Alcohol, dairy products, sugar, artificial sweeteners, caffeine, salt, chocolate, processed foods, chemicals and nicotine are all unbalanced products lacking in food value. They are poisons that rob your body of the vital nutrients it needs to be healthy and lean. They rob you of your best appearance by creating excess body fat, wrinkles, unhealthy hair and skin, and by eliminating the spring in your step and the sparkle in your eyes. They rob you of money by costing more and generating medical and weight-loss expenses. They rob you of sexual drive and performance, the energy and desire to accomplish worthwhile goals, your ability to handle stress and to think clearly and see the positive side of life, your sense of humor and your ability to smile and enjoy the many wonders of life. They even rob you of years of healthy and vital life. They are truly your worst enemies.

Some of these items are drugs. The others are not labeled as drugs, but because they are unbalanced and concentrated they act like drugs in your system and cause negative side effects. The ones causing only minor negative effects may seem harmless but the mild damage accumulates until it finally causes big problems. Add one straw to a camel's back every day for ten to twenty years and you will finally break the camel's back. Most people know that alcohol and nicotine will kill you long before your time but do not realize that salt and sugar will do the same. These and most of the other unbalanced products discussed in this chapter are addictive and control the eating and other behaviors of many people. But, like drugs, each can be cleansed from your body until no more physical craving remains. Then your emotional addiction must be gotten rid of or you will start using these unhealthful products again. You will learn how to eliminate your addictions later in this book. Remember that my goal is to help you find *and* put together all the pieces of *your* permanent fat-loss puzzle. Banishing these products are large and vital pieces of that puzzle.

It is difficult to completely avoid all of these harmful products, but the less you use of each the better off you will be. You may be thinking about using them in moderation. This is certainly better than using them to excess, but is the same as saying you will use only a little arsenic, a bit of strychnine and moderate amounts of a few other poisons. Small to moderate amounts of a number of different poisons will still kill you. Moderation also often stimulates more want and can easily lead to excessive use. *Make the decision* to avoid them all as much as possible. They are like termites eating away at your house (body) each time you use them. Keep in mind that if you are already low in the nutrients caffeine depletes, just one cup of coffee may be enough to create a deficiency and serious health consequences. You may also be extra sensitive to one or more of these unhealthful products.

Think seriously for a moment about the last paragraph. Would you want someone slowly poisoning you and prematurely robbing you of your youthful looks and vitality and shortening your life by perhaps decades? I doubt if you would, but you may be doing it to yourself with alcohol, caffeine, sugar, salt, and processed foods, and by overeating. *Everything you ingest is either building health or destroying it.* Keep this in mind as you make your food and drink choices.

You may be wondering why Nature created such things as tobacco and coffee if they are so bad for us. Remember that we have been given the freedom of choice and that almost anything can be used for a positive and healthful purpose as easily as for a destructive and unhealthful one. I have heard that tobacco makes a great healing poultice for sick cattle. It is used in homeopathic medicine and probably has a few other positive uses as well. I believe that

Nature intended it to be used only for its healthful purposes. Coffee may have been meant as an herbal remedy for spider or snakebites in the regions where it grows. Remember that a coffee plant produces only one pound of beans and grows in only a few parts of the world. That is not enough to supply coffee to very many people. Also, many plants and foods that can be eaten by some animals are toxic to us. Both tobacco and coffee may have been intended as food for certain insects. Mankind, not Nature, turned coffee and tobacco into the booming businesses they are and by doing so, has made billions of dollars but ruined the health of millions of people. Unfortunately, this is true of numerous others things as well. For example, many illegal drugs and most of the enemies discussed in this chapter.

Be Kind to Your Pet

Most pets are loving companions that bring tremendous joy into people's lives. They need good nutrition just as much as we do and rely on you to get it. If you want your pet to live a long and healthy life you must avoid feeding it these harmful products. Look at all the fat animals around today and look at the diseases they get—cancer, heart disease, degenerative joints and other health problems seen in humans who live modern lifestyles. Do you think wild dogs and cats hundreds of years ago got cancer? Do you think that wolves, tigers and other animals that eat the way Nature intended die of cancer today? Do you think that humans eating as Nature intended will greatly reduce their chances of getting cancer and other diseases?

Because most pets are fed processed, lifeless foods filled with chemicals, it makes sense that they get heart disease and cancer just like the people who eat these types of foods often do. *Natural Health for Dogs and Cats* by Richard H. Pitcairn, D.V.M., Ph.D. and Susan Hubble Pitcairn, is an excellent book about feeding dogs and cats natural foods for good health. I highly recommend it if you have a dog or cat you love. You will be appalled at what pet food producers are allowed to put in the food. There are other good books available that explain how to keep your dogs and cats healthy with nutritious meals, snacks and nutritional supplements. Use what you learn in this book to help you to choose one.

My beloved dog Caitie was fed raw ground beef and turkey along with brown rice and other whole grains, steamed vegetables, and various supplements like bone meal. I daresay she ate far better than most of the people of this world who can afford good food. She was even given most of the same nutritional supplements that I use.

Remember that a great way to prolong the length and improve the quality of your pet's life is to keep it from getting fat. Good nutrition, adequate exercise, mental stimulation and love are the primary keys, just as they are for you. Keeping your pet healthy saves money on veterinarian bills and keeps them alive longer for you to love and for them to share their divine love with you.

The Choice is Yours

Numerous diseases have been conquered with improved sanitation and advances in medical knowledge and techniques. Unfortunately, many new diseases have replaced the old ones. If you greatly reduce your consumption of the items discussed in this chapter, you will minimize your chances of getting most diseases. You will also eliminate many of the physical causes of excess body fat and possibly even get rid of your emotional reason for being fat.

It never ceases to amaze me how the people who would never put low quality gasoline or oil in their cars or cheap, poorly built furniture in their homes think nothing of putting worthless and harmful foods and drinks into their bodies. You can buy a new car or chair but you cannot buy a new body. Think about this for a moment. You cannot put inferior fuel in your car's gas tank if it is already full of good fuel and you will not want to once you feel the performance from the good stuff. Likewise, if your body is getting good nutrition, there will not be room for or the desire to eat empty, lifeless foods. You may have forgotten what it's like to feel good, but once you start to experience it, you will probably not want to go back to feeling the way you had been.

Have you ever noticed that white sugar, salt and white flour look like cocaine and other addictive and harmful drugs? Unfortunately, they are perhaps even more harmful than the drugs because most people do not perceive them as threats to their mental and physical well-being. You have probably brought the enemies right into your home and do not even realize it. They are like spies undermining all your other efforts. Dare to keep yourself and your children from ingesting these harmful products. Say no to them and yes to good health.

The decision to eliminate these enemies could make the other steps necessary to achieve your victory over fat extremely easy. They are your biggest obstacles to success next to eliminating the cause. Because one or more of them may even be *your* cause, eliminating them could take you two giant steps at once.

Develop the awareness now that your choices at every meal have a tremendous impact on your future. You can create a bright, healthy, energetic and loving future or a dismal, unhealthy and pain-filled one. *The choice is yours—now and always.*

The more light you allow within you, the brighter the world you live in will be.
Shakti Gawain

The invariable mark of wisdom is to see the miraculous in the common.
Ralph Waldo Emerson

Consider your origin; you were not formed to live like brutes,
but to follow virtue and knowledge.
Dante

The moment past is no longer; the future may never be;
the present is all of which man is the master.
Jean Jacques Rousseau

The chains of habit are generally too small to be felt
until they are too strong to be broken.
Samuel Johnson

The problem is not the problem.
The problem is one's attitude about the problem.
John Harrigan

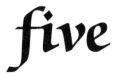

five

From Food to Function

In chapter two you learned the four steps required from ingestion to proper utilization. Here now are the details of these steps that will maximize the efficiency of your body, so it can extract and use as many health-building nutrients as possible from everything you ingest. The more nutrition you get from what you eat, the less food you need to live a healthy and active life. Eating less means lower expense, decreased build-up of energy-draining internal waste, more efficient bodily functions, reduced fat deposits and chances of living a much longer and healthier life. The benefits of eating less have been proven over the years. Researchers in one study regularly underfed a mouse and it lived to be the human equivalent of one hundred years old. In fact, systematically eating less is the only thing proven to extend the length of life.

Achieving Maximum Digestive Efficiency

You now know about the friends (foods) that will supply your body with the nutrition it needs. Here are the primary steps necessary for getting these foods effectively converted into usable forms.

Full-Strength Digestive Enzymes

Our bodies use digestive enzymes to break down foods into their usable forms. Liquids ingested with meals or soon afterward dilute these enzymes, making them less efficient. Imagine how the effectiveness of a chemical such as acid or cleaning fluid would be diminished if diluted with water or other fluids. Because the quantity of digestive enzymes is relatively small, diluting them with one or two glasses of liquid makes a tremendous difference in their effectiveness.

One example of why this is important can be seen when you consider the process of eating meat. It will be broken down poorly if the enzymes of the stomach are diluted. The pancreatic enzymes of the small intestines will have to do more in an attempt to finish the job. This allows for the possibility of some undigested meat to pass through your system. As it travels through your intestinal tract it can putrefy, creating toxic and perhaps carcinogenic waste. You will also not get the amino acids and other nutrients the meat contains.

The key to allowing enzymes to work at full strength is to not drink anything too soon before, during or for a certain time after each meal. The quantity of food at each meal must be considered as well. The larger the meal, the more time the enzymes need. The texture of meat determines how fast it is broken down; fish is lighter in texture than fowl, which is less coarse than red meat. One hour may be sufficient after eating fish, where three hours is best with red meat. I suggest waiting at least two hours after a protein meal before drinking anything. Wait one to one-and-a-half hours after a complex-carbohydrate meal and after eating a mixed meal of protein and complex carbohydrates, wait approximately two hours before drinking anything. When taking supplements with your meals, use the smallest amount of water necessary.

If you drink sufficient water prior to eating, you will not feel thirsty during or for a few hours after your meal. Your body creates thirst when you are eating if it does not have enough water to make the digestive enzymes necessary to process that meal. Eating bread, crackers and salty foods will stimulate more thirst, but these are not foods you should be eating. The natural foods you will be eating contain water and enzymes.

You should drink water throughout the day, but at the appropriate times. Everyone has heard of the importance of drinking enough water, but few people know when the best time to drink it is. Timing is everything. A good habit to develop is to drink one to two glasses of water between 45 and 60 minutes before each meal. It helps you get the amount of water you need each day and your body will be well hydrated prior to eating. If you forget or are unable to drink at that time, do it as long before eating as possible. When you go out to eat, drink some purified water before leaving home or from a bottle in your car before going into the restaurant. If you forget but know they serve purified water at the restaurant, you can drink a glass of water as soon as you are seated. Have some bottled water or a glass of tomato juice if they do not serve good water. By the time you order and get your meal, 15 to 20 minutes may have passed. Say no thanks to the wine, regardless of what you have heard about it aiding your digestion. If you follow my dietary guidelines, you should not need anything to aid your digestion and the negative effects of the alcohol are not worth it.

Many years ago I was explaining to someone in a health club the principle of when to drink water. A week later, a woman approached me at the club and said she had overheard the explanation. She had followed the guidelines during the previous week and had already lost five pounds. The only change she had made in her lifestyle was *when* she drank water. One patient recently lost three pounds in a week and another lost more than 20 pounds in about six weeks. I have often seen this happen. These examples demonstrate the significant benefit that drinking water at the proper time has on good digestion and your health. Please do not let a doctor or anyone else convince you to abandon this vital health habit.

One exception to the rule of not drinking with meals is while eating only fruit. Because fruit does not need digestion, you will not be diluting any enzymes. Drinking water with fruit dilutes the fructose content to some degree so the sugar level of your blood stays closer to normal and your pancreas works less. Drinking water with a fruit snack also helps you to supply your daily needs.

Some "diet" programs recommend drinking one or two glasses of water just prior to eating. The goal is to fill you up so you will eat less and lose weight. This is a gimmick that backfires, because it reduces your digestive efficiency, creating the need to eat more in an attempt to get the nutrition your body requires. Follow my guidelines so the water is absorbed into your system prior to eating. If you were to eat some fruit and drink a glass or two of water about an hour before dinner, you would normally eat less, because the fruit supplied your body some nutrition, not because you tried to trick it into feeling full.

Drinking with meals is also unhealthful, because the diluting effect causes your body to produce more enzymes in an attempt to increase the potency. This continual stimulation to make more enzymes than necessary could overstress the body's production ability and may be part of the reason why many people's digestive systems become less effective as they age.

After eating a high-protein meal or an excessive amount of food, you will often feel tired and drowsy because your body is channeling more energy to your digestive organs, leaving less available for your brain and muscles. If you feel weak and drowsy after other meals, it is most likely because you did not drink enough water prior to eating. Do not reach for a stimulant (caffeine, sugar or tobacco) to wake you up, just drink some water and your energy level should increase. Then make sure you drink enough water prior to your next meal.

A common problem affecting normal digestion is a deficiency of hydrochloric acid (HCl). If you have a burning sensation in your stomach, noticeable gas, cracks or sores at the corners of your lips, sore mouth or tongue and feel full for a long time, especially after eating meat, you might have this problem. Other symptoms include burping, bloating, indigestion and bad breath after eating. You may crave pickles or other foods pickled in vinegar. It is best to avoid white vinegar and foods processed in it. If you suspect low HCl output, add a teaspoon or two of apple cider vinegar to a quarter cup of water and drink it just prior to a protein meal. If your symptoms are relieved, it indicates a low HCl output. After that, find a competent nutritionist or holistic doctor to help you choose the best HCl supplement for you and to determine the correct dosage. Just think, something as simple as this could be the primary reason why you have excess fat. This is why some people lose body fat when taking apple cider vinegar with meals. If you have difficulty digesting fat or have had your gallbladder removed, you need supplemental bile salts and pancreatic enzymes. Your digestive symptoms should be gone after a few days of taking the correct supplements.

Having adequate HCl is important, because it activates the protein-digesting enzyme pepsin, improves the absorption of protein, iron, calcium and a variety of other nutrients, kills most bacteria entering the stomach, prevents bacterial or fungal overgrowth in the small intestine, and deactivates plant and animal hormones. It also affects other phases of digestion. For example, if food entering the small intestine is not acidic enough, the pancreas and gallbladder are not stimulated to release their digestive juices. Antacids diminish the body's digestive functions and can cause headaches, diarrhea and stomach pain. People sometimes trade their heartburn for these three problems.

A chronic lack of HCl can cause food and environmental allergies, pernicious anemia, loss of taste for meat and other proteins, emaciation (extreme thinness), iron-deficiency anemia, and flabby flesh under the arms. It can make you prone to osteoporosis, skin problems, liver and thyroid gland trouble, and many other health conditions.

Eating excess amounts at one time reduces your digestive efficiency. A normal stomach holds only about one liter (four cups) of food. Excess food can cause indigestion, bloating and other discomforts, and can lead to fewer nutrients being absorbed.

Chew Foods Thoroughly

The next step to achieving efficient digestion is to chew all foods thoroughly. This is easy if you eat whole foods as close to their natural states as possible. For example, a whole grain cereal is difficult to swallow without chewing it well, but it is almost impossible to thoroughly chew a piece of white bread or spaghetti. Chewing whole foods helps keep your teeth and gums healthier and maintains normal bone mass in your jawbone. Chewing also stimulates the flow of digestive enzymes. People often drink liquids with meals to wash foods down, but this reduces the amount they chew. This is another good reason not to drink liquids with meals.

Chewing foods well is important, because it gives your body a chance to signal you when it has had enough. When people eat a meal of greasy processed foods that require almost no chewing, they can easily overeat before getting the message they have had enough. They then get the discomfort, lethargy, indigestion, fat gain and anger at themselves that often accompanies overeating.

Many people say they derive a great deal of pleasure from eating, but few of them chew enough to experience much enjoyment. A large number of them keep eating in an attempt to get some satisfaction. What they usually get instead is more excess body fat. Chewing well extends the pleasure of eating and reduces the desire to overeat. Chewing all types of foods is important, but for different reasons.

Chewing protein foods

Protein foods need thorough chewing, because they are among the tougher foods to digest. If your stomach is functioning normally, protein foods stimulate HCl that converts the pre-enzyme pepsinogen into the active protein-digesting enzyme pepsin. Protein foods stay in your stomach for hours and are mixed thoroughly with pepsin. The smaller the particles, the larger the surface area exposed to the digestive juices of the stomach and the faster the digestion. When the food is released into the small intestine, protease and other pancreatic enzymes further break down the protein into the amino acids your body can absorb and use.

Chewing complex-carbohydrate foods

When a complex-carbohydrate food is eaten, it is important to chew it well, so more surface area is exposed to the digestive enzymes, but carbohydrates undergo minimal digestion in the stomach because they are not broken down by pepsin. Digestion of complex carbohydrates starts in the mouth. Saliva contains the enzyme salivary amylase or ptyalin and chewing increases the amount of enzyme released. As you chew, the food is mixed with your saliva and digestion begins. To experience this, eat a whole grain. As you chew, you will notice it getting sweet. This is because the salivary amylase is converting the complex carbohydrates into simple carbohydrates or sugar. The more you chew, the more the enzymes work, and the sweeter it gets. Chewing breaks the indigestible cellulose membranes in many of these foods so their nutrients can be released. Chewing well also prevents the cellulose from irritating your digestive tract.

After complex-carbohydrate foods are swallowed, your stomach simply mixes them more completely with the saliva. These foods stay in your stomach for less time than protein foods and are released into your small intestine where the enzyme pancreatic amylase continues the conversion of complex carbohydrates into simple carbohydrates.

Chewing simple-carbohydrate foods

Simple-carbohydrate foods such as fruits do not need digestion, because they are already in a usable form. Nevertheless, it is still important to chew them thoroughly, because many have indigestible cellulose membranes that must be broken before the nutrients can be released. I have read that some fructose is absorbed inside your mouth. This is done more effectively if fruit is chewed well, so the fructose is released slowly. This appears to be true, because when you hold fruit juice in your mouth it becomes less sweet.

Relax and Digest

It is important to feel relaxed and peaceful before, during and for a few hours after eating. You will derive more satisfaction from your meals and it improves the function of your stomach and other digestive organs. Anger is the main thing to avoid, because it has been shown that even nutritious foods, if eaten when you are angry, can produce harmful toxins in your body. Anger also undermines our health by making us temporarily stop caring about the consequences of our actions. This is when words are spoken that we do not mean and foods are eaten that we do not want. Let's examine why being calm during and after eating is so important.

Your brain controls your body primarily through the autonomic (automatic) nervous system that is composed of two complementary parts— the sympathetic nervous system and the parasympathetic nervous system. The sympathetic is known as the "fight or flight" nervous system and is activated during times of stress or physical activity. Its function is to prepare the body for physical action by increasing blood flow to the brain, muscles, heart, lungs and adrenal glands. Because we do not have enough blood to have full blood flow to all parts of our body at the same time, it must decrease blood flow to the organs of digestion and elimination. The function of the parasympathetic nervous system is essentially the opposite. It increases blood flow to the organs of digestion and elimination and reduces it to the areas needed for physical action. It can be called the "rest and digest" nervous system. When you eat, the parasympathetic nervous system normally takes control and channels more blood (via the enteric (intestinal) nervous system) to your stomach and other digestive organs. You feel tired after a heavy or large meal because less blood is going to your muscles and brain. This is why most people want to take a nap after stuffing themselves on Thanksgiving. The tryptophan in the turkey has absolutely nothing to do with making you tired. The amount is too small and it takes quite a few hours for the turkey to be digested and converted into tryptophan and other amino acids.

You may have heard the admonition to not go swimming after eating. That is good advice, but now you often hear that you should take a walk after eating. Walking is less intense than swimming but still directs blood away from the digestive organs. After you eat, it is best to rest until the food has been digested efficiently. Swim or walk *before* you eat, not after. In some countries people often rest after eating lunch and many even take a siesta. This is a healthy habit because it allows for good digestion and then the energy from the meal is used during the afternoon. Eating late and then going to sleep is an unhealthy habit because most of the energy from the food is not used so it gets stored as fat.

Whenever you are stressed, angry or upset, the sympathetic nervous system is activated and blood flow and nerve stimulation to your digestive organs is reduced. They will not get enough blood to supply them the energy needed to do their jobs properly. You will also over-breathe, reducing oxygen to your cells, causing more stress and creating a negative cycle. These are the main reasons why your stomach feels tied up in knots if you are angry or stressed while eating. When you are upset, you and your digestive efficiency will suffer. If you eat to cope with stress, you will compound your problems and make yourself feel terrible while getting fat at the same time. The fastest way to resolve this problem is to take slow and shallow breaths.

If your sympathetic nervous system is chronically overactive you will experience an increased gag reflex and a dry mouth. If your parasympathetic nervous system is chronically overactive you will not have a gag reflex and you will tend to drool.

A connection also exists, via two vagus (tenth cranial) nerves, between the emotional centers of the brain and the organs of digestion and elimination. These nerve connections are a major reason why your thinking has a large influence on numerous bodily functions. It is why just the thought of food can stimulate acid or saliva secretion or why a man may get "butterflies in his stomach" if apprehensive about speaking before a large group of people. This is another reason why fear, anger and other negative emotions have such detrimental effects on digestive efficiency.

Our bodies communicate with individual cells using protein messengers known as ligands. When a ligand attaches to the receptor of a cell, it can change the state of that cell. Immune cells are able to send information to the brain and receive information from it. Various systems of the body can communicate via these chemical messengers and dramatic changes in behavior, mood and physical activity can occur. High concentrations of receptors are found where information from the five senses—sight, sound, smell, taste and touch—enters the nervous system. Thoughts, feelings and all five senses affect the body's receptors and have a tremendous impact on our mental and physical well-being. This is why you are going to learn how to improve your thoughts and feelings, and how to supply balanced stimulation to all five senses to help you accomplish your goals.

Because being calm and relaxed is so important for good digestion, here are two emotional balancing techniques that are easy to learn and use. Both are capable of calming you down and clearing your head.

Emotional center clearing

This method for calming your mind is part of a healing technique known as Neurovascular Dynamics (NVD). This therapy can rebalance the sympathetic and parasympathetic nervous systems and normalize blood flow to glands, organs and even the brain. Some of my patients are also treated with NVD if they need it. The procedure for clearing the emotional centers is simple.

To calm down, clear your head and get a truer perspective on what is happening, you need to reestablish normal blood flow to the emotional centers of your brain. There are bumps on each side of the upper outside edges of your forehead. These bumps are known as the frontal eminences. Gently place the fingertips of your left three longest fingers on your left eminence and your right three fingertips on the right eminence. Hold them there and you should soon feel a pulsation in your fingertips. When the pulsations on both sides synchronize, the treatment is completed and you can remove your hands. It generally takes only a minute or two. During times of stress or emotional upset, people often put their hands on their foreheads, instinctively doing essentially the same thing. When you do this procedure, you may want to think or talk out loud (in private) about what is bothering you.

The writing method

This method of calming yourself down and seeing the reality of your current circumstances is also simple but takes a bit more time. First, answer this question. If you had your choice of fighting an alligator or an invisible monster, which would you choose? You most likely chose the alligator, because you can see what you are dealing with and develop a plan. You can avoid the teeth and tail and position yourself to grab and defeat it. On the other hand, an invisible monster is impossible to fight, because you cannot see it. This is why many people have such difficulty dealing with their problems. They usually have no idea what the problem really is. Many spend years and pay others thousands of dollars to help them define and see their invisible monsters. After people see the problem, they can often easily see its solution. The writing method is highly effective at helping you to see your invisible monster so you can determine how to deal with it. Your invisible monster (problem) may seem like King Kong or Godzilla, when in reality it is only six inches tall and has no teeth. In other words, your problem is rarely as large, or as difficult to solve, as you believe it is.

The writing method is simply sitting down at a table with a pen and paper and writing out your feelings. Hold nothing back and continue for as long as you have something to write. Do not worry about what you are writing or if it is legible. The key is to get the words out so you can see clearly what the problem is. What you write will not be read or analyzed by you or anyone else. Simply write it, tear it up and throw away the pieces. You may already know how to start dealing with your problem before you stop writing. Even if you do not determine the answer to your problem, you will at least be calmer. This is like explaining a problem to a good friend who makes no suggestions or judgments. By clearly defining it, you can then determine how to deal with it. If you still do not have the answer, sleep on it and you will often wake up with an idea about how to solve the problem.

Cooking for Best Digestion

The best way to eat many foods is not to cook them at all. Heat destroys many vital nutrients, so eating as many raw foods as possible is best. Fruits should always be eaten raw and many vegetables are delicious raw. Legumes, grains and vegetables can be sprouted and eaten raw. Some people advocate eating all raw foods, but it is extremely difficult to get certain nutrients or adequate amounts of protein and complex carbohydrates from all raw foods. Also, I doubt if many people would eat raw meats and eggs. A combination of raw and cooked is best.

How long your food is cooked is a factor in getting good digestion. This is especially true for meats. For example, raw meat is broken down much more easily into usable amino acids than well-done meat, but this does not necessarily mean you should eat raw meat. Some people eat raw fish (sushi and sashimi) and raw steak (tartar steak), but generally it is important to cook fish and fowl to kill various illness-causing microorganisms. Red meat is the coarsest meat and therefore the most difficult to digest. If red meat is cooked rare or medium rare, it is broken down faster and more efficiently than if it is cooked more. Fish and fowl are digested easier than red meat even when they are well cooked.

Another important consideration to get optimal digestion is how your food is cooked. Primarily, you can boil, broil, roast, poach, bake, fry, deep fry, smoke, microwave, steam or barbecue. It is best to avoid barbecued foods, because the smoke contains harmful substances that are ingested with the food. I do not recommend eating smoked foods. Almost everyone knows that fried foods should be avoided, because the food absorbs fat from the cooking oils. Deep fat frying is the worst and is often done in rancid oil that can cause serious health problems. Quick stir frying using a minimal amount of oil is not a bad alternative, but I prefer boiling, broiling, baking, steaming or poaching. For example, if a chicken is boiled in water, much of the fat goes into the water and can be discarded instead of ingested. I encourage you not to make soup from the fat-filled water. Poaching fish or red meat also causes some of the fat to go into the water instead of accumulating on your waistline. Broiling, roasting or baking are good ways to cook meats. Boiling or poaching eggs is the best way to cook them. Beans and grains are usually boiled, but it is not a good way to cook vegetables because they lose nutrients into the water.

Steaming is an excellent way to cook vegetables. It is fast and destroys only about 10 percent of the many vital nutrients in vegetables. This is far fewer than the 40 to 60 percent of some nutrients that are lost with boiling. Steaming is also how I recommend warming up most foods. Cook your vegetables to suit your taste and texture preferences, otherwise you will not eat them. Experiment some, because you will be amazed at the difference that the size of the piece and the amount of time cooked make in the taste. You may really like rutabaga when it is cut into thin slices and lightly steamed but dislike it if the slices are thicker and cooked longer. Baking vegetables is a good way to cook them but takes more time. Quick stir-frying is also a healthful alternative. You should also eat plenty of raw vegetables as well.

A slow cooker made of crockery is a great way to cook many different foods and is timesaving, easy to use, and the low heat destroys fewer vital nutrients. Slow cookers are inexpensive, so I suggest you purchase a good one. Your entire dinner (except for the salad) can be cooking while you are away all day. There will be a nice hot meal waiting for you, so you should not be tempted to stop and eat some unhealthful and fattening fast food.

Microwave ovens are found in most modern kitchens, but I do not recommend using them. Most forms of cooking expose the outside surface of a food to a source of heat. The food cooks from the outside inward and the center gets less heat. Microwaves vibrate the molecules of a food at a very fast rate and this produces heat. This starts from the inside and moves outward. I believe that the life force is at the center of many foods to reduce the heat it gets. Microwave cooking generates excessive heat in the center of the food thereby destroying most of the life force. Close to 100 percent of some nutrients are destroyed when vegetables are cooked in a microwave. Microwave cooking may have other harmful effects that are yet undiscovered. To thaw out a food fast, put it in a plastic bag in a pan full of hot tap water. Do not use a microwave oven.

I recommend using only stainless steel or ceramic cookware. Avoid non-stick and aluminum pots and pans. As non-stick cookware wears out, the chemicals go into your foods, and you will learn later why aluminum is bad.

The main points to remember when cooking are to destroy as few nutrients as possible and to prepare the food so it can be easily broken down into usable forms.

Food Combining

Food combining can be described as including foods in the same meal that are digested in a similar way and not including foods that digest differently. The goal is digestive efficiency. The main rules are to avoid mixing complex carbohydrates and proteins in the same meal and to not eat simple carbohydrates (fruits) with other foods. It is also best to eat just one type of meat at a time. Fish and other seafood would combine well, but it is best not to combine different types of meat. This is because of the difference in the time it takes to digest them. As you have learned, red meats take longer to digest than poultry and poultry takes more time than most fish.

Other rules say it is best to not combine different melons with each other or with other fruits. The same holds true for berries. Sweet fruits such as nectarines, plums, pears and peaches can be combined and eaten together. Apples can also be included in this combination. It is best not to combine citrus fruits with other fruits, but they can be combined with each other. Eating an orange and some pineapple together is a nutritious treat.

The two main rules are the most important. Following them will supply more nutrients to your body and generate less internal waste. It should also stimulate your body to start cleansing, thereby becoming more efficient even faster. It is equally helpful for people wanting to lose excess body fat or people wanting to gain muscular weight but whose systems are so inefficient that they cannot get the nutrients necessary for growth.

Because protein undergoes more digestion in the stomach, it is best if it stays there longer than other foods. Fruits pass through the stomach quickly and complex-carbohydrate foods are churned and mixed in the stomach for a longer time. Because fruits pass through fast, it is best to eat them separately so they do not stay in the stomach and ferment, forming gas. You can eat a protein or complex-carbohydrate meal 20 minutes after you eat some fruit, because the fruit will be out of your stomach by then.

The food-combining theory says that if you eat protein and carbohydrates (simple or complex) at the same time the foods are either released from the stomach too quickly for efficient protein breakdown or stay in the stomach too long causing the carbohydrates to form gas. If these foods are eaten at different times, the protein will stay in the stomach long enough for efficient digestion and the carbohydrate foods will be released into the small intestine faster so their digestion can be completed. Also, when protein foods are eaten alone, the pH of the stomach is more acidic and this improves the digestion of the protein. If complex carbohydrates are eaten alone, the pH of the stomach is more alkaline, which improves the digestion of the carbohydrates. When protein and complex carbohydrates are eaten together, the pH is somewhere in between and both foods will digest more slowly and less efficiently.

Another important guideline is to avoid ingesting oils with meats or other protein foods. Oils coat the pieces of food and prevent the pepsin from breaking down the protein. Therefore, it is best to not use oil on your salad when eating protein. This works out well, because oil is best ingested during the day and complete protein foods should generally be part of the evening meal. Most protein foods contain some fat but it is not in liquid form, so will not cause a problem.

Some nutritionists believe that the food-combining theory is nonsense, but I have seen and experienced so many positive results from adhering to its guidelines that I highly recommend following them as often as possible. It is especially important in the beginning of your program, because these guidelines are remarkably helpful for increasing your body's efficiency and getting a positive cycle started. These rules should be followed closely if you have a great deal of excess body fat or have temporarily weakened or naturally weak digestive capabilities.

When following the food-combining rules, you will feel hungry much sooner, because your digestion is faster and more efficient. It will be easy to eat five or six smaller meals each day, which is the best way to stay lean and healthy. Smaller meals do not stretch and overload your stomach and they help ensure that a meal is not eaten when the stomach still contains the previous one. You will also feel more satisfied, because your body is getting better nutrition.

Numerous authors and nutritionists recommend eating five or six meals a day, but few explain what kinds of meals to eat. Some tell their readers that every meal should contain a combination of carbohydrate, fat and protein. By following this advice, you will have to constantly eat when you are not hungry and this is a very bad habit to develop. Eating five or six mixed meals also leads to each meal being eaten when the previous one is still in the stomach.

This causes poor digestion and can overwork your stomach and other digestive organs.

You now have the main food-combining rules and the only ones you need to understand and use. Various books and charts are available if you want to learn more about it, but be advised that some people advocate being extremely strict with food combining. This is impractical and unnecessary except in extreme circumstances.

Sometimes combining heavy complex carbohydrates (starches) and proteins in the same meal is advantageous. For example, if you are not going to be able to eat for four or five hours, you will not feel hungry as soon if you combine protein and complex carbohydrates in the same meal. This keeps your body satisfied until you can eat again. If you often go hungry, your body will store fat for the anticipated famine so it is *extremely* important to eat whenever you feel hungry, especially if fat loss is your goal.

Proper Function of Digestive Organs

Your digestive system consists primarily of your salivary glands, stomach, liver, gallbladder, small intestine, pancreas, and your brain, which controls the function of all the other parts. The gastrointestinal tract is controlled by a system known as the enteric nervous system but sympathetic and parasympathetic nerve signals can strongly alter its degree of activity. Therefore, the nerves exiting from between the vertebrae of your spine have a large impact on how your digestive system functions. Nerves branching out from the spinal cord at approximately the level of the bottom of your shoulder blades allow your brain and stomach to communicate. The nerves going to and from the liver are one level higher and the nerves connected to the pancreas are one level lower.

If the spinal vertebra where the nerves go to and from your stomach is misaligned, it causes inflammation that puts pressure on one of the nerves and impairs the normal function of your stomach. This is like having a short circuit in your car's wiring. For example, if the wire to your headlight is shorting out, the headlight will work intermittently or perhaps not at all, even though nothing is wrong with the headlight. Similarly, your brain communicates with your stomach through a nerve, and if the correct message is not received, your stomach will not function normally. There is also a nerve going from the stomach to the brain that communicates what is happening in the stomach. If this nerve has interference, your brain will not know what is happening in your stomach and will be unable to determine an accurate response. Faulty communication in either direction leads to abnormal function of your stomach. I have seen patients' gastric reflux pain end within minutes after the pressure was taken off this nerve and the signal finally got through for the lower esophageal sphincter valve to close. Also, if your brain is unaware a problem is developing, it will not do anything about it. A disease could go undetected until it becomes such a large problem that the body cannot deal with it. Similar nerve communication applies to the pancreas, liver, other organs of digestion, muscles, blood vessels and all other parts of your body.

For optimal function of your digestive organs, your spine must be aligned properly so there is normal two-way communication between your brain and digestive organs. This can be done effectively with Precision Muscle Balancing Technology^SM (PMBT^SM) treatments to realign the bones of the spine. These treatments are by far the most long-lasting and usually restore permanent balance. PMBT is currently available only in southern California from me and Mark F. Cornett, D.C. To learn more about it and of any new practitioners, go to my Web site at <u>DrAlexander.com</u>. If you do not have access to PMBT treatments, Directional Non-Force Technique (DNFT) chiropractic treatments are recommended as an alternative. These treatments do not create damage and can realign the spine better than numerous other chiropractic techniques. PMBT can usually establish permanent balance unless new muscle injury occurs, and DNFT can sometimes produce long-lasting relief but requires periodic treatments. If normal nerve flow is not reestablished permanently or for long periods, the glands and organs will not function normally. Do not be discouraged if you cannot get these treatments. Most people will make amazing progress by following the guidelines in this book but I want you to be aware of possible reasons why your progress may be slower than normal.

Chewing stimulates the release of certain digestive enzymes and triggers other digestive processes. If your teeth do not hit together properly, these processes could be inhibited and your digestion negatively affected. If crooked teeth are causing this problem, the teeth need realignment with braces. A far more common cause is a temporomandibular joint (TMJ) misalignment. This usually develops from compensating for skull and upper neck misalignments. I developed a severe TMJ problem from the muscle damage caused when my wisdom teeth were removed. The "specialist" I went to had me wear braces on my teeth for four years to make them crooked to match my misaligned jaw. It helped somewhat but I still had problems for ten more years until I realigned my jaw using my PMBT therapy.

Most doctors believe stress causes bruxism (teeth grinding) that then leads to TMJ pain and dysfunction. I believe that the jaw being misaligned causes the grinding. It is simply the body's way of attempting to realign the jaw, like moving and contorting your neck around if it feels slightly out of place. Another reason I believe emotional stress is not the cause is because my PMBT treatments have successfully realigned the jaws of many patients and eliminated the bruxism and the TMJ pain and dysfunction. The jaw misalignment was the only stress eliminated. Numerous patients, including me, have been able to throw away the dental splints and mouth guards that treat the symptoms instead of eliminating the cause of the problem. Even if you use these mouth guards at night, your teeth will still not hit together properly when you chew and send the normal stimuli to your digestive system.

A problem that can affect normal stomach function is known as a hiatus (or hiatal) hernia. Like many other conditions, the medical community has not yet figured out what causes it. For legal reasons, I am not allowed to say that I treat this problem, but my PMBT treatments have resolved a number of them by eliminating what I believe to be the cause. The cause generally occurs in older people and that is where this condition is most commonly seen.

Eating smaller meals is another way to improve your digestive efficiency. Eat five or six meals a day instead of two or three. This way, your body has less to deal with at each meal. You will not eat more each day if you eat nutritious foods. You will most likely eat less, because of improved efficiency. Eating more meals also has a stimulating effect on your metabolism. If you follow the main food-combining rules, it will be easy to eat more meals because you will feel hungry sooner. Instead of three large meals, you may end up eating three moderate meals and two or three snacks. Listen to your body. If it tells you it is hungry, give it some nutritious food. This is an extremely important guideline to follow if losing body fat is your goal. Also, eat slowly and give your body a chance to tell you it is satisfied. That's *satisfied*—not ready to burst. You will soon learn the difference. When you get the message you have had enough, stop eating. It is as simple as that once you get rid of abnormal emotional and physical cravings and get in touch with and start trusting the wisdom Nature programmed into your body and mind. If you are having problems, simply stop eating a while before you think you are full. Then wait for 10 minutes. If you still feel hungry, you can eat more.

Assimilate Those Nutrients

Your digestive tract is isolated from your body. It is like a tube running from your mouth to your anus. Nutrients not assimilated into your bloodstream simply pass through and are eliminated.

After foods have been ingested and broken down into their usable forms, they are then absorbed into the bloodstream through the small intestine. This third step (assimilation or absorption) on the way to utilization is important, but is often overlooked in dietary programs and books on nutrition. A vital key to good assimilation is the proper breakdown of foods into their usable forms. You learned how to achieve that goal in the preceding sections about improving your digestion.

Enzymes are necessary for efficient assimilation and utilization of your foods. Your body produces some, but others come from raw foods. This is why it is important to eat raw foods with each meal and to not overly cook other foods and destroy all their enzymes. A good way to get some enzymes with your meals is to eat a large salad with most of them. This gets the "live" enzyme-containing foods in your diet; foods containing life force. This is the force that gives life to everything. When people are alive they are animated with this force. When it leaves the body, the body then becomes a lifeless thing. The life force I speak of is a vibration and is recognized by many scientific disciplines as a real thing. It is seldom talked about when discussing foods, but every food has its own special vibration. That is why I refer to cooked foods that have lost their life force as "dead" foods.

It is important to have a balance between live and dead foods in your diet. If your diet contains primarily dead foods, you will not get enough of the life force your body needs to assimilate and use the nutrients found in those foods. The vibrations from live foods create the balance necessary for your body to use the nutrients from the dead foods. Eating all raw foods is helpful for reestablishing lost balance, but normally a combination of live and dead foods is best. The dead foods supply certain nutrients difficult to get from raw foods. Vitamins are important, because they often act as coenzymes working in conjunction with enzymes to cause the chemical reactions necessary for life to occur.

If your body has a naturally low production of digestive enzymes, you may need supplemental enzymes to make up the difference between what your body produces and what it needs. This could be part of the reason why you have excess body fat. Eating more enzyme-rich raw foods should also help. If your system is functioning below par because of excess fat and internal waste, supplemental enzymes will be helpful until your body gets more efficient. You may then no longer need the extra digestive support. Digestive enzyme tablets can be taken or you can drink raw vegetable juice between 15 and 30 minutes prior to eating. The best juice to use is made from green vegetables like celery, lettuce, spinach, parsley and others.

Excess body fat and internal waste can make your digestive system less efficient at absorbing nutrients. As you lose fat and waste, your assimilation of nutrients should improve. Cleansing the small intestine can be helpful. Abnormal nerve flow to your small intestine could have tremendous impact on how well nutrients are absorbed and an imbalance between your sympathetic and parasympathetic nervous systems could also adversely affect normal assimilation. You will learn more about these topics in upcoming pages.

The Right Food at the Right Time

Here we are at the bottom line—utilization. The three previous steps are necessary just to get us to this point. Utilization is a vital step, because everything else can be perfect, but if your body does not need what you are giving it, it either eliminates it or stores it as fat or internal waste. Most dietary programs and books on nutrition also fail to mention this step.

During the day, when most of us are physically active, our bodies primarily need carbohydrates (simple and complex) and fats to supply energy for our mental and physical activities. At night when our bodies are sleeping, we need mostly amino acids for the repair and rebuilding of tissues. About an hour after you go to sleep, your body releases growth hormone. The function of growth hormone is to stimulate the breakdown and use of body fat for energy and to increase protein synthesis for rebuilding and repairing various body structures. It makes sense then that most of the repair to muscles that have been broken down during work or exercise, or the normal replacement of worn-out cells, is done at night when your body is at rest. Your body has the time and energy to do this repair when you are sleeping. It can burn stored fat for the energy needed for growth and repair. Your brain also sorts and files the experiences of the day at this time.

It is logical for your evening meal to consist primarily of protein so the raw materials for growth and repair are readily available. This is also the most natural time to eat protein, because most people relax after their evening meal. This makes more energy available to the digestive system, so protein digestion is improved. Protein uses far more energy for digestion than carbohydrates and fats, and gives much less energy in return. This is part of why a high-protein diet helps people lose body fat. I do not recommend a high-protein diet, however, because it is stressful and can lead to numerous health problems. Protein should be used for growth and repair, not as an energy source. The tissues of a human body prefer carbohydrates for energy to fats and proteins. Because your body's primary need is energy, your diet should consist mainly of carbohydrate foods. The key is to eat *whole* and *natural* carbohydrate foods, not processed grain products.

Research indicates that one-and-a-half to two hours after strenuous exercise is when the body uptakes many of the nutrients used for rebuilding. Exercise stimulates the release of growth hormone and increases the demand for nutrients to repair the muscles. Therefore, eating some protein soon after heavy exercise may be beneficial for repair of muscles. I do not recommend a large amount of protein (more than 20 to 25 grams), unless you have time to rest and allow for good digestion. It is also important to replenish the glycogen (energy) stores in your body soon after exercise. This is best accomplished by eating simple or complex carbohydrates. Eating some fruit and taking some amino acid tablets right after exercising and then eating a protein and complex-carbohydrate meal 15 to 20 minutes later will work well for most people.

Start your day with some fruit and water. The water and the energy from the fruit will wake you up and get you going. This eliminates the need for stimulants such as caffeine, donuts or other refined sugar products that are used by many. Stimulants deplete their bodies of energy and start a roller coaster ride for their blood sugar levels. This in turn often causes the release of excess insulin, which causes fat storage. It is easy to see why so many people complain of fatigue. How do they expect their bodies to be energetic if they do not supply them with the nutrients necessary to produce energy? Do you expect your car to run without gasoline?

Next, have a good breakfast that will keep your blood sugar stable and give you long-lasting energy. It is common to hear fat people say they usually skip breakfast because they are not hungry. This is usually true, because they ate an excess amount the night before. Lean people usually eat breakfast and eat less at night. If you do not feel hungry for breakfast, eat earlier in the evening or eat less at night until you do feel hungry in the morning. Eating more in the evening and skipping breakfast is a bad habit that needs to be replaced with a good habit.

The rest of the day's meals until dinner should consist primarily of non-processed complex carbohydrates and healthful fats. Fruits can be eaten as between-meal snacks or even as a meal. Healthful fats are best eaten early in the day, either at breakfast, lunch or as part of an early afternoon snack. Fats and heavy (starchy) complex carbohydrates will most likely be stored as fat if eaten in the evening, when not much energy is usually needed. Many fat people starve themselves all day and then eat at night. They expect to drive a car all day with an empty gas tank and then put gas in it at night. Does that make any sense? What these people should do is eat more during the day and less in the evening.

Eating late at night is a very bad habit that usually leads to fat gain. Having your evening meal before 6:30 p.m. is a good guideline. When this is not possible, adjust *what* and *how much* you eat according to *how late* you eat. Follow my 3L rule: If you eat Late, eat Lighter and Less. In other words, the later you eat, the smaller and lighter your meal should be. Do not eat heavy carbohydrate foods if you eat late. If you eat after 9:00 p.m., just have a small meal of chicken breast or fish with a salad and some peas or string beans. Also eat lighter (fruit, instead of whole grains) and less the next morning.

If you eat dinner too early you may get hungry and want to eat something shortly before going to bed. This is a bad habit. When you go to bed you should not feel full, nor should you feel hungry. If you are full, it may disrupt your sleep, and chances are that the food will be stored as fat. It may also keep you from being hungry in the morning. You want to feel hungry in the morning when you "break the fast." Experiment a little and adjust the time of your dinner until you can go to sleep feeling satisfied and content. If you are occasionally hungry before bedtime, eat a small, low-fat, high-protein snack (one quarter of a chicken breast) or a bit of fruit (ten grapes, a plum or an apple).

Ingest olive oil and other good fats with complex-carbohydrate foods, but not with protein. Fat entering the small intestine releases a substance that inhibits gastric secretion and motility. This is detrimental to good protein digestion. Fats are not broken down much in the stomach so, as you have learned, oils consumed with protein will coat the protein and block the digestive action of pepsin. When fat enters the small intestine, bile is released to emulsify it so fat-digesting enzymes can further break it down.

Ingesting good fats along with vegetables, grains or legumes is best, because they are all efficient energy foods that should be eaten during the day. Providing your body with essential fatty acids also reduces cravings for bad fats like fried foods, fatty meats, cheese and pastries.

An exception to these general rules occurs when you are going to be physically active in the evening. If you work at night you should eat carbohydrates and fats prior to and while you are working and a protein meal about four hours prior to going to sleep. If your plans are dinner and dancing, supply your body with a small amount of protein and some complex carbohydrates at dinner so you will have energy for the dancing and other enjoyable activities. Eating a high-protein meal or an excess of food will make you tired and sluggish and could ruin a good time.

You have learned that eating smaller meals throughout the day improves your digestive efficiency. It also leads to greater usage and decreases the chance of eating more than you need. Give your body a nutritious meal and when it needs another one, it will let you know.

When your goal is fat loss, you should eat a variety of and larger amounts of alkaline foods—fruits, vegetables and legumes. Your energy needs will be met by these nutritious carbohydrate foods and the stored fat your body will burn to balance the pH of your blood.

Glycemic Index

The glycemic index (GI) expresses how fast a particular food is converted into glucose. The GI of a food is defined as the blood glucose response for two hours after it is eaten. It is expressed as a percentage of the two-hour response to an equivalent amount of ingested glucose. Glucose is rated at 100 percent and various foods are rated at lesser or greater percentages relative to the glucose. The lower the GI is, the smaller the glycemic response. But numerous differences exist based on each person's glucose tolerance that is determined by variables such as age, fitness level, fat percentage, genetics and nerve flow to various digestive organs. The glycemic response also averages out when foods are eaten together. This index can be somewhat helpful for someone with a glucose-handling problem such as diabetes, but a diabetic should be under the care of a competent doctor who is familiar with the GI of various foods.

Here are the glycemic index ratings of a few of the foods recommended in this book. Toward the higher end: red potatoes and parsnips are rated at 80 to 90 percent; millet and rutabagas at 70 to 79 percent and pineapple; cantaloupe and beets at 60 to 69 percent. Buckwheat, sweet corn, brown rice, yams, bananas and frozen peas are rated at 50 to 59 percent and carrots, grapes, peaches and oranges at 40 to 49 percent. Toward the lower end: butter beans, chickpeas (garbanzo beans), navy beans, lentils, pears and apples are rated at 30 to 39 percent; kidney beans and fructose at 20 to 29 percent; soybeans at 10 to 19 percent; and raisins and watermelon at less than 10 percent. Basically, a parsnip will release its energy and raise your blood glucose quickly and lentils or an apple will raise it at a much slower rate. More comprehensive charts are becoming available as more foods are tested for their glycemic index.

Knowing the GI of foods can help you plan out certain meals to fill a specific need. For example, eating some rutabaga and potatoes would supply relatively fast energy, but eating chickpea, lentil and soybean soup would supply long-lasting energy.

Some people recommend never eating foods with a high GI because it raises your blood sugar fast, but they fail to consider that we almost always eat a few different foods at the same time. This generally supplies a gradual release of energy. For example, you may eat some brown rice (GI of 55) with a few chopped dates added. Even though dates have a GI of 103 the quantity is so small that the total GI for the meal is only about 57. I have heard recommendations to eat an unhealthful food with a low GI instead of a healthful food with a higher GI. This obviously makes no sense. You will find more information about the glycemic index in chapter thirteen. Unless you are a diabetic, you should not need to concern yourself with GI ratings. Most of the meals recommended in this book will supply a balanced release of energy.

How Much Food Do We Need?

Giving your body the nutrition it needs—when it needs it—helps your system to normalize and lets you take control of your appetite. Binges will be rare, because your body will feel satisfied most of the time. We will deal with your emotional satisfaction later. If you eat foods with minimal nutritional value, you are literally starving your body. It needs nutrition, not just food. If it gets the nutrition it needs from a small amount of food, you will feel satisfied. Until your body gets the nutrition it needs, it will continually ask for more food. You could eat worthless food all day long and never feel satisfied. Meanwhile, your body will keep asking for more. Never mistake "food" for nutrition.

Would you believe me if I told you it is possible to lose fat and stay lean by eating more food than the amount necessary for getting or staying fat? Probably not. But let's take a closer look at this concept. If a person with excess fat eats a large amount of alkaline-forming foods, those foods will stimulate the burning of stored body fat. The quantity of food and nutritional value would be substantial but the calorie content low. As you know, the fat being burned would supplement the caloric needs of the body. After the person loses the excess body fat, more acid-forming foods could be eaten to supply those calories and a healthy body weight could easily be maintained even though the person continued to eat a large quantity of food. On the other hand, a person eating a relatively small amount of acid-forming foods would get fat. The calorie content would be high but the quantity of food and amount of nutritional value small. Even less food would maintain this excess fat. Therefore, the quantity of food needed to get and stay lean could be much greater than the amount for getting or staying fat.

The story of a former nutritional client comes to mind. She was counseled on a Saturday evening, and thought I was crazy when I told her she could eat as much as she wanted and eat ten times a day if she wished. All she had to do was eat whole, natural foods at the right time of day and in good combinations. She purposely tried to overeat in an attempt to prove me wrong, but when we spoke the following Thursday she had already lost four pounds. She was now a believer and continued to lose rapidly until her body weight normalized. It is difficult to overeat with whole, natural foods if they are eaten in good combinations and at the appropriate times.

In chapter fifteen you will learn some basic guidelines on how to exercise to gain muscle and shape your body. When the *proper* exercise program is completed, the appetite of a thin person is stimulated so more food is eaten to supply the increased need. On the other hand, the appetite of a fat person is decreased, because the body burns more stored fat to supply the additional energy needs. Proper exercise has a normalizing effect on the metabolism. When you give your body nutritious foods, it will tell you when it needs more and when it has had enough. Abnormal cravings and excesses should gradually be eliminated as your metabolism and internal systems become more balanced. You could end up eating much more food than you have been but burn body fat at a rapid rate. A combination of fruits, vegetables, legumes and some meat could weigh three pounds but contain only 600 calories. You could eat six to eight pounds of these foods a day and still lose body fat fast.

The metabolism of glucose, fatty acids, triglycerides, and amino acids is controlled by cellular enzymes, coenzymes (mostly B vitamins), cofactors (mostly trace minerals) and hormones. This is why it is so important to eat whole, natural foods containing these nutrients or their building blocks.

How much you eat depends on your activities and your body's needs and efficiency. As your body becomes more balanced, your metabolism and appetite should normalize. Then all you have to do is eat something nutritious when you are hungry and do not eat if you are not hungry. That is the simplicity of Nature's health plan. It is important to eat when you are hungry, but it is always better to undereat instead of overeat. Think about the 100-year-old mouse. Eating less creates fewer free radicals, keeps you cleaner inside, and helps reduce aches and pains, illnesses, allergies and many other problems. Because digestion uses a considerable amount of energy, eating less also gives you more energy to feel good and enjoy life.

Now that you understand the purpose of various foods and how to get the most from them, you should be getting an idea of what to eat at different times. In chapter seven I provide numerous sample meals to further help you determine what to eat and when to eat it.

six

For Your Body Only

"**O**ne man's meat is another man's poison." That saying can have many meanings. Nutritionally it can be taken literally, because our digestive capabilities, activity levels, unique needs and personal tastes are as varied as our outward appearances. This is why the information in this chapter is crucial to your success. Most nutritional plans assume that if we all eat the same, we will all get the same results. Chances are, you have already figured out the error of this way of thinking.

You inhabit a one-of-a-kind body that responds to various foods differently than anyone else's body does. This is why it is imperative to determine the unique dietary program your body needs to maintain balance once you achieve it. As you have learned, you must first eat in an unbalanced way to reestablish the balance you have lost. Because stimulating fat burning is the same for all of us, your initial program may be similar to what it should be for other people. It will vary primarily because of personal tastes in fruits, vegetables and legumes and in the quantity of food.

A few dietary programs address individual differences and how to develop custom eating plans to help people achieve and then maintain normal body weight and optimal health. I will give you my guidelines for developing the best nutritional program for you, but first I want to familiarize you with the works of Dr. William Kelley and Dr. Elliot Abravanel. The purpose of explaining their programs is to teach you about metabolic profiles, oxidation rates and body types, which I will be referring to later. I also want you to understand the drawbacks and complications of their programs, if you should ever hear about them. Other programs are discussed in chapter thirteen.

Dr. Kelley's Program

Dr. William D. Kelley, a dentist from Texas, developed a program of various metabolic profiles based on the belief that the autonomic nervous system is the main thing that determines our biochemical individuality. He believed that people are controlled primarily by either their sympathetic or parasympathetic nervous systems. Using a complex method involving blood and urine tests, and 3,200 questions about health and lifestyle, he developed twelve profiles with various physical and metabolic differences among them. The most common one, where both nervous systems play an equal role, he labeled type eight. Dr. Kelley considered this a balanced metabolism and it was found in most reasonably healthy people.

His idea was to determine a person's metabolic profile and then specify a diet based on those findings. As people followed the program, their metabolisms usually changed, and their diets were gradually modified until most achieved the balanced state where neither the sympathetic nor parasympathetic nervous system was dominant. Some people never attained balance, but stayed relatively healthy by eating as recommended for their particular profile.

Dr. Kelley found that the problems of some of his patients worsened when they followed his dietary guidelines. His assistant, William L. Wolcott, eventually discovered that people's oxidation rates also had a significant influence on their health. Oxidation is the process through which your body turns the foods you eat into energy. Mr. Wolcott determined that people are fast, slow or mixed oxidizers. He noted that a sympathetic dominant person was normally a slow oxidizer and a parasympathetic dominant person a fast oxidizer. Later he learned that sympathetic dominant people could be fast oxidizers and that parasympathetic dominant people could be slow oxidizers.

Normally, a slow oxidizer or a parasympathetic dominant person experiences hypoactivity, depression and alkalinity. Fast oxidizers and sympathetic dominant people experience hyperactivity, anxiety and tend to be acidic. Generally, the autonomic type and the oxidation rate are in balance, so they work in a complementary manner.

Besides recommending different foods, Dr. Kelley's program uses specific nutritional supplementation. Certain supplements are used to move a sympathetic dominant person closer to balance or to increase someone's oxidation rate. Different supplements are used to move someone of parasympathetic dominance closer to balance and a fast oxidizer back to normal. These supplements are used until the body achieves balance and then a well-rounded supplementation program is used.

The goal of Dr. Kelley's program is to achieve balance by restoring a person's digestive function to normal so the foods being eaten can be processed efficiently. This is a primary goal I stress throughout this book. Health is balance and a large part of our health comes from the internal chemical environment created to a large extent by what we eat. Keep in mind that nerve flow to various glands and organs, nervous system balance, exercise, when you eat, your thoughts and other variables can all have a tremendous impact on your internal chemistry and what your body gets and utilizes from the foods you eat.

I believe Dr. Kelley's program restored many people to balance because they had been balanced before but had created imbalance by following poor dietary habits. He believes in cleansing the body, but his program is quite complex because it has numerous categories and deals with a large number of variables. His recommended dietary programs also include many foods I advise people never to eat.

Dr. Abravanel's Program

Elliot D. Abravanel, M.D., developed a method to determine how different people should eat to lose excess fat and stay lean. He believes that people are controlled primarily by one particular gland in their bodies. Men are considered to be predominantly pituitary, adrenal or thyroid types, and women to be any one of the preceding three or a fourth he calls gonadal. The body type is based on how food is metabolized by someone's body.

A person's body type is determined by the answers to thirty-three questions about specific physical and emotional characteristics. Dr. Abravanel believes that you will lose weight and be healthier if you eat a certain way based on your body type. Typically, people crave foods that have a stimulating effect on the dominant gland of their particular body type. Dairy foods stimulate the pituitary gland; starches stimulate the thyroid gland; meat, butter, eggs and salt stimulate the adrenal glands; and spices, fats and oils stimulate the gonads. Frequently eating the foods that stimulate your dominant gland in an attempt to get the lift this creates will eventually weaken the gland. The foods have similar effects to those of stimulating drugs.

Restricting your intake of stimulating foods gives your metabolism a chance to normalize and eliminate the cravings. This places you on a program that supplies your body's nutritional needs in a balanced way instead of constantly stimulating it. Once again, the goal is to restore balance.

Out of curiosity I answered Dr. Abravanel's questions and came up with an equal number of answers for two of the types and some answers that matched the third. Perhaps this means I am fairly balanced, but based on his questionnaire, I do not know which type I would be considered or how to eat based on his program. It was impossible for me to answer some of his questions because I do not eat any of the foods he gave as choices. Dr. Abravanel's program is relatively simple, but his sample meals are poor food combinations. They also include drinking coffee or tea and consist of numerous foods I consider unhealthful.

I do not totally disagree with Dr. Kelley and Dr. Abravanel. In fact, I applaud them for the ability to see that it is ridiculous to think that a generic nutritional program will work for everyone. Both of them focus on determining the right foods for you and restoring balance. Unfortunately, they recommend foods that are unhealthful and leave out many key pieces of the puzzle, including the most important—determining and eliminating the primary reason why you have excess body fat. Sometimes it is simply about eating the wrong foods, but usually physical and emotional imbalances must be eliminated or a nutritional program will fail. The bottom line is simply this: *the best nutritional plan for you will not work if you have certain physical problems or if you do not follow it.*

My *Victory Over Fat* Program

Now that we have explored the programs of Drs. Kelley and Abravanel, I will explain my method to determine your unique nutritional needs. It is simple and costs nothing (beyond the price of this book). My method is extremely effective because it is based on Nature's laws and because it gives control to the person who is ultimately responsible—YOU. You do not become dependent on a doctor, consultant or group, but learn how to develop and improve your own program. This independence and control over how your body looks and feels creates a sense of accomplishment, increases your confidence and improves your self-image. You will discover that you have tremendous power to control how your body looks and feels. All you have to do is assume the responsibility and apply the knowledge found in this book.

A large number of variables affect how your body reacts to foods. We all have different strengths and amounts of digestive enzymes, unique nerve and blood flow to our glands and organs, varied activity levels and distinctive body temperatures and metabolisms. We also have different amounts of body fat and internal waste, unique normal strengths and weaknesses in bodily functions, distinct body types, individual thoughts and we live in different environments. Are you starting to understand why it is vital to determine the right foods for you and you alone?

An easy way to get to the truth is simply by experimenting and observing the results. This experimentation is by no means random but is based on an educated guess of what foods will make you feel your best. Start by following the nutritional guidelines in this book. If you do not get great results, simply vary your program one way and then another to determine what changes are necessary to help *you* to be lean and healthy. In other words, if you are eating a low amount of fat, try eating more fat and fewer carbohydrates. If you are eating quite a bit of meat, reduce the amount. Replacing sugar, salt, dairy products and processed grains with legumes, vegetables and fruits is all you may need to do. You will learn more about how to develop your program later. Chances are, you already know many of the best foods for you—you just have unique reasons why you do not eat them. You will also learn how to discover and eliminate those reasons.

To determine your ideal nutritional program as fast as possible, the following steps should be completed.

Cleanse Your Body

Cleansing your body of mucus deposits and other internal wastes helps restore balance and efficiency quickly. Remember that restoring normal function to your digestive and other systems is a primary goal. Cleansing your body has many positive effects. It eliminates the mucus and wastes that rob your internal systems of energy and efficiency. Removing internal wastes that disease-causing germs are attracted to should also greatly reduce your chances of contracting many illnesses. If your internal environment is clean, nothing is available to attract these scavengers. I believe that many germs are similar to roaches that are attracted to, and live on the waste in unclean kitchens.

During the final stages of sewage treatment, water that has had most of the waste filtered out is trickled over thousands of stones contained in large tanks. Bacteria live on these stones and as the water runs over them, the bacteria eat the remaining microscopic particles of waste. This is how Nature purifies the water in many streams and rivers.

If the internal environment of your body is polluted, germs can go in and have a field day. I believe your body eliminates the internal waste in an attempt to get rid of the invading germs. You already know that I believe a cold is simply Nature's way of eliminating excess internal wastes. This is why a cold is self-limiting (stops by itself) and lasts about a week in most people, if they do not inhibit the cleansing process. A cold is a self-preservation mechanism your body uses to prevent worse problems. If internal waste continued to accumulate, your body would be more susceptible to serious health problems. To prevent this, one of the many different cold viruses will go into your body and start the cleansing necessary to reduce the toxins to a healthier level. Remember that your body was designed to be self-healing and that cleansing is an important part of healing.

Let's compare your body to a dam on a river. If the water is kept at a safe level (your body is free of excess waste), all will be well. If the water rises to an unsafe level (excessive amounts of internal waste accumulate), spillways are opened to drain off the excess water (a cold occurs to eliminate excess waste). This prevents the dam from overflowing or breaking (keeps your body from being damaged or destroyed).

Your body is not completely clean inside after a cold. A cold is merely a safety mechanism to prevent more serious illness. It cleans out only enough waste to get you back on your feet again. Essentially, the water is not far below the top of the dam. If your diet causes waste to build up quickly, you could get another cold within a few months. Frequent colds are one way your body uses to tell you that you are eating foods that are not right for you. To regain more of your lost energy and improve internal efficiency, you must do a thorough cleanse and then avoid the foods that are causing mucus, waste and fat to accumulate. Most of the waste being eliminated comes from unhealthful foods you ate in the past. This waste is not doing you any good and you will be happy to hear that most of it is coming from fat cells.

Think about how perfect Nature's cleansing system is. Your thirst is stimulated to get extra liquid to clean with and your appetite is reduced so there is less input and less energy used for digestion. This energy can then be used for output. The organs of elimination—skin, kidneys, lungs and bowels—work overtime to get rid of the waste. Because these organs get more blood flow and energy, your brain and muscles get less. This is why you usually feel weak and tired and should rest as much as possible. Think about what animals do when they are sick or injured. They stop eating, drink more water and rest. They do this instinctively so their bodies can cleanse and heal. Nature knows that many diseases are caused by excess waste (or fat). If you did not get a cold to cleanse out excess garbage, as more waste accumulated, you would be susceptible to influenza (the flu) or even more serious illnesses. For example, if the additional waste gets stored in the lungs, you may develop pneumonia to cleanse the lungs. Preventing a cold with drugs, high amounts of vitamin C or other means just sets you up for worse problems down the road. Colds are common, because people commonly eat improperly, and the cold has not been conquered, because it is a natural cleansing function. If researchers ever do find a "cure" for the common cold, it will be disastrous for the health of anyone who uses it.

When a cold starts, instead of attempting to prevent it, give your body some assistance. By speeding up the cleansing, you can recover in just a few days instead of a week. This generally makes the symptoms worse, but reduces the toxins to a healthier level much faster. It is like opening two spillways on the dam instead of one. You can speed things up by resting as much as possible and drinking large quantities of water. You've heard this before and it is helpful.

Another thing you can do is stop eating heavy foods like starchy vegetables, grains, and complete proteins. Do not believe anyone who tells you that you need to eat to keep up your strength. If you stop putting these foods in, your body will have more energy to clean out the excesses already there. Drinking vegetable juices or fruit juices (diluted 50 percent with water) or eating fruit will supply energy for cleansing but require hardly any for digestion. This will give your digestive system a well-deserved rest and your sluggish organs a chance to rejuvenate. The digestive energy saved may also be used to heal wounds or resolve other unhealthy conditions. We would normally stop eating when we are sick but have been conditioned to think and act contrary to our instincts. This leads to confusion and frustration. We need to observe and learn from Nature. As you cleanse, you should find yourself getting more in touch with your natural instincts and more aware of your body's needs.

Another way to cleanse out toxins faster is by sweating in a sauna or steam bath. If you do not have access to one of these, put a teaspoon of powdered gingerroot herb or one-quarter teaspoon of cayenne pepper in a hot bath. This will make you sweat profusely and flush out toxins fast. Do not use a steam or sauna for more than 15 minutes at a time and drink plenty of water before and after. You can stay in the hot bath for 20 to 30 minutes if you desire. Do not use exercise to cause sweating, because this uses energy your body needs for the cleansing process. After your body has reduced the internal waste to a healthier level, the cleansing will stop. You will learn later how to do deeper cleansing to get your body's toxin levels much lower.

The next step is to prevent internal waste from accumulating by eating the natural, clean-burning foods you have determined are best for you. At this point, you have in essence found the elusive "cure" for the common cold. After that, if your nose runs or is plugged up in the morning, take a look at your diet for the previous day or two. When your body is clean inside, it will react quickly to eliminate the waste products of foods you should not be eating. These reactions will help you fine-tune your program and discover foods your body does not want. Remember that dairy and processed grain products are the worst offenders.

When someone's body is cleansing out nicotine or other drug residue, various side effects, or withdrawal symptoms, will occur as the toxins travel through the bloodstream on the way to being eliminated. (I believe that this is what causes LSD flashbacks.) A craving for the drug will also be stimulated, and if more of the drug is ingested, the residue will be forced back into storage. This will stop the cleansing process and the unpleasant side effects. The more drug residue that is stored in the tissues, the sooner the body starts the cleansing process. This is why people usually use the drug more frequently as their bodies get saturated with the drug. They have to use it to stop the cleansing and avoid the uncomfortable side effects.

Withdrawal from eating unhealthful foods is similar to drug withdrawal, so be aware that as your body is cleansing, you will most likely crave foods you know are not good for you. You must resist these abnormal cravings long enough for the residue to be eliminated. After that, your *physical* cravings will stop. If you crave chocolate, fatty meats, sugar, salty and greasy potato chips, or other unhealthful foods, clearly your body is not telling you that it needs them. Your cravings are usually for unhealthful foods you have eaten in the past. The waste residue of these foods traveling through your bloodstream on the way to being eliminated is what stimulates the cravings.

Sometimes cravings for unhealthful foods are your body's attempt to get a nutrient it needs. This should alert you to the presence of some kind of imbalance. Your diet may lack the variety it needs, your supplements may be incomplete or poorly absorbed or your body may have a gland or organ that is functioning abnormally. These abnormal cravings are usually for excessively sweet, salty, fatty or sour foods. Seek out the healthful foods that will supply the nutrients your body needs. If you crave a greasy hamburger or donut from a fast-food restaurant, you most likely need more good oil in your diet. This is a common problem because low-fat diet programs often make people afraid to eat *any* fat. Your body needs a certain amount of the right kinds of fat every day.

Another common craving is for sugar. This is usually caused by overconsumption of processed foods loaded with this concentrated substance. A sugar craving usually indicates a deficiency of the mineral chromium. I have seen many people lose the physical craving for sugar within a week of starting to take a chromium supplement.

Salt craving is another common problem, especially before the body is thoroughly cleansed. It is usually not a problem afterward. If you cleanse your body, but find yourself still craving salt, increase your intake of kelp or saltwater fish for a while. This will usually resolve it. If not, eating a little unprocessed sea salt may help. Extra salt will compensate if you have a nerve or blood flow imbalance causing your body to excrete excess sodium, but it is best to restore your body to normal function with correct treatment. The best solution to any problem is to find and eliminate the cause, not just treat the symptoms.

Cleansing your body helps you to get more in touch with its needs. In other words, after you have cleansed your body and are eating a relatively balanced diet, if your body needs more of a particular nutrient, you will crave a food containing it. This is why some women have unusual food cravings when they are pregnant. Their bodies are asking for the nutrients needed by the growing fetus. Your cravings should be for natural, healthful foods. If you are eating a vegetarian diet but crave a lean steak once or twice a month, chances are that you need the iron, vitamin B12 or other nutrients it contains. Listen to your body and give it what it needs. If you crave steak five or six times a week, either an internal imbalance exists or your body is attempting to treat a problem that needs to be discovered and resolved.

It is easy to know the difference between a good, wholesome, natural and instinctive craving based on your body's needs and a craving for food you know is detrimental to your health and weight. Resist your unhealthy cravings and they will soon be gone, and use your healthy cravings to learn more about your body's needs. You will learn more benefits of cleansing your system and various ways to do it in an upcoming chapter. You will also be taught ways to eliminate your emotional cravings.

After thoroughly cleansing, you should rarely get sick if you keep yourself clean. I have read about numerous people who kept their bodies clean inside and did not have a cold or other illness for scores of years. Because I cleansed my body thoroughly and have kept it clean, I have not had a cold for almost thirty years. Almost eleven years of that time was spent in a house with children and in a climate where the winters are cold and snowy. I have also been exposed to patients with colds thousands of times. During all those years, I used herbs on two occasions to induce deep lung cleanses. These were done in an attempt to cleanse out a toxin I was exposed to on a job many years ago. During both of these cleanses, I coughed frequently and felt quite badly for five or six days.

I have also experienced four or five mini-cleanses, when I started eating a new food my body does not digest and utilize well. During these, I felt fine, but had a runny nose for a few days. Now I avoid those foods to keep my body clean.

You may be wondering about the old "I got wet or chilled and caught a cold" syndrome. Getting cold and wet constricts your tissues and often causes shivering. Either of these can start a cleansing process early by shrinking the waste storage space or by shaking the waste loose. You would have "caught the cold" before long anyway. I have often been cold and wet in the past thirty years and not one cold was triggered. I have read about people in their sixties, seventies and even eighties swimming in the ocean off New York during the winter. They are members of the Polar Bear Club and rarely, if ever, catch colds from doing this.

Most people know that viruses cause colds and the majority of these people have been conditioned to believe that they should take a drug or use some other method to attempt to prevent one. Colds are caused by the viruses that Nature created to stimulate the cleansing reaction. More than one hundred different rhinoviruses have been identified. Why? Because Nature does not want our bodies to develop immunity and block the cleansing that is so vital to survival. Also, man-made drugs are almost useless against viruses. Nature did not use bacteria to cause colds, because they can be killed easily. This would make it easy to block the cleansing reaction and Nature does not want that to happen. For the same reason, no two influenza viruses are the same, because we need these viruses to protect us from polluting ourselves to the point where our bodies would actually drown in their own internal waste.

You have been told you will get a cold if your immune system is weak and you will not get one if it is strong. I disagree with this idea. Think about it. We are exposed to different cold and flu viruses every day. Why wouldn't people with weak immune systems have one cold after another or get the flu every few weeks? They are constantly being exposed to a different virus and the last cold or flu has supposedly weakened their immune systems even more. They are not always sick, because the cold or flu has reduced the amount of internal waste to a healthier level. This decreases (as Nature intended) the chance of getting another cold. These people will not get another one until the waste builds up again to an unhealthy level. If they block the cold they will increase their chances of getting the flu. If they keep the amount of waste at or below a healthy level, they should not get a cold or the flu.

I have not had the flu or a cold for almost thirty years and I do not feel like my immune system is particularly strong. My immune system has been stressed many times by overwork, fifteen years of chronic and severe lower back pain, other joint problems, loss of jobs, loss of loved ones, back and knee surgeries, financial stress, hypoglycemia, the extreme mental demands of becoming a doctor, emotional stress and numerous other influences that are believed to weaken it. And for more than ten years of that time I lived in an environment where it gets cold and snowy in the winter and, as I said before, I was wet and cold on numerous occasions—especially while riding my motorcycle for fifteen years during the fall and winter. Why then have I not been sick? Because I keep my internal waste level far below the point where a virus would enter my body and trigger the cleansing process.

The flu is worse than a cold, because more internal waste needs to be eliminated. Remember that if you block a cold, the waste will continue to accumulate and then the flu or something worse will eventually get you. If you prevent the "little brother" cold germ from doing his job, he will tell his "big brother" flu germ to go after you. Because more waste needs to be eliminated, the flu has worse symptoms and generally lasts longer than a cold. They both stop on their own (as Nature intends) when their jobs are done.

Because the body has more waste coming out during the flu, a fever will often be created. This happens when waste is removed from the cells faster than the body can deal with it. If the elimination system cannot keep up, internal heat is generated, causing the fever. Fevers are less common and not as severe with colds, because fewer toxins are being expelled and the elimination system can usually keep up. Children may have a fever during a cold, because their elimination systems can be overloaded more easily. I have read of children whose fevers were gone within a few minutes after being given an enema to help get things moving. Adults with poorly functioning elimination systems may also experience fevers during a cold.

The timing of when people get colds varies based on certain differences like body fat percentage, speed of metabolism, physical activities, efficiency of digestive and elimination systems and fitness level. If someone's body is able to cleanse out waste almost as fast as it builds up, then that person will not get colds very often. Most of the variables that influence body efficiency can be improved and are important, but the biggest key (one that anyone can do) is to simply not eat foods that create much waste. If it is not put in, it does not have to be cleansed out. A strong immune system is not the key to preventing colds or the flu. The immune system stimulates the cleansing process but the real secret is to prevent the need for cleansing by keeping internal waste levels low.

Many wild animals are forced to fast periodically simply because they cannot always get food when they want it. This is Nature's way of keeping them lean and healthy. Fasting or eating light one day a week is a great way to help keep your body clean and lean. For example, if you often go out to dinner on Saturday night, eating a small breakfast and then only fruit until having a light to moderate dinner is an excellent way to eat on Sunday. Doing this will eliminate fat and waste build-up from a dinner that may have been excessive and eaten late. It will also give your digestive system a rest and you or a loved one a break from food preparation and cleanup. Eating this way on Sunday is a healthy habit even if you eat more healthfully on Saturday.

Internal cleansing is also a good first step for someone who is underweight, because the underweight condition may be due to digestive inefficiency caused by excessive internal waste. After cleansing itself, the body will be better able to use the foods that are eaten and body weight may increase to normal. Force-feeding an underweight person usually makes matters worse by generating more internal pollution. Many underweight people resist cleansing, because they are afraid of losing more weight. This should not be a concern, because healthy tissue should not be lost during a proper cleanse.

If an underweight person follows a good cleansing program but does not experience any cleansing reactions, the underweight condition is due to either a lack of proper exercise to stimulate muscular growth or an internal imbalance that must be discovered and corrected. Overactive thyroid function would be a possible suspect. Some people are naturally ectomorphic (slender, fragile body type) and being thin is normal for them. Keep in mind that most fat people are underweight in the lean muscle mass vital for good health and maintaining a normal metabolism.

I have been a fitness trainer and nutrition consultant to many underweight people. Prior to our meeting, most of them were extremely afraid to eat any fats and spent most of their time doing inefficient exercises in an attempt to keep their waistlines trim. None of them knew how to train to stimulate muscular weight gain. They also did not know that, because of their fast metabolisms, they needed more good fats to supply the extra calories necessary for their workouts and for their muscles to grow. The last thing they needed to worry about was getting fat. Some might add a few pounds of body fat if they ate excess fats and did not exercise correctly, but any fat gained would be simple to lose. Chapter fifteen has guidelines about how to exercise and eat to build a strong shapely body.

Eat a Clean, Balanced Diet

The second step in my program is to eat a well-rounded diet of clean-burning whole foods. This will supply most, if not all, of the nutrients we all need. If your unique body does best on carbohydrates, it will be getting some carbohydrates. If your body does better on proteins or fats, you will also be getting some of each of these. You will not be getting an excess of anything. Therefore, no matter what your metabolic profile, dominant gland, oxidation rate or other variable, you will be getting a fair amount of everything you need. You will soon learn how to make any necessary modifications.

Eating an excess of certain foods and poor combinations of processed and unbalanced foods are the primary causes of most people's imbalances and distorted needs. Cleansing your body should move you closer to being able to do well on a balanced nutritional program. Then by following a balanced diet of natural, whole foods, your body should be able to stay lean and healthy. If Dr. Kelley's belief that most Americans are a balanced type is correct, the odds are good that a balanced diet will be right for you. If your body has moved away from balance, you will need to make a few modifications to develop your ideal diet. After your body function is closer to normal, you can then eat in a more balanced way. Eating right for you should restore or maintain balance and produce natural energy. You should not need to stimulate a particular gland by eating an excess of the foods Dr. Abravanel believes causes imbalance.

If you have excess fat, remember that you initially will have to eat in an unbalanced way to lose it and reestablish lost balance. You should eat more of the alkaline foods that stimulate the burning of stored fat. Eat mostly the alkaline-forming fruits, vegetables and legumes along with a meat entrée for dinner. Use fish and fowl mostly. Eat red meat no more than once a week. Reduce your consumption of grain products as much as possible. Any grains you occasionally eat at this time should be whole grains. I mean the *whole* grain, not bread, pasta or cookies labeled "whole grain."

Eating a well-balanced diet and taking a good multivitamin and mineral supplement should be right for most people to maintain a healthy body weight. By now you should have a fairly good idea of what a well-balanced diet is. If you are still losing excess fat, keep doing some cleansing every few weeks. You will stop having cleansing reactions after your body is fairly clean inside. Then, by eating clean-burning foods and doing one or two thorough, three to five day cleanses each year, you should maintain your internal cleanliness.

Initially, during the two or three week intervals between cleansing programs, start making minor changes to your nutritional program. If you are underweight, do not attempt to gain by eating butter, fatty meats or weight-gaining supplements. Instead, eat more foods containing good fats, such as avocados, eggs, seeds and nuts. Also use more olive and coconut oil and occasionally some sesame, grapeseed or sunflower seed oil. These healthful fats supply your body more calories without overloading your digestive system. Eat the additional fats before two or three o'clock in the afternoon and remember that this should be done only if you are stimulating the need for muscular weight gain. No benefits come from gaining excess body fat. If you do start gaining body fat, reduce your fat consumption until you find the right amount to help you gain muscle mass only.

If you are eating properly you should not have to worry about overeating. You will find that the more naturally you eat, the less you will eat, naturally. This is because your body will be getting the nutrition it needs, so it will stop asking for more food. You will feel satisfied and it will be difficult to overeat. If your goal is fat loss and you are not losing any excess, eat more fruits, vegetables and legumes, and fewer grain products. Also reduce the amount of meat you eat at dinner. You may do best eating more fruit and fewer vegetables, or eating more vegetables and less fruit may be better for you. Make sure you are eating a minimal amount of salt, because it is extremely detrimental to any fat-loss program. Reread the salt section in chapter four if you cannot remember why. You should get plenty of sodium from the natural foods you are eating. If these changes fail to speed up your fat loss, it may be because you are a fast oxidizer, even though your body has excess fat. Eating more meat and healthful fats may be the key to helping you lose body fat. Do not judge the type of metabolism or digestive capabilities you have simply by something you have read or by looking at your body type. Your metabolism and body type may have become distorted.

Everyone is born of two parents. The parents inherited different digestive capabilities that they have passed on to their children. Genetics is a major cause of the wide variety of metabolic capabilities among people. Your body may put out far more or far less stomach acid than average. Your pancreas may produce strong digestive enzymes or weak ones. This may be an inherited characteristic, it may be caused by spinal nerve interference, or your sympathetic and parasympathetic nervous systems could be out of balance. Inherited function, spinal nerve flow and blood flow are three of the six primary components that determine your unique digestive capabilities.

Your thoughts (the fourth component) also have substantial influence on your health and metabolic capability. As I explained in chapter five, besides the link from your brain to most parts of your body through the spinal nerves, another connection exists between the brain and many areas through the vagus nerves. You have learned that this connection and chemical ligand messengers are how your thinking can affect the function of your stomach, pancreas, liver and many other glands and organs. Your thinking can create improved health or cause disease. Mental, emotional and certain physical stresses can have tremendous negative impact on your health. Stress can be caused by your thinking, from other imbalances, or from a combination of one or more. You will learn more about stress later.

Stress can irritate an ulcer by stimulating excess production of stomach acid. As you have just learned, a nervous system imbalance or excess nerve stimulation can do the same. Impaired nerve flow to a section of the stomach lining could inhibit secretion of the mucus needed to protect the stomach from its own digestive juices. This is the most likely cause of ulcers and explains why they stay a certain size. Some doctors believe that the bacteria *Helicobacter pylori* cause ulcers but I think the bacteria just live there once the ulcer forms. If bacteria were the cause of ulcers, they would grow larger in diameter and could be easily cured with antibiotics. But they do not get larger and they are not always easily cured, so the bacteria idea does not make sense. Also, billions of people are infected with the bacteria but only 12 to 25 percent of them will get an ulcerative disease. I believe it will be the people with impaired nerve flow to the stomach lining.

Diminished function of your internal systems can result from insufficient nutrients or excess fat and internal waste. These are the fifth and sixth primary components affecting your digestive capabilities. (Excess fat and internal wastes are not usually seen separately so I grouped them as one component.) The timing of when you drink water could also be included, because of its significant influence on proper digestion. Correct exercise is another we could add. The good news is that all of these components except your genetic inheritance can be improved to varying degrees. The digestive capabilities normal for your body may possibly be improved with exercise, and some weaknesses can be compensated for with supplemental digestive enzymes. If all else fails, you may just have to avoid the foods your body has difficulty digesting.

Take a look at your heredity and think about what your ancestors have eaten for thousands of years. For example, if you are of East Indian descent, your ancestors did not eat much meat. Therefore, you may do best as a vegetarian or by eating meat only occasionally. You may have inherited a poor capability for digesting and using it. If you eat an excessive amount of meat, you could easily get fat and develop internal imbalances and metabolic problems. Someone of Japanese descent will do much better eating fish, brown rice and vegetables for dinner than eating spaghetti, meatballs and garlic bread with butter. Of course, the spaghetti, garlic bread and butter are not good for anyone. If your ancestors were big meat eaters and you start eating a vegetarian diet, chances are that you will become sickly and weak and develop internal problems. This will happen because your body lacks the digestive capabilities necessary to break down and use some of the vegetarian foods that you need to be healthy. You may do best eating a "meat and potatoes" diet. The key is to determine and eat the foods that your body digests and utilizes the best.

Your goal should be to get in touch with your body's inner knowledge or instincts. As you start to eat in harmony with Nature, you should become more aware of your instincts and develop an inner "knowing" of what is right or wrong for your body. You will trust your instincts more and more as you experiment with various foods and determine the best ones for you. The cleaner your body becomes internally and the more balanced and efficient your system gets, the easier it will be to know what to eat, when to eat it, and how much to eat.

Getting in touch with your inner self will improve the emotional, physical, mental and spiritual aspects of your life. You will be more in tune with the truth of who you really are and able to enjoy life more fully knowing you are being who you should be and doing what you should do. There is a good possibility that you will experience an inner satisfaction and peaceful feeling from this. Remember that you have emotional, spiritual, mental and physical aspects and that each one affects the others. Just as your thinking affects the function of your body, so does the function of your body influence your thinking. Internal cleansing in particular has a noticeable effect on improving your thinking. You will learn more about improving your thinking in chapter fourteen.

Our bodies are able to digest and use most whole, natural foods. It does not make sense that our bodies would have the capability of breaking down and digesting meats if we were not intended to eat some meat. We are also capable of using fruits, vegetables, legumes and grains. Dairy products are the main foods most of us are unable to use well. A few races have used milk for hundreds or even thousands of years and their children are capable of using milk products fairly well. But the milk of today is nothing like what these people's ancestors used. It is low fat, no fat, homogenized, pasteurized, and completely distorted and unbalanced. Also, most of them used milk that was similar to human milk. They did not use cow's milk. You have already been given many reasons why you should avoid all dairy products.

In the beginning of your search, it will be extremely helpful to keep a diary of the dietary changes you are making. As you experiment with different foods, write down what you eat and how you feel after each meal. Try each food alone and in good combinations with other foods. If you have not learned what good combinations are, refer back to the section on food combining in chapter five. Find new foods you like and that make you feel good. Also record your weight, measurements and body fat percentage. Observe if you are gaining muscle, losing fat, or both. You will soon start to see patterns. If you get tired and irritated or energetic and emotionally uplifted every time you eat a certain food, you will see it recorded in your diary. You will learn how different foods affect you. You can then stop eating the foods that make you feel poorly and gain fat, and eat more of those that make you feel good and stimulate fat loss.

As you determine your right and wrong foods, make sure not to overdo it with any of them, especially concentrated acid-forming foods like grains and complete proteins. Eating excessive amounts of a food that makes you feel good and gives you abundant energy may not be healthful if it is acting like a stimulant. This causes stress, internal imbalance and fat gain. The right foods for you will give you long-lasting energy, make you feel good *and* help you stay lean or lose excess fat.

An excess of one food can overload your system and create a sensitivity or allergy to it. You would then experience unpleasant symptoms after eating it. You can be tested for allergies in various ways. The scratch test is commonly used. Others include applied kinesiology (AK), a type of muscle testing, and electroacupuncture. I recommend using these tests only to point you in the right direction. Avoid the suspect foods for a month or two and then eat each one by itself and observe your reaction. If you have always gotten hives from eating strawberries, you should not eat them unless the internal imbalance that triggers your reaction has been eliminated. Avoid all foods you know cause serious reactions. What I am talking about here are foods that make you tired, depressed or otherwise negatively impact your fat-loss program. After avoiding a food for a while, you may find that you can eat it occasionally with no negative effects. Cleansing your body of the residue of certain foods may be helpful for eliminating any unhealthy reactions to them. If you seem allergic to many foods, you either have a low output of hydrochloric acid or nerve or blood flow imbalances affecting the normal function of your digestive system. Low HCl production could be caused by a nerve or blood flow imbalance or it may be normal for you. Whatever the cause, it can be compensated for with an HCl supplement.

Keep searching for more foods that make you feel happy and healthy. Remember that eating a wide variety of foods will help ensure that your body gets the nutrients it needs to maintain good health and a normal amount of body fat. It will also keep your system from becoming unbalanced by being overloaded with a few foods. Greater variety will also make your meals more enjoyable. Look at your program occasionally to make sure that you have not fallen into an eating rut.

Thinking about a "diet" that was relatively successful for you in the past may help you determine some of the best foods for you. If a high-protein diet helped you lose body fat, it may be that you need a bit more protein or possibly more fat. Do not follow a high-protein diet; just use it as a guide to help learn your unique needs. If a vegetarian diet worked well for you, eating less meat may be best for you. If a low-fat diet did not work well, you may stay healthier and leaner by eating healthful fat, because your body is good at using fat for energy.

If a food is keeping you lean and physically healthy, it should also make you feel good emotionally. You should have less stress and feel better about yourself and your life. You should be energetic and want to do the creative things in your life you have been postponing because of a lack of energy and enthusiasm. Your mental attitude should be greatly improved, because your brain is getting the nutrients it needs to function normally.

Continue your food diary until you find the best nutritional program for you. As time goes by, experiment with new foods to see how they react in your body and how they make you feel. Get more in tune with your inner self as it guides you to find more of the whole, natural foods that are best for you.

The Ultimate Program

I know that most people will not have access to the following treatments but I want you to be aware of what they can do. If you have extreme problems or want the fastest possible results, you may want to get treatments from me before spending a fortune at some "famous" weight-loss center or having a radical surgical procedure to remove most of your stomach.

Precision Muscle Balancing Technology (PMBT), the unique musculoskeletal balancing technique I have developed, realigns joints and eliminates the aches and pains of tendinitis, bursitis, osteoarthritis and neuritis. Its success rate in treating headaches (muscle tension and migraines) and other musculoskeletal conditions is greater than 99 percent. By aligning the vertebrae of the spine, it can reestablish normal nerve flow between the brain and internal organs, glands, blood vessels, muscles and all other parts of the body. More than 90 percent of my patients with internal health conditions have recovered. High blood pressure has normalized and gastric reflux, chronic coughs, irritable bowel syndrome, insomnia, asthma, constipation, hypothyroidism, snoring and many other conditions have been resolved. I explain to my patients the reason why pressure on certain nerves can cause these problems. Gallbladders and colons have been saved from surgical removal, and women who had suffered miscarriages got pregnant and had babies after normal communication between the brain and uterus was restored. Keep in mind that PMBT eliminates the *cause* so the bones *stay* in alignment. This is the key to lasting results.

Patients who need it are also treated with Neurovascular Dynamics (NVD). Practitioners of this therapy (myself included) believe that an imbalance between the sympathetic and parasympathetic nervous systems can cause ill health and that the imbalance is usually created from a trauma. Because of this imbalance, normal blood distribution is disrupted and the body cannot function properly. Patients are first treated to reestablish balance between the two parts of the autonomic nervous system. Then all glands and organs are tested and those functioning abnormally are treated to restore normal function.

The two therapies just discussed can restore someone to balance much faster than any dietary methods. The person would then be able to eat a balanced diet right away. Even though an improved diet is always helpful, it cannot reestablish normal nerve flow. Over time, Dr. Kelley's program may be able to balance the nervous systems and improve blood flow, but someone could still have severe problems if normal nerve flow was not also reestablished. These imbalances explain why Dr. Kelley's program was unable to restore everyone to balance and why people eating the right foods for them may still have problems.

My experience during the last 29 years has shown that most forms of spinal manipulation are ineffective at restoring the permanent alignment necessary to restore normal nerve flow and internal function. Getting your spine forcefully adjusted usually makes matters worse. Periodic Directional Non-Force Technique chiropractic treatments are sometimes long-lasting and will not cause damage, but forceful manipulations are not recommended. You may be able to find an NVD practitioner to treat you and balance your nervous systems. This would be helpful if you have a nervous system imbalance, but is unnecessary for success.

The ultimate program would be to balance the body using PMBT and NVD treatments and then follow the preceding nutritional steps. Using applied kinesiology, I can test people for their needs for, or sensitivities to, various foods and nutritional supplements. This can also speed up the balancing process tremendously, but is not necessary for success.

If you do not have access to any of the therapies of the ultimate program, your progress will be slower and you may have to eat fewer acidic foods to maintain your fat loss. Do not be discouraged, because the chances are excellent that you will still be successful if you follow the guidelines in this book.

The spirit of melancholy would often take its flight from us if only we would
take up the song of praise.

Philip Bennett Power

Do not wait for extraordinary circumstances to do good actions;
try to use ordinary situations.

Richter

What lies behind us and what lies before us are tiny matters
compared to what lies within us.

William Morrow

The people who live long are those who long to live.

Anonymous

A man who does not think and plan long ahead
will find trouble right at his door.

Confucius

The man who stops learning is as good as dead.

Robert M. Hutchins

seven

Making the Change

A number of questions must be answered before you start your new nutritional program. These questions include how fast to make changes, whether to cleanse prior to or along with changing, how much to change, and how frequently to follow good nutritional guidelines, especially when dining out.

Naturally, everyone will answer these questions differently. You may want to jump right in with both feet or you may choose to change a little at a time. The way that best suits your personality is the right way for you. It doesn't matter how you do it; it matters only *that you do it*. To get and stay lean you must make some permanent changes in your thinking and behavior. It's simple. Just replace your poor eating habits and food choices with good ones. Then the power of habit will start working for you instead of against you. Let's explore some of these questions in detail and see what can be expected from different ways of changing.

How Fast to Make Changes

Deciding how fast to change depends on how soon you want to reap the benefits of healthier eating. Changing fast creates more rapid results but can cause some uncomfortable effects, because of the accelerated cleansing it stimulates. This is easy to deal with if you remind yourself that your body is eliminating the residues of unhealthful foods that have been polluting your body, making it fat and inefficient.

Gradually replacing the unbalanced foods you have been eating with nutritious foods is a slower but easier method of changing. This has worked for many people and may work best for you. You can make one change at a time over a period of a few weeks or a few months. Some of them may be a bit challenging for you but most will not be difficult. Your first change might be to replace your morning coffee with a piece of fruit and some water. Be prepared for the coffee withdrawal symptoms. Headaches are common, but should not be a problem for long. After a week, you could then replace your cold, processed, sugarcoated breakfast cereal that is drowned in milk and sugar with a nutritious and delicious vegetable omelet or a whole grain cereal dish I describe later in this chapter. Even if you make only one change a week, it will not be long before you are eating much more healthfully. You can also vary how fast you make changes.

As time goes by, your body will be able to cleanse itself and become more efficient. The nutritious foods will supply more energy for cleansing and your body will be able to gradually eliminate accumulated waste. Progress will be made, because you will be putting less waste in than your body can eliminate. It is like doing five or ten minutes of housecleaning every day when no new messes are being made. It will take some time to clean the entire house, but because less additional new dirt or dust is accumulating, you will make progress and eventually have a clean house.

Some of the other simple changes you can make are drinking water at the right times, taking a good multivitamin and mineral supplement, chewing foods more thoroughly, visualizing your new body and lifestyle, eating the right food at the right time, eating breakfast every day and eating dinner earlier. It will take time to develop some new meals but you may make substantial progress just by implementing the changes just mentioned.

You may notice in the beginning that some of the healthful, natural foods taste bland or completely tasteless. This is common and usually happens because the taste buds on your tongue have been desensitized from eating excess salt. Your taste buds may be so deadened that unless a taste is extremely strong, such as sugar, salt or some other spice, you cannot taste anything. Many people eat an entire meal and all they taste is the salt, sugar, ketchup (with sugar and salt), or other seasonings they put on it. They cannot taste the less potent flavors of the natural foods. Some people even need salt or sugar on fruits or they taste almost nothing. Do not judge your healthful meals too soon and then pledge never to eat a particular food again, because as you eat more healthfully, your taste buds will rejuvenate. After a few months, try some of the foods that you may not have liked in the beginning. Many of the initially bland-tasting foods will make your mouth water just thinking about them. Eliminating salt is the main key to rejuvenating your taste buds. Many fat people say they love food, but most of them never taste anything except salt, sugar or fat. Processed foods like crackers, pretzels and chips would be completely tasteless if the salt and fat were eliminated.

I do not recommend eating foods that you dislike, but some nutritious foods you have never eaten before may not initially strike your fancy. These are the ones you can easily learn to like and, with all the new choices available, you should find plenty. If you do not find many foods that you like, but you want to eat some foods you know are healthful for you, combine them with something you really like. For example, if you do not particularly like broccoli but you love corn, eat them together and soon you may like the broccoli by itself. If it does not happen, nothing is wrong with always combining them. Try mixing some mashed rutabaga or acorn squash with some mashed potatoes. You may find you like certain combinations better than potatoes alone or that you like a particular type of squash mashed, but not in bite-sized pieces. Adding a little olive oil or a bit of cinnamon to some mashed squash may be the trick to making it taste great to you. When I was a child, I disliked eating zucchini squash by itself but I loved it when my mother mixed it with some scrambled eggs. I still enjoy it with eggs but I also like it with other vegetables.

If you are eager to reap the benefits of a dramatically improved nutritional program, by all means go for it, but realize it may be tough in the beginning. It is far better to change gradually and be successful than to change fast, get discouraged and quit. If you have been eating relatively well based on what you have read so far, making the necessary changes may not be a big deal. It should be easy for you to eat a clean, balanced diet, because you will experience few cleansing reactions.

If you want to start immediately on the entire program, I recommend first completing a body-cleansing program. This gives your body the opportunity to do extensive cleansing in a short time. Besides getting rid of the waste and blockages that are over-stressing your digestive organs, it also gives them a rest, allowing them to get stronger and more efficient. After the cleanse, your taste buds will be rejuvenated so most of your new and healthful foods will taste good to you.

It is important to keep your body free of toxic waste. Many health problems are created, because germs are attracted to and live in toxic environments. They live on the waste. Internal waste also creates friction in your body. This is like operating your car's engine with thick and dirty oil. The parts are subjected to more stress so the engine uses more fuel, performs poorly, breaks down more often and wears out faster. The same thing can happen to your body. Clean the engine and change the oil regularly and you will feel the difference in your car's performance. Cleanse your body and then eat clean-burning foods to keep it clean and you will also feel the difference. After all, your body is simply a vehicle, just like your car.

Most people think the energy level they currently have is the best they can experience. They envy the energy of youth. They have forgotten that they once had the same abundance of energy and have not noticed the gradual decline or simply believe it is a part of "natural" aging. If it is natural, why are there people in their seventies, eighties and even nineties with abundant energy? Could it be that they exercise, keep their bodies clean inside and supply it with nutritious foods? Our bodies produce a certain amount of energy. The more we use carrying excess weight and overcoming internal friction the less we have available for work and play. Professor Arnold Ehret's formula is V=E - O, where V stands for vitality, E for energy and O for obstructions. Simply put: the more obstructions you have, the less vitality you will have.

Children have an abundance of energy because they are relatively clean inside and the energy-robbing friction is low. Maintaining, or regaining, most of the energy of youth can be accomplished by internal cleansing and following a nutritional program that supplies the nutrients your body needs to stay clean and operate efficiently. Resolving musculoskeletal imbalances and tight muscles and ligaments with my PMBT therapy can eliminate aches and pains and restore youthful flexibility. This is an important key to having more energy for your activities, because less energy is needed to move your joints if tight muscles and ligaments are not restricting their movements. Stronger muscles also help and, of course, not wasting energy carrying excess fat leaves more energy for productive pursuits.

Various cleansing programs have helped many of my former nutritional clients. The type and length of cleanse you start with should be determined by the diet you have been eating. If your diet has been poor in comparison to what you have already learned, start out with a short cleansing program and a gradual change of nutrition. I recommend starting with a one-day fruit cleanse on a Saturday, so you can deal with the cleansing reactions on a day when you are off work and you can use Sunday to transition back to more normal eating. Cleansing is best done when you are not working and are free to deal with the waste being eliminated. Also, more energy is channeled to your organs of elimination during a cleanse so less is available for your brain and muscles, reducing your work efficiency.

As previously stated, a good first step is a one-day fruit cleanse. Bananas do not work well, but otherwise you may use any fruit you enjoy. The most cleansing fruits are berries, cherries and grapes. Apples, peaches, pears and melons are also great. You can eat different fruits throughout the day but it is best to eat only one kind at a time. Make sure to drink water with the fruit and more between meals. You already know that it is important to eat whenever you feel hungry and this also applies during a cleanse. If you experience any of the moderate to severe cleansing reactions I describe later, wait a week or two and do it again. When you have only minor reactions from a one-day fruit cleanse, wait one to two weeks and eat only fruit for two days in a row. Friday and Saturday would be the best days if you work Monday through Friday. If you have a reaction from this cleansing, wait another week or two and repeat it. When you have hardly any reaction from a two-day fruit cleanse, wait one or two weeks and do a three-day apple juice cleanse. Apple juice is excellent for cleansing, because it contains malic acid that helps break up hardened mucus deposits so they can be eliminated. Normally it is best to eat the whole fruit but drinking juice is effective for cleansing.

A three-day apple juice cleanse is done using pure natural apple juice without sugar or additives. Buy a few gallons and dilute them 50 percent with water to reduce the sugar concentration. This way your body gets the fructose in similar amounts to eating the fruit. Carry a container with you and whenever you feel hungry, drink some of this diluted juice. Drink it a few sips at a time and savor the flavor instead of gulping it down.

Between cleanses you should be eating cleaner-burning foods so less internal waste will accumulate. Once you have determined the diet that is best for you and are eating balanced and clean-burning foods, hardly any waste should accumulate. Paul Bragg, Dr. John R. Christopher, and a number of other health pioneers have written good books about fasting and cleansing, if you wish to learn more. I do not recommend excessively long fasts (more than ten days) and they are normally unnecessary. I believe it is better to do shorter fasts more frequently. This is Nature's way. Fasting with just water is too intense for most people and also not recommended. A three-day diluted apple juice fast is the most intense cleanse many people will ever need. It usually needs to be done a few times to get the body cleaned out well. A diluted apple juice fast can be extended to five days if desired. After any cleanse, be sure to transition gradually back to normal eating.

Chemical and herbal cleansing products are effective for eliminating internal waste. Some contain bentonite and others use psyllium seed hulls or various herbal combinations. Some combine all three. Cascara sagrada and other herbs are good for deep cleansing the colon. Some products contain herbs that help the body cleanse the liver, kidneys and lungs. These are available at most health-food stores and by mail order. You may want to try a few different kinds to find the one that works best for you. This could be helpful in the beginning of your program, especially if you feel you have a large amount of internal waste you want to get rid of fast.

You can stimulate a cleansing of mucus from your body using unrefined Celtic Sea Salt. Put one teaspoon of this salt in eight ounces of warm (preferably distilled) water and drink it just before going to bed. This can be done for up to two weeks and may be repeated after a few months. Once the cleansing process stops feeling refreshing and stimulating or any phlegm coming out tastes salty, you should end the cleanse. Never do this cleanse using any other type of salt.

Some people say that after your colon is clean you will have a bowel movement shortly after each meal. This is not true. We are all unique and will have only the number of bowel movements each day that our bodies require for good health. Cleansing the colon should improve anyone's bowel movements, but if you have only one a day, do not think something is wrong with you. If your colon has normal nerve flow, the fiber and other nutrients from your whole food diet will keep your colon clean and your bowel movements healthy and regular. Water and fruit in the morning often stimulate a bowel movement.

When you give your body a chance to "take out the garbage" it is important to understand the various reactions you may experience. Your sinuses will drain large quantities of mucus, so have plenty of tissues on hand. Usually one nostril drains for a few days and when it has finished the other one starts to drain. This is your body's way of keeping one side clear to breathe through. Waste is eliminated through your skin, so be prepared to sweat more and have a stronger odor. Waste is also eliminated through your urine, stool and lungs. You will urinate more frequently and may have bad breath. You may experience mild diarrhea. Because you understand why these reactions are happening, there is no need to worry about them unless they are unusual and persist after your cleansing program has ended. You should then consult a healthcare professional, preferably one who understands cleansing and natural health. Remember that cleansing reactions will feel like you have a cold. You may feel weak, tired and dizzy at times, because your elimination system is getting some of the energy that normally goes to your brain and muscles. You have already learned how to help your body cleanse faster, but remember that the faster it cleanses the worse you will feel. If you choose to cleanse intensely in the beginning, pick some days when you can rest most of the time. The cleaner your body gets internally, the deeper you can cleanse with less discomfort.

Your body can store waste for many years, so get ready for some reminders of the past. A man I used to know was in his thirties when he did a cleansing program. For two weeks, his body odor smelled like a dirty ashtray. He had smoked cigarettes for a few years, but had stopped more than ten years before his cleanse. The nicotine residue had been stored in his tissues for all those years.

Attaining internal cleanliness requires a different amount of time and effort depending on your age, former eating habits and other minor influences. Normally, the younger you are, the fewer toxins and waste you will have accumulated. Youth may have left you with a cleaner system or perhaps age and experience have given you more desire and determination to get and stay healthy.

Sometimes during a cleanse your bowels can get overloaded, causing constipation. This happens simply because stored waste is being eliminated faster than it can be excreted. If you get constipated during your cleanse, herbal laxatives usually work well to get things moving again. The internal heat generated because of the blockage can cause a fever to develop. Get rid of the blockage and everything should be fine. Small children often get fevers when they are constipated and most often get that way because of the unhealthful foods they are eating. If this is the cause, a child's temperature could be back to normal within minutes after the blockage is eliminated.

Another way to clear a blockage and get the waste moving out is to take an enema. Some people believe that enemas are unnecessary. I do not believe Nature intended us to have to internally flush our colons with water, but it can be helpful during a cleansing program. Most people have waste in their colons that needs to be flushed out for good health. An enema is an unnatural method that is helpful for undoing the problems created by eating unnaturally.

It is just a way to clean out our colons faster. Our bodies should then be able to keep our colons clean if we eat as Nature directs us.

If you should choose to take an enema, this is the procedure I recommend. Fill the enema bag with warm water and hang it a few feet above you. Lie on your back and insert a well-lubricated nozzle into your anus. Slowly release some water and stop the flow when you feel slightly uncomfortable. Now, massage your abdomen upward starting at the lower left and working up to just under your ribs. Raising your hips by placing a pillow underneath them helps the water move up. Release more water and work it across from left to right underneath your rib cage. What you are doing is moving the water backward through your colon. Keep releasing more water but stop when it gets uncomfortable. Next, lie on your right side and massage the water down into your ascending colon which extends from your right lower ribs down the right side of your abdomen for about six to eight inches. Put in one to two quarts of water. Knead and massage your colon for a few minutes and then pull out the nozzle, sit on the toilet and eliminate the water and waste. Repeat this procedure three or four times or until the water comes out relatively clear. In the beginning you may not be able to hold much water. Do not worry, just do what you can and you should be able to put more water in as your colon becomes cleaner and you get more comfortable doing it. If you have never taken an enema, read the basic instructions that come with your enema bag and then reread this paragraph before starting.

Adding certain substances to the water can increase the cleansing effect of an enema. Lemon juice works well, as does garlic juice. Add the juice of one fresh lemon or the juice of one clove of garlic to the final bag of water. Regular coffee (warm only) can also be used for your enema and this is the only time that I recommend its use. It has the effect of drawing waste into the colon so it can be eliminated.

Another method of flushing the colon with water is called colonic irrigation, or a colonic. Getting one requires locating someone with a colonic machine and paying for the service. During a colonic, water is put into the entire colon, circulated and eliminated. This is done a number of times, flushing out more waste each time. The procedure is done while you lie comfortably on a table. Sometimes cold water and warm water are alternated to contract and expand the colon to break loose more toxins. Colonics do a good job of deep cleaning the colon. Old, nagging aches and pains are often eliminated as if by magic. After an enema or colonic it is important to replace the friendly bacteria in the colon that may have been washed out. Purchase some capsules that contain a variety of these good bacteria and take one or two a day (orally) for a few days.

I counseled a couple about eighteen years ago who were in a hurry to lose fat, so I had them do some cleansing in the beginning of their program. The man lost 27 pounds and his wife lost 20 pounds in just three weeks. They did this without any exercise. They did weekend cleansing and ate a whole-food diet of mostly alkaline-forming foods during the week. They never went hungry. My record-holding client lost 33 pounds in just three weeks. He did it the same way except he was also exercising for strength and fat-burning. All three of them lost stored body fat and internal waste.

Many of my nutritional clients had read books on healthful nutrition and had begun to make healthier food choices. But they did not understand that they would feel cold, weak, dizzy and tired because of their bodies channeling energy internally for cleansing. Some of them believed their cleansing symptoms were negative side effects being caused by the more nutritious foods they were eating. What they did not understand was that the elimination of the residue of previously eaten foods was the true cause of their uncomfortable symptoms. Many had gone back to eating those unhealthful foods, because this stopped the cleansing symptoms. Some of them assumed they were better off eating junk food, because they felt better than when they were eating the healthful foods. This, of course, is not true and why you must understand that you may go through some of these uncomfortable reactions periodically until your body is well cleansed and working efficiently again. You should then feel far superior to how you felt with your old ways of eating and be much less likely to develop health problems.

Keeping your body clean inside is an important decision. I have read of people having up to 40 pounds of waste inside their colons. This waste hardens on the intestinal walls and forms rings like those seen in the cross section of a tree. This build-up of waste gradually decreases the diameter of the colon. This is a common reason constipation becomes a problem for many people as they age. Waste build-up in the small intestine can inhibit nutrient absorption. This is one reason why it is more difficult for most people to get adequate nutrition as they get older. In both the small and large intestines, excess waste can inhibit normal peristaltic action, reducing the normal transit time of foods and waste traveling through the intestinal tract. You should be able to reduce or avoid these problems if you keep your intestinal tract clean.

Being cleaner inside usually brings additional benefits, such as the reduction, or total elimination, of body odor and bad breath. Many aches and pains will also vanish. After a cleanse, your thoughts are generally more positive and uplifting and your thinking more clear. For this reason, I believe that the saying "Cleanliness is next to Godliness" refers to internal cleanliness of body and mind, not to taking a daily shower. You cannot be close to your Creator if you defile your temple with unbalanced and unhealthful foods and drinks. Cleansing your body gets you more in tune with Nature and your true self. Healthier actions create healthier reactions and lead to health benefits.

You have just learned the biggest secret to having a flat stomach—cleansing. Correct abdominal exercises along with fat loss are important, but the real key is cleansing out internal waste. Have you ever felt the stomach of someone with a potbelly? Most of the time it is fairly hard without much fat on the outside except for some love handles on the sides. Many people with protruding stomachs have small arms and legs and not much subcutaneous body fat. Why do they look like that? They look that way because the weight of internal fat (under the muscles) and waste is pushing out against their abdominal muscles, making them tight and hard. Excess weight in this area places stress on the lower back and can cause chronic problems to develop there. It is also stressful on the heart. Cleansing the colon and reducing the fat around the abdominal organs eliminates the weight that is stretching the muscles. During and after cleansing, safe and efficient exercises are important to tighten the abdominal muscles and keep them strong. The excess weight may have caused some of the internal organs to prolapse (drop down lower than normal). Sometimes these organs can be repositioned and will stay in place.

Most forms of abdominal crunching exercises (crunches) push the internal organs downward and doing these exercises intensely can strain the upper abdominal muscles. This strain can negatively affect the nerves of the solar plexus and inhibit normal function of the digestive system. An upper abdominal strain will also make the muscles tighter than normal, causing them to pull the sternum (breastbone) downward and create poor posture. Crunches have other negative effects, and sit-ups and leg raises primarily stress the hip flexor muscles, not the abdominal muscles. Overdeveloping the hip flexors can stress the lower back and perhaps cause a chronic back problem. Many people believe that sit-ups and leg raises are effective because the abdominal muscles burn while doing them, but because they are mildly isometrically contracted during the exercise, blood flow is reduced to the abdominal muscles. The muscles burn due to a lack of oxygen not because they are being trained effectively. I do not recommend any of these exercises. To learn how to train the abdominal muscles safely and effectively, see my planned book about proper exercise. I hope to have it published soon after this one.

After you have thoroughly cleansed your body and are regularly eating as recommended in this book, you should stay clean inside. There may be times, however, when you eat things your body does not handle well or that are not particularly good for you. This will be especially true when you are developing your personalized program and learning the best foods for you. Therefore, you may gradually accumulate some internal waste, especially if you are dining out often. I highly recommend a periodic cleanse for a few days using fruit or apple juice during this learning period. This gives your digestive system a good rest and eliminates any accumulated waste. Some health advocates recommend doing a one-day cleanse as often as once a week. They usually suggest doing it on Sunday to clean out excesses and poor food choices made on Friday and Saturday. This is a healthy habit but a bit extreme for most people.

For everyone, I recommend a three- to five-day fruit or juice cleanse once a year. Springtime is best, because the most cleansing fruits are in season. This cleanse lets your body do some spring-cleaning and get rid of the residue of the heavier foods normally eaten during the winter. It also gives your digestive system a well-deserved rest. After that, all the great fruits and vegetables available in the summer will help keep you clean and cool.

Most of my nutritional clients have needed what I call a "pig-out" meal occasionally, especially in the beginning of their programs. The less you do it the better, but if you feel you must, it is best to limit it to two or three times a month. So, if you feel the need, go ahead and indulge yourself. The morning after a pig-out meal, you should have fruit and water only. Then have a light lunch of steamed vegetables or more fruit. Finish the day with an early dinner of fish or chicken. Doing this should give your body the chance to cleanse out the excesses or unhealthful foods so they will not accumulate in your digestive tract or around your waist.

A patient gave me a newspaper article (dated March 2002) saying that the "experts" say that fasts do not detoxify the body. These so-called experts were most likely medical doctors who I am sure have no personal or clinical experience with fasting. It was obvious from reading the article that they are not even aware of a fast's purpose. I have seen cleansing reactions and dramatically improved health in hundreds of people who have fasted. I have also experienced the positive effects in my own body. Fasting to rejuvenate and cleanse your body is extremely important, so please do not let someone with little knowledge of health, or experience in restoring it, stop you from doing something with the potential to dramatically improve yours.

How Much to Change

How much you choose to change your eating habits is entirely up to you. It is necessary to follow the program in its entirety if you want to reap the maximum benefits. After completing this book and doing a bit of experimentation, you should know how to enjoy as many of them as you want and to whatever degree you want. The choice is always yours. You may not want to give up eating dessert entirely or will occasionally eat other foods you know are not good for you. That's all right. Nothing is written in stone. The key is to follow the program as much as you can and get the powers currently working against you to start working for you. Doing just a few of the things suggested can increase your body's efficiency tremendously and may be all you need to eliminate the excessive waste and fat you now have and keep it gone without effort.

As you follow the program and start enjoying some of the benefits, you may be inspired to follow it more completely so you can look and feel even better. Following more of the guidelines also gets easier as time goes by and good habits replace bad ones. Once the residues of chemicals and unhealthful foods have been purged from your body, your physical cravings for them will disappear. Many emotional cravings will also cease to be, as unhealthful foods become less appealing. Your increased energy level makes it easy to eliminate the use of stimulants, such as caffeine. You will not feel the need for the quick caffeine pick-me-up that you know will be short-lived and drop you down hard. You may find it easy to stop smoking, if you have that habit. Also, your improved appearance and self-image will most likely give you even more incentive to progress further. Always keep in mind that the goals you set are your own. If losing 40 pounds would be optimal for you, but you are happy after losing 30 pounds, be content and give yourself credit for your accomplishment. If you later set a goal to lose another 10 pounds, that's great. Worrying and getting emotionally stressed about what you have not done yet are detrimental to your success.

Meal Planning

Eating healthful meals is just as easy as eating unhealthful meals. All it takes is some simple planning. Many people assume that eating healthfully is complicated or takes tremendous will power and sacrifice. All that is needed is the knowledge of how to change to eating well, how to break free of cravings and other negative cycles, and how to get organized. It takes more energy to prepare a healthful meal than to order a pizza delivery, but most of the additional energy will be expended in chewing the natural foods. Learn what is best for you, develop some nutritious meals and buy yourself a present with the money you save.

To stay on track with your nutritional program, you must first lay down some tracks. Planned meals are the tracks. Planning your meals also makes the transition period go smoother. How often have you arrived home from work and asked yourself the question, "What am I going to eat?" That question creates a great deal of stress in many people's lives and some people repeat it three to five times a day. To eliminate this stress and the years of wasted time and effort put into it, planning is essential. Reducing emotional stress is always a good thing and is helpful for eliminating many causes of overeating. Planning also prevents you from stopping off at a fast-food restaurant because you have nothing to eat at home. If your kitchen is stocked with good nutritious foods and you know what you are going to eat, you can eliminate that temptation. If you do not feel like eating what you have planned, however, you are free to change and eat something else. The main thing is to be prepared by always having adequate nutritious foods available.

A helpful and healthy habit to develop is to have only good, nutritious foods in your house. If you have cookies, candies and other similar products in the house, you will be tempted to eat them. Instead, have nutritious fruits available as snacks. Avoid looking at pictures of desserts in magazines or going down the bakery and cookie aisles of the supermarket. Your plan should be "out of sight, out of mind." You will think less about unhealthful foods if you reduce your exposure to them. Instead, think about new healthful meals or about other pursuits that will add positive value to your life and the lives of others.

If possible, all members of your family should eat healthfully. If you are easily tempted by lifeless, empty foods left around by others, it will be detrimental to your fat loss progress and health. Your family members should not be eating these foods either. It is an easy and enjoyable experience if you support each other. If one person is getting healthier and more vital and the others are not, the gap created can negatively affect their relationships.

Create a Weekly Schedule

After you have finished reading this book, tried some sample meals, experimented with different foods and created some of your own favorite meals, sit down and create an eating schedule. It is not difficult and will not take long. A one- or two-week schedule is adequate. Simply sit down and plan out your meals for the period you choose. After the week or two is over, just repeat the same schedule. Remember that none of this is absolute. You are always free to try new meals and change or expand the schedule as you discover new meals you love. Having a schedule is essential and, as previously mentioned, eliminates an enormous amount of stress and wasted time thinking about what to eat and what to buy when shopping. You will always know what to defrost for your evening meal and you will stop wasting money on fast foods.

As you plan your meals, keep in mind that meats, other complete protein foods and whole grains are highly concentrated. For this reason, it is best to cycle them. In other words, do not eat the same grain more than two days in a row. Likewise, do not eat chicken more than two days in a row. If possible, do not even eat them two days in a row. Cycling these foods every three or four days is healthier, because concentrated foods eaten too frequently can cause your body to develop a sensitivity to them. Your body simply gets overloaded with the nutrients in these foods and starts rejecting them, because it needs different nutrients from other foods. It needs more variety. Too much of the same food can become an irritant. When planning your dinners, you may schedule chicken on Monday and Thursday evenings, salmon on Tuesday, cod on Friday, turkey or duck on Wednesday and red meat on Saturday. On Sunday you could eat another species of fish or have an early dinner of legumes and vegetables. This should give you an idea how to space out these concentrated foods. You will be given more examples later.

If you know what you are going to eat tomorrow, it is easy to prepare for it. You can have some whole grains cooked or eggs already boiled for breakfast. I often prepare unleavened bread with raw almond butter and maple syrup, and take some boiled eggs out of the shell so my breakfast is ready when I get up in the morning. Sometimes I cook the eggs in the morning so they are warm when I eat them. While you are making your dinner salad, make your lunch salad for the next day. Just add different entrees and tonight's dinner and tomorrow's lunch are both ready. Some mornings, you can put your dinner entree in a slow cooker to cook during the day. This way, it will be warm when you get home from work. It will be quick to get ready and you will not be tempted to stop for fast food on the way home. Occasionally I do not have any whole grains or vegetables cooked, but I need a lunch for the next day. I put some pecans, cashews and figs or dates in a container and have a great-tasting, nutritious lunch in less than one minute.

Back-up Meals

What if you forgot to thaw out your dinner entree, did not turn the slow cooker on, or just do not want to spend five minutes to steam some fresh or frozen vegetables? The answer is back-up meals composed primarily of relatively healthful canned foods. For example, dinner could be half a can of salmon, half a can of string beans and a salad. Occasionally, when you just do not feel like spending the five to ten minutes needed to make your meal, you can throw one of these back-up meals together in about two minutes. How's that for fast but healthful food? I keep my pantry stocked with no-salt canned corn, string beans, Italian beans, canned chicken breast, salmon, sardines, oysters, clams, pinto beans, black beans, kidney beans and artichoke hearts. I go to a regular supermarket about every six months to get these items and use them as needed or desired. These foods can also be used to feed unexpected guests.

Shopping

If you are like most people, grocery shopping is not the highlight of your week. The solution to this problem is at hand, because after you have an eating schedule you can easily write your shopping list. If you know what you want, you just go to the store, buy it and you are done. More stress is eliminated and you save time by not wandering around being tempted by all the processed food labels screaming "Buy me! Buy me!" Food manufacturers pay a fortune to advertisers who know a great deal about how to entice you into buying products that are not good for you.

Because many people enter a store and go up and down each aisle, supermarkets are set up in a specific way. The storeowners understand psychology extremely well. The candy, pastry and other junk foods are located at the front so you will be tempted to buy them when your shopping cart is empty. If you already have a cart full of nutritious foods, chances are you will buy fewer of these items or, dare I say, none of them. The healthiest foods, fruits and vegetables, are usually located at the far end of the store. If you want to eat better and save a substantial amount of money, reverse shop. Start at the aisle farthest from the front door and work backwards. Better yet, go around the periphery and then down a few aisles to get the other items you need. Do not even go past the junk food. The colors and wordings on the packaging are designed to be tremendously tempting. Avoid temptation by using the "out of sight, out of mind" concept. Be wary, because stores are now putting candy and other junk food in the centers of aisles and on the ends. Keep in mind that the lower-priced foods are on the highest and lowest shelves. By reaching and bending, you will not only save money but will get some stretching and exercise as well. Avoid purchasing any food products found at the checkout section.

Shopping as just described could save the average family hundreds of dollars a month. Even a single person may save more than a hundred dollars a month. Investing the money you save on groceries has the potential to make you a millionaire. Here is an example: If a thirty-year-old woman saves $70 a month and invests it in mutual funds at an average return of 15 percent a year, she will have *one million dollars* at age sixty-five. This is more than most people have when they retire and chances are she will also have the good health to enjoy it. All just from money saved by wise grocery shopping. Most people spend more than $70 a month on junk food that makes them fat and unhealthy. Then they spend even more money on doctors, drugs and weight-loss programs in an attempt to feel better. These are many of the same people who will retire on a few hundred dollars a month from social security. Which path would you rather travel?

Because you will be eating more fresh foods, you may have to go shopping twice a week—once to get produce, meats and other foods that keep longer and perhaps another quick trip to grab some fresh produce. If you know you are going to eat chicken on Monday and Thursday, simply buy enough chicken for those two meals when you go shopping. The only thing easier is hiring someone to do it for you. If you live alone, you may get by shopping only twice a month. I spend only one hour every two weeks.

As you are planning and shopping, do your best to avoid the rut of eating the same things all the time. You may eat chicken every Monday night but you can cook it differently, vary the vegetables you have with it and even use a different variety of lettuce for the salad. Experiment with something you have not eaten with chicken in the past. When you are shopping, look for foods you have never eaten. Try them to see if you like them and to see how your body reacts.

You may buy most of your food at a health-food store. I highly recommend buying organically grown fruits and vegetables, fertile eggs, and meats that are free of antibiotics, growth hormone and steroids. These cost a bit more but are still less expensive than eating fast foods and processed foods. Organic fruits and vegetables have labels with a code number that starts with the number nine. Be aware that most of the processed foods these stores sell are not much better for you than their counterparts found in supermarkets. The definition of health food is "any natural food believed to promote or sustain good health." Many of the foods found in health-food stores are not natural and will not promote or sustain good health. Just because a food is sweetened with honey instead of sugar or says "natural" on the label does not mean it is good for you. Health-food stores are often filled with processed "whole-wheat" breads, cereals, crackers, cookies, pasta and more, along with products made from wheat gluten designed to simulate a meat product. It is absurd to think that these products are healthful, because wheat—especially processed wheat—is a common allergen that can cause excessive mucus build-up, fat gain and even lower back pain. I have counseled many fat and unhealthy vegetarians whose diets consisted largely of processed whole-wheat products and dairy foods. If you want to eat wheat, eat only the whole grain or an unleavened, sprouted wheat bread. Health-food stores also sell numerous other processed foods full of preservatives, artificial flavors and artificial colors. The bottom line is: "If you want *real* health, eat *real* food."

Favorite Meals

To give you some ideas and help you get started, here are some of my favorite meals. They are listed by category: breakfast, lunch, dinner, late night snacks and other snacks. They are also divided by season. Try them out and see how you like them. Follow them as shown, use them as examples to help you create your own special meals or modify them to suit your own tastes. They are simple meals, not a bunch of fancy recipes few people would make. Complex recipes are time-consuming and time is one reason so many people eat processed or fast foods. Remember that eating healthfully must be simple and easy, otherwise few people would do it. Most of these meals take minimal time and effort to prepare and are difficult to eat fast, which leads to better digestion and greater enjoyment.

If you think you will be giving up all of your favorite foods by eating healthfully, I think you will be pleasantly surprised by the foods you won't be giving up: hamburger and fries, fish and chips, spaghetti (squash) and meatballs, chiliburger and even a healthful Thanksgiving dinner!

Summer breakfasts

Any type of melon

Bowl of berries (any type)

Combination bowl of sweet fruits (e.g., plums, peaches, nectarines, grapes or others)

Any kind of individual fruit

Unleavened, sprouted bread with natural jelly

French toast made from unleavened, sprouted bread with natural jelly or pure maple syrup

Omelet with three to five steamed summer vegetables (with or without steamed potatoes)

Eggs (cooked any style) and beans

(Remember that it is a good habit to drink water with fruit.)

Summer lunches

Baked potato
Three to five steamed summer vegetables (e.g., zucchini squash, leeks,
broccoli and artichoke hearts)
Salad of dark green lettuce, radishes, cucumber, bean sprouts, seed sprouts
and other raw vegetables
Olive oil or grapeseed oil with apple cider vinegar (if desired) or grapeseed
mayonnaise

Three to five steamed summer vegetables (e.g., onion, yellow squash, red
potatoes, Brussels sprouts or okra)
Salad of dark green lettuce, radishes, cucumber, bean sprouts, seed sprouts
and other raw vegetables
Olive oil or grapeseed oil with apple cider vinegar (if desired) or grapeseed
mayonnaise

Three to five steamed summer vegetables
Grated cabbage (any type or combination)
Natural soy and flaxseed oil mayonnaise or grapeseed mayonnaise

Homemade soup made from a combination of summer vegetables (with
or without beans, grains or tofu chunks)

Homemade soup or salad made from either a single type or a variety of
two or three different beans (with a small amount of chicken, if desired)

Homemade chili (red meat, chicken or turkey) (with salad, if desired)

Fruit (like summer breakfasts)

Summer dinners

Fish (fresh or salt water)
Salad of dark green lettuce, radishes, cucumber, bean sprouts, seed sprouts
and other raw vegetables
Peas, green beans, Italian beans, mixed vegetables or steamed zucchini or
broccoli
Lemon juice with or without apple cider vinegar

Stew made with chicken, turkey or red meat and a variety of vegetables

Fowl (e.g., chicken, turkey, Cornish game hens, duck or other; ground or whole)
Salad of dark green lettuce with sprouts, radishes, cucumbers, tomatoes and other raw vegetables
Peas, green beans, Italian beans, mixed vegetables, corn or steamed summer squash
Lemon juice with or without apple cider vinegar

Red meat (e.g., beef, lamb, buffalo, venison or other; ground or whole)
Salad of dark green lettuce with sprouts, radishes, cucumbers, tomatoes and other raw vegetables
Peas, green beans, Italian beans, mixed vegetables, steamed summer squash or broccoli

(A healthful taco)
Chicken, turkey or beef
Salad of dark green lettuce with sprouts, radishes, cucumbers, tomatoes and other raw vegetables
Kidney, pinto or other beans
Corn or a few baked, no-salt corn chips
Brown rice or another whole grain can be included if desired

(A healthful burger and fries)
Lean ground beef
Baked french fries (low or no salt)
Salad of dark green lettuce with sprouts, radishes, cucumbers, tomatoes and other raw vegetables
Peas, green beans, Italian beans, mixed vegetables, steamed summer squash or corn

(A healthful chiliburger)
The above meal with kidney, black, pinto or no-fat refried beans instead of french fries

(A healthful fish and chips dinner)
Poached or baked fish
Baked french fries (low or no salt) (kidney, pinto or other beans may be used in place of the fries)
Salad of dark green lettuce with sprouts, radishes, cucumbers, tomatoes and other raw vegetables
Peas, green beans, Italian beans, mixed vegetables, steamed summer squash or corn

(A healthful "spaghetti" and meatballs dinner)
Meatballs (any kind)
Spaghetti squash
Salad of dark green lettuce with sprouts, radishes, cucumbers, tomatoes
and other raw vegetables
Healthful tomato sauce (no salt, sugar, white vinegar or other unhealthy
ingredients)

Homemade chili (like summer lunch)

During the summer it is generally best to eat fish and fowl more often and red
meat less often. Rarely include grains or starchy vegetables as part of your
summer dinners unless you will be using the calories for dancing or other
relatively intense physical activities after dinner. Beans may be added to meals
that do not include french fries.

Note: If you eat the foods of the preceding dinners at the same time, there will
be no need to put dressing on the salad to flavor it, but you may use various
herbs, apple cider vinegar and lemon juice if desired. Do not use any oil when
eating complete protein foods but do use some on your complex-carbohydrate
lunches.

Summer daytime snacks

Fruit (like summer breakfasts)

Raw vegetables (e.g., carrots, broccoli, raw zucchini or others)

Summer late-night snacks

A small amount of fruit

A small piece of chicken, turkey or fish

Winter breakfasts

Here are five healthful grain combinations:

1. 70% brown rice, 20% wild rice, 10% millet
2. 70% oat groats, 20% quinoa, 10% buckwheat
3. 70% pearled barley, 20% spelt or kamut, 10% amaranth
4. 70% rye, 20% millet, 10% amaranth or teff
5. 70% kamut, 20% quinoa, 10% buckwheat

A single whole grain or a combination of two or three grains
Raisins, chopped dates, date crystals or chopped figs

A single whole grain or a combination of two or three grains
Coconut, sesame, grapeseed or sunflower seed oil (with or without one of
the following liquids)
Amazake (or another brown rice drink), grain drink or soymilk (with or
without one of the preceding oils)
With or without raisins, chopped dates, date crystals or chopped figs

Unleavened, sprouted bread with sesame or nut butter (not peanut butter)
and pure maple syrup or natural jelly
Boiled or poached eggs
Steamed potatoes

Omelet with three to five steamed winter vegetables (e.g., yam, banana
squash, yellow onion and rutabaga)
Steamed potatoes

Omelet with three to five steamed winter vegetables. Tofu chunks can be
added
Unleavened, sprouted bread with sesame or nut butter (not peanut butter)
and pure maple syrup or natural jelly

French toast made from unleavened, sprouted bread. Spread with sesame
or nut butter (not peanut butter) and pure maple syrup or natural
jelly

A single whole grain or a combination of two or three grains (with or
without pine nuts)
Amazake (or another brown rice drink), grain drink or soymilk
Boiled or poached eggs or an omelet (with or without added vegetables)

Oatmeal (with or without pine nuts)
Coconut, sesame, grapeseed or sunflower seed oil (with or without one of
the following liquids)
Amazake (or another brown rice drink), grain drink or soymilk (with or
without one of the preceding oils)
(Oatmeal is not a whole grain, so you should eat it only in restaurants or
when time is short, whole grains are not prepared or whole grain bread
is unavailable.)

Two or three seed combination soaked in water overnight in the refrigerator
(e.g., pumpkin, sunflower and sesame; with or without pine nuts)
Amazake (or another brown rice drink), grain drink or soymilk

Unleavened, sprouted bread with sesame or nut butter (not peanut butter)
Amazake, or another brown rice drink or grain drink poured over the
bread

Apples, pears or a combination of the two

Orange, pineapple or a combination of both

Pecans and dates

Almonds and figs

Raisins and walnuts or hazelnuts (filberts)

Sunflower seeds, pumpkin seeds, hemp seeds or a combination

Winter lunches

A combination of three to five steamed winter vegetables (with or without
some beans, a combination of whole grains or both)
Salad of dark green lettuce with radishes, cucumbers and other raw
vegetables
Olive oil or grapeseed oil with apple cider vinegar (if desired) or grapeseed
mayonnaise

A combination of three to five steamed winter vegetables (with or without
a baked potato, brown rice or other whole grains)
Salad of dark green lettuce with radishes, cucumbers and other raw
vegetables
Olive oil or grapeseed oil with apple cider vinegar (if desired) or grapeseed
mayonnaise

A combination of three to five steamed winter vegetables (e.g., sweet potato,
banana squash, yellow onion, rutabaga and peas)
Salad of dark green lettuce with radishes, cucumbers, alfalfa (or other)
sprouts and other raw vegetables
Pumpkinseeds, sunflower seeds, hemp seeds, sesame seeds or sliced
Jerusalem artichoke
Olive oil or grapeseed oil with apple cider vinegar (if desired) or grapeseed
mayonnaise

Homemade soup made from a combination of winter vegetables (with or
without beans or grains; tofu chunks can be added)

A combination of three to four steamed winter vegetables
Grated cabbage (any type or combination)
Natural soy and flaxseed oil mayonnaise or grapeseed mayonnaise
Tofu chunks, some avocado, or both

A single whole grain or a combination of two or three grains
Salad of dark green lettuce with radishes, cucumbers and other raw vegetables
Avocado (whole or part)
Peas or string beans
Tofu chunks (if desired)
Sesame, sunflower seed, grapeseed or coconut oil

A single whole grain or a combination of two or three grains
Salad of dark green lettuce with radishes, cucumbers and other raw vegetables
Kidney, black, pinto or other beans
Peas or string beans
Sesame, sunflower seed, grapeseed or coconut oil

Unleavened, sprouted bread
Avocado
Dark green lettuce, tomato, and alfalfa, radish or clover sprouts
(This meal can be prepared as an open-faced sandwich or the bread can be broken into pieces and put in the avocado salad. String beans or peas can be added.)

Homemade soup made from either a single type or a variety of two or three different beans (with chicken, if desired and with or without grains)

Boiled eggs (cooked as you like)
Fresh-roasted cashews (do this in a toaster oven)
Spinach salad with cucumbers, radishes, tomatoes and other raw vegetables
Lemon juice with or without apple cider vinegar
(This also makes a good Sunday brunch)

Pecans and dates or figs

Almonds and figs

Raisins and walnuts or hazelnuts (filberts)

Sunflower seeds, pumpkinseeds, hemp seeds or a combination

Winter dinners

Same as summer dinners but use seeds and beans instead of seed and bean sprouts

(A healthful Thanksgiving dinner)
Turkey
Salad of dark green lettuce with radishes, cucumbers, tomatoes and other raw vegetables
Steamed sweet potato and peas
Lemon juice with or without apple cider vinegar

(This is pseudosushi using cooked fish.)
Fish (fresh or salt water)
Salad made with seaweed (a green salad may be included if desired)
Brown rice
Lemon juice with or without apple cider vinegar
(It is best to eat this dinner relatively early and only occasionally.)

During the winter you will want to eat some fish, but have fowl and red meat more often than in the summer. In the winter you can have potatoes, banana squash or other starchy vegetables more often as part of your dinner. Eat grains as part of dinner only occasionally. Foods eaten during the winter will naturally supply more of the good fats that you need during cold weather.

Winter daytime snacks

Pecans and dates

Almonds and figs

Raisins and walnuts or hazelnuts (filberts)

Apples, pears or a combination of the two (whole or blended)

Orange, pineapple or a combination of both

Unleavened, sprouted bread with sesame or nut butter (not peanut butter) and pure maple syrup or natural jelly (or use amazake, another rice drink or grain drink poured over the bread)

Avocado

Pistachio nuts, pine nuts or both

Sunflower seeds, pumpkinseeds, hemp seeds or a combination

Any type of nut (except peanuts) with or without dates, figs or raisins

<u>Winter late-night snacks</u>

An apple or pear

A small piece of chicken, turkey or fish

Spring and fall meals will be transitional. Spring breakfasts will be like summer breakfasts but with the fruits that are in season in the climate where you live. Refer back to my food pyramids in chapter three for ideas about what to include in your spring and fall meals. Your lunch and dinner meals should include a salad instead of bread, pasta or other processed wheat products. Eat chicken salads instead of chicken sandwiches, hamburger salads instead of hamburgers on a bun and so on.

When eating out in restaurants (not fast-food restaurants), you should be able to get lunches or dinners similar to a few of the examples given. Oatmeal, potatoes, fruit and eggs are usually available for breakfast. Eat fruits separately or 15 to 20 minutes before eating other foods.

You should have the knowledge by now to determine the pH balance of the sample meals and the meals you develop. If a meal is primarily alkaline foods, it will stimulate fat burning. Therefore, most of your meals should be alkaline if fat loss is your goal. If a meal is mostly acidic foods, it will cause fat gain if not balanced with alkaline meals. You have learned that the majority of most fat people's meals are acidic. If you are thin and training correctly to gain muscular weight (which you will learn about in chapter fifteen), more of your meals should be slightly acidic (primarily more good fats), because acidic foods are more concentrated sources of calories. Some meals will be a relatively balanced pH and will cause neither fat loss nor gain. Do not worry about each meal being pH balanced. Your fat-to-lean ratio should stay the same if most of your meals are balanced or alkaline and some are acidic.

Healthful Alternatives

In chapter four I recommended reducing or eliminating the consumption of processed foods, milk, sugar and certain other products. You have learned many foods to eat in place of them, but you may still want meals that are similar to what you are used to eating. The preceding meals have given you some ideas. You already know some healthful alternatives and with your newfound knowledge, it should not be that hard to exercise your mind a little and come up with more. Here are a few examples to get your creative (and digestive) juices flowing.

Instead of cow's milk with chocolate syrup, try some soymilk with carob powder or a little blackstrap molasses, rice milk or other "milks" made from brown rice and other grains or from nuts and seeds. Some great-tasting combinations are now available. You can even make your own special blends by combining soymilk with rice milk, for example. Replace that candy bar with some sunflower seeds, hemp seeds, pumpkinseeds or dates and pecans, figs and almonds or raisins and hazelnuts. Experiment to find your favorite seed, nut and date, fig or raisin combinations. Create your own healthful trail mix and eat these nutritious foods instead of protein bars, meal replacement bars or even commercially available nut and date bars. All of these bars are processed and expensive and most of them are unhealthful. In place of a soft drink, have some water (you can sometimes use sparkling mineral water) with lemon, lime or cranberry juice, some diluted apple juice or a blended fruit smoothie. Try blending up two apples with a little water and a dash of cinnamon. I usually use hot water if the apples are cold. For a unique taste treat, use a Granny Smith apple with another variety. Blend up an apple and a pear in the winter, an apple, nectarine and plum in the summer or numerous other proper fruit combinations. Replace peanut butter and honey on refined white bread with cashew or almond butter and pure maple syrup or natural jelly on unleavened, sprouted grain bread.

Put raw sunflower seeds, pumpkinseeds, pine nuts or sliced Jerusalem artichoke (sunchokes) in your salad instead of croutons. The seeds can be whole, freshly ground or sprouted. Egg whites and toast are incomplete and bland but a mixed vegetable omelet made with whole eggs is a nutritious and appetizing meal. Forget about french fries deep fried in unhealthful oil and covered with salt. Buy the unsalted fries or potato logs that you can bake in a toaster oven in about 15 minutes. Some brands have a small amount of olive oil and sea salt and others are available without oil. You can also easily slice up a potato (organic preferably) into the shape of fries or logs and bake them in a toaster oven. I sometimes put sliced and previously steamed potatoes in the toaster oven for five to ten minutes to heat them up and make them crispy.

You can replace your evening animal protein entree occasionally with a soy product that has had some of the fat removed. Soy products have been widely recommended in recent years but I advise using them in moderation unless your ancestors have been eating soy products for hundreds of years. You may be sensitive to soy products or may not digest and use them well. Edamame (whole soybeans), tofu and soymilk are the soy foods I recommend using.

When you want something sweet, eat some fruit. You can also eat dates, figs and raisins with nuts or whole grains. Date crystals, date sugar, and pure maple syrup can be used to sweeten things. Use grade C maple syrup if you can, because it contains more nutritional value than grade B or A. Grade A contains the least amount of nutrients, because it is processed the most. When I was a child, my favorite dessert was chocolate cake in a bowl with milk poured over it. Now I sometimes put unleavened rye bread with nut butter on it in a bowl and pour amazake over it. Every ingredient is nutritious and the taste is better than I remember the cake being. These alternatives not only have much more nutritional value, but better taste as well. Once you try a few, I think you will agree.

Let's analyze a simple alternative for calorie content. An apple as a snack between lunch and dinner compared to a piece of pie for dessert after dinner. A slice equal to one seventh of a 9-inch apple pie contains 345 calories. An apple weighing about one third of a pound has 80 calories. A big difference but easy to see why. The piecrust made from enriched flour and other unhealthful ingredients contains 1,485 calories, so one slice has 212. Now add about 2 1/2 tablespoons of sugar containing about 112 calories and you are up to 324. The final 21 calories are from the apple. Remember that because the apple was cooked, most of its nutritional value was destroyed. Now you have something close to 100 percent worthless at creating health, and a large number of calories added to the dinner meal. On the other hand, the 80-calorie apple not only tastes great but is nutritious and health building. It will help you lose excess fat instead of gain it because it is alkaline, supplies good nutrition and because it will decrease your appetite at dinner. Chewing it also helps keep your jawbone and jaw muscles strong.

Iceberg lettuce does not contain much chlorophyll, an important nutrient that helps keep your digestive system clean and healthy. During a nutritional seminar I attended many years ago, it was stated that iceberg lettuce contains a chemical that inhibits the peristaltic action of the intestines. You will be healthier if you use a variety of the dark green lettuces and other greens that are rich in chlorophyll and other important nutrients. Another reason I do not recommend iceberg lettuce is because its lack of taste causes people to smother it with dressings that are high in fat and loaded with salt and sugar.

I have heard that black pepper can irritate your digestive tract; therefore, I recommend using cayenne pepper (capsicum) instead. Cayenne is nutritious and has numerous health benefits. It improves your circulation and metabolism, stimulates the production of gastric juices and can even help relieve gas. All are helpful for fat loss and maintaining good health. The late Dr. John R. Christopher, a famous herbalist, once told me that cayenne contained many nutrients beneficial for the heart. He said that a small amount of cayenne pepper in a teaspoon of water given to someone having a heart attack could often relieve the condition, at least until medical help arrived. I have never attempted this and am not necessarily recommending it; I just want to emphasize the importance of this nutritious herb.

What if you are resistant to the idea of eliminating salt? I recommend using only a natural unrefined sea salt. If you are unable to get it, products are available that contain some sea salt (possibly refined) along with kelp and other herbs. If you feel the need to use something, this is less harmful, because it contains less sodium. I suggest using this only in the beginning of your program and then using kelp powder, other herbs or herbal combinations.

There are also a wide variety of spices available. Cinnamon, cumin, sage, dill, marjoram, mint, mace, oregano, paprika, thyme, garlic, nutmeg, saffron, cloves, turmeric, ginger and others can enhance the taste of some of your meals. Avoid spices that have had unhealthful ingredients added. Limit or stop using hot condiments like horseradish and hot mustard, because they can irritate the stomach lining, and be aware that some spices may cause negative reactions. Once again, you must learn what works best for you. It is best to buy herbs and spices in small containers so they will be used before they lose potency.

If you enjoy cooking you will want to make some of your favorite meals and others that you read about. Sometimes you may be able to eliminate an unhealthful ingredient. When this is not possible, just substitute a healthful ingredient for an unhealthful one. Substitute Celtic Sea Salt or kelp powder for processed salt, cayenne pepper for black pepper, carob flour for chocolate or cocoa, and seed butter or another nut butter for peanut butter. Instead of butter, use coconut butter or oil, or a nut or seed oil. Replace refined sugar with pure maple syrup, date sugar or Rapadura Sugar® that is made by evaporating the water from sugar cane juice. It is available from the same company that sells Celtic Sea Salt. With a little creativity and experimentation, it is simple to make nutritious *and* delicious meals.

Create Your Own Meals

It is important to learn what foods you enjoy, what combinations of foods you like and how you prefer them prepared. Like my sample meals, the ones you plan for yourself should be simple. This makes preparation easier and digestion more efficient. It is important to make meals you enjoy so you will not get bored and tired of eating them. With seasonal differences and the wide variety of natural foods available, this should never be a problem. By using your imagination and experimenting a bit, you will soon find the combinations of foods that taste extra special to you. Most of your personalized meals should make your mouth water just thinking about them.

When you want something crunchy, eat some raw vegetables, seeds, nuts, Jerusalem artichoke or other healthful foods that crunch. When you want something sweet, have some fruit. If you want something sweet and crunchy, eat a crisp juicy apple or some almonds and figs. If you crave a fatty pastry or greasy fried food, you need to eat some good fats. If it is after three or four o'clock in the afternoon, eat a small amount and start providing your body with good fats earlier in the day.

Eat to Live

Many people "live to eat" but Nature tells us we should "eat to live." But just because you are eating to be as healthy as you can does not mean your meals have to be tasteless, dull and boring. Unfortunately, this is how many people who have never eaten simple, healthful meals view them. If the meals are not high fat, high sugar, loaded with salt, spicy or poor combination conglomerations, they do not think they will like them; and with their deadened taste buds and polluted bodies, a nutritious meal would not taste good to them. People have been telling me for years how great my meals look and smell. I look forward to and enjoy each and every one, because they taste great too. Many of them taste like most people's desserts. Nature created the healthful foods we should eat to taste good, but few of us like every natural food. Eat only the whole, natural foods that taste good to you. Never eat something you dislike just because it is healthful.

You will find your simple nutritious meals tasting better and better as your body gets cleaner inside and your taste buds more sensitive. A peach or nectarine will soon taste much sweeter and be more satisfying than a candy bar or ice cream. As your body gets cleaner and more efficient, you will find yourself gradually getting more in tune with the needs of your physical body. You will know if it needs red meat, citrus fruit, fish or another type of food. As you become more aware of your body's needs and learn more about customizing and fine-tuning your nutritional program, you will design new meals to enjoy. As you get more in touch with your instincts, you will gradually develop an inner knowing of what is right for your body. As your body gets cleaner and more balanced, you will probably also find yourself getting more in touch with your mental, emotional and spiritual needs. You should also start to feel more deserving of getting your needs filled in all four areas.

I am often asked how I have been able to resist pastries, candy, soft drinks, chocolate and thousands of other unhealthful "foods" for more than thirty-seven years. Most people believe it takes tremendous will power and effort, but it is actually effortless. After enjoying the variety of great tastes, physical and emotional satisfaction, improved health, greater energy, more attractive body and the other benefits of eating whole, natural foods, why would I want to return to eating foods that cost more and cause the opposite results? Why would anyone? Would you want to go back to paying more to drive an old, junky car than you had been paying to drive a new Rolls Royce or Mercedes? Would it take will power to drive the luxury car instead of the junker? Of course not, but you won't do it unless you feel you *deserve* the nicer car or the benefits of healthful eating.

Dining Out

How you view dining out and how you eat when doing so are important thinking and behavioral habits you may need to change. Unfortunately, when you choose to eat in a healthful, simple way, it is sometimes difficult to find nutritious meals in restaurants. Many meals are poor food combinations and contain sugar, salt, white flour, chemicals such as MSG and various other unhealthful ingredients. Most of these enemies are in sauces, so you should order your meals without sauce or with sauce on the side. Then use it sparingly if at all. Learn to taste the foods you are eating, not just the sweet or salty sauce. Remember that the sugar in the sauce will combine with the meat and form oxalic acid, which has numerous negative health effects. Sugar also causes cholesterol-containing foods to elevate your blood cholesterol. Most restaurant meals consist primarily of acid-forming foods.

Restaurant patrons are often offered breads, crackers and other unhealthful fillers made from processed white flour. And there is always butter to put on them. This allows the main course, which may be fairly healthful, to be smaller, saving the restaurant money but also reducing the amount of nutritious food you get. If you eat the fillers, it adds unhealthful (and acid-forming) foods to the meal. Some restaurants furnish raw vegetables prior to your meal. If you find one that does, it may have potential. Sometimes I have to order two meals or something extra on the side to get enough good food to supply my needs. Getting a nutritious meal when dining out is frequently challenging but can be accomplished if you understand and follow the guidelines in this book. It is easy once you find a few good restaurants.

You may enjoy the foods of other cultures. Depending on where you live, your choices will be numerous or few. You can eat foods of Thailand, Japan, China, India and many others. I enjoy eating out occasionally and having Indian food, Thai food, Greek food or sushi made with brown rice. Restaurants that serve the foods of different cultures often offer many healthful and nutritious meals. You will most likely do best eating in restaurants that serve the foods of your, or your ancestors', country of origin.

Avoid going to most fast-food franchises. You will rarely find anything that will build health and keep you lean. Eating at the majority of them will make you fat and deaden your taste for healthful, natural foods. A few of these restaurants offer steamed vegetables, baked chicken and other healthful foods from which to choose. Some are offering salads and foods that they consider healthful. You may be able to find something that is good for you, but most people will end up eating unhealthful foods along with it or only the unhealthful foods. It would be better to go to a restaurant that offers a larger variety of healthful foods.

I do not recommend most of the salads sold at fast-food outlets because they are often made from iceberg lettuce, the quality of the meat used is questionable and the meats are often processed, breaded or deep-fat fried. People also usually get a large number of unhealthful calories from the salt- and sugar-laden dressings that they add. The oil in these dressings can also inhibit efficient digestion of the meat. It is also best to avoid eating meat for lunch unless your lunch is eaten right after doing strength training.

Occasional Dining Out

Dining out may be a part of your job, your social life or just a way to get out of the house and take a break from meal preparation and clean-up. Whatever the reason, eating in restaurants once or twice a month is not a big problem. You may even choose to include this in your eating schedule. Even once a week is all right if you follow my upcoming guidelines.

You can approach occasional dining out in a few different ways. You can eat as healthfully as possible every time you go out, eat healthfully on some occasions and unhealthfully the rest of the time, or eat unhealthfully every time. Most of my clients and patients have chosen to have their pig-out meals when they eat out. Some people feel they need to do this as a psychological release, especially if they feel at all restricted or bored eating a natural foods diet. Most of the time, however, they do not feel good after pigging out and are happy to get back to their clean, balanced meals. It reminds them that they are not really missing anything (except indigestion, less energy and excess fat and waste) by avoiding those foods and poor combinations. The best thing to do is to eat a variety of great-tasting, nutritious meals so you do not get bored and to discover some healthful restaurant meals. If you find yourself wanting to eat out more than usual, you must make sure it is not an abnormal psychological condition—perhaps the one that made you fat. You have already learned how to eliminate physical cravings for foods that are detrimental to your health. Later you will learn how to recognize and eliminate unbalanced and unhealthy psychological cravings and feelings. If you do pig out occasionally, make sure you eat as previously suggested on the following day to prevent the pig-out meal from having any major detrimental effects on your body.

What about eating at the homes of friends or relatives? The best solution is to simply let them know what foods you like and how you like them prepared. This way you will not have to worry about offending them if you do not eat much of what they have. If they really care about you, they should not have a problem cooking your chicken without barbecue sauce or serving the salad dressing on the side. This is sometimes a problem, because when you are eating to be lean and healthy, your worst enemies are often your friends and relatives. You may be tempted to make this a pig-out meal, but it would be detrimental to your self-image (and progress) to compromise your values in front of friends and relatives. It can become a frequent habit and will make you look wishy-washy in front of them. It will also make you feel like you have betrayed your principles and goals. A better idea is to be a good example and perhaps inspire one or more of them to improve their eating habits and health.

Frequent Dining Out

If you dine out frequently, the best thing to do is find some restaurants where you can get simple, healthful meals. Some meals may not even be on the menu, but they will often accommodate special requests. Go to a few different restaurants and figure out the most healthful meals you can get at each one. Do not be afraid to ask about the quality of their meats, what additives they use in sauces and how they cook things. You may eat a fish special every Friday night at one restaurant and chicken every Monday evening at another. Lunch can be steamed or baked vegetables with a salad, or perhaps brown rice and legumes with a salad. You can sometimes have vegetable or legume and vegetable soup. Because it is best to have oil at lunch, you should usually avoid eating meat or other complete protein foods at that time. Remember that complete protein foods are acidic, high in calories and can make you feel tired, causing you to look for an unhealthful pick-me-up.

There may be some "health-food" restaurants near where you live. They sometimes have better foods than average, but not always. Their definitions of healthful meals are often much different from what you have been learning. Some of them include cheese and "whole-wheat" flour products in every meal—foods that will make you fat, constipated and sick. Restaurants with salad bars, allowing you to choose from a variety of foods and season it the way you want, can be good places. For example, a steak house where you can get steak, chicken or fish along with a variety of vegetables may have what you need to put together a relatively nutritious and appetizing meal. Avoid the prepared foods that are full of salt, sugar and unhealthful fats. If you go out for lunch frequently, take your own dressing of grapeseed oil, olive oil or apple cider vinegar and olive oil to put on your baked potato, steamed vegetables and salad; or take some grapeseed, sunflower or sesame oil for your brown rice and legume salad.

It is best, whenever possible, to prepare and take your own lunch to work each day. A small ice chest can keep it fresh if you do not have access to a refrigerator. You will get better nutrition, and it is faster and much less expensive than going out for lunch. Read a good book with the time you save and invest in your future or buy something you want with the money you save. Some of my college classmates spent more money on lunches and snacks from the school cafeteria than I spent for my entire monthly food supply. What did they get for their money? Excess body fat and poor health, of course.

Whenever you dine out, it is especially important to follow the rules of good digestion, assimilation, and utilization. Following the guidelines in this book helps your body get the most from your meals and causes the least amount of internal waste. If you eat out frequently, you may want to take extra nutritional supplements to make up for the nutrients you may not be getting. I also suggest completing an internal cleansing program more often.

eight

Health "Insurance"

I often hear about medical doctors telling their patients that it is unnecessary to take nutritional supplements; as long as they eat a good diet, they will get all the nutrients they need. Unfortunately, the patient (and usually the doctor) has no idea what a "good" diet is. You will know after reading this book that few people—especially most doctors—know much about eating healthfully.

In this day and age, nutritional supplementation is necessary for almost everyone. It is especially important if you live in a city and eat foods—even whole foods—from a supermarket. Many foods are grown in soils that are deficient in vital nutrients, therefore, even though a food is supposed to have good nutritional value, it may not. Some foods have fewer nutrients because they are not allowed to ripen naturally. This also reduces their tastes tremendously. Shipping and shelf time deplete nutrients from the whole, natural foods you should eat and other nutrients are lost in cooking or canning. It is getting more difficult every day to find foods with adequate nutritional value. Most of us refrigerate foods and reheat them the next day, causing the loss of even more nutrients. Because our modern lifestyles tend to create more mental, physical and emotional stress, we need more of certain nutrients to maintain health and normal function. Add to that the extra vitamins and minerals needed to protect us from the numerous chemicals in our environment and personal care products, and you will see why it is extremely important to take at least a daily multivitamin and mineral supplement.

Vitamin and mineral supplements should be just that: supplements. They are not food. Many of them have special functions related to digesting and using food, so taking them without eating nutritious food is like having four brand new tires but no car. I have known people who wake up in the morning and take a handful of vitamins with some coffee. They do not eat until later. Some people eat junk food and take supplements to fill in the gaps. Doing this helps a little but still falls far short of good nutrition. This is like putting brand new tires on a beat up old car that barely runs. If you want your car to perform well, you have to maintain it entirely. A car with new tires but a bad engine will not go very far. Junk food creates imbalance and a greater need for certain nutrients, so even with supplementation you may still easily end up being deficient in one or more vital nutrients. These deficiencies will have negative physical and emotional consequences. Even with supplements, junk foods are not used well by your body because they lack enzymes and other nutrients your body needs to use them. Junk foods also contain a large amount of unhealthful ingredients. Remember that natural foods contain many ingredients scientists have yet to learn how to put into a pill. If the food is not used, it will be stored as fat, create allergic reactions or build up as excess waste. Many vitamins and minerals help us use other nutrients, so the foods we eat must contain these nutrients or we will not get the benefits from the vitamins and minerals.

Whole, natural foods contain enzymes, vitamins, minerals and other nutrients known as phytonutrients. A few of these have been discovered and nutrition companies are isolating and selling them. Once again, the balance and wholeness of Nature's foods are being destroyed. Hundreds or even thousands of these phytonutrients may be yet undiscovered, so putting them in a pill is a difficult task. Remember that the beneficial effects of whole foods come from the synergistic action of everything in the food, not just one or two ingredients.

I doubt if scientists will ever be able to put into a pill the "life force" that is found in natural foods. Some believe that supplemental enzymes are this life force, but I do not. Enzymes can be helpful and create wonderful changes sometimes, but I believe that they still fall far short of the elusive life force that only Nature can create.

Do not trust your health to mankind's limited knowledge and greed. Instead, put your trust in the infinite knowledge and balance of Nature. Nature has created food for all creatures on earth, from microscopic organisms to elephants and whales. Eat what Nature provides, in the way Nature teaches, and you should enjoy optimal health and a lean, attractive body.

Through processing, cooking, chemical additives and poor combinations, people distort what Nature has created and in doing so, distort their own behaviors, physical appearances and emotional and spiritual well-being. They create imbalances that lead to more imbalances and a declining spiral of poor health. People also often give distorted and unbalanced foods to the cats and dogs they keep as pets. The imbalances created cause disease, low energy and shortened lives for these trusting and loving creatures. If you care about your four-legged companions, feed them whole, natural foods so they can be lean and healthy. Make sure they also get adequate exercise and plenty of love.

Years ago, most mineral supplements were poorly assimilated into the body. Then a process known as chelation was developed that bound the minerals to amino acids. Amino acids are easily absorbed and they carry the minerals into the body, greatly enhancing mineral absorption. Minerals are now sometimes combined with vitamin C, creating their ascorbate forms, because this also improves mineral absorption.

Many multivitamin and mineral supplements release their nutrients at approximately the same time. This causes your body to get more of certain nutrients than it can use at one time; therefore, much is eliminated from the body before being used. And, some nutrients can reduce the effectiveness of others. For example, synthetic iron diminishes the effects of vitamin E if they are taken at the same time. In an attempt to solve these problems, some companies have developed what they call "time-release" or "sustained-release" tablets or capsules. These are often just terms that mean they are large tablets that dissolve slowly. They are generally better than regular vitamin and mineral supplements but there will still be decreased utilization and negative interactions between some nutrients.

Anthony Pescetti, Ph.D, originally developed the best multivitamin and mineral supplement I have ever used. He was the innovative biochemist who invented the time-release process used in them and in some medications. He was also the co-developer of the chelation process. A company named Super Spectrim® currently markets his supplement. The nutrients in the Super Spectrim multivitamin and mineral supplement are coated with substances that dissolve at different rates and release nutrients at varying times throughout a 12-hour period. Because of this timed release, the utilization rate is stated to be close to 95 percent. Nutrients that reduce the effectiveness of others are released at different times. After more than twenty years of nutritional study and experimentation, it was the only vitamin and mineral supplement to cause any difference in how I felt. I had more energy and greatly increased strength in my bodybuilding workouts. It is available in regular, no yeast and vegetarian formulas. Super Spectrim products are not sold in stores but can be ordered by calling toll-free (888) 772-6398.

Some companies market supplements with extremely high amounts of certain nutrients. This may be done to sell more vitamins to those who think more is better. Remember, the amount your body *uses* is what counts, not what is written on the label. Some supplements are so poorly absorbed you may get less than 10 percent into your system. Others may be absorbed well but supply much more than your body can use at one time. Some nutrients can be stored in the body but most excesses are eliminated. Your money and potentially improved health literally go down the toilet. It is better to take a smaller dose of vitamins and minerals with each meal than to take a large amount all at once. This is why a true time-release supplement supplies far more nutrients that are actually used.

If you choose not to use the Super Spectrim time-release multivitamin and mineral, I recommend alternately using two different brands of a sustained-release multivitamin and mineral supplement. Ask friends or acquaintances if they have found one that makes a difference for them. Try the ones they recommend and others until you find two brands that create a noticeable improvement in how you feel.

Alternately using two different brands helps ensure that your body gets the nutrients it needs. Because sources of nutrients vary, your body may easily absorb a certain nutrient in one product but get hardly any of the same nutrient from another. The two brands may also have slightly different nutrients. If you used only one brand, and it was lacking chromium, you may become deficient in this vital nutrient. At least one of the two brands should contain chromium and selenium.

The source of the nutrients is important for another reason. If one brand of supplement has a natural source of beta-carotene and the other a synthetic source, you will get most, if not all, of the benefits from the natural source. There has been considerable debate about whether natural sources are better than synthetic ones. I'm sure you can guess which one I recommend. The natural, of course, because it usually has other elements scientists have not yet isolated or even figured out if the nutrients have any positive health benefits. Numerous studies have shown that various natural source products create health benefits their synthetic counterparts do not. For example, synthetic beta-carotene has no positive effects on cancer or heart disease. In fact, it increases the risk of lung cancer. This is most likely because it is unbalanced due to the fact that it contains only one of the four isomers of beta-carotene found in natural foods. An isomer is a different arrangement of the same kinds and numbers of atoms. Each isomer has unique properties and therefore different effects in our bodies. Nature supplies all four isomers in perfect balance and science provides only one.

Vitamins and Minerals in a Nutshell

In general, vitamins work as coenzymes to assist enzymes in causing the chemical reactions constantly occurring in your body. Vitamins assist in the formation of new cells, help your body convert fat and carbohydrates into energy and help regulate your metabolism. They are vital to building lean tissue, burning fat and having vibrant health.

Vitamins are either water-soluble or fat-soluble. The B-complex vitamins, vitamin C and bioflavonoids are water-soluble. It is best to get a daily supply of these vitamins, because they are excreted if not used. On the other hand, the fat-soluble vitamins A, D, E, and K can be stored in the body. Vitamins A and D can have toxic effects but only after extremely high dosages for a long time. Excess vitamin E can elevate the pressure in someone with high blood pressure and can cause serious problems, even death, in someone with chronic rheumatic heart disease. Vitamin K is produced in the intestinal tract by friendly bacteria and is also found in certain natural foods. Natural vitamin K does not seem to have any toxic effects, but excess synthetic vitamin K can cause a form of anemia.

All of your tissues and bodily fluids contain minerals of varying types and quantities. Minerals are vital to your mental and physical health. They help maintain proper water and acid/alkaline balance and assist in the production of antibodies. Minerals are also necessary for normal nerve and muscle function, hormone production, and the proper digestion and utilization of foods. Like vitamins, they are essential for good health and fat loss. Minerals are believed to have other functions that have yet to be determined.

Minerals account for four to five percent of your weight. There are a total of twenty-six minerals believed essential to good health, although one well-known medical doctor and author claims there are twenty-eight. Unfortunately, he does not include their names in his book. Regardless, if you eat as you are learning, you should get them all and perhaps others necessary for good health.

The minerals that your body contains in relatively high amounts are known as macrominerals. These are calcium, chloride, phosphorus, potassium, magnesium, sodium and sulfur. Most of these function as electrolyte minerals, because they are found in their ionized forms and carry electrical charges. They are all used in other ways as well.

The minerals that your body contains in small amounts are known as trace minerals. Those deemed essential are arsenic, boron, chromium, cobalt, copper, fluorine, iodine, iron, lithium, manganese, molybdenum, nickel, selenium, silicon, strontium, tin, tritium, vanadium and zinc. Others may someday be determined to be essential.

Trace minerals are extremely vital to normal health. For example, zinc is necessary for normal function of the prostate gland and low levels reduce the senses of smell and taste. Get adequate zinc and your taste for whole, natural foods should come back faster. Not much is currently known about the functions of most trace minerals. As more research is done, there will surely be many important functions found for these minerals. What we do know is that many enzymes need trace minerals for full activity. Because of their interactions with enzymes and hormones, a small deficiency of even one trace mineral can have a tremendous impact on the entire body.

Products containing trace minerals are available through multi-level marketing and from other companies. The benefits people get from these products most likely come primarily from the trace minerals. Positive effects are experienced, because most people are deficient in trace minerals. The trace minerals in whole foods are usually all stripped away during processing. Fatigue is a common complaint and the primary result of getting adequate trace minerals is an increase in energy. This is helpful for everyone, especially those people who never have the energy to even think about exercising. Some of the products being marketed are good, but I believe many of them are extremely overpriced. The Super Spectrim multivitamin and mineral supplement that I use and recommend contains trace minerals.

Foods of animal origin are the best sources of all trace minerals except manganese. Concentrations are higher and the minerals are more available for absorption. You will most likely get an adequate supply of trace minerals if you eat seafood and sea vegetation. If you want to be sure, add a capsule or two of kelp to your daily diet or use kelp powder to season your food. Kelp absorbs the minerals from seawater that contains them in similar balance and kind as your body. Kelp is inexpensive and contains a substance called algin that helps carry lead (a toxic trace mineral) out of your body. Kelp also supplies iodine for normal thyroid function.

Some people recommend avoiding supplements that contain iron. They believe taking them may cause iron to build up to toxic levels and cause health problems. Excess iron can cause certain side effects, but I think that toxic levels will rarely occur. I believe this for two reasons—iron is usually poorly absorbed and it is found in a large variety of foods. Why does Nature supply it in abundance if it is going to harm us? Also, the absorption rate of iron increases dramatically if someone is deficient. This seems to indicate that the body will absorb only the amount it needs. I have taken a multivitamin and mineral supplement containing iron for many years and have none of the symptoms of an overdose. People who have excess iron in their systems have probably used a type of iron supplement that is stored in their tissues because it cannot be used properly. Usually after you are told to avoid using an iron supplement, you are given a long list of foods containing iron. This does not make sense.

Understanding all the functions of vitamins and minerals is unnecessary. Many people know numerous nutritional facts and figures, yet have excess body fat and no idea how to eat well. I will explain later how to determine if you need special supplementation beyond the basic foundation I recommend. We each have our own unique and varying needs determined by our age, gender, body size, physical and mental activities, environment (climate, air quality, chemical exposure, light exposure and others), genetic variations, stress, fitness level and current health status. Most people will get all the vitamins and minerals they need following the program of eating and supplementation explained in this book. If you want to learn more about the specific functions of different vitamins and minerals, numerous books are available with this information.

Heavy Metals

Some minerals are toxic even in small amounts. The primary offenders are often referred to as heavy metals. The degree these metals affect us varies based on the amount in our systems and our individual tolerance to them. Heavy metal intoxication is the cause of a large number of mysterious symptoms that many people treat with drugs. It would be better, of course, to eliminate the toxin than to use drugs to mask the symptoms. Essential trace minerals taken to excess can also cause imbalances that create health problems, but this rarely happens.

Lead is one of the most well-known heavy metals. It causes fatigue in adults and hyperactivity in children. Many of us have it in our systems because of the leaded gasoline emissions in our air pollution. Some people believe that lead intoxication from water carried in lead pipes and containers caused the fall of the Roman Empire. Ancient Romans also used copper cooking pots and became overloaded with copper as well.

Many people have toxic levels of mercury, another heavy metal. You may have heard about mercury from dental fillings being absorbed into the body and causing problems. Eating contaminated fish is probably how most people get mercury into their systems. Methylmercury is one of the most highly toxic forms of this metal and is a pollutant found in many rivers, lakes and oceans. It can cause numbness, sore mouth and gums, diarrhea, tremors, vertigo, irritability, memory loss, moodiness, hair loss, headaches, depression, and loss of coordination, vision and hearing. At high levels it can cause birth defects, kidney and brain damage and other serious health problems. It most likely causes numerous other problems yet undetermined.

Some people believe that the mercury found in some vaccines can cause autism in children. I recommend that all women who want to have children be tested for mercury before getting pregnant. If your levels are high, stop eating fish for four to six months. This will usually allow your body to reduce your mercury to a safer level. Mercury can be passed to infants through breast milk. Some doctors believe the body overgrows *Candida albicans* (a yeast-like fungus found in the body) in an attempt to have the yeast absorb the mercury. Dr. Hulda Clark believes that mercury in the joints is the primary cause of rheumatoid arthritis. See chapter ten for more on rheumatoid arthritis.

Because mercury is found in many fish and shellfish, I would recommend eating these foods only two to three times a week. The safest ones currently are salmon, sole, sardines, tilapia, farm-raised trout, shrimp, clams, oysters and scallops. I suggest limiting the consumption of sea bass, orange roughy and mahi mahi to about once a month and avoiding or rarely eating other fish, especially large predators like sharks and swordfish.

Cadmium is a toxic mineral that can be kept under control if adequate zinc is included in the diet. Cadmium is found primarily in refined foods like white flour and sugar. Coffee and tea also contain high amounts of this toxin. The total body concentration of cadmium generally increases with age and some researchers believe it is a possible cause of hypertension. Patients with high blood pressure have far more cadmium in their urine than those with normal pressure, and when rats are given cadmium they develop hypertension. Drinking coffee or tea and eating many refined foods can easily disturb the important cadmium/zinc balance and cause toxic symptoms. Cigarette smoking dramatically increases cadmium intake. Is the gradual accumulation of this toxin why many older people have high blood pressure? It certainly seems like it could be at least part of the cause for some people.

Other toxic metals are gold, which can cause tingling throughout the body; platinum, which can cause numbness in the spine and extremities and silver, which can cause a heavy feeling in the feet and hands and a cold numbness in the heart region. Still others are graphite, which can cause numbness all over; beryllium, which can deplete the body's magnesium and interfere with normal function of enzymes and internal organs; bismuth, which can cause arterial congestion; and aluminum, which has been linked to Alzheimer's disease. Other metals considered toxic are antimony, thallium, thorium, uranium and titanium. Keep in mind that the symptoms listed in this section are by no means complete. I just want to make you aware of these toxic substances that may be negatively affecting your health.

The following trace minerals are considered essential in small amounts but can create problems if excessive levels occur. Cobalt can cause increased bleeding and tin can cause numbness of the feet and a cold feeling throughout the body. Arsenic can cause spasms in the back muscles, enlargement of the tonsils and a hot burning sensation in the eyes, throat and chest. Copper can cause a burning in the throat and the desire to open and close the hands frequently. Nickel is often used in the hydrogenation process that makes oils remain hard at room temperature. Peanut butter is usually hydrogenated so the oil does not separate. Margarine is made through hydrogenation and many foods are cooked in, or contain, hydrogenated or partially hydrogenated oils. These foods are the most common sources of excess nickel and are not recommended. Nickel poisoning can cause paralysis and perhaps even epilepsy.

Because high levels of lead and mercury are common and cause fatigue and other conditions detrimental to getting and staying lean, I strongly recommend being tested for heavy metal intoxication. An excess of heavy metals can be determined by analyzing the amount stored in the hair. A small sample of hair is sent to a lab and a report is obtained. For many metals, the amount found in the hair is an accurate reflection of the quantity found throughout the body. After the hair analysis, other laboratory tests can be done to confirm the results.

It is extremely important for a pregnant woman to be free of excess heavy metals and to avoid exposure to them during pregnancy. Numerous birth defects have been linked to these toxins. Pregnant women deficient in certain vitamins and minerals also increase their chances of having babies with physical or mental defects. If you have any children with learning disabilities or severe behavioral problems, I highly recommend getting them tested for heavy metal intoxication.

Good nutrition and certain foods in particular can protect our bodies from these heavy metals and even help the body to cleanse them from our systems. You already know that the algin in kelp can help purge lead out of the body.

Poppy seeds help rid the body of nickel. Chelation therapy and certain homeopathic and other supplements claim to cleanse heavy metals from the body. These have varying degrees of effectiveness. Consult a holistic physician for testing and treatment.

Banish Free Radicals

Free radicals are oxygen or other molecules with an unpaired electron in their outer shells or orbits. An oxygen molecule unbalanced in this way is known as a superoxide. It is highly unstable and goes in search of an electron so it can become stable again. Even molecules need balance. When a superoxide comes in contact with hydrogen peroxide, it forms an even more toxic free radical called a hydroxyl. When free radicals come in contact with certain parts of your body, they steal electrons from the atoms of your cells. This starts a chain reaction that damages your cells.

Your body contains enzymes capable of neutralizing free radicals. The two main ones are superoxide dismutase (SOD) and catalase. Two others are glutathione peroxidase, which protects against peroxide free radicals and methione reductase, which neutralizes the hydroxyl radical. These enzymes can sometimes stabilize most free radicals if you live in an environment without an excess of them. But because of our modern surroundings and lifestyles, we are exposed to a greater number of free radicals than we would be if we lived in a more natural environment. We can easily be exposed to many more free radicals than our bodies can neutralize. These enzymes need particular vitamins and minerals to act as coenzymes. Any deficiencies will decrease the number of free radicals that can be eliminated. Free radicals are created during cellular energy production when oxygen and food nutrients are used to make ATP, the basic energy molecule of the body. Therefore, the more you eat, the more free radicals your body produces. Some of the other causes of free radicals are:

Air pollution	Asbestos	Alcohol
Cured meats	Carcinogens	Chemotherapy
Trapped ozone in the atmosphere	Radiation from sunlight & X-rays	Infection Excessive exercise
Phenobarbital	Physical trauma	Heat
Stress	Toxic herbicides	Toxic pesticides
Tobacco smoke	Oxidized oils	Manmade pollutants
Water pollution	Household chemicals	High-fat diet

Following the recommendations in this book will tremendously reduce your exposure to free radicals. You will not be exposed to alcohol, cured meats, numerous carcinogens, tobacco smoke, fried foods, excess fat, and many toxic herbicides, pesticides and other chemicals. Your physical and emotional stress levels will be lower and you should rarely get infections.

Some of the other causes can easily be avoided and you can use an air purifier to improve the quality of the air you breathe at home and perhaps at your office as well. By learning to exercise safely and efficiently, you can get all the benefits of exercise without overdoing it. You will not be overeating and should be getting more of the nutrients that neutralize free radicals. Certain supplements can also be taken to protect against free-radical damage.

Free radicals are destructive to all parts of the body and are especially damaging to our cell walls. They are linked, at least in part, to more than sixty diseases, including Alzheimer's disease, Parkinson's disease, AIDS, cancer, arthritis, rheumatism, cataracts, retinitis, kidney and liver disorders, all vascular diseases including angina and heart disease, stroke, sickle cell anemia, senility, collagen deterioration, edema, phlebitis, swollen extremities, cold toes and fingers, and even jet lag. Many researchers believe they are a major cause of aging, because they can alter DNA codes and damage so many areas of the body.

Free radicals are produced under your skin when it is exposed to sunlight. This damages the collagen connective tissue fibers supporting your skin and causes wrinkling and premature aging. Because so many symptoms of aging are associated with free-radical damage, it is very important to protect yourself against these unstable molecules. Supplements containing vitamin E, vitamin C, beta-carotene, selenium, glutathione, zinc, sulfur-containing amino acids like cysteine, and various other nutrients are sold as antioxidant complexes or free-radical-quenching formulas. These nutrients stabilize the free radicals by donating an electron to them. Foods containing these nutrients help protect you from free-radical damage as well as provide numerous other benefits.

Another product with strong free-radical-fighting ability is Pycnogenol™. This is a form of bioflavonoid derived from the bark of the maritime pine tree. It is fifty times more potent than vitamin E and twenty times more powerful than vitamin C at protecting you from free-radical damage. This product seems to be more powerful at fighting free radicals than the vitamin and mineral products. I have seen and heard about many amazing health benefits from using various pycnogenols. Pycnogenol seems to also have the ability to repair previous damage. I have seen a woman's legs with many blue veins scattered throughout the back of them improve dramatically in just a few weeks. Pycnogenol is now often replaced with the terms proanthocyanidins, oligomeric proanthocyanidin complexes (OPCs), or procyanidolic oligomers (PCOs).

Numerous antioxidant products are currently on the market. The one made from grape seeds claims to be more effective than the pine bark pycnogenol and is usually less expensive. It is generally recommended to saturate the body with these products during the first week by taking two or three daily doses of 200 mg. This gives a total of 400 to 600 mg a day. After the first week, a daily dose of one milligram per pound of body weight should maintain the saturation level that has been established. Some products combine pycnogenol with various free-radical-fighting vitamins and other nutrients. You may want to alternate using two or three different products. Do some research and use the ones you feel work the best for you. Reduced glutathione is another antioxidant I sometimes use. Green tea contains a powerful antioxidant, but also contains caffeine. If you use green tea, I recommend using only a decaffeinated brand or a caffeine-free green tea extract. I highly recommend using a potent free-radical-quenching product daily to help prevent and perhaps even reverse free-radical damage.

I believe that Nature intended us to get additional antioxidant protection from eating the seeds of grapes and various other fruits. The seeds of fruits are concentrated with nutrients. Unfortunately, many of them have absorbed chemical pesticides and other pollutants from the soil and water. Therefore, it is best to avoid eating fruit seeds unless you know they have been grown free from exposure to pollutants.

Special Needs

Just because a nutrient is good for you does not mean a large amount is necessary. Excesses of many vitamins and minerals are simply eliminated from the body, but some minerals and fat-soluble vitamins are stored and may accumulate to toxic levels. Problems develop from the internal imbalances excessive amounts create. The ratio of various nutrients, especially certain minerals, is very important. You may be aware of the calcium to magnesium ratio of approximately two to one. This is why most calcium supplements contain about half as much magnesium. Because taking an excess of a particular nutrient can sometimes create more harm than good, using nutritional supplements indiscriminately is not recommended.

Special nutritional supplementation can be extremely helpful when someone has an internal imbalance. It is important to take the required nutrients in the right amounts and at the appropriate times until normal internal chemical balance has been restored. A good multivitamin and mineral should then be able to maintain balance for most people. Some people may need large amounts of certain nutrients if their bodies naturally need more than normal or are unable to use a particular nutrient effectively.

Numerous books have been written about which nutrients may help resolve various health problems. But knowing what your body needs can be complicated, especially if you do not know what the problem is. If your doctor performs tests and diagnoses you with iron-deficiency anemia, the solution is usually simple. But because most doctors know hardly anything about nutrition, they are seldom much help if the problem is more complex. You may be able to learn what you need, but the best course of action would be to consult a holistic doctor or nutritionist with experience in helping people restore internal chemical balance using nutritional supplements.

Some nutritionists and doctors (including me) use applied kinesiology to test for nutritional needs. If done correctly, two primary tests are done. The first is to see if the supplement is good for you and contains no harmful additives or fillers. The second is to see if your body has a need for it. If the second test is positive, it means your body is already getting enough of the nutrient being tested. Someone using only the first test can make you believe you need every supplement under the sun when in reality you need only a few. All people will test strong with vitamin C, but that does not mean that they need an additional amount. You should also be tested with some of the supplements together to make sure no duplications or conflicts exist. After establishing what your body needs, a third applied kinesiology test should be done to determine correct dosages.

Another way to test for needs and dosages of nutritional supplements is electroacupuncture. This method can also test for numerous imbalances. It can help determine physical causes for having excess fat. When testing for supplements, the same three tests used in applied kinesiology should be done.

People often use nutritional supplements to treat the symptoms of a health problem while the true cause goes undetected and untreated. Covering up symptoms by any means creates the illusion that the problem is resolved, when in reality it is almost always getting worse. And, you are usually doing things to make it worse but do not know you are because the symptoms are masked. You remain unaware of the progression until the condition gets so severe that the supplements or drugs can no longer mask the symptoms. Unfortunately, by then it is often too late to successfully resolve the problem. Always strive to eliminate the true cause of an imbalance, not just treat the symptoms it creates. What you can learn from this book is how to eliminate your true causes for being fat, not just how to treat the symptoms by occasional (or constant) dieting.

You may need to take a certain supplement regularly if your body does not use it effectively or needs more of it than you can get from a good diet and multivitamin and mineral supplement. You also need more of certain nutrients if you deplete them by smoking, drinking alcohol, taking certain drugs or have excess stress. Keep in mind that using the wrong nutritional supplements can make current problems worse or create new ones. For all of these reasons, it is important to know why you are taking a particular supplement along with a way to test for need, dosage and interaction with medications or other supplements you are using.

Some Current Nutritional Notions

The mineral chromium has gotten extensive publicity in recent years and is often marketed as a fat-burning product. Its primary benefit is helping to normalize the blood sugar level, which is a common problem thanks to increased use of sugar, processed grain products, alcohol, caffeine, nicotine and many drugs. I believe that these items increase our need for chromium to unnatural levels. We should eliminate the enemies not take extra chromium.

Only certain forms of chromium are biologically active. One is called GTF (glucose tolerance factor) chromium. I prefer this form to the currently popular chromium picolinate.

Another often seen benefit of chromium is a reduction of cholesterol and triglycerides in the blood. Is a deficiency of (or unnatural need for) chromium why so many people (and pets) have unhealthy levels of cholesterol and triglycerides? Many whole foods contain chromium but the refining process removes most of it. Mankind strikes again and eliminates the substance necessary to effectively use the food being eaten. I believe that the abundance of processed foods Americans eat is why chromium is such a common deficiency in the United States. Chromium is processed out of the whole foods, leading to a deficiency and sugar craving. This often leads to excess fat and low energy due to blood sugar problems. Then more sugar, flour products, caffeine, alcohol, nicotine or other drugs are used in an attempt to get some energy. This is one of the many negative cycles created by processed foods.

Because chromium helps balance your blood sugar level and reduces your cravings for sugar and other sources of empty calories, taking chromium may help you to stop eating the harmful foods recently listed. The Super Spectrim Tri-Mineral supplement contains chromium and works well to balance and maintain a normal blood sugar level. Supplementing your diet with chromium may be helpful, but do not expect a miracle. You may have other imbalances that need to be corrected. After your body is more balanced and efficient, you should get all the chromium you need from whole foods and a good multivitamin and mineral supplement.

Many people, especially women, take extra calcium and magnesium out of the fear of osteoporosis. It is often poorly absorbed or utilized, however, and is sometimes combined with unhealthful products like chocolate. Most of these people need supplemental calcium because their unhealthy eating habits have increased their needs to unnatural levels. The over-consumption of protein and processed grains (both acid-forming foods) causes a loss of calcium. It is also depleted in other ways and this increases the need. A lack of the correct type of exercise decreases the amount of calcium stored in the bones, and without this exercise the body has no stimulus to replace the calcium in the bones. The osteoporosis section in chapter ten contains more information on this subject.

Vitamin C is another supplement commonly used to excess. Some people take it to prevent colds, but do nothing to improve their diets and reduce the build-up of internal waste. Remember, preventing a cold is truly done only by keeping your body clean inside. Blocking the cleansing reaction with drugs or vitamin C just makes the problem worse. Wouldn't it be better to let your body take out the garbage instead of leaving it inside to cause problems?

If we needed high amounts of vitamin C every day, don't you think Nature would have put large amounts of it in almost every food? Instead, few foods contain large amounts of vitamin C and most of them are the foods many people do not get enough of—fruits and vegetables. Some "experts" recommend taking five or more grams of vitamin C a day. One orange has about 66 mg, so to get the amount they recommend without taking a supplement you would have to eat about seventy-six oranges. Do you think Nature intended us to eat seventy-six oranges every day?

I believe that most of the beneficial results obtained by Linus Pauling and others who recommend massive doses of vitamin C come from its antioxidant properties. It is much easier and more effective to get these benefits from pycnogenols and other strong antioxidants instead of excessive vitamin C that can cause gastrointestinal and urinary dysfunction. I used large amounts of vitamin C many years ago and it made almost every joint in my body ache. High dosages of vitamin C or other supplements may help reestablish balance in certain severe problems but should not be needed once balance has been restored. I do not believe vitamin C should be used in high dosages otherwise.

I received an advertisement in the mail for a daily supplement to improve your eyesight. It supposedly contained the nutrition found in more than forty cups of orange juice, hundreds of carrots, and many pounds of tomatoes, Brussels sprouts and romaine lettuce. It is absurd to think that Nature intended us to have poor eyesight unless we take this pill. Balanced light is the best nutrition for the eyes and is free if you use Nature's source and inexpensive using full-spectrum lights.

"Eat bananas for potassium." You hear this frequently and many people believe they need a banana every day. Who do you think started this one? I feel that bananas are a good food if eaten occasionally during hot weather, but not at other times. Do you see bananas growing outside in the snow or even in the summer in Montana? Most fruits and vegetables contain more potassium than a banana. Avocados, available from late summer to late winter, contain four times the amount of potassium as a banana along with the good fat needed for energy and warmth in the cold winter months. Equivalent weights of most red meat, poultry and fish also contain more potassium than a banana. Are you surprised?

Some nutritional supplement companies do not understand balanced nutrition. They market incomplete processed products, poor combinations of nutrients, unbalanced amounts of nutrients and others that just cater to the current nutritional fad. Be aware that there are hundreds of unbalanced and unhealthful food supplements on the market.

Eat based on the truth of what is in a food and what it can do for you, not what some television commercial tells you. Do not let yourself be brainwashed by advertising hype, and do not let your children tell you what to feed them based on the sugarcoated breakfast cereal or cookie advertisements they see during Saturday morning cartoons.

Observe and learn from the wisdom of Nature if you truly want to know how to eat properly. If you feel you need more of a particular nutrient, find out which foods are good sources of it and eat a variety of those in season. Most people will not need anything extra if they eat in the balanced way explained in this book.

Mysterious Ailments

A large percentage of people's stress, lack of energy and other emotional and physical problems come from minor vitamin and mineral deficiencies. Yes, *minor* deficiencies. The ones that go unnoticed by most doctors. For example, did a medical doctor ever ask you what you eat or if you use nutritional supplements or drink enough water? I doubt it. The effects of these minor deficiencies are most easily seen in children and the elderly. Most of the people not in these groups believe that being stressed and feeling terrible is normal, because most of the people they know feel the same way. How badly would your car run if it had one or two spark plugs missing? Sadly, millions of people are taking drugs or even having surgeries for symptoms caused by minor nutritional deficiencies, and the drugs and surgeries almost always make the problems worse or cause new ones.

Minor nutritional deficiencies have *major* influences on how we look, think and feel. They can cause or contribute to the primary physical or emotional reason why you have excess fat. Therefore, it is imperative that deficiencies are corrected. A negative cycle is often created, because inadequate amounts of certain nutrients can cause us to be too tired to exercise or to not care if we overeat or make poor food choices. These both lead to more physical and emotional deficiencies. Many of the symptoms caused by these minor deficiencies are covered in the upcoming chapters that deal with physical and emotional reasons for being fat. Taking an effective multivitamin and mineral supplement may make a world of difference for you.

If you are eating well and taking a good multivitamin and mineral supplement, but have mineral deficiency symptoms, chances are you are not absorbing the nutrients due to low hydrochloric acid production. Either get tested for need by a competent professional or experiment as explained in chapter five with apple cider vinegar or HCl supplements. Often, only HCl is needed but most HCl supplements contain pepsin. These can be used, but I prefer those without pepsin or just using apple cider vinegar.

Some people say that glandular supplements are just expensive protein supplements that have no special effects on our health. My experience with them has been different. I have seen dramatic improvements in people who have used them and have experienced positive results for myself as well. When people used to raise or hunt animals for food, they often ate the glands along with the muscle meat. I believe that the glandular meats provided nutrients that could not be gotten from other sources. Because most of us do not eat glandular meats, taking supplements made from them can be beneficial. A multiglandular supplement taken once or twice a week would be adequate for most people. Make sure the supplement is made from the glands of healthy animals. If your pancreas is your weak link, a pancreas supplement may be extremely important for keeping yours functioning normally. It is best to be tested for need and dosage.

Miracle Supplements?

People spend millions of dollars a year on the latest "miracle" supplement and new ones are popping up all the time. Many of them are designed for weight loss but few of them work even in the short term. Remember octacosanol? Years ago it was discovered that wheat germ gave people endurance, so wheat germ and wheat germ oil became miracle energy supplements. Eventually the ingredient in wheat germ that was creating the energizing effect was isolated. Now you can spend even more money to get the supplement octacosanol. The only reason these supplements are beneficial is because the people using them are eating diets deficient in the nutrients contained in the supplements. Eat some whole-wheat grain and you will get the octacosanol along with proper amounts of the other synergistic parts of the grain. Some supplements are made from the juice of fruits and vegetables. These are expensive, processed, lack wholeness and supply none of the stimulation your five senses need for balance and good health. Eat fruits and vegetables, not junk food and these supplements. Beware of expensive products having miracle health claims. Many of them are like the snake oil of the past and are rarely necessary if your diet is composed of nutritious foods and a good vitamin and mineral supplement. Doesn't it make more sense just to eat the real miracles—whole, natural foods? I recommend trusting in Nature and buying yourself something nice with the money you save.

Products have been developed to replace certain things naturally made by the body. These can be beneficial for people whose bodies are not producing normal amounts, but many of them are unnecessary and they can cause other imbalances. One that is currently popular is DHEA (dehydroepiandrosterone), a hormone produced by the adrenal glands. One problem with taking this (or others) in supplemental form is that getting more than needed may put excessive demand on the body to produce something else. This could overstress another gland or organ, or create an imbalance among other hormones. Both of these can cause health problems. Difficulties are more likely if a person's body is inefficient and lacking in good nutrition. Someone may need other nutrients for the DHEA to have an effect. If those nutrients are missing, then no positive effects will be experienced.

Always remember that if you supply your body with an excess of something it is supposed to make naturally, it will usually stop producing it. If you stop using the supplemental form, your body will have a large deficiency until it starts making it again. It may never be able to regain normal production. If you want to take DHEA or similar supplements, make sure you are eating well first. Then get tested for your levels and if they are low, supplement only what is needed. Know that you may have to continue supplementing for the rest of your life to maintain normal levels. Before using DHEA or similar products, be sure to read and adhere to the warnings printed on the label. It is best to work with a professional who is knowledgeable in nutrition and able to test you for need and dosage.

Some people take DHEA, growth hormone stimulators and similar products in an attempt to enjoy benefits unearned by correct exercise and good nutrition. They are trying to cheat Nature, but doing this is like putting expensive paint on a house made of rotten wood. The benefits are often temporary or fall far short of what could be enjoyed. It's not nice to mess with Mother Nature, but people often do just that instead of learning and following Nature's laws. Unfortunately, a price is *always* paid when any of these immutable laws are broken.

Special supplements can sometimes be beneficial in certain extreme situations. But, you must remember that your first need is a strong foundation built from a variety of whole, natural foods and a good multivitamin and mineral supplement. If a deficiency still exists, supplementation can be used to restore balance faster or to supply the body's daily needs. For example, a man may have a low production of digestive enzymes. If he supplements his diet with enzymes, he will get more of the nutrients from the foods he eats and perhaps achieve balance. He may need them only until his body begins to produce more on its own. If his normal production is naturally low, he will need supplemental enzymes for the rest of his life.

Herbs are a hot topic these days. Various herbs have been used for thousands of years and are supplied by Nature when certain nutrients are needed. I have used and recommended herbs for many years. St. John's Wort is used for depression in place of various antidepressant drugs. In those that it helps, it is most likely just supplying the missing nutrients that are causing the depression. Using this herb is certainly better than taking a drug, but to restore true health the cause of the depression must be determined and eliminated. Many people just treat their symptoms with drugs or herbs instead of getting rid of the source of the problem.

I believe most herbs were intended for temporary use to restore lost balance faster than through normal eating. Get your body balanced in as many ways as you can and ingest a nutritious diet. Then see if any herbs you may be taking are still necessary. Many of them will no longer be needed. Some people have inherited a body incapable of functioning normally and will need a particular herb daily. If you do need or just want to take an herb regularly, I feel it is best to find two or three with similar functions and alternate them. For example, two good herbal tonics for the body are ginseng and fo-ti. Alternate taking them every other day to avoid possibly getting an excess of something one contains or not enough of what the other does. Remember the variety principle.

Some authors of health newsletters claim that you "probably" will not die of cancer, diabetes, heart attack or numerous other diseases if you subscribe to their newsletters and get their special free reports. All you have to do is use certain herbs from India, Egypt, Japan or some other country. They sometimes have good information and I am glad to see a few medical doctors finally studying health instead of disease. They often write about herbs that help treat certain symptoms. Most of these newsletters seem to be advertisements for products that the doctor is selling. If you have a particular condition, there may be a product that can help restore you to balance. That would be wonderful; however, do not be lulled into a false sense of security. If you are eating foods with little nutritional value that are creating serious deficiencies and imbalances in your body, these herbs are not going to cure you. If you are obese, your chances of getting diabetes or a heart attack will still be extremely high. The problem may also have a different cause, so treating the symptoms with a nutritional supplement may help but is not eliminating the cause.

Do you think Nature intended everyone living outside the country where a so-called "cancer-curing" herb grows to die of cancer? Do you think Nature intended millions of women to get osteoporosis until some root vegetable was discovered in Mexico? A variety of herbs (and foods) grow in many different countries. You can find an herb in China, another in India and yet another in America that all have similar effects. For example, the herb ginseng is used in China for vitality and longevity and the herb gotu kola is used in India for the same purpose. I believe Nature placed what we need for good health in the environment where we live. If you live in Texas, you should not have to use an herb found only in Brazil to prevent or cure a particular disease. Being healthy and maintaining a lean body is not complicated. Exercise for the body and mind, a variety of whole, natural foods, a worthwhile purpose, adequate soul food and feeling loved. That's really all there is to it.

A Balanced Plan

Much of the nutritional research that has been done, including figuring out the recommended dietary allowance of various nutrients, was done on rats, not humans. Therefore, I believe that many recommendations, especially those giving the amount of nutrients we need, are inaccurate. The best way to supply your body what it truly needs is to eat as balanced and in harmony with Nature as possible. This gives you the best chance of getting the right amounts of each vitamin, mineral, enzyme and other vital nutrients your body needs to function at peak efficiency.

If you eat a variety of whole foods, both cooked and raw, you should provide your body with a good base of nutrition. Add to this a good multivitamin and mineral supplement and a potent antioxidant supplement every day and you should do well. Because our livers must detoxify numerous chemicals and pollutants in our modern environment, I also recommend taking the herb milk thistle or a product made from it every two or three days. Using this herb to help keep your liver strong may be extremely beneficial for preventing almost every disease.

If you live in a clean and natural environment, taking an antioxidant and milk thistle is not as important, but most of us need them to protect us from the harmful effects of toxins in our environment. Another key step is to be tested for, or experiment with, various digestive supplements and take them if they are needed. These are important to assist your body in getting the nutrients it needs from your foods and other supplements. This can be especially helpful in the beginning of your fat-loss program. Remember that proper digestion is the second vital step on the way to the bottom line of utilization. You may need digestive aids only until your body starts producing normal amounts. As you have learned, adequate HCl is vital.

If you are planning to gradually transition into a better nutritional program, I recommend taking a B-complex supplement every day. This is in addition to the multivitamin and mineral supplement you will be taking in the morning. Take it with your evening meal for a month or two or until you run out of it. These vital nutrients will help restore your brain and body to normal function faster. After that, you should need extra B vitamins only during times of increased stress.

Finding Help

If you have a problem you believe is coming from a nutritional deficiency, it is best to consult someone knowledgeable in nutrition. Unfortunately, many college-trained nutritionists do not know how to design a healthful eating program or use supplements correctly. Most are still schooled in the four food groups and know little about how to eat for efficient digestion, assimilation and utilization. The majority of them primarily use supplements to treat deficiency symptoms. They usually do not know how to find and eliminate the causes of these deficiencies. This is the true key to restoring health, because treating symptoms with drugs *or* natural methods can be extremely dangerous. For example, if the symptoms of a kidney problem are masked by a drug or supplement, as the condition worsens you will be unaware of it until it is extremely severe and perhaps life threatening. Look for a nutritionist or holistic doctor who has learned from years of experience and study and who has been successful at helping others.

Be wary of nutritional consultants who sell supplements. Sometimes they sell specialized products that are not readily available elsewhere or other products that they believe are the best. A good consultant may offer to sell you a few products at or below the price you would pay elsewhere. In other words, you are being sold what you truly need, not a bag full of over-priced products you do not need. If you are told that you need $250 worth of supplements that the consultant sells, chances are you are being taken for a ride. Most of these people believe that you need what they are trying to sell to you. Unfortunately, they lack the means to determine your real (and less expensive) needs. It has happened to me so I want you to be aware of the possibility and exercise some good sense.

When looking for a nutritionist or holistic doctor, if you can, find one who has experience with your particular condition. If your problem is iron-deficiency anemia, go to someone who has had success helping people resolve it. If your condition is unusual, look for someone who has helped many people with a variety of ailments. That person will probably have the knowledge and skills to determine and help you eliminate your particular imbalance. The people you consult should be honest enough to tell you if they feel they cannot help you and be willing to refer you to someone they know who may be able to help you.

Good nutritionists will ask you what your diet is like, what supplements and medications you are using and emphasize that eating a varied diet of *whole* foods (excluding dairy) is the foundation of good health. They should have a means of testing you to determine your specific needs so time and money are not wasted in trial and error experimentation.

If you like to do things yourself, or have an extensive nutritional background, books are available to help you determine your special needs. I still recommend sharing your beliefs with and getting tested by a competent professional so you do not just treat your symptoms. Chapter ten deals with some of the more common problems that can be helped with a natural diet and nutritional supplements.

nine

Complementary Health Habits

This chapter contains information about some powerful health habits that complement your new nutritional program and improve the balance of your entire life. Some of them increase your body's efficiency and help you achieve your physical improvement goals faster. Most of them make you feel better emotionally and physically, and this can help you eliminate emotional reasons for overeating or making unhealthful food choices. Space limitations prevent me from going into a great deal of detail on these various subjects but most of them are covered more in upcoming chapters. You will find that getting and staying lean includes far more than just eating well. In this chapter you will learn how these health habits complement and support each other to make reaching your goals easy and natural.

Exercise

We all know that exercise is good for us, but few people even know about the different types of exercise. Even many of those who do know have limited knowledge of how to exercise safely and for maximum benefit. Millions of people have started exercising, but due to lack of knowledge, most quit because they obtained little or no results. If people knew how much of a difference exercise can make in how they feel, many more of them would exercise regularly. Only about 30 percent of Americans exercise regularly and most of what they do is unsafe, inefficient, unproductive and often even counterproductive.

An important benefit of exercise comes from the positive cycle it creates. Here is how it works. Correct exercise done regularly increases the efficiency of your body by improving its ability to process and absorb the foods you eat. This supplies better nutrition to your body and improves your health. You can then progress to a higher level of fitness, which increases your body's efficiency even more. Like good nutrition and internal cleansing, exercise improves your body's efficiency and your ability to work or play harder, handle stress better and enjoy life more fully.

Some of the most important benefits of exercise are emotional. These are often of greatest value to the person struggling with excess body fat. One benefit is the release of chemicals (endorphins) that can lift your spirits and produce what is called a natural or runner's high. This may be all some people need to eliminate their chronic depression. Exercise also increases blood flow to your brain, improving its function and usually your thinking. It is easy to comprehend the importance of this when you understand that even though your brain is only about two percent of your body weight, it uses approximately 25 percent of your energy. It is also responsible for controlling the rest of your body. If it is not functioning properly, the other parts of your body won't either.

Physical activities requiring coordination and skill like tennis, racquetball and basketball keep your brain function sharper. Exercising with dumbbells heavy enough to challenge you also improves your coordination along with maintaining or increasing your strength.

Exercising often places you in a healthy environment where other people with similar goals can be found. This gives you an opportunity to improve your social skills and meet new people. You may make some new friends or even find a mate with a similar interest in living a healthy lifestyle. These environments can be stimulating and inspiring, and this can help motivate you as you pursue your physical goals.

Your self-image and confidence should improve with exercise, because you will start feeling stronger physically and emotionally. You have tremendous control over your physical appearance and can improve it once you make the choice. You just have to eat well and exercise correctly. Using these tools, you can dramatically improve the shape of your body and then maintain it for many years. I have seen men in their late seventies who looked about the same as they did when they were twenty and they looked great then.

Reduced stress is another valuable benefit of regular exercise. When your sympathetic nervous system is stimulated, it triggers the release of epinephrine and norepinephrine, hormones that increase your metabolic rate, constrict your blood vessels and increase the activity of your heart. They make your body tense and ready for physical action. These hormones have similar effects and are usually released at the same time, so throughout this book the word epinephrine will refer to both of them. For most of us, emotional conflicts, commuting in rush-hour traffic, most advertising, type A personality, excess noise, sexual fantasies and numerous other things can stimulate a release of epinephrine when we do not have a physical way to use it and release the tension. The effect of epinephrine is long-lasting because it is removed from the blood slowly. Exercise uses the epinephrine in a natural way so your muscles can relax.

The best time for most people to exercise is after the commute home from work. Unwind in a healthy way with exercise instead of sitting and having an alcoholic drink, eating to excess, or venting your stress on your family or yourself. Stop off at the gym three days a week and do something physical at home on the other days. Taking your dog for a walk, playing catch with your child or making love with your mate reduces your stress and gives you some soul food as well. It is always best to exercise before you lose your momentum. Do not sit down first, because it is extremely difficult to get back up. Use the powers of inertia and momentum to work for you instead of against you. If you cannot exercise, lying on a slant board (with your head at the low end) inclined at 20 to 45 degrees for 10 to 15 minutes or meditating for 15 to 20 minutes can help clear your head and get you ready for an enjoyable evening. You could slant and meditate at the same time. Both exercise and meditation increase the carbon dioxide levels in your blood, which increases oxygen to your brain and body.

If you still think you do not need to exercise, here are a few more benefits you will get from regular exercise, primarily strength-building exercise:
- Decreases insulin levels
- Stimulates glucose to be stored in muscles as glycogen
- Fat cells are smaller than with just dietary reduction
- Increases glucose tolerance
- Increases sensitivity to insulin
- Often decreases appetite and the desire to overeat
- Increases HDL cholesterol (the good kind)
- Usually decreases LDL and VLDL cholesterol (the bad kinds)
- Improves sleep
- Increases stamina and energy
- Stimulates a more balanced breathing pattern
- Increases interest in healthful pursuits
- Helps eliminate cellulite and fat interlaid within muscles

A long list of good reasons to complete a regular exercise program, wouldn't you say?

There are three main types of exercise—anaerobic (without oxygen) exercise for muscle strength, size and tone, aerobic (with oxygen) exercise for cardiovascular fitness and aerobic exercise for burning body fat. Few doctors know much about health or fitness, but I still recommend getting a physical checkup prior to beginning any exercise program.

Strength-Building Exercise—the real secret to staying lean

Training for strength and muscle size increases your lean body mass, which raises your metabolism. This means your body will burn more calories 24 hours a day, every day, helping you to stay lean and also to lose excess body fat faster. The average adult loses five to seven pounds of muscle every ten years after about age twenty-five. A loss of lean body mass is very likely part of the reason why you have excess fat. Each pound of muscle raises a moderately active person's metabolic rate by approximately 40 calories a day. If you regained just five pounds of lost muscle, your body would burn about 200 more calories a day. If your diet and activity level stayed the same, you would lose a pound of fat about every eighteen days. That's 20 pounds in a year.

An effective strength-building program takes hardly any time but yields many valuable benefits. I call one of them the "basic-training" effect. People who enlist in the Army spend the first eight weeks in basic training. The thin recruits gain muscle and shape up their bodies and so do the fat ones. The only difference is that the fat recruits lose excess body fat at the same time. At the end of the training, their bodies all look remarkably similar. The identical physical training increases the appetites of the thin recruits, thereby supplying more nutrients to grow with, but decreases the appetites of the others so stored fat is burned. It has a normalizing effect on their metabolisms and restores the balance Nature intended. Proper strength training has the same balancing effect on your metabolism.

Building muscle strength, size and tone can be accomplished using a variety of resistance exercises. The resistance comes from your body weight in exercises such as push-ups, squats, pull-ups and others like those done in the military. It can also come from exercise machines and free weights (barbells and dumbbells). Strength- and muscle-building exercise is more efficiently done with weights and exercise machines, because the resistance can be easily varied. You can start with less resistance than your body weight and, as you progress, possibly use more than your body weight in certain exercises.

Isometric exercise can be used for strength building, but is ineffective for building muscle size and shape. It is done by contracting a muscle as hard as possible for six seconds against an immovable object. Nothing moves during this type of exercise. Isometric exercise builds strength by training the nervous system to contract more muscle fibers at the same time. You learn to use more of the muscle you already have, but do not increase the size of the muscle. It can be useful if done correctly and may be the only form of exercise some people can do. I do not recommend it for most people, because it is not as productive as other forms of exercise.

It is far more productive and beneficial to exercise your muscles through their full ranges of motion. During this form of exercise, your bones and joints move as your muscles contract and stretch. It is called isotonic and is the type of strength-building exercise I will be referring to throughout this book. This is what most people should do, because regaining and then maintaining lost muscle is an important part of staying lean and healthy. Isotonic exercise done *correctly* builds strength *and* increases flexibility.

Many people believe that aerobic exercise is necessary to lose fat. It is not. Proper fat-burning exercise will increase the amount of fat burned, but correct strength training and proper nutrition can produce fast results. This is good news for busy people (most of us) who can spare only two or three hours a week for exercise. With all the aerobics classes and videos that have been around for many years, you would expect to see more lean people but, as you know, the number of fat people is increasing. This is because strength training is the real secret to getting and staying lean. I have seen many people at the gym get on an aerobic kick to lose weight. Because few of them do strength training, or use a low intensity level when they do, they get smaller but not necessarily leaner. Whatever they lose is primarily the result of dieting, because the intensity of most aerobics classes is so high that no fat is burned. The aerobics is ineffective at helping people maintain their lean body mass, and because of improper nutrition, most of them lose muscle tissue along with some fat. Losing the muscle mass slows their metabolisms, making it easier to gain fat. Before long, most of them are right back to the same body weight but with an even higher fat percentage.

Follow a regular schedule of strength training and add a couple of weekly cardiovascular training sessions to it. Cardiovascular training is explained in the next section. If you like them, aerobics classes or videos are fine for your cardiovascular training, but they must be done only in addition to your strength-training program. Even with good nutrition, the latest aerobic fad will do almost nothing to help you get and stay lean. You must regain and then maintain your muscle mass with strength training. Besides adding muscle to increase your metabolism 24 hours a day, strength-building exercise has by far the most dramatic effect on increasing your metabolism during and after exercise.

In 1986 I moved to California and began working at a health club prior to starting my own fitness training and nutritional counseling business. The health club management wanted all male instructors to have body fat levels of 15 percent or less. Because I had lived initially in a motel for a number of weeks, I had no choice but to eat most of my meals at less-than-ideal restaurants. (No fast food, of course.) When my body fat was tested, it was 17 percent. Not bad but higher than it had been. I completed three to four hours a week of strength training, along with cutting back slightly on meats and grains and eating more fruits and vegetables. The exercise program and minor dietary changes reduced my body fat level to 7.3 percent in just three months. I did not use any "fat-burning" supplements or do any aerobic or fat-burning exercise. This is an example of why strength training is by far the most important and productive form of exercise to do if you want to get lean and stay that way. Currently my body fat percentage is less than 10 percent.

Correct training for strength and muscle size has numerous other health benefits. It can reverse many of the symptoms often attributed to old age. It increases the transit time of food through the gastrointestinal tract. This, along with the dietary fiber from legumes, whole grains, fruits, vegetables and other natural foods, improves elimination and decreases the risk of colon cancer. Strength training stimulates the production of testosterone and growth hormone. These hormones increase your metabolism and have powerful anti-aging effects. Testosterone plays a major role in sex drive and performance for both men *and* women (an important benefit you should be happy with). A study comparing the muscles of lifelong swimmers and runners with those of bodybuilders found that only the older bodybuilders' muscles looked like the muscles of young people. William Evans, chief of the human physiology lab at the Human Nutrition Research Center on Aging at Tufts University, believes strength training to be the single most important step for retarding the aging process. I agree.

In some areas of the world, people consistently stay healthy for more than one hundred years. Their diets vary widely so it is not the yogurt or other "miracle" food. The nutritional similarities they have are that they do not overeat and they eat simple meals of whole, natural foods available in their environment. Does this sound familiar? Something else common to all these people is the "vigorous" labor they do regularly.

Strength training strengthens the heart muscle so it has more contractile force when it beats. Increased muscle strength and tone decreases stress on your heart, because once blood has circulated to your feet and hands there is no pressure to move the blood back to your heart. It is squeezed back up by muscular contractions in your arms and legs. Those who do not keep their calf and thigh muscles strong often have edema (pooling of fluid) in their feet and ankles. Walking is ineffective for keeping the muscles strong enough unless perhaps it is up steep hills and done frequently. Varicose veins can also be prevented by keeping the muscles of the lower body strong and toned. During strength training, even the muscles of your arteries are exercised and get stronger. This may reduce your risk of aortic rupture and other forms of vascular failure.

Every physical activity is easier and less stressful if you have greater strength. Increased strength enables you to do many of the same activities you did when you were younger. If you are as strong at seventy as you were at forty (excluding joint injuries), you should be able to be just as active. I am stronger now than I was twenty years ago and I was exercising regularly then. The shape of my physique is also better now and it was good then. Most of the people barely getting around with the help of canes and walkers could throw them away and walk normally if they just strengthened a few muscles with a month or two of proper exercise. Even studies using minimally effective exercises have proven this. Strength-building exercises also put stress on your bones, supplying the demand for your body to keep them strong. This is helpful for preventing or reversing osteoporosis. To stay strong, bones need exercise just as regularly as muscles.

Another important benefit of strength training is that it makes your muscles more resistant to damage from repetitive stress or trauma. Your body repairs muscle damage with fibrotic adhesions (scar tissue). This shortens your muscles and can eventually cause joint imbalances, pain and reduced flexibility. It is the cause of almost all musculoskeletal conditions. Proper resistance training increases your flexibility along with your strength and can sometimes help certain joint problems. Increased flexibility also makes your muscles more resistant to injury. On the other hand, aerobic exercise almost always exacerbates joint imbalances. This has happened to hundreds of my patients prior to them coming to see me.

When body fat is lost, the skin often gets loose because the excess fat has stretched it. This can make people feel flabbier and perhaps think they look worse than before they lost the fat. Some people let this discourage them, so they abandon their goals and gain fat to tighten the skin. Exercising to build some muscle size and shape, and improve circulation helps your body tighten the skin faster. Exercise also helps smooth out the distribution of subcutaneous fat and reduces cellulite. The good nutrition your skin will be getting is also helpful. There is a special supplement that I believe helps the skin tighten faster. It is a liquid protein made from pre-digested collagen. This product contains the nutrients your body needs to form the collagen necessary to tighten the skin. A tablespoonful after each strength-training session and another just prior to bedtime should be helpful. The herb gotu kola is also good for the skin and is claimed to prevent and help rid the body of cellulite.

Eventually you will experience another valuable benefit of strength training. As your physical strength increases, you will start seeing yourself as a stronger person mentally and emotionally as well. This may help you to resolve your emotional reason for being fat. You may become motivated to get a better job or start challenging yourself mentally and end up accomplishing far more in life than you otherwise would have.

Many people go to gyms and health clubs with the goal of building muscle strength, size and tone. Sadly, few of them have even the slightest idea of how to train to achieve their goals. Many push and pull and grunt and groan for years with little, if anything, to show for all their time and effort. Lack of results is the main reason why so many people quit. I have had hundreds of fat people tell me they *used* to exercise. In my experience, few of those who call themselves fitness trainers know how to train efficiently or safely. They just teach inefficient methods they have learned. The primary keys to successful strength training are described in chapter fifteen.

Cardiovascular Exercise

Cardiovascular (CV) exercise trains the body to uptake and use oxygen more effectively. Providing more oxygen to your body keeps your normal cells healthy and helps prevent the development of an unbalanced environment where abnormal cells can grow. Cardiovascular exercise enlarges your heart chambers so more blood is pumped with each beat, thereby requiring your heart to beat fewer times to pump the same amount of blood. This is why your resting heart rate will decrease when you get in better cardiovascular condition.

Aerobic fitness is developed by doing a repetitive activity such as walking fast or running (outdoors or on a treadmill) for approximately 30 minutes at a time. Bicycle riding (outdoors or on a stationary bike), swimming, aerobics classes, using a stair-climbing machine, cross-country skiing machine, climbing machine or similar types of aerobic-training equipment are also good. Hiking would be excellent. New types of aerobics classes are being marketed regularly. I recommend the exercises that put low impact on the weight-bearing joints, but people tend to do what they enjoy the most. It is better to do a variety so it is more interesting and your joints get less of the same stress. This is known as cross-training.

High-impact exercises can cause new muscle and joint injuries or aggravate existing ones, especially if you have structural imbalances in your feet, ankles, knees, hips, pelvis or lower back. A joint problem may force you to stop doing any form of exercise, so it is usually best to do high-impact exercises infrequently, if you do them at all. I do not recommend running more than once or twice a week. Some people carry weights in their hands as they walk in an attempt to make the exercise more beneficial. I advise against doing this, because it is stressful on the shoulder joints and muscles. A safe way to increase the intensity of walking is to wear a weighted vest or belt or a backpack with weights or books in it.

The most efficient way to train for cardiovascular fitness is to make the exercise strenuous enough to get your heart rate into what is called the "training zone" for about 20 minutes. Your training zone is between 70 and 85 percent of your maximum heart rate, which is determined by subtracting your age from 220. For example, if you are fifty years of age, your maximum heart rate would be 170 (220 minus 50) beats per minute (bpm). Therefore, your training zone would be between 119 bpm (70 percent of 170) and 144.5 bpm (85 percent of 170). Round those figures to 120 and 144 and divide them by 4 to determine how many beats in 15 seconds. Take your pulse for 15 seconds while you are training. It should be between 30 (120 divided by 4) and 36 (144 divided by 4).

Start your CV training with a low intensity warm-up for about five minutes. Then increase the intensity to get your heart rate in the training zone. Train at that level for 20 minutes and then decrease the intensity and do a five-minute cool-down. The first time you train, you should do only about five minutes at your lower training zone heart rate. Gradually build the time up over a few weeks until you reach 20 minutes. After that, increase the intensity each session from the lower (70%) level to the upper (85%) level. Give yourself at least three to six weeks to build up to 20 minutes at your upper level. Training this way three or four times a week will increase your CV fitness quickly. Training twice a week should then be sufficient to maintain your fitness level.

Unless you are training for some sport or endurance event, more than 60 to 90 minutes of intense aerobics each week is essentially a waste of time. Using your time for strength training has numerous benefits, but excessive aerobics has hardly any and may even lead to an overstress injury or slower progress because it can lower your testosterone levels.

You now know the basics of training for CV fitness. This is all most people will ever need. If you want to train for specific aerobic activities, I suggest reading a book on the subject or consulting with a competent physical trainer. The advice should be similar to what you have just learned. Look for help elsewhere if it is not. Cardiovascular fitness will be covered in my book about proper exercise along with how to do strength training, bodybuilding/shaping, and fat-burning exercise safely and efficiently. I was a personal fitness trainer for ten years and have been training with weights for more than thirty-seven years. I was a karate instructor for two years and have taught productive and safe exercise programs to patients for more than eleven years. For information about my planned exercise book, get in touch with the publisher of this book.

Millions of aerobics classes have been attended and millions of aerobics videos purchased and followed by people who believed that these things would help them lose weight. Disappointment is what most of these people have gotten for their time and money. There are aerobics instructors out there who teach ten or more classes a week and have fat bodies. What do you think two or three classes a week are going to do for you?

Cardiovascular training makes you feel better physically and emotionally but burns little, if any, fat in most people. It will increase your metabolism for an hour or two after doing it but that will burn almost no fat. Many people and some fitness "experts" believe that CV training burns fat, but this has not been my experience. Numerous women have asked me why they have not lost any fat after months or even years of doing four to six hours a week of intense aerobic exercise. They wondered why burning all those calories did not result in any lost body fat. They also asked why their buttocks had not gotten firmer and shapelier. I explained to them that strength training is necessary to firm and shape muscles, and that during intense aerobic exercise the body usually uses glucose for energy, because it is a fast-burning fuel. All the calories they had burned were replaced with their next meal. On the other hand, fat is a slow-burning fuel the body can burn for energy only when the intensity of the exercise is low enough. People often assume more is better but this is not always true. Now let's discuss how to exercise to burn fat.

Fat-Burning Exercise

Fat burning can be done using most of the same exercises as CV training but at a lower intensity. Examples are walking instead of running and riding a bike at a lower intensity. Riding a stationary bicycle has tested as the most result-producing fat-burning exercise with walking a close second. Swimming is ineffective for this purpose and can even cause a gain in body fat to insulate you and increase your buoyancy. This is how your body attempts to protect you or make the activity more efficient. Some aerobic training machines are difficult to use at a low intensity. Experiment with different ones and use some variety if you can.

As a general rule, a heat rate of 110 to 120 bpm is best for burning body fat. You may burn fat at a slightly higher intensity, but I do not recommend exceeding 120 bpm if losing fat is your goal. If your heart rate is more than 60 percent of your maximum, the body starts using more carbohydrate for energy and less fat. Body fat burning can be done five or six times a week or even more if you have the time. If your body fat percentage is at a healthy level, you do not need to do any fat-burning exercise.

Fat-burning exercise takes more time than CV training, because your body needs 15 to 20 minutes to shift into the fat-burning mode. Because of this delay it is usually recommended to spend at least 60 minutes at each session. Fat-burning exercise is best done immediately after your strength-training workout, because your body will start to burn fat for energy much sooner. It saves time if scheduled this way. Forty minutes of fat-burning exercise done after your strength program will burn about the same amount of fat as a one-hour session done at another time. Fat-burning exercise also has cardiovascular training effects. Therefore, strength training and fat burning (if desired) would be the best combination to get lean. To stay lean you only need your strength training, but I would recommend also doing some CV training. It is usually best to do CV training on a different day than strength training. Your strength training will be more productive and you will end up doing some form of exercise five or six days a week.

Many people believe running is a great way to lose body fat, but as you have just learned, it is not. It is good cardiovascular exercise but the intensity is usually too high to burn any fat. People have asked me, "Why then is the marathon winner so thin?" The best runners are extremely thin, because they are ectomorphic and naturally built to be good long-distance runners. It is the same reason why a well-built seven-foot-tall man makes a much better basketball player than jockey. Watch the Los Angeles or New York marathon sometime and you will see that many people who run in marathons are not that lean. Some runners are lean because the body gradually adapts to the activity being done. For example, someone who swims often will usually develop a streamlined body shape and may even gain fat for better buoyancy. As you have learned, this is why swimming is ineffective for fat burning even though it is fine for CV training. Frequently running long distances stimulates the body to get lighter so the activity can be done more efficiently. The body loses fat *and* muscle to accomplish this goal. This is why you do not see good long-distance runners with large muscles. In contrast, sprinters have large muscles to give them the power necessary to run fast for short distances.

If you have a large amount of body fat to lose and you have the time, doing strength training six days a week with 45 minutes of fat burning after each session would give fast results. Most of us cannot spare the time to do this much exercise. Completing three or four strength-training sessions a week is best for most of us but good progress could be made with only two sessions a week. Fat-burning exercise can be added if time permits. Remember that fat-burning exercise will help you lose fat if you are eating an alkaline or balanced pH diet, but I have seen many people spend years doing fat-burning exercise with no results. The way they ate countered any progress they may have made. You can easily lose fat without exercising if you eat properly but will usually experience minimal results with fat-burning exercise alone.

Structural Balance

Structural balance plays a vital role in your health. For example, vertebral misalignments in your spine cause inflammation that puts pressure on the spinal nerves that carry messages between your brain and internal organs, muscles, blood vessels and all other structures. If a nerve is irritated, it can over-stimulate an area causing excessive function or increased sensitivity. This can create problems such as allergies, colitis (inflammation of the colon) and miscarriages. Sometimes pressure on a nerve acts like someone stepping on a water hose and decreasing the flow. This leads to diminished function of the organ, muscle, gland or other structure that the nerve innervates. Abnormal nerve flow can dramatically affect the digestion, assimilation or utilization of the food you eat. If the nerve to your colon is affected, it can cause constipation. Digestive and elimination problems can cause a build-up of waste and toxins in your system. You may also be stimulated to eat more to get the nutrients your body needs.

Decreased nerve flow to your thyroid gland can reduce its function, making it difficult to lose and easy to gain excess fat. If your thyroid gland is over-stimulated, it can speed up your metabolism and make you thin and nervous. A structural imbalance in a joint of your body, such as your spine, hip, knee or shoulder, causes either tendinitis, bursitis, osteoarthritis, or neuritis. All structural imbalances increase stress and cause an energy drain that robs you of vitality and uses up certain nutrients more rapidly. This can possibly cause nutritional deficiencies and decrease any desire to exercise. Many structural imbalances make it impossible to exercise.

I have discovered that the cause of almost all structural imbalances are muscles and tendons (sometimes ligaments) that have been damaged by either an injury or repetitive overstress. As mentioned earlier, your body heals the damage with fibrotic adhesions to prevent further injury. The accumulation of adhesions causes the muscle to become shorter than normal. When it reaches a threshold level, it gets tight enough to either pull the bone it is attached to out of normal alignment or cause stress at the muscle's attachment points. This leads to inflammation, pain and abnormal joint function. Joint misalignments and tight muscles irritate bursae, tendons, cartilage or nerves, and cause tendinitis, bursitis, degenerative joint disease (DJD, a.k.a. osteoarthritis) and neuritis. Prior to reaching the threshold level, muscles just feel gradually stiffer and tighter.

I have experienced many injuries and misaligned joints. I suffered with my first injury for more than twenty-three years and with the last injury for fourteen years. The various treatments I received (approximately 1,500) sometimes gave me temporary relief, but for the most part did nothing but tear the muscles more, thereby making the existing problems worse and creating new ones. I have even had surgery to both knees and my lower back. In 1990, driven by pain and frustration, I developed my Precision Muscle Balancing Technology[SM] therapy. Using it I was able to realign my joints and eliminate the pains I had endured for so many years. Since then I have relieved the chronic pain and suffering of thousands of patients and straightened out scoliotic spines, dowager's humps, arthritic fingers and resolved many other conditions most doctors believe impossible to correct. Some patients lost fat rapidly after a particular neck vertebra was realigned and normal nerve flow was restored to the thyroid gland. Their metabolisms increased and this quickly burned off the excess body fat they had been fighting to lose. Often, few changes were made to their diets or activity levels.

Some people do not have major structural misalignments but almost everyone has areas of chronic tension. The lower back and the area between the neck and shoulders are the most common and most people have tight hamstrings and calves. These can all be resolved by restoring the muscles back to their original lengths. Improper sleeping and sitting postures are the most frequent causes of these muscles getting tight. Sometimes people have an injury or postural habit that causes muscle damage on one side of their bodies. After compensating and striving to achieve balance, their bodies gradually develop damage on the other side as well. This is often how chronically tight areas develop. The physical tension created can dramatically increase stress levels and may cause some people to overeat. My PMBT treatments can make people feel thirty or forty years younger than they are. I hope to train doctors worldwide someday so that more people can get the treatments and pain relief they need.

Because the key to structural alignment and balance is normal length of muscles and ligaments, stretching can be beneficial to keep your joints healthier. Proper strength training increases your flexibility dramatically but additional stretching can be done. See chapter fifteen for information on the best time to stretch. Yoga is excellent and is especially good for stretching the muscles of the spine. If you choose to practice it, learn from a qualified instructor or progress gently and slowly after learning from a book or video. You can cause muscle damage attempting to become more flexible too quickly.

Develop an awareness of your posture and body usage. Notice if you hold the telephone between your shoulder and ear, or if you stand or sit in odd positions. Poor postural and body usage habits cause a gradual build-up of muscle damage until enough finally accumulates to cause chronic misalignments. Essentially, the last straw has been added to the camel's back. Books give instruction in, and people teach a method called the Alexander Technique. This technique was developed by F. M. Alexander (no relation to me) and is about sitting, standing, lying and moving with good body balance and posture. It teaches how to put the least amount of stress on your joints and muscles during repetitive activities. This is an extremely valuable thing to learn. Practicing the Alexander Technique reduces your stress and helps prevent repetitive stress muscle damage that can eventually cause musculoskeletal imbalances and impaired nerve flow.

Stretching cannot eliminate the fibrotic adhesions that cause structural misalignments but frequently gives some temporary relief. Because of this, it should be obvious that the cause is tight muscles. The only thing I know of that can permanently correct almost all joint imbalances is PMBT. Other deep-tissue therapies may help your condition to varying degrees but most of them are extremely limited and too generalized to produce effective and lasting results. Also, after getting these therapies you will rarely be taught how to prevent the muscle damage from recurring.

If you do not have any major structural misalignments, stretching and good body usage should keep your body in relatively good alignment. Prevention is of prime importance and this is what my patients need after their joints have been realigned back to normal. They are instructed in proper body usage and stretching, because this reduces their chances of new muscle injuries. They are also taught the importance of strength training that makes their muscles more resistant to traumatic or overstress injury. Many are taught safe and efficient exercises for all of their major muscles. This information will be in my exercise book.

Emotional Health

Your emotional health is vital to the health of your body, because your mind and body are interconnected. What affects one affects the other. You have already learned about the nerves that travel from your brain through the spinal cord and out at different levels between your vertebrae to your internal organs. These nerves are affected by spinal misalignments. Other nerve and hormone connections from your brain to your internal organs are affected by emotions. You have learned that these connections are what cause "butterflies in your stomach" when you are afraid and poor digestion if you eat when you are angry or upset.

Your emotional health is tremendously influenced by the physical nutrients your brain and body get. Neither can function normally unless adequate nourishment is received. Your self-love, self-image, self-confidence, continued learning and sense of doing something worthwhile in the world also influence your mental and physical health. Your thoughts feed your mind and, like food for the body, cause health or disease. Every thought and feeling has a positive, neutral or negative effect on both your mind and body. Therefore, it is vital to get daily feedings of uplifting, loving thoughts and feelings. Keeping stress to a minimum is also helpful. Here is a brief explanation of the different components of emotional health.

Self-Love

Self-love is in no way selfish, egotistical or narcissistic. On the contrary, loving yourself opens you up to express the true beautiful being you are. Loving yourself is the master key to happiness and peace of mind. All other necessary things (like a lean body) are added relatively easily after this is achieved. The more you love yourself the more your worldly life will blossom. You will be able to truly give love to others and fully accept it from them. Until you love yourself, you will not believe that anyone—even your Creator—really loves you. Until you feel you deserve a lean and healthy body, it will never happen and then only to the degree that you love yourself. I am referring to true divine love.

Divine love is simply accepting yourself 100 percent unconditionally as you are now without any judgment, self-condemnation or need to change. The beauty and simplicity of divine love is that it is unconditional. You can love yourself even if you dislike everything about yourself and the life you have created. Once you truly love yourself, it is easy to see *and* change things about yourself that you dislike. Loving yourself is the first step to improving any part of your life and the greatest thing you can ever learn. It is the number one need we all have.

You cannot love yourself until you learn to stop judging, because after judgment comes punishment. If you judge yourself unworthy to live in a lean and healthy body, you will punish yourself by sabotaging any progress you may occasionally make. Do you love any friends or family members with fat bodies? At least love yourself as much. Realize now that you are not any of the roles you play in life (employer, employee, parent, spouse, son, daughter, sibling, uncle, aunt, grandparent, colonel, lawyer, doctor, janitor, mayor and others). In reality you are much, much more. You have a purpose for being here and you deserve to inhabit a lean and healthy body as Nature intended. Being in touch with Nature helps you to fulfill your purpose and to help others fulfill theirs as well. Eating well, losing excess fat and internal waste, and enjoying improved health helps you get more in touch with your true inner nature. Stop wasting time with futile weight-loss attempts. We were not intended to spend our lives on such pursuits. It is time to get on with the important things of life.

You are also not your past thoughts, feelings or actions. They have influenced how you have labeled, judged and punished yourself, but they are not who you are. You are a being with the power to change your thinking, feelings, actions and perceptions whenever you choose. The power was given to each of us; all we have to do is feel worthy to use it to create the benefits we deserve. When you love yourself, you feel worthy to experience joy in your life, and feelings of joy create positive vibrations that attract what you want. The secret is to let our true inner spirit constantly create what we need instead of letting our worldly programmed ego create what will never really satisfy us. This will happen naturally when you stop focusing your attention on what you don't want and start enjoying the gift of life you have been given.

Self-Image

Your self-image is how you view yourself. It has nothing to do with your true capabilities or how others see you. You may be extremely capable at something and others may see you that way, but you may feel like a dismal failure. You must realize that you live your life based on who you think you are—your perception—not who you really are. To have a healthy self-image you must eliminate the labels you have placed on yourself as a child and throughout your life. This will move your perception closer to the truth, because labels create limitations and prevent expression of your true self and capabilities.

Experiencing your true self-image requires being extremely objective and completely honest with yourself. You must see yourself truly as you are and not as you falsely believe you are. You have programmed (hypnotized) yourself into believing you are something other than what you really are. Once you start to look honestly at yourself, you will easily see the past programming that is controlling your negative behaviors. As your thoughts and actions improve, your past programming will gradually fade away and your self-image will become closer to the truth. A better self-image is important to help you learn and follow a healthful nutritional program and is a vital part of the permanent fat loss process. More about self-image is included in chapter twelve.

Self-Confidence

Self-confidence is the number one quality people look for when searching for a mate. It is important for success in all areas of life. Self-confidence is built on the foundation of a good self-image and is further developed by regularly stepping out of your comfort zone and pushing yourself to do more than you have done in the past. Strength training is a good example of this and an excellent way to learn this habit you can then apply to different areas of your life. Start experiencing more of life by doing things yourself instead of watching others. An entire chapter about developing self-confidence can be found in my book, *How To Be Macho*, written under the pseudonym T.R. Llove. Do not let the title fool you. It is about balanced personal development for men and women. You can learn more about its contents on my Web site.

Self-confidence improves your mental and physical health by helping you gradually change your dietary habits as you get more attuned to your needs and develop the best nutritional program for you. It also helps get you to the gym or health club regularly to complete your exercise sessions.

Creative Expression, Learning and Change

Another vital key to happiness and emotional health and well-being is creative self-expression. Some people have occupations where they can regularly express creativity, and for this reason, they usually enjoy their work. Unfortunately, many people are unable to express creativity through their occupations. It is imperative that these people develop a regular creative outlet. It may be playing a musical instrument, woodworking, photography, ceramics, painting, woodcarving, drawing, writing, gardening or other pursuits. We all need healthy and positive ways to express our creativity. If this need is not being met, we usually feel depressed and unhappy, and our lives seem unfulfilled. Another way to express this need is by developing your own special meals. You can create unique taste treats and make eating healthfully an even more enjoyable experience.

Learning is another pursuit that creates joy and gives meaning to life. It exercises your mind and gives you something new and exciting to look forward to each day. Learning new things helps keep us young and celebrating the adventure we call life. You can learn a countless number of things and millions of books and classes are available to help you do it. The more you learn, the more your confidence, self-image and creative ability will improve, leading to greater emotional health and happiness. Study and learn about things you truly enjoy and you will never be bored.

Learn to see the truth of what is happening in your life and *act* accordingly. Do not *react* using false thinking and behavioral patterns created in the past. This causes you to live your life like a robot instead of expressing your true self in each new moment. Various ways to free yourself from past programming are explained in an upcoming chapter.

Many people fear change so they constantly resist it. The fear prevents them from learning and growing and experiencing the joy and excitement life has to offer. Resisting change causes them to become rigid in their thinking and behaviors. This makes them feel isolated from others, bored and unhappy. These people often create excess fat, poor health and rapid aging for themselves. Life without change is boring and boredom is a major cause of depression and overeating. Sadly, many people create unhappiness, fat bodies and ill health simply because they lack the joy and excitement that learning brings. Some are literally bored to death. Never stop learning about life and love and continue discovering what foods and combinations of foods you enjoy and the ones that give you the most energy and vitality.

Get excited about and embrace change. Realize that your life is constantly changing. Change makes life new and exciting and keeps you growing and adapting. Accepting change is an exciting and wondrous learning experience.

Embrace and enjoy change and you embrace and enjoy life. If you have this attitude about life, yours will constantly be changing for the better.

Feed Your Mind Healthy Thoughts

Just as your body needs nutritious foods to keep it lean and healthy, your mind needs positive and uplifting thoughts to keep it healthy. Learning new positive things and expressing your creativity are two other nutrients your mind needs to stay strong and healthy.

Think positive. You have heard this before, but when I say it, I mean something different from what is commonly thought. Many people believe that positive thinking means attempting to fool themselves into believing something they know is not true. This "positive thinking" is not believed by your mind and usually backfires, creating more negativity. You may say a positive affirmation ten times a day but if you do not feel you deserve it, you will not believe it and will subconsciously affirm the opposite a hundred times. Besides not working, this way of thinking is detrimental to your self-image, because it makes you feel like a liar—pretending to be something you are not.

True positive thinking is simply seeing the positive value in everyone (especially yourself), everything around you, every incident and every other part of your life. It is seeing and focusing on all the wonderful positive things being done by you and others. Always find the positive value in whatever happens to you. You are being given a learning experience. Learn your lesson the first time and you can move on to better things instead of repeating the same lesson over and over. No matter how tragic an event may seem, a seed of positive potential always exists. Every cloud has a silver lining. It just takes practice to learn how to see, appreciate and learn from it.

As you feed your mind more positive thoughts through what you see, hear and do, your thinking will become more balanced and healthier. All things in your life will become easier. Your healthier mind and body will improve your self-image, which will lead you to make better food choices and to think more positive and uplifting thoughts. I believe that thoughts are the most powerful creative force in the universe. Every action starts with a thought and everything ever created started with a thought. Thoughts create the feelings that create the vibrations that attract what you are thinking about. Your thoughts are the secrets to your success in all areas of life including being healthy, strong and lean. Do not waste your time (life) with negative, destructive thoughts. The moment you waste will never come again.

Another important key to having a healthy mind is to stop feeding it garbage. Just like your body, if you feed your mind garbage, it creates problems and accumulates waste. Garbage thoughts lead to garbage behaviors that waste your time and attract unhealthy things into your life. Any garbage you put in your body or mind is doing you harm and taking up space where good foods or good thoughts could have been. Be extremely selective about the people you associate with, the books and other material you read, and the movies and television programs you watch. They all have either a positive or negative influence on you and your life. Seek out the positive influences that help create emotional health and happiness and aid you in accomplishing your goals.

Reduce Stress

Stress comes in three forms: physical, mental and emotional. Many physical stresses like manual work and exercise are good for us, because they release tension and stimulate our bodies to adapt and get stronger. But some physical stresses like poor posture, carrying things on one shoulder or hip, sitting or standing excessively, wearing high-heeled shoes, sleeping on the stomach, holding a telephone between the ear and shoulder and many others cause excessive stress and strain to our muscles and joints. The resultant muscle damage and scar tissue formation leads to tighter muscles and even more stress. This often leads to chronic problems, as you have already learned. Physical imbalances and tight muscles drain your energy. This affects your daily activities and makes it harder to exercise at all and less effective if you do. You accomplish less and avoid activities you would enjoy. You may eat more, use stimulants or do deep breathing exercises in an attempt to fight your fatigue. These just add to the problem. Fatigue and sedentary living (often caused by the fatigue) are common stressors that often lead to overeating.

Ingesting the substances discussed in chapter four (your enemies) creates a tremendous amount of physical stress. First, they stress your internal organs when you ingest them and then they make your organs work harder in an attempt to eliminate them from your body. This also creates fatigue and possibly overeating, increased use of stimulants and a lack of desire to exercise. Second, because these substances do not supply good nutrition, your body is forced to work without proper fuel and raw materials. This causes more fatigue. Third, these enemies deplete nutrients you already have and this compounds the second problem. Fourth, without proper nutrition your brain's ability to cope with physical, mental and emotional stresses is greatly reduced. Fifth, these substances create imbalances (illness) your body must expend energy to attempt to resolve. This causes even more fatigue. Can you see how these substances create a negative cycle that can make you fat and feel terrible physically and emotionally?

Some psychologists and psychiatrists who do marriage and family counseling believe that poor nutrition is involved in 75 percent or more of all their patients' problems. They saw relationships improve dramatically in a short time after those involved stopped eating refined flour products, sugar and caffeine. They believe that many of them were affected with hypoglycemia, which can cause irritability, fatigue, apathy, bad temper and numerous other symptoms detrimental to a happy life and harmonious relationships.

If the ninth thoracic vertebra of the spine is misaligned, it can affect the nerve flow to the adrenal glands and possibly stimulate an excess release of epinephrine. This will make someone feel tense most of the time. Some of my patients' stress levels were greatly reduced after this bone was aligned correctly by removing the cause of why it was misaligned.

Fortunately, most harmful physical stresses can be reduced or avoided with a little knowledge and desire. For example, if you sit for long hours on your job, make sure you sit up straight in a good chair with a firm foundation and a lumbar support. Keep your head up by tilting your work up 30 to 40 degrees and your eyes down. Position your computer monitor directly in front of you and high enough so the center of the screen is at eye level or slightly higher. Make sure it is close enough so you do not have to lean forward to see it. Sleep on your back on a firm mattress and use a good cervical pillow to maintain the normal curve of your neck. This is by far the best sleeping position. If you sleep on your side, learn how to do it with the least amount of stress on your body. Avoid sleeping on your stomach. A tremendous amount of stress will be eliminated if you do not ingest the substances discussed in chapter four.

Mental stress comes from things that require us to think excessively. This is the stress we have when learning large amounts of information or solving complex problems. This stress is not harmful and usually just requires sleep or a change of activity so the brain can organize what is being learned. Like strength training, it is a healthy stress that helps us grow and get stronger. Boredom, on the other hand, is an unhealthy mental stress that often leads to overeating.

Another form of stress is emotional. This is the big bad boogeyman most of us fear. Let's take a look at how big and bad this boogeyman really is. Most emotional stress comes from the difference between what you have and what you want. Think for a moment. You have the power to change what you want, thereby eliminating the difference and your emotional stress. You also have the power to change what you have, although you may not believe it or know how to do it yet. And remember, you have to feel you deserve something better before you will have it. Emotional stress should be relatively easy to eliminate. You can change either what you have to match what you want or what you want to match what you have. Please do not get the wrong idea. I am not proposing that you resign yourself to what you have now. That is the opposite of what I am suggesting. By accepting what you have, like accepting who you are, you free yourself from fighting the stress boogeyman. Now you have the time and energy to focus on and create the things you want. Remember, just because you accept (and appreciate) what you currently have does not mean you are not working toward achieving greater goals.

Perfectionism is another source of emotional stress. Because perfection is unattainable, constantly attempting to achieve it is stressful and negatively affects your self-worth, because you or anything you do will never be good enough. Learn to differentiate between what needs to be done well and what doesn't and then *strive for excellence* in the important areas of your life.

An important key to progressing in life is setting goals. The trick is to set goals with your heart (true self) instead of your worldly programmed mind. Some people have created wealth, power and fame using their minds but have ended up being miserable and feeling empty inside. Your worldly mind does not know what will make you, a spiritual being, happy, but your inner self does.

Another cause of emotional stress comes from not differentiating between real and imagined threats to your physical and emotional safety. Whenever you have a fear, your breathing intensifies, leading to more stress and less ability to cope with it. This problem can usually be resolved simply by breathing less so your carbon dioxide level increases and more oxygen goes to your cells. Your thinking will then improve and you will be better able to deal with your current situation.

An extremely powerful way to eliminate emotional stress is to count your blessings and accept and be thankful for what you have (and for who you are). If you do this, your inner self will set the right goals for you and create more blessings for you. Unfortunately, what most of us do is complain about what we do not have. In this instance our mind creates more lack and more problems for us to complain about. Ask and you shall receive. Complain and attract more reasons to complain, or give thanks and attract more blessings to be thankful for and enjoy. The choice is yours.

Each different form of stress influences the others, so do not underestimate the power of a simple physical stress reliever like a hot bath or taking a walk. Relaxing can help you get in touch with your inner spirit and help you see and appreciate what you have. Improving your thinking and finding something positive in everything is also a great stress reducer.

Eliminate or reduce sources of negative stress such as excess noise, advertising pollution, disorder, over-breathing, information overload and negative stories and people. Avoid watching the evening news. It is mostly bad news that will prevent you from sleeping well and does not generate uplifting thoughts for your mind to think about all night. Do not focus on the negative events happening in the world. This creates more negative energy and makes situations worse. Think about how you want your life and the world to be and your positive thoughts will send out energy that will improve them both.

Mute out commercials when watching television—especially the ones for soft drinks, drugs, alcohol, fast foods and junk foods. Be selective and reduce the amount of television you watch. This will give you time to exercise, express your creativity or learn something. Be a more active participant in life instead of watching others act out true or fictional stories. When traveling in your car, listen to tapes or CDs with inspiring messages or to those that teach you something. This reduces the stress of driving in traffic and makes you feel good about using your time wisely. You can even do this if you are riding the bus or using another form of transportation. Read to learn new things and for entertainment. The book is always better than the movie, because reading exercises your imagination. Develop the habit of reading positive, inspirational messages prior to going to sleep each night.

If you cannot eliminate an emotional stress, an effective way to reduce it is to exercise. Stress activates our sympathetic nervous systems. Unfortunately, most of the time we are unable to dissipate the tension this creates. Exercise eliminates the tension so we can relax. It also stimulates the release of endorphins and other chemicals that make us feel better. Exercise helps us get more in touch with our bodies' needs and makes us feel more alive. It helps normalize our appetites and metabolisms.

We all have emotional and mental stresses. After all, we are not supposed to lead dull lives devoid of challenges and problems to solve, because that is how we grow and progress. The secret is to balance these stresses with the physical stress of hard physical work or exercise. Once again, balance is what we need. Without this balance, the other stresses will have negative effects on our bodies, minds and lives.

If you are shooting raging rapids or nearing the top of a waterfall in a boat with no motor or oars, water can be intensely stressful. Most often, however, water is soothing and relaxing. A bubbling hot tub or a warm bath or shower can all reduce tension and stress. Jump in a pool and swim or exercise and you get the additional benefits of exercise. Listening to or watching a babbling brook or the endless waves at the beach can also reduce stress, whether you are there in person or experiencing it with audio or video recordings.

Music can be a wonderful stress reliever. A beautiful operatic aria or classical music piece can be relaxing while supplying a large portion of soul food. Soul food is explained in the next section. You may sometimes prefer the upbeat music of your youth. The kind that makes you feel positive, alive and like singing or dancing. If possible, go dancing and get the additional benefits of exercise. Go ahead and sing in the shower even if your singing would make a dog howl. Make yourself a few customized cassette tapes or CDs of some of your favorite feel-good music. Listen to them when driving or doing tasks where the words of the songs will not distract you. You can listen to classical or instrumental music when doing things requiring more concentration. I often listened to my classical favorites while editing this book. Avoid discordant, depressing or excessively loud music.

Get outside more and surround yourself with the many wonders of Nature. Observing the beauty and wonderful balance of Nature helps you to get more centered and balanced. It also helps you to realize that you are an important part of this incredible adventure we call life. Being in beautiful natural surroundings helps slow your vibrations down to normal. The rhythm of the earth is approximately 8 cycles per second. Unfortunately, the majority of us are surrounded by energy fields of 60 cycles per second created by the electrical wiring in the walls of the buildings where we work and live. We are also exposed to lights and electronic equipment pulsating at that accelerated rate.

These faster vibrations cause unhealthy stress. I recommend keeping your electric alarm clock at least two feet away from you when sleeping.

Sitting by a stream in the woods is peaceful and relaxing, because it reestablishes the natural vibration and rhythm of your body. It usually also slows your breathing rate and, if you are not blocking it, you will get the health benefits of natural light. Another reason it is relaxing is the rhythmic sound and lack of discordant noise. Even listening to the sounds of nature on a recording can be relaxing.

Televisions, some computer monitors and certain other electronic devices create positive ions in the air that can cause us to feel tired and depressed. Having a negative ion generator nearby can balance out the excess of positive ions and reduce your stress level, fatigue and depression. Negative ions are what make the air seem fresh and clean after it rains or when you are near a waterfall. Many air filters and purifiers produce negative ions.

Sex is always a physical stress release and when shared with the right person, for the right reasons, can reduce emotional stress and supply a healthy dose of soul food. This is when it is appropriately called making love. But sexual union with the wrong person or for the wrong reasons can cause a great deal of emotional stress. Like everything else, sex can produce positive or negative results depending on how it is used.

Do your best to determine what causes the most stress for you. If it is anger turned internally, learn how to express it in a positive way or at least disperse it. Exercising to release the physical stress created can be helpful, but the best thing to do if possible is to calmly communicate your feelings to the person that you feel made you angry. Keep in mind that you are the only one who can make you angry. It all comes from your thoughts and feelings about yourself and what is happening in your life. Also know that it is a good thing to express anger in positive ways.

Repressed anger causes tremendous emotional stress and can create physical pain or cause you to gain fat as a punishment for having those feelings. It also negatively affects your digestion. Therefore, it is important to rid yourself of any repressed anger. You may be able to eliminate it by talking with a friend, counselor or therapist. The writing method may help you to define the anger and see how to deal with it in a loving way. Then you must forgive the person that the anger is directed toward. I believe that almost all anger is primarily directed at ourselves, so look first at your own thinking, feelings and actions—the only things you have control over.

It is important to learn how to change the way you deal with stresses you cannot eliminate. If your normal reaction is to eat when you feel stressed, walk around the block a few times, dance around the house or do something creative or mentally challenging. *Act* instead of *react* or at least replace the harmful reaction with a healthy one. After you eat, your parasympathetic nervous system directs more blood to your digestive system and less to your brain. Your brain function will decrease and you will not think about your problems as much. This treats your symptom (stress) temporarily but does nothing to get rid of what is causing it. You have learned that eating when stressed leads to poor digestion and a greater chance that the food will not be used. Even good foods can become toxic. Stress eating usually just creates more negative stresses like guilt, self-judgment and feelings of despair or decreased self-worth. This leads to more eating, gaining more fat, more negative emotions and the creation of a negative cycle that works against you.

The best thing to do is eliminate the cause of the stress. If that is not possible, at least learn to dissipate it in a healthy way. Write down all you have to be thankful for, take a soothing warm bath, exercise or read something uplifting. These and other positive actions decrease your stress, improve your self-image and feeling of self-worth. They create a positive cycle that works for you. It is just as easy to create a friend to work for you as it is to create an enemy to work against you.

Keep learning more about yourself and the sources of your emotional stress. Much of it may be caused by poor nutrition and will disappear as you start eating better. Once you determine the root of a problem, you can then develop a plan to eliminate it and its negative effects on you. I plan to write an entire book about the reduction and elimination of stress and achieving emotional health. For information about its availability, get in touch with the publisher of this book.

Do not forget two of the most important stress reducers—controlled slow and shallow breathing and balanced light. The nutrients obtained (full-spectrum light, carbon dioxide and oxygen) have such a tremendous influence on our health and well-being that I cannot emphasize them enough. They do not cost anything. Correct breathing can be done continually and natural light is available daily from either the sun or full-spectrum lights.

Soul Food

Perhaps the most important food on your new dietary program is what I call soul food. Just as organic food, water, air and sunlight feed your physical body and the thoughts you think feed your mind, your feelings feed your soul—the real you who never dies. Your soul is the life energy that just changes form when it leaves your physical body. The health of your soul (spirit) has a tremendous effect on your emotional and physical health. If your soul is starving, you may create physical death from alcohol, drugs, excess fat, or suicide from faster methods. Keeping your spirit well fed may prevent you from being depressed, having a poor self-image and condemning yourself to a life of ill health or being fat. Your spirit contains the divine love you need to succeed and be happy.

How do you feel when you hug someone you truly love? No words or thoughts can express what you feel then or when you see a beautiful flower, incredible sunset or your own baby being born. You cannot describe these feelings, you can only experience them. Loving and positive feelings are what feed your soul and keep it healthy. We are that we might have joy; so keep your soul well fed and your life joyful.

Some people experience many unpleasant and negative feelings that poison their souls. This is detrimental to their emotional and physical health and can create beings so out of touch with their inner spirits that they become capable of terrible, distorted behaviors toward themselves and others. Some feel they deserve to be punished but cannot do it to themselves, so they commit crimes against others and then let society punish them. It is still self-punishment based on a lack of self-love or feeling unworthy of something better.

Other people may not have many negative feelings but are lacking in positive feelings. These people generally experience depression, loneliness, isolation and other feelings that make their lives miserable. They feel an emptiness inside that makes it difficult for anything in life to produce any joy or satisfaction. Some feel unwanted and unloved. Many of them turn to drugs, alcohol, unhealthful foods, overeating or other ways to deaden their feelings. If they cannot feel good, they do not want to feel at all.

Some people overeat because they feel empty inside. Their souls are starving, but because they do not know how to feed them, they attempt to fill their emptiness by feeding their bodies. Sadly, as long as their souls are undernourished, they will keep overfeeding their physical bodies. This is like storing food in the trunk of your car when *you* are starving. It is vital to feed your soul with positive, uplifting and loving feelings. What's great is that you can feed your soul as many good feelings as you want and it will only get healthier, never fat.

Being physically and emotionally healthy, reading uplifting material, listening to beautiful music, enjoying Nature's beauty and socializing with healthy, giving and loving people all give you opportunities to experience feelings that nourish your soul. What you feel when you really "hear" a beautiful piece of classical music cannot be described in words. Its beauty can sometimes bring a tear of joy to the eye or send chills up the spine. The positive lyrics of some of the music you grew up with may give you a great feeling inside and make you feel like all is right with the world and your life. Feelings of joy that lift up your spirit and make it soar cannot be described, they can only be experienced. Enjoy as many as you can. They generate positive vibrations that attract more positive experiences and opportunities.

Laughter is good for the soul if it is positive and based on true humor. It's the amusing stories and events you keep thinking about and do not regret laughing at later. Laughter is good for you emotionally and physically, because it reduces cortisol (hydrocortisone) and epinephrine levels in the blood. Excess amounts of these chemicals suppress the immune system. Laughter can help relieve depression and improve numerous other emotional imbalances. Laughter makes you feel good and when you feel good you send out positive energy vibrations that attract positive things to you. I believe that it increases the carbon dioxide in your blood and stimulates more oxygen uptake by your cells. Get some joke books and videos of comedians or movies you find amusing. Find as many as you can that make you laugh so hard it hurts. One of my friends watches the dinner scene from the 1996 version of the movie *The Nutty Professor* whenever he feels down and needs a good laugh. Associate with people who make you laugh. A good sense of humor and someone who makes them laugh is high on the list of what people look for in a mate. Don't take yourself so seriously. Learn to laugh at yourself and the silly things you (and the rest of us) do every day. Instead of getting upset with yourself, laugh. Get at least a few good laughs every day.

Meditation can help you commune with your true inner self and get to know who you really are. The more you know yourself, the more you will love yourself and the easier it will be to be happy. Your inner spirit will help you learn how to eliminate the mental programming that causes you to behave in negative ways, overeat or punish yourself in other ways for real or imagined sins. Some people starve themselves (their souls) to death as the punishment they feel they deserve. As their souls starve so do their bodies. They may literally eat themselves to death or ingest alcohol, nicotine or other drugs until their bodies are destroyed. You must realize that no matter what you have or have not done in the past, it is not your job to judge. If you judge yourself, you will then pass sentence and carry it out. You will be your own judge, jury and executioner. If your punishment is to live in a fat body, you must pardon yourself or you will never permanently lose your excess fat. The body and mind reflect the spirit. If your body and mind are in bad shape, start feeding your spirit and watch your emotional and physical health improve.

Prayer is another great way to get in touch with your true inner spirit that is linked to the Infinite Intelligence of the universe. Whenever you hit a stumbling block in life, pray to be shown how to turn it into a stepping stone. Pray to find your reason to be lean, to discover and eliminate your reason for being fat or to find the right person to help you. Pray as often as you want for everything your heart desires. Because none of us consciously knows what we really need, it is best to pray for what you need to be healthy and happy. Your spirit knows what you need in precise detail and will create it for you unless you block it by focusing on what you don't want or reject it by feeling unworthy. Always be grateful for what you get and add it to your appreciation list—the things for which you give thanks. Be careful what you pray for, because you will get it but usually not in the form your conscious mind wants. For example, if you pray for strength, expect to get an obstacle to overcome, because that is what makes us stronger. I think it is best to just pray to give thanks and to ask for guidance to know what is right for you.

I believe that service to others is the best way to learn who you really are and to feel worthy to enjoy the positive feelings that feed your soul. Giving love or sharing a part of yourself with someone else is perhaps the greatest feeling you can ever experience. Do some volunteer work helping people or animals. Because all we have is time, when you give yours in selfless service, it gives back to you loving feelings. It makes your heart rise up and sing for joy. This is especially true with raising children, because a parent's time is the most important thing a child wants. Spending quality time with their children feeds the parents' souls by giving them the joy having children was meant to bring. It also feeds the child's soul and creates a good self-image and a great start in life. If you have children, learn to really listen to their hopes, dreams, concerns, fears and thoughts about their accomplishments. Do not forget to lovingly touch them physically and with what you say and do. This is soul food for both of you.

Doing something for someone who is incapable of doing it, or teaching people how to do something they can do are two of the best ways for being of service to others. Your personal discovery and positive feelings will more than outweigh the time you use to do these loving acts. You get more than those you are being of service to get. For more information about learning how to know and love yourself, contact the publisher of this book about my planned book tentatively titled, *The Greatest Love of All.*

Loving and caring for an animal can be especially rewarding and supplies your soul with much nourishment. Saving an animal from the pound can be a great gift to you and the animal. Animals are divine beings that are generally in tune with Nature. They have much love to give and can bring a tremendous amount of joy into a person's life. Special programs sometimes allow people in prisons and hospitals to partake of the soul food that the divine love of an animal can give. Many of these people are there because their souls are undernourished.

Planting and tending a vegetable or flower garden can supply a healthy portion of soul food. You are helping Nature to create nutritious food or beauty for you and others to enjoy and appreciate.

I believe that many people fail to take advantage of the positive feelings that come from a job well done. This is something that can be done whether people like their work or not. If you like your work, these feelings will help you to excel and be more successful. If you do not like your work, they will make you feel deserving of something better and guide you to work you will enjoy. If you feel worthy, I believe your spirit will lead you to the best work for you.

No matter how bad the job, doing it well has a positive effect on your self-image. I have had numerous low-paying jobs with less than ideal working conditions, but I always worked hard and did my best to go the extra mile. When I delivered used appliances, I was careful not to scratch people's walls or the product; when stacking boxes of explosives in trucks, I made sure it was done correctly; and when working as a janitor I took pride in making the floors and toilets shine. This always took more time than I was being paid for but I knew that I was getting other benefits. I believe that the positive feelings I experienced from doing my best helped me to enjoy the jobs more and kept me progressing to more lucrative and enjoyable work. It is still happening to this day.

Life is made up of relationships—with family members, friends, co-workers, spouses, strangers, children, pets, the earth, activities, Nature, self, possessions and even food. To achieve permanent fat loss you must change how you think and feel about yourself, food and your responsibility for your own health. Your relationship with food is especially important, because it affects all of your other relationships to some degree. Many ways to improve this vital relationship are included in upcoming chapters. Use your time to cultivate and nourish all your relationships so they are healthy and happy. Appreciate them for the joy they bring into your life. The more of them you can make positive, the more soul food, joy, fulfillment and health you will enjoy.

Use your sense of touch by physically hugging and touching the people and animals you care about. Touch their hearts and minds with the loving things you say and do. Make sure you get your own share of handholding, hugs and gentle touches every day. If you are alone, do things for yourself that uplift your mind and spirit. Do not wait to share quality time with those you love and care about. And do not postpone giving yourself the time you deserve to do the things in life you enjoy. If you wait too long, it will be too late.

Getting more in touch with your true self makes it easier to know what you need to learn, your creative outlets, the foods best suited for your body and what you should do with your life on this earth. Take the time to get to know who you really are.

Make a soul-food list of at least ten activities that make you feel happy and content. Think about the pursuits that lift your spirit and create positive feelings about yourself, your life and your future. Your list should include things like cuddling with your sweetheart, playing with your pet, painting a picture, playing golf or pool, reading a good novel, gardening, listening to your favorite music, completing a work task well, skiing, playing a musical instrument, singing, hiking, or reading your child a story. Be sure to include those special activities you may not have done for many years. Most of us get so busy we stop doing many of the things that make us happy. Some of us have created such deep ruts for ourselves that we rarely do any. This leads to a malnourished soul and an unbalanced life. You may get a lot of satisfaction from doing different types of work and it is fine to have them on your list, but make sure you have a number of light-hearted and fun activities as well. Add to your list as you think of more soul food. My minimum recommended daily allowance is three of these activities for at least 10 minutes each. No matter how busy you are (or think you are) you can make time to do at least three. This small time expenditure may contribute most of the satisfaction you derive from living each day. It will also make your other activities more enjoyable. For a happy and truly satisfying life, get as much soul food as you can. The more positive feelings of joy you experience, the more success and happiness you will attract to all parts of your life.

ten

Special Cases

This chapter deals with some major health problems and how they can possibly be prevented or helped through nutritional and other natural methods. I will explain how vital the nutritional program you have been learning is for preventing them and why it is so important to eliminate certain foods from your diet and toxins from your environment. I hope that what is presented here will help you prevent any of these serious conditions from developing. I believe that, with the exception of osteoarthritis, they are all "man-made" diseases caused by exposure to toxic chemicals, lack of correct exercise and not nourishing the body as Nature intended. Discussing these topics in great detail is not the focus of this book, but enough information is given to get you started in the right direction and furnish much food for thought. This chapter also has advice on the healthful feeding of infants and children.

The information contained here is not intended to diagnose or offer complete treatment plans for these diseases. If you have any of them, you should seek guidance from at least one health care professional. This help should consist not only of a complete nutritional program but other natural methods of reestablishing normal bodily function. You should, of course, be under the care of a competent physician who believes in the body's ability to heal itself and does not discourage you from using natural methods to help your body restore lost health. Because your health is ultimately *your* responsibility, developing a natural course to balance, strengthen and restore normal function to your body should be undertaken in conjunction with the advice of your physician. You must determine and eliminate the causes of all imbalances if you ever expect to fully regain lost health. Treating the symptoms will not eliminate the cause; it will just mask the problem as it continues to worsen. I have studied most of these diseases extensively and have developed methods of helping the body restore balance and normal function. I believe that proper breathing and an abundance of natural light (and less exposure to unbalanced light) are among the most important things that you need to prevent or improve these problems and others. Because almost all of them can be resolved or improved with diet and exercise, they can usually be prevented by the same methods. Another vital key to preventing these diseases (or helping the body to heal them) is to make sure that the brain and internal organs have proper nerve and blood flow.

Most, if not all, of the diseases discussed in this chapter are affecting people at an earlier age than they did in the past. Why is this happening? Simply because people are getting fat and eating nutrient deficient diets starting at younger ages. If you are obese, your chances of dying early are increased by 40 percent. The combination of obesity and inactivity is second only to cigarette smoking as a preventable cause of death and it is estimated that it will soon overtake smoking as the leading cause. Good reasons to avoid smoking and to get and stay lean, wouldn't you say?

Numerous books have been written telling us how to eat in order to treat or prevent osteoporosis, hypoglycemia, diabetes, this cancer or that cancer, heart disease and other life-threatening conditions. The question these books raise is, "How are we supposed to follow all of these different diets and protect ourselves from all these diseases?" Should we follow one program on Monday, another on Tuesday, a third on Wednesday, and so on? The answer is simple. We need only one diet plan. Remember Nature? The same diet that keeps you lean also keeps you healthy by protecting you from *all* diseases. Many diseases have been conquered with improved sanitation and other means, and most of the current ones would be rare if we lived more natural and healthier lifestyles. In essence, many people are following a diabetes-, heart disease-, cancer-, or other disease-*causing* diet. Clearly, the first step to better health is to stop doing this.

Other people will attempt to sell you "magic" supplements that will prevent or cure these diseases. The question is the same. Do we need the cancer-preventing supplement on Monday, the diabetes-preventing supplement on Tuesday, and so on? People selling these products would prefer that we took all of them every day, but you are learning that most of these supplements are unnecessary except in extreme cases.

Certain diseases can have other causes, but even if we are exposed to one of them, good nutrition gives our bodies the best chance at protecting us from them. Do not drive yourself crazy attempting to follow every new "miracle" healing diet you read or hear about. Just follow the same dietary principles that have kept many people healthy in the past. After all, most "new" scientific discoveries—like certain foods that protect us from cancer—were written about more than a hundred years ago by nutritional researchers who were in tune with and believed in the wisdom of Nature.

Why do most people's bodies age excessively fast and die prematurely? I believe it is caused by a combination of malnutrition and slow poisoning.

Malnutrition comes from not getting enough of the health-building nutrients found in whole, natural foods and the other sources we have discussed (e.g., water and sunlight), lack of proper exercise, insufficient mental stimulation and inadequate amounts of soul food. The poisoning comes primarily from the enemies discussed in chapter four and our negative thoughts and feelings. Realize now that you can control both of these causes and subsequently the health of your body.

Because most physical ailments develop gradually, the easiest and best thing to do is to prevent them, and the best time to start is now. A balanced and healthy lifestyle gives you the greatest chance to avoid the conditions that can reduce the quality of your life and end it prematurely.

Your Weakest Link

A well-kept secret to staying healthy throughout your lifetime is to keep your weakest link strong. Most of us are born with one particular gland or organ that is hereditarily weaker than the rest of them. This is our natural weak link. You have learned that the function of our glands and organs can be negatively affected from pressure on nerves exiting and entering along the spine, or from decreased blood flow from a nervous system imbalance. Either one of these imbalances can cause any gland or organ to become our weakest link. If our genetic weak link has decreased nerve or blood flow, it will be extremely vulnerable to stress and disease. Your weak link may be a gene that can cause a particular problem. If you never do anything to activate or "turn on" that gene, then it should not be a problem. If a gene is activated, proper health habits may be able to deactivate it and resolve the problem.

A chain is only as strong as its weakest link and will break at that point if enough stress is applied for a long enough time. The glands and organs of your body are the links in your internal health chain. If one is weaker than the others are, as you stress your body throughout life, it will most likely be the gland or organ that breaks down or develops disease before any others. Following the guidelines in this book will help keep the stress on all links in your health chain low, thereby decreasing the chance of even the weakest link breaking. Another important thing you can do is determine your weakest link and then make special efforts to protect it from stress.

Your genetic weak link can frequently be determined by looking at your family health history. Did your father and grandfather both die of heart attacks at a relatively early age? Did your uncle and your mother both have diabetes? Many doctors look at your family history to see possible hereditary weaknesses. Unfortunately, they usually wait until a person already has a problem and then it is more difficult or impossible to resolve. The real key is to prevent health problems or detect and treat them when they are just starting.

A thorough blood test can sometimes help determine someone's weakest link. For example, if all of the markers for kidney problems are higher than the average range, someone may have early kidney disease, inadequate nerve or blood flow to the kidneys or perhaps it is that person's genetically weak link. Yearly blood tests can provide signs that an unhealthy condition is developing or getting worse. Unfortunately, many doctors do not take the time to read them carefully and compare them with previous years to detect a trend. They usually wait until something has progressed to an extreme before they pay any attention to it. Then it is more difficult or impossible to treat successfully.

A rarely used health secret is to determine your weak link and then do everything you can to keep it strong. For example, if you believe your heart is your weakest link, you should exercise and eat in ways that will strengthen your heart and reduce stress on it. You do not need a special heart-disease-prevention diet, but you should avoid certain foods and start using certain additional supplements. Taking antioxidant supplements to reduce damage to the inner walls of your arteries can help prevent the development of atherosclerosis, and limiting salt consumption and staying lean decrease stress on the heart and help prevent high blood pressure. You may still die younger than someone with a stronger heart, but chances are that you will add many healthy years to your life that you would otherwise not have enjoyed.

We have all heard stories of people who drank and smoked all their lives and lived to be ninety years old. That does happen occasionally. But you seldom hear the part about how these people did not recognize anyone for the last ten years of their lives or were hardly able to do anything physical for the last twenty years because of breathing problems and an oxygen tank by their sides. Living to an old age does not describe the quality of life. What you want is quantity *and* quality. Some people live into their eighties and nineties, yet the quality of their lives is so poor they enjoy almost nothing and are unable to do much of anything.

Do not look at people who abused themselves in the past as examples, because many variables can play a part. The person you heard about who abused himself all his life and stayed relatively healthy may have worked hard physically, breathed cleaner air, drank chemical-free water, was not fat, had less exposure to toxic chemicals and had eaten fewer processed foods. If you live in a large city, the air you breathe may be stressing and polluting your lungs as much as the smoking did to that person; therefore, additional smoking would be far more damaging. If you are not eating fresh and natural foods, you will not be getting the enzymes and other vital nutrients that help protect your body from free radicals and other damaging influences in your environment.

After you determine your weakest link, or if you develop a problem in a particular gland, organ or system in your body, you should learn all you can about it and do everything possible to maintain or reestablish balance and normal function in the affected area. This will give you a good chance at keeping your weakest link strong and preventing a serious health problem.

The guidelines in this book are major steps toward helping you live a longer, healthier and more active life.

Some people are blessed with a strong constitution where even their weakest link is unusually strong. If you were born with a body like this, make sure you appreciate it and take care of it, because it does not give you the ability to constantly overstress your body without the possibility of a breakdown. Even if your weakest link is strong, any area can develop problems if normal nerve communication is disrupted or if there is imbalance between the sympathetic and parasympathetic nervous systems.

The first three diseases we are going to cover claim the most lives. They are the first, second and third leading causes of death in the United States. If you can prevent these three, you will greatly increase your chances of living much longer. It is also important to prevent the other diseases, because they can diminish the quality of your life and possibly shorten it. Remember that the goal is to live a long *and* healthy life, not just stay alive for a long time.

Heart Disease

The most common heart problems come from the heart muscle not getting enough oxygen. This leads to the conditions angina and myocardial infarction (heart attack). The cause of both of these problems is blocked coronary arteries that supply oxygen-rich blood to the heart. So, the logical question is "Why do these arteries get clogged?"

You have no doubt heard a great deal about cholesterol levels and may think that the amount of cholesterol in your blood is what determines whether you develop hardening and blockage of your arteries. But you now know that cholesterol is a natural substance in everyone's bloodstream and has numerous functions vital for good health and well-being. You have learned that egg yolks, which many people avoid, are a good source of lecithin that helps protect against hardening of the arteries and heart disease along with having other health benefits. It makes no sense that an organism such as the human body, so perfectly designed and constantly striving for balance and health, would have a substance running through its blood vessels that would deposit on the walls and clog them, perhaps killing the organism. This is contrary to everything the body constantly strives for and opposite of its prime directive—self-preservation. I believe cholesterol levels have some importance but play a minor role in most heart disease and other arterial problems. If excess cholesterol is not the main problem, then what is?

The beginning of arteriosclerosis (hardening of the arteries) is damage to the tunica intima (inner lining) of your arteries. When damage occurs, your body uses cholesterol and other lipids to repair the injured area. This makes perfect sense, because if the artery has a damaged section, it will be weaker and also hazardous to the red blood cells, platelets and other cells constantly going past. Sharp or rough areas pose a threat of tearing these sensitive cells;

therefore, your body does what it can to smooth out the rough sections and protect the cells from damage. These rough sections may also cause life-threatening blood clots to form. The initial condition after the damage is repaired is called atherosclerosis. The damaged areas later become fibrotic and eventually calcify. This makes the arteries hard and the condition is then called arteriosclerosis. As atheromatous plaques (cholesterol deposits) build up, they narrow the artery and when blood flow is blocked to a particular part of the body, the cells there die. This is what happens in a heart attack. Part of the heart muscle dies when it does not get oxygen, and if enough of the muscle dies, the heart can no longer beat. If these plaques are inflamed they can burst open, creating a blood clot that can block the coronary artery. Some doctors now believe that this is the cause of most heart attacks.

If the second thoracic vertebra of the spine is misaligned, it can put pressure on the nerves that enervate the heart and the coronary arteries. If a person with this misalignment gets in a position that increases the pressure on the nerve enough, it could cause the coronary arteries to spasm and cause a heart attack. Most doctors would be unable to find any explanation for the heart attack.

Because arterial damage is what starts the whole process of arteriosclerosis, preventing injury to the arteries seems like the obvious key to keeping the arteries healthy. If little damage occurs to the arterial lining, then there should not be much build-up of plaque. I believe that the patches are larger if an excessive amount of cholesterol is present when repair is necessary. High blood pressure appears to accelerate the rate at which cholesterol is deposited. It makes sense that the body repairs the artery with a larger and stronger patch because of the greater pressure. What causes the arterial damage? I believe that free radicals, sugar and various chemicals are the primary causes, although unbalanced light wavelengths may be a contributor.

When a free radical comes in contact with your inner arterial wall, it steals an electron in an attempt to stabilize itself. This sets up a chain reaction that leads to inflammation and damage. You have learned that free radicals are constantly created in our environment by natural and unnatural mechanisms. I believe heart disease has increased because more people live in modern environments, breathe polluted air, eat poorly and are exposed to numerous chemical products, greater stress and other sources of free radicals. Oxidized oils generate free radicals. This is why avoiding fried foods (especially deep fat fried) is such a good idea. Chlorine either creates free radicals or damages the intima of the arteries directly. A study I read many years ago indicated that the people of a city without chlorinated water had much less atherosclerosis than the people of a nearby city with chlorinated water. Those who moved from that city to the city with chlorinated water began to develop more atherosclerosis. There are other chemicals and possibly even certain organisms that can damage the inner lining of our arteries.

High blood sugar levels are extremely injurious to the blood vessels. This is why diabetics often have a great deal of vascular damage. Eating refined sugar regularly subjects your blood vessels to higher blood sugar levels than normal. This can cause vascular damage and contribute to the development of atherosclerosis. High blood sugar levels can also cause cataracts. Two more good reasons to avoid refined sugar.

Some doctors believe that a primary cause of the inflammation and subsequent damage to arteries is an excess of homocysteine, a waste product of protein digestion. Normally, particular B vitamins quickly break down homocysteine. Sadly, because most B vitamins are lost during the processing of foods, the people who eat mostly processed foods are deficient in these vital nutrients. This deficiency allows homocysteine levels to build up and damage the arteries.

You have learned that when the cells of animals were subjected to red light they weakened and finally ruptured. This effect was more dramatic when heart cells were used. Is the excessive amount of red color spectrum from incandescent lights damaging to our heart or other cells—perhaps the cells of the tunica intima? I believe it is.

Our bodies make a substance called C-reactive protein (CRP) in response to inflammation. A super-sensitive CRP blood test can check for inflammation in the coronary arteries. A level of 3 or more is considered high risk for a heart attack, a level of 1 to 3 indicates moderate risk and less than 1 is considered a low risk. Dr. Richard M. Fleming is a cardiologist who believes that a diet high in calories and saturated fats can cause inflammation in our arteries. In his book *Stop Inflammation Now!* he states that the best way to treat the condition is with a healthy lifestyle. He has his patients eat primarily fruits and vegetables for a few weeks to quickly lower the inflammation. Then he has them start eating other foods, including healthy fats. Do these recommendations sound familiar?

If your goal is to prevent heart disease and other vascular problems like strokes and kidney dysfunction, you must prevent as much arterial damage as you can. The best way to do this is to follow the dietary recommendations in this book and in others that explain ways of preventing arterial damage.

Have you ever wondered why the arteries harden but not the veins? Because veins do not carry oxygen there are few free radicals to cause damage. Veins also do not carry sugar and other substances that can create inflammation and damage. They do, however, carry unused cholesterol and other fats back to the liver.

Current estimates indicate that more than fifty million Americans have hypertension. This condition increases the risk of heart disease and other health problems. I believe that excessive pressure in the arteries is another possible source of damage, but the main problem hypertension creates is that it causes more plaque to form when the body repairs any arterial damage. People with hypertension are usually prescribed medication in an attempt to control it.

Some are told to reduce their salt intake. Not much is usually done to discover and eliminate the cause or causes, which is unfortunate, because many of them can be eliminated relatively easily. One cause is a constant pattern of vascular constriction from hyperstimulation of the sympathetic nervous system or from an overproduction of epinephrine. This can be the result of a nervous system imbalance, pressure on certain spinal nerves, mental patterns of imaginary stress, or from using drugs, alcohol, caffeine, nicotine and other nonfoods that distort normal function. Various nutritional deficiencies or imbalances can also be the cause. A lack of calcium has been indicated in some studies and potassium has lowered blood pressure in some people, probably because it reduces the negative effects of sodium. Other nutritional imbalances can interfere with the normal water balance and osmotic pressure of the blood. Excess salt is most likely the main culprit. Stiff arteries due to arteriosclerosis or a lack of heavy exercise may also contribute to hypertension.

Obesity is correlated with high blood pressure even more than an excess intake of sodium. But, research indicates that the relationship is with body fat mass, not just weight. This seems to confirm excess body fat as the problem, not total body weight. This is another reason why my program focuses on losing body fat, not weight. About 50 percent of obese Americans have high blood pressure. This is because their hearts have to pump blood to the fat and against the greater resistance that the excess fat creates. Lean body mass is healthy and improves blood flow back to the heart, thereby reducing stress on the heart muscle—another good reason to keep your muscles strong with regular strength training. Keep in mind that excess salt is a major cause of obesity.

Another possible cause of hypertension is misalignment of the first cervical vertebra. This is the one at the top of your neck that is commonly called the atlas. A misalignment of this bone affects the nerves that control blood flow to the brain. If the brain is not getting adequate blood flow, it signals the body to increase the pressure in an attempt to get the amount of blood it needs. The brain then gets what it needs, but blood pressure is increased in the rest of the body. If the pressure was also high in the brain, everyone with hypertension would have a constant headache, but this rarely happens. Most people with hypertension do not have any symptoms and many do not even know that they have it. When the misalignment of the atlas vertebra is permanently corrected, the arteries supplying blood to the brain open up to normal. This causes excess blood pressure in the brain, so the brain then signals the body to lower the pressure back to normal. Correcting this misalignment has resolved hypertension for almost all of my patients who had it. I believe that an atlas misalignment is a common reason for this condition, especially in people who are not obese. Because the adrenal glands and kidneys play a major role in regulating blood pressure, I have seen spinal misalignments affecting their normal nerve flow contribute to, or cause this condition.

Excess cadmium is believed to be another possible cause of hypertension. Why do so many people get high blood pressure when they get older? It makes a great deal of sense when you learn that cadmium levels usually increase with age and that it is found in refined foods, coffee and tea. Studies indicate that only about 9 to 20 percent of the population is genetically susceptible to developing hypertension. It also seems that if many of these people consumed less sodium (salt) they would not have problems. Genetics is a common reason given to people by doctors who do not know how to discover or eliminate the true cause of the patient's condition. They simply treat the symptoms with drugs while the cause continues to worsen. Treating symptoms with food, supplements and herbs is certainly better than using drugs, but still often does nothing to eliminate the cause. If you have high blood pressure, chances are excellent that the cause can be eliminated.

We have all heard that maintaining healthy cholesterol levels is helpful for preventing heart and vascular diseases. You may have genetically high levels, but if you prevent arterial damage, it should not make much difference. If you follow even a few of the guidelines suggested in this book, there is a good chance that you will maintain normal cholesterol levels for your body. The fruits, vegetables, legumes and whole grains Nature has created all contain fiber that not only helps keep your colon clean and your bowels regular but also keeps cholesterol levels normal. Here is how: bile gets trapped in the fiber and is carried out of the body, then cholesterol is used to make more bile. Otherwise most of the bile is just recycled. Do not eat a processed breakfast cereal to reduce your cholesterol. It may have some fiber in it, but so does cardboard. Eating that would have about the same effect as eating the processed cereal. Eat foods that have fiber *and* an abundance of health-building nutrients.

Eating good fats instead of bad ones is important to keep cholesterol at a healthy level. The mineral chromium can help reduce cholesterol levels, so eating foods containing it is helpful. Nicotine raises cholesterol levels, so avoid this toxic drug. Cholesterol levels are usually elevated in people with diabetes, and an inadequate amount of thyroid hormone can increase cholesterol concentration in the blood. Exercise helps reduce total cholesterol levels while increasing the HDL (good) cholesterol and lowering the LDL (bad) cholesterol. Current estimates indicate that more than 102 million American adults have high cholesterol levels. Unfortunately, most of them are just given drugs (with unhealthy side effects) to lower it but are not educated in proper dietary habits or how to prevent free-radical damage.

Many severe health problems can be caused by imbalances in other parts of the body and may not be purely chemical imbalances from poor nutrition. Nevertheless, nutritional methods can improve most abnormal health conditions to varying degrees. Occasionally, a nutritional deficiency is the entire cause, so other balancing techniques are unnecessary. Following the guidelines in this book should keep your cholesterol level low and blood pressure normal unless you have a genetic predisposition or an imbalance in your body that is causing them to be excessively high.

Cardiovascular exercise contributes to the health of your heart and blood vessels, but is a minor factor compared to preventing damage to the arteries, maintaining normal blood pressure and having a healthy cholesterol level. You can be in great shape, but still die of a heart attack. CV exercise increases the size of the heart chambers so the heart can pump the same amount of blood with fewer beats. Therefore, it does not have to work as hard. Another thing CV exercise can do is to stimulate new blood vessels to form. This creates collateral circulation that can supply blood to a particular area if another artery to that area is blocked.

During strength training, blood must be pumped against a high pressure. This makes the heart muscle and the muscles of the arteries stronger. I believe this is an important part of keeping the cardiovascular system healthy. The groups of people who consistently live to uncommonly old ages perform vigorous labor that keeps their hearts and arterial muscles strong and toned. A combination of strength and CV training makes your heart able to pump greater volume and to do it with less effort.

Be aware that exercise creates free radicals and may contribute to developing atherosclerosis if adequate nutrition is missing. For example, someone eating poorly and doing an excess of cardiovascular training could cause arterial damage. The people in the United States who live into their nineties or beyond are usually not in good cardiovascular condition, so CV training is not the primary key to preventing vascular problems. Most of these people have good mental attitudes, are fairly lean and eat small amounts of food.

Losing excess body fat is important for preventing heart disease, because the heart has to work harder to pump blood through the fat. Men are more at risk for heart problems than women are, because they generally store fat around their waistlines and this puts more pressure on the heart causing it to work harder. Men probably also gain more fat on the heart itself than women do.

Some people take a baby aspirin every day because it thins the blood, decreases inflammation and reduces the chance of heart problems and strokes. I believe this is unnecessary if you eat well and exercise regularly. Remember that the long-lived peoples of the world do not take aspirin every day. They simply eat naturally and stay physically active. They do not ingest foods that cause arterial inflammation so they do not need a drug to reduce it. Because aspirin can cause gastrointestinal bleeding and other damage to the body, I recommend using the herb white willow bark to people who are afraid (not a good way to live) and want to thin their blood, because it is a balanced product created by Nature. Vitamin E and garlic have a similar blood-thinning effect along with other healthful benefits.

Emotional distress and imbalance can contribute a great deal to the development of heart disease. Depression and sadness are bad for the heart, as is excessive mental and emotional stress. These emotions are also damaging to other parts of your body and your life. In general, men are more competitive and aggressive, and often feel more stress from being in the role of breadwinner, so it is easy to see why men have more heart attacks. This is not to say women are uncompetitive or have less stress in their lives. If you are a man, try running a household and raising a few children and see how much stress is created. Women are better able to handle certain stresses than men and are usually far better at expressing their feelings and venting stress than men are. But because more women are getting involved in stressful, competitive occupations, the incidence of heart disease in women is increasing. Anger can be an extremely destructive emotion. You must learn healthy ways of expressing your anger, reducing your stress and finding happiness. You have already learned how important good nutrition and exercise are for restoring balance. You will find other keys to doing this throughout this book, and many other good books are available to help you.

Following my nutritional guidelines will supply you with plenty of vitamins A, E and C, and other antioxidant nutrients that help protect you against free-radical damage and keep your body healthy and youthful. Numerous other things besides regular exercise and good nutrition can be done to stay youthful or even reverse many of the symptoms of aging. These will be covered in a book I plan to write about natural longevity. Other things can be done to keep your heart healthy, but losing excess body fat, getting adequate balanced nutrition, taking antioxidant supplements, keeping blood pressure normal, maintaining healthy cholesterol levels, eliminating salt and foods that contain cadmium, and doing strength-building and cardiovascular exercises are the main things.

Cancer

In *The Cure for All Cancers*, Dr. Hulda Clark writes that the cause of cancer is the pollution of the liver with isopropyl alcohol (commonly called rubbing alcohol). If enough of this pollutant builds up in the liver, intestinal flukes (a common parasite) travel to the liver, where they are normally not found. Adult flukes and the alcohol in the liver produce a cancer cell growth factor called ortho-phospho-tyrosine. This growth factor stimulates cancer cells to multiply rapidly.

When abnormal or mutated cells are created, your body can usually eliminate them. For example, if you smoke, the nicotine causes cells in your lungs to mutate. Your body can usually eliminate these mutant cells before they mutate a few more times and become cancer cells. This is fairly easy for your body—much like if someone dropped a lit match on your floor, you could easily stamp out the flame. But if the growth factor is present, the cells can sometimes mutate and then multiply faster than your body can eliminate them. This can cause the cancer to get out of control just like dropping a lit match in a puddle of gasoline.

Dr. Clark states that she always finds a heavy metal in the cancerous tissue and has never seen isopropyl alcohol without aflatoxin being present. Aflatoxin is a mold by-product known to be highly carcinogenic. The isopropyl alcohol may accumulate in the liver because of aflatoxin. She states that if the flukes are eliminated, the growth factor can no longer be created. The cancer will stop growing and is essentially cured. This is like the fire finally being brought under control. Now the body has a chance to gradually eliminate the cancer just like a fire being extinguished when it is no longer growing faster than it can be put out. You must, however, then supply your body with the nutrients it needs to eliminate the cancer, along with the raw materials to repair damage to normal cells.

To prevent cancer from developing again, it is necessary to periodically kill any new parasites and to stop polluting your body with aflatoxin and isopropyl alcohol. A good way to do this is to eat natural foods. Does this sound familiar? Dr. Clark's research and successes make sense to me and I am following her program. I suggest that you read her book. New discoveries and updated information can be found in her book *The Cure for All Diseases*. Dr. Clark's research explains why people can smoke for fifty years and never get lung cancer. They will have other serious lung diseases but will not get lung cancer if their livers are free of isopropyl alcohol and parasites. For decades, I have felt that the chemicals in our air, water, environment, personal care products and foods are the primary causes of many diseases. Dr. Clark seems to have determined the one that causes cancer and the different chemicals that cause numerous other diseases.

I wrote the following information about cancer prior to reading Dr. Clark's books. My previously developed beliefs do not conflict with anything she says, but give you more ideas about how to strengthen your body, help it repair damage from cancer and stay clean from isopropyl alcohol and other pollutants.

Is obesity a major risk factor for developing cancer? It certainly is. It is easy to see why, because the lifestyle and foods that keep us lean also protect us from cancer. For example, research shows that exercise reduces cancer risk and eating whole grains and vegetables reduces the risk of many cancers. On the other hand, the foods that cause obesity create an acidic environment where cells can mutate and multiply. Think about it for a moment. The foods that make us fat contain chemicals and artificial additives that can cause cancer but contain hardly any of the nutrients that protect us from it. These foods are also loaded with salt, sugar and other substances that cause cancer cells to multiply faster and because these processed foods lack nutritional value, people eat more of them. Fat cells produce excess estrogen, which increases the risk of breast cancer. Medical books even state it to be generally accepted that as much as 90 percent of human cancers are caused by environmental or nutritional influences—chemical and drug exposure, dietary habits and smoking. I would add unbalanced light and not enough oxygen to these causes.

These books indicate that the remaining 10 percent of cancers are caused by radiation, viral or genetic abnormalities. Even the medical community is saying we have tremendous control over up to 90 percent of all cancers. Unfortunately, they do not know much about how to improve our environmental or nutritional status. This is why the obesity and cancer rates are both increasing.

In 1996 I visited someone in the cancer ward of a hospital. I found a brochure in a rack in the hallway that listed certain foods as carcinogenic. Then I looked at the list of foods from which the patient could choose. About half of them were on the list of cancer-causing foods. Bacon was one that comes to mind. I heard almost forty years ago that the nitrite additive in bacon is converted in your body into carcinogenic nitrosamines. This is another example of the unhealthful meals given to hospital patients. The hospital's dietitians either have not read the pamphlet put out by the American Cancer Society or believe it is safe to eat carcinogenic foods if you already have cancer.

The cause of cancer seems the same as most, if not all, other diseases— some form of imbalance creating abnormal vibrations. Certain substances create tremendous imbalance in our bodies when we are exposed to them. Radiation and toxic chemicals create severe abnormal vibrations that cause normal cells to mutate. I find it strange that the medical profession uses radiation and toxic chemicals as their primary treatments against cancer. It is sad that they persist in going down a dead-end street with these ineffective treatments.

About fifteen years ago I heard about researchers who destroyed cancer cells using tuning forks set to certain vibrations. A laboratory petri dish containing both normal cells and cancer cells was touched with the tuning fork, causing it to vibrate at the same frequency. The normal cells were unaffected but the cancer cells broke into pieces. If you can create an environment in your body that vibrates in tune with your normal cells, it may cause abnormal cells to break up and then be eliminated by your body.

I have known a few people who cured their cancers using nutritional means alone. Their diets reestablished balance by restoring the normal vibratory rate to their bodies. I believe that healthy cells vibrate at a particular frequency and cancer and other abnormal cells vibrate at different frequencies. If the foods and drinks you are ingesting create an abnormal vibratory environment, then cancer cells can develop and thrive. An environment healthful for cancer cells is unhealthful for normal cells, so the body is less able to eliminate the cancer cells, because the normal cells are weakened. You can change the vibratory rate of your internal environment with foods and nutritional supplements. By creating a normal vibratory rate, your healthy cells should thrive and the cancer cells should die. Most people have heard that eating fruits and vegetables reduces the risk of cancer. One way these foods help is by making the internal environment less acidic and closer to a normal pH. They also supply the nutrients our healthy cells need to be strong and function normally. It is the same diet that stimulates healthful fat loss. Another reason why the people I knew recovered was because their nutritional programs helped their bodies to cleanse aflatoxin, isopropyl alcohol and other harmful chemicals from their livers.

Medical doctors surgically remove cancerous tissues every day, but they rarely know the cause so usually do nothing to eliminate it. If some of the cancer cells still remain, chances are high that the tumor will start to grow again. If all the cancerous tissue is removed but the cause is still there, new cancer cells will eventually develop and start to multiply.

If people with lung cancer have the diseased tissue removed entirely, they may do well if they stop inhaling the carcinogenic chemicals that originally caused it. Even if they have an unhealthful internal environment and the growth factor is present, chances are that they will not get lung cancer again. They will, however, be extremely susceptible to developing cancer in another area if cancer cells develop there for some reason.

All of the people with cancer that I have treated for musculoskeletal problems had impaired nerve flow to the part of the body with the cancer. For example, if the cancer was in the left lung, there was pressure on the nerve going to the left lung and if the cancer was in the right lung, the pressure was on the nerve going to the right lung. The fourth lumbar vertebra is where the nerves exit the spinal cord and go to the prostate gland. It was always out of place in my patients who had prostate cancer. Normally, the body can easily eliminate mutated or cancerous cells. I believe that the bodies of those patients did not eliminate the mutated cells because there was insufficient communication between their brains and the affected areas. Their brains did not know there was a problem, so did nothing to correct it.

I believe cancer cells can possibly develop from eating an excess of processed foods that cause abnormal vibrations and starve your healthy cells for nutrition. This creates conditions for mutations (cancer cells) to develop. The cancer cells can then multiply in this abnormal environment. If the growth factor is present, the cancer can grow and spread rapidly. I have explained how to achieve balance in your diet so a healthful internal environment can be established and maintained. This greatly reduces the chances of cancer cells developing or creating an environment where they can thrive.

Why do children get cancer? Various possibilities exist. I believe cow's milk or infant formulas can possibly cause cells to mutate. Carcinogenic toxins could also be passed to a developing infant from the mother's bloodstream or perhaps through the breast milk. Children may be exposed to cancer-causing chemicals or isopropyl alcohol. Many children are not getting adequate nutrition to help their bodies eliminate these toxins. Secondhand smoke increases the risk of cancer, as does obesity. Overcooked meat contains carcinogens, and the nitrite additive in cured and processed meats is converted into carcinogenic nitrosamines. The diet of Americans seems to be deteriorating with each generation while the exposure to toxic chemicals is increasing. Therefore, people with inadequate nutrition or internal toxins may pass on weak or abnormal genetic material to their offspring. This may make their children's bodies more susceptible to developing mutant cells and less able to dispose of them. Children can also have spinal misalignments that inhibit normal nerve communication between the brain and the area with the cancer. These misalignments can occur during birth or be caused by a trauma that knocks the bone out of alignment. The body of a child cannot realign the bone by contracting a muscle to pull it back into place because the ends of the vertebrae where the muscles attach are still cartilage that just bends when the muscle contracts. These misalignments can be easily fixed with an extremely gentle non-force chiropractic adjustment that I and a small percentage of chiropractors do. I have successfully resolved constipation and other problems for infants and children in just a few minutes.

After eliminating isopropyl alcohol, parasites, or both, people with cancer should restore balance to their bodies as soon as possible. Most of them have eaten excessive amounts of processed and cooked foods and created an internal environment conducive to cancer development and growth. To reestablish a normal environment as quickly as possible, they should eat in an unbalanced way that is the opposite of how they had been eating. To counteract the effects of an excess of acid-forming and dead foods, an abundance of alkaline-forming and live foods is needed. This is what the people I have known who cured their own cancers did. They ate raw fruits, vegetables, nuts and seeds, and drank large quantities of water and green vegetable juices. They ate no processed or cooked foods until after the cancer was gone. Make sure you drink good water and remember that bottled water may be contaminated with isopropyl alcohol. Salt, caffeine, nicotine, alcohol, sugar and artificial sweeteners should be avoided completely.

Eating all raw foods and drinking vegetable juices is an unbalanced way of eating and is insufficient to maintain good health for the average person. But when a severe imbalance has been created, eating opposite to the way that caused the imbalance reestablishes homeostasis faster. A pH balanced diet of raw and cooked foods should maintain the balanced environment and help prevent further problems. Returning to old dietary habits will re-create the internal imbalance and lead to new problems.

Other things can be done to help the body regain normal balance faster and aid it in cleansing out cancerous cells. The internal cleansing programs explained in chapter seven accelerate the elimination of diseased cells, chemical toxins and other waste matter. Colon and blood cleansing herbs can also help restore balance more quickly. Be aware that a diet of raw vegetables, fruits and their juices will create a severe cleansing reaction in many people. The most intense cleansing will occur in those with the worst imbalances and the most internal waste. These cleansing symptoms have caused many sick people to abandon healthful dietary programs that may have resolved their conditions. This is why you must understand the cleansing reactions so you will not become afraid and stop. It is best if you work with a qualified professional who can advise you and answer questions as they arise.

If the diet of raw foods does not create any cleansing symptoms, then short cleanses should be undertaken. Longer cleanses can be done as the body gets cleaner and the reactions less intense. Remember that it is extremely important to eat properly following a cleanse. Refer back to chapter seven for how to do this. Most cleanses cause some weight loss but what is being lost is excess body fat and internal waste. Because weight loss is a common symptom of cancer, this can be especially frightening for cancer patients if they do not thoroughly understand this. Be aware that cancer causes a loss of healthy, normal cells but cleansing does not.

Living and working under artificial lighting is a part of our unnatural modern lifestyle that also creates an imbalance of vibrations in our bodies. Therefore, another thing that can help restore the normal vibratory rate of your internal system is to get the balanced light from the sun through your eyes. Get outdoors as much as possible or sit near an open window. You do not need to be in direct sunlight and you should never look at the sun. You merely need to be outdoors without glasses that block the ultraviolet light from entering through your pupils. This natural light seems to feed and strengthen the pineal gland, which then normalizes endocrine balance and internal vibrations. It is also important to reduce your exposure to the unbalanced light sources mentioned in chapter three. In *Health and Light*, John N. Ott cites examples of how sunlight helped cancer patients and those with other diseases. In a study of fifteen cancer patients, fourteen of them showed no advancement of their tumors and some even seemed improved. The patient whose condition did not stop progressing had misunderstood the instructions and had continued to wear eyeglasses that blocked the UV light. Another story told of tribes of African natives who had no history of cancer until after they began to wear sunglasses as a status symbol. Their lifestyles were otherwise unchanged. I believe it is best for everyone to get as much natural light as possible and to reduce exposure to unbalanced light sources.

Walking is a good exercise for someone with cancer. It does not break down muscle tissue, which would require the body to use energy for repair, and it helps the cleansing process by increasing circulation. It also helps strengthen and tone certain muscles and internal body systems to some degree. Walking outdoors is best, because balanced light can be obtained and the beauty of natural surroundings enjoyed. After the cancer has been eliminated, strength-building exercises can be done to regain and then maintain lost muscle mass.

Some nutritional supplements seem to have cancer-fighting properties. This is most likely because they help restore a more normal vibratory environment in the body. Shark cartilage is a supplement that some believe has cancer-fighting properties and Pycnogenol is another. Some of these products may either destroy cancer cells directly or help indirectly by restoring balance to the internal environment. I doubt if any would be able to resolve the problem if the growth factor is stimulating the cancer to grow at a rapid rate. They may be helpful for someone who has eliminated the growth factor.

Some herbs are claimed to help prevent or even treat cancer. Red clover, ginseng and ginkgo biloba are a few. Milk thistle is an herb known for helping the liver cleanse out toxins and regenerate its cells. This may be helpful for eliminating isopropyl alcohol and preventing more from accumulating. It may also help cleanse aflatoxin from the liver. I take a milk thistle supplement once or twice a week, because no matter how careful we are, most of us are still exposed to toxic chemicals the liver has to detoxify. Keep your liver healthy and it will help keep the rest of your body healthy.

Our thoughts are another vital component in the prevention and treatment of cancer or any other disease. Abnormal vibrations can easily be created if someone is judgmental, lacks self-love, or is expressing anger, regret or other negative emotions. These vibrations can depress the immune system, weaken normal cells and even cause abnormal cells to develop. Learn to deal with negative emotions and feelings in a positive way so they will not continue long enough to create physical problems. If this is part, or perhaps all, of the cause of someone's cancer, it must be eliminated before full recovery can be enjoyed.

Louise Hay has written books about how she cured her own cancer just by changing her thinking and learning to love (accept) herself. Norman Cousins did not have cancer but greatly reduced the pain of his chronic inflammatory disease (ankylosing spondylitis) using laughter. Jesus and other great healers have used the power of love and faith to heal for centuries. Never forget how powerful your thoughts are at generating the feelings that will attract what you want. Use yours to create a life filled with health and happiness.

Current estimates are that one in every eight women will get breast cancer, and the rate has been increasing right along with the obesity rate. This is because obesity more than doubles the risk, as does breathing secondhand smoke. Even *small* amounts of alcohol increase the risk as does major depression and psychological stress. The synthetic estrogen many women use for hormone replacement therapy (HRT) also increases the risk. Why? Because it is an unbalanced product that contains only one (estradiol) of the three forms of estrogen naturally produced by the body. It is now included on the list of known carcinogens. If a woman needs HRT, I recommend that she use a natural product containing a balance of all three forms (estradiol, estrone, and estriol) along with a natural progesterone product. Some women may also need a small amount of testosterone. Before starting any HRT, women should be properly tested for need and dosage.

When Dr. Hulda Clark tests women with breast cancer, she often finds many of the chemicals found in makeup stored in the breast tissue. These chemicals could be what caused the normal cells to mutate. I have heard of other researchers who believe that the brassieres worn by many women restrict the normal drainage of toxins through the lymph vessels and this allows the chemicals to accumulate to toxic levels. I believe that abnormal nerve flow to the breast (usually just one) can also reduce the elimination of toxins, as well as affect normal communication between the breast and the brain.

Dioxin is a toxic chemical that can cause cancer. It has been linked primarily to breast cancer. If you freeze water in a plastic bottle, this carcinogen is released into the water. It might also be in ice cubes frozen in plastic trays. This is another reason why I recommend avoiding iced drinks. Using a microwave oven to heat foods (especially fatty foods) that are in plastic or foam containers can also release dioxin. Even covering a tempered glass container with plastic wrap when heating foods in a microwave can release dioxin. I recommend against heating foods in a microwave for this reason and because of the destruction of vital nutrients that occurs.

What can reduce your chances of getting breast cancer? The main things are a good fat-to-lean ratio, a healthful diet and attitude, natural light, regular exercise, normal nerve flow and function of the breasts, hypothalamus, pituitary glands, liver and ovaries, and of course, elimination of the causes—most of what you are learning in this book.

Stroke

A cerebrovascular accident (CVA) or stroke occurs when part of the brain is deprived of oxygen long enough to damage or kill brain cells. Preventing this condition is the same as preventing heart disease and most others—maintaining a healthy body fat percentage, getting adequate balanced nutrition, taking antioxidant supplements, keeping cholesterol levels low and blood pressure normal, and doing strength-building and cardiovascular exercises.

Osteoporosis

Osteoporosis is an abnormal condition that is becoming more common in the United States and other countries where people lead similar lifestyles. According to recent statistics more than twenty-eight million Americans currently have it, but it most likely affects a much larger number. The estimated cost for treating it is more than $14 billion each year and predictions are that it will affect more than fifty million Americans by the year 2020. If you understand the causes, it is easy to see why it is becoming more prevalent.

Osteoporosis occurs when bones lose density and strength. This makes them more susceptible to being fractured. It is more common in women by a ratio of about four to one, and postmenopausal women are the ones most affected. Complications arising from this condition make up the twelfth leading cause of death in the United States.

Osteoporosis can lead to fractures of the spinal vertebrae in the upper and middle back. Most of the people this happens to have tight muscles causing their upper backs to curve forward. This puts excess pressure on the weight-bearing part of the vertebra. This causes it to collapse in the front, which leads to a compression fracture. The vertebra ends up being normal height in the back and much shorter in the front. Because the top of the vertebra is now slanted forward, the vertebrae above it tilt creating a hyperkyphosis (excessive bending forward) of the spine between the shoulder blades. Many people have this excessive forward curvature, but tight muscles are the cause of it in most cases. I have restored normal spinal curvatures for hundreds of patients using my PMBT therapy. Reducing a hyperkyphosis relieves the forward pressure and decreases the chance of a fracture occurring. Carrying something in front of the body or bending forward can also contribute to a vertebral fracture. An estimated 700,000 of these fractures occur each year due to osteoporosis.

The two other areas most affected by osteoporosis and therefore more susceptible to fracture are the distal radius (near the wrist in the forearm bone on the thumb side) and the neck of the femur (upper area of the thighbone). This is the broken hip you often hear about. An estimated 300,000 occur each year due to osteoporosis. Gum disease and tooth loss can also be caused by osteoporosis.

I believe osteoporosis is preventable and even reversible to a large degree, because it goes against the body's prime directive of self-preservation. Why would a mechanism designed to heal itself and maintain health create conditions where its bones get weak and easily fractured? It makes absolutely no sense and is completely unnatural.

Because osteoporosis is unnatural it has to be caused by unnatural actions, unnatural conditions, or a combination of the two. Two main questions must be answered in determining the cause of osteoporosis. We must determine why the bones lose calcium and, once lost, why it is not replaced when calcium is ingested. Research suggests that bone formation stays the same as we age but resorption (bone loss) increases. Therefore, to prevent the problem we need to determine and eliminate what causes the loss of bone mass to be greater than the bone formation. If we can keep the bone loss at the same rate as the bone formation then the bones should stay strong. This is what I believe Nature intended and what happens in countries where people eat natural foods and do physical labor. The human body is designed to stay healthy by maintaining the best homeostasis it can. It is this striving for balance that causes calcium to be lost from the bones. When the pH of the blood is acidic, the body takes calcium from the bones to restore equilibrium to the blood.

There is more to preventing or successfully treating osteoporosis than taking a calcium supplement. First, we have to determine approximately how much calcium we need. Second, the balance between calcium and other minerals must be maintained. Third, anything that increases or decreases calcium absorption must be taken into account. Fourth, anything depleting our body of calcium needs to be understood and eliminated if possible. Fifth, we have to regularly do activities that retain or replace calcium in our bones.

And finally, we need to consider other influences that can cause bones to fracture more easily. Don't worry, none of this is difficult.

Calcium needs vary from person to person. The main thing, however, is not how much is ingested but how much is absorbed and utilized. Remember the final two steps necessary for all nutrients? Body size and composition, gender, activity level, age, diet, digestive efficiency, medications used and other variables all influence need as well as play a part in how much is absorbed and used.

Calcium absorption is influenced a great deal by your diet. To be absorbed, it must be present in a water-soluble form in the small intestine. Usually only about 20 to 30 percent, sometimes less, of ingested calcium is absorbed. So, how much do we need? Studies have shown that given a little time to adjust, humans can maintain calcium balance on only 200 to 400 mg a day. The recommended dietary (daily) allowance in 1980 was 800 mg and is currently 1,000 to 1,500 mg for women over age fifty. The RDA for children four to eight is now 800 mg, 1,300 mg for children nine to eighteen and 1,000 mg for adults. The RDA has been increased to compensate for the high levels of protein and phosphorus (and dairy products, refined sugar and sodium fluoride) contained in the typical American's diet. The World Health Organization (WHO) and the health authorities of many countries recommend much lower amounts.

Most whole, natural foods contain calcium. Dark green leafy vegetables, almonds, Brazil nuts, sesame seeds, dates, dried figs, oysters and canned salmon, mackerel and sardines with the bones are especially high. It is difficult, however, for most people to get 800 to 1,500 mg of calcium daily without using milk and milk products. Because Nature does not want us to drink milk, I believe it is telling us we do not need that much calcium. Is the message that we should eat less protein and other foods that contain phosphorus? Most grain products contain high amounts of phosphorus, as do colas and certain other soft drinks. Reducing our intake of phosphorus-containing foods makes more sense than ingesting more calcium and disrupting our body's mineral balance.

Acid-forming foods (complete proteins and grains) have more phosphorus than calcium, and alkaline-forming foods (fruits, vegetables and legumes) have more calcium than phosphorus. If you eat mostly fruits, vegetables and legumes and some complete protein foods and grains, you should maintain a normal pH in your blood and not lose calcium from your bones. You will also maintain your normal weight with a healthy body fat percentage. This is another example of how the diet that keeps you lean also keeps you healthy.

The mineral balance in our bodies is very important for maintaining normal function. The body wants a particular ratio between phosphorus and calcium. If excess phosphorus is ingested, the need for calcium increases. If insufficient calcium is available from the diet, it will be taken from the bones and will not be replaced unless certain conditions are met. Excess phosphorus seems to be the primary cause of osteoporosis but I believe other minerals play a part.

Sodium is the main culprit and most Americans eat too much salt. Excess sodium disrupts the balance by increasing the need for other minerals. It also causes calcium to be pulled into the kidneys and excreted in the urine. If you follow the dietary guidelines in this book, your body should easily be able to maintain normal mineral balance without taking calcium from your bones.

What increases the amount of calcium that is absorbed? A highly acidic pH in the stomach is one example. As you have learned, an acidic medium in the stomach is stimulated by protein foods. Eating protein also makes calcium more soluble and increases absorption. A high-protein diet, however, seems to impair the ability of the kidneys to reabsorb calcium. Because many older people have decreased acid production, it is easy to see why they also have less calcium being absorbed. When a moderate amount of fat is present, it slows the transit time through the digestive tract, allowing more time for minerals to be absorbed. Isn't it interesting that most protein foods also contain some fat? Is this part of Nature's plan? It sure seems so to me.

Vitamin D stimulates intestinal absorption of calcium. This vitamin is formed (from cholesterol) when the skin is exposed to sunlight but, as you know, I prefer to limit sun exposure and get this vitamin from foods or supplements. The body even absorbs calcium more efficiently when exposed to UV-containing full-spectrum lights. The herb horsetail helps the body absorb and utilize calcium. If someone has the lactase enzyme (like almost all babies) then lactose enhances calcium absorption, but if a person is lactase deficient (like most of us after age three or four), the lactose acts to inhibit calcium absorption. This is how Nature ensures that growing babies get enough calcium. It also gives the rest of us another good reason to avoid dairy products.

The amount of calcium we absorb is dependent on need. It is a matter of supply and demand. If you create the need, the body naturally absorbs more. Need is increased primarily during times of growth. An example of this is when babies are growing rapidly in their first few years. Calcium need may be slightly increased when people are doing intense strength-training exercise, primarily because most of them will be eating an excess of complete protein.

Based on the preceding information, I believe that the best time to ingest calcium is with meals consisting of foods containing protein and some fat such as meats, eggs, seeds or nuts. This is one reason why I often eat green leafy vegetables and other calcium-containing vegetables when I eat meat. Remember that the essential fatty acids found in these foods work with vitamin D to make calcium more available to our tissues. Vitamin D is found in egg yolks and liver. Canned salmon, mackerel and sardines (with the bones) contain protein, calcium and vitamin D. Many wild animals chew on bones when they ingest meat. This gives them the calcium they need to balance the phosphorus in the meat. Because we usually do not chew on bones as our distant ancestors probably did, an excellent calcium supplement is microcrystalline hydroxyapatite (finely ground bone meal). This supplement should also contain at least magnesium and vitamin D, and be taken with your protein meals. The trace mineral boron seems to enhance calcium absorption. Unfortunately, because of the diseases found in many cattle these days, even supplements made from their bones may be hazardous to your health. For this reason, vegetarian sources of calcium such as calcium citrate may be the best supplement to use. This form is absorbed fairly well on an empty stomach and some doctors recommend that it be taken just before bed. I suggest taking it with the evening meal when complete protein foods are eaten.

A person could have progressively worsening osteoporosis even though quite a bit of calcium is being ingested. For example, if a woman ate mostly acidic foods during the day and took a calcium supplement at night, she would lose calcium from her bones during the day but most of it would not be replaced at night. This is another example of the principle of timing. She could most likely improve her condition or keep it from worsening if she did correct weight-bearing exercise but she would get better results if the calcium was taken with the acidic meals.

Some evidence suggests that excess calcium may be harmful. If you are eating a pH balanced diet and taking a multivitamin and mineral supplement, it is unlikely you will need much extra calcium. It is important to be tested for need; otherwise your calcium supplement may be doing you more harm than good. Many of my female patients were taking excess amounts of calcium, because when I tested them their bodies indicated a much lower need. Because of their lack of knowledge and fear of osteoporosis, they were creating imbalance in their bodies. Most of them were also not doing the correct exercises to maintain strong bones.

What decreases calcium absorption? Obviously, both a vitamin D deficiency and a fast transit time through the intestines will reduce calcium absorption. Because essential fatty acids work with vitamin D to make calcium more available to the body tissues, a low-fat diet may contribute to the development of osteoporosis. Some fruits and vegetables and, if you recall, chocolate, cocoa, and a combination of sugar and meat, contain oxalic acid that combines with calcium to form calcium oxalate, a non-absorbable compound that is the primary component of most kidney stones. I believe that the small amount of oxalic acid found in a few whole foods is necessary for balanced nutrition and is not enough to cause any health problems. But the excess amounts people get from unnatural sources can overload the body and lead to unhealthy conditions. In an alkaline medium, calcium and phosphorus join to form calcium phosphate, another non-absorbable compound that is a part of most kidney stones. Another substance, phytic acid, makes calcium non-absorbable by combining with it to form calcium phytate. Phytic acid contains phosphorus and is found primarily in grains. Some studies have shown a high-fiber diet to reduce the absorption of calcium and other minerals. I would guess, however, that these studies did not have the participants ingesting the calcium at the appropriate times. I also doubt if they had a proper balance of soluble and non-soluble fiber. My nutritional program is rich in fiber but the high-fiber foods and complete protein foods are usually eaten at different times.

Numerous drugs can cause malabsorption of calcium. Here are a few: prednisone and other glucocorticoids, phenobarbital, Dilantin® (phenytoin), neomycin, phenolphthalein, diphosphonates, glutethimide, and primidone. The long-term use of thiazide diuretics also results in decreased calcium absorption. Alcohol, salt, tobacco, caffeine and high-fructose corn syrup interfere with normal calcium absorption. Lack of exercise and particularly lack of weight-bearing exercise on the legs decreases your ability to absorb calcium. Mental stress also decreases absorption, as does age. It should be easy to determine what you are doing (or not doing) that is decreasing the amount of calcium your body absorbs.

Here are a few things other than excess phosphorus that can cause a loss of calcium. Processed sugar depletes calcium from your body, and drugs containing aluminum result in a loss of calcium and a loss of bone. Salted foods and caffeinated sodas leach calcium from your bones. Drugs such as corticosteroids (cortisone), tetracycline, thyroid preparations, heparin, Dilantin, isoniazid, ethacrynic acid, triamterene, furosemide and alcohol can induce calcium loss. You should check any drug you may be taking to see if it decreases absorption of calcium or has a calcium-depleting effect. Smoking increases the loss of calcium from the bones and mental stress causes increased excretion of calcium.

What you have just learned indicates that we should avoid ingesting grains (they contain fiber and phytic acid), sugar, salt, caffeine, alcohol, nicotine, high-fructose corn syrup and foods containing oxalic acid when we eat a protein meal and take a calcium supplement. Remember that sugar eaten with meat causes oxalic acid to form. This is why it is important not to eat desserts or other foods containing sugar (sauces and salad dressings) or to drink anything with sugar added when eating meat. You have learned that regular weight-bearing exercise and maintaining a calm mental attitude are helpful in many ways. Now you can see that they are both extremely important for absorbing and retaining enough calcium for good health and strong bones.

When excess protein is eaten, the blood pH becomes acidic and the body acts to correct this imbalance. You have learned that our bodies have ways of reestablishing the pH back to normal. One way is to put calcium in the bloodstream to neutralize the excess acidity. The bones act in part as an emergency storehouse for calcium. Later, the calcium will be replaced only if normal conditions exist and the *need* to replace it is there. Acid-forming grain products create a similar condition. I believe that an excess of acid-forming foods is the most common cause of calcium loss. Other methods are initially used to achieve a normal blood pH, but if they are inadequate then calcium is taken from the bones or, as you also know, the acidic nutrients are stored as fat.

Our bodies have other storehouses besides calcium in the bones. For example, skeletal muscles are about 70 percent water. Our internal organs have priority for water, because they are more important for good health and self-preservation. If insufficient water is ingested to keep the internal organs healthy and functioning normally, water will be taken from the muscles to supply their needs. Another example is fat. Fat cells are designed to store energy for use in times of famine or other periods when adequate amounts of food are unavailable. Fat also insulates our bodies to keep us warm. Our ancestors needed this, because they did not eat on a regular schedule and were often subjected to a cold environment. Most of us do not need to store excess fat on our bodies now, because we live in warm houses and can store food in the refrigerator or buy it fresh at the supermarket.

I believe that the majority of people in the United States and other developed countries ingest excessive amounts of acid-forming foods. This creates the need for abnormally high amounts of calcium. Few people, however, get enough calcium to deal with the high amounts of protein, processed grain products and other phosphorus-containing foods they eat. Most of them ingest things that cause calcium to be lost or that inhibit the absorption of this vital mineral. Calcium is necessary for numerous bodily functions, so if you do not get enough, you can become deficient or your body may take it from your bones to supply your needs.

I do not believe our bodies need much calcium each day, because if you eliminate milk products, as you should if your goal is good health, you will not find many foods high in calcium. This seems to be Nature's way of telling us we do not need large amounts. Many of the calcium-containing foods you do find do not contain much protein. If you eat a wide variety of natural foods, you should get all the calcium your body needs to balance out the *normal* amounts of phosphorus you will be getting from other foods.

Mother's milk contains 340 mg of calcium per liter and cow's milk contains 1,220 mg per liter. That is about three and a half times as much. Cow's milk also contains about three and a half times as much protein. Do you see the ratio of calcium to protein Nature puts in the food? Human milk contains what is right for a human infant and cow's milk contains what is right for a calf. Even college textbooks on nutrition say that cow's milk is inappropriate for human infants. All animals (except humans) stop drinking milk after they are weaned. They are not fully-grown at this time but their bones and teeth keep growing rapidly and then stay strong without milk or calcium supplements. This happens because they eat the way Nature intended—unless humans interfere and feed them unnatural foods. Animals do not do things that inhibit calcium absorption and use, or that pull calcium out of the bones. No reason exists why the human animal should be different and have weak bones if they do not drink milk. Women do not keep producing milk for everyone to drink. Also, what would happen to an entire race or tribe of people who did not have access to cow or goat's milk? Would they all have stunted growth and weak osteoporotic bones? No, they would get mother's milk when young and later eat a natural adult diet. Their bones would stay strong, because they stress them with use and do not ingest foods and other products that leach calcium from the bones or inhibit absorption or use.

If you still think you need dairy products to protect you from osteoporosis, here is some additional information. North American and northern European nations where the people consume the most dairy products have the highest rates of osteoporosis. Asian and African countries where the least amount of dairy products are consumed have the lowest rates. Studies have shown that when people ingested more calcium, the susceptibility to hip fractures increased. Another study done on a large number of nurses found that the ones who drank the most milk broke more bones (especially the hip) than the others did. This information does not make dairy products look effective at preventing the problem, does it? Dairy products do contain calcium but they contain almost as much phosphorus. Cottage cheese has more phosphorus than calcium. The protein in milk products can cause a loss of calcium and the lactose may be inhibiting the absorption of even other sources of calcium. Are dairy products contributing to the development of osteoporosis? It sure seems that way when you consider the facts.

Because so many people are afraid of developing osteoporosis, numerous products now contain added calcium. Unfortunately, some of the calcium comes from cheap sources and is added only to help companies sell their products. Chances are that hardly any of this calcium is being absorbed or used. A popular antacid product now has added calcium. Supply calcium while reducing the acid necessary to absorb it. Does that make any sense? Some people even eat chocolate with added calcium. This makes no sense either. Remember that chocolate contains oxalic acid that combines with calcium in the digestive tract, making it unavailable for use. Even if a woman with osteoporosis takes a good calcium supplement that is well absorbed, the most she will usually do is stop or slow down the progression of the condition. Calcium will not be redeposited in her weakened bones unless she also creates the need.

Our bodies are born with the programming to do what is believed necessary to maintain balance, to protect against injury, or for self-preservation. For example, if your body believes it is being starved because you eat only one meal a day in the evening, it will live on stored glycogen and muscle tissue all day and store much of the meal as fat. If you do not drink enough water, your body may retain water in your tissues as a way of storing extra. To rebuild bone mass, you must give your body a reason to put calcium back into the bones to strengthen them. Like exercising to strengthen your muscles, you must create a need for the body to make the necessary changes. Let me explain muscle adaptation first. When people start strength training, their muscles adapt to the stress placed on them by getting stronger and usually larger as well. If they stress their muscles against increasingly greater resistance, their muscles will get stronger and larger up to their genetic potentials. If they exercise with less resistance, their muscles will *reduce* in size and strength, to be able to handle only the current demand. If they stop their strength training, their muscles will get much smaller and weaker, because the need to be strong is gone.

Your bones also get stronger only if you create the need. If you put regular physical stress on your bones, they adapt by getting stronger. But, as with your muscles, you must keep doing it if you want them to stay strong. If a woman rarely stresses her upper thigh, wrist or spinal bones, her body has no reason to deposit the calcium she may be ingesting back into her bones to restore lost strength. The thoracic (mid and upper back) vertebrae, the wrist bones and the neck of the femur are the areas most frequently fractured, because the body seems to remove calcium from them first. If they are osteoporotic, excess stress on them can easily cause a fracture. Correct strength-building exercise is the key to keeping these and other bones strong or for restoring lost density and strength. Of course, adequate calcium and other necessary nutrients must be available. Your body cannot build a brick house without the bricks.

Studies have proved that weight-bearing exercise can stimulate increased bone mass. If the rate of bone formation stays the same, this seems to indicate that the exercise slowed down the loss of bone, allowing the body to catch up. With balanced nutrition and regular strength training, the rate of bone loss and bone formation should be the same and the bones should stay strong. Remember that weight-bearing exercise also increases the absorption of calcium. Our bodies are the vehicles we inhabit so we can function in a physical world. If they are not used, they weaken and start to break down. The adage "Use it or lose it" applies. This is why regular strength-building exercise should be as natural a part of everyone's life as eating and sleeping. It is absolutely essential for keeping your bones and skeletal muscles strong. It also helps keep many other parts of your body strong and functioning efficiently.

After a woman goes through menopause she is more susceptible to osteoporosis. Why? Many health professionals believe that decreased estrogen production is the primary reason. I am not convinced it is, because it makes no sense. Why would a body with self-preservation as its highest priority start to self-destruct after menopause? I feel the answer more likely lies in the estrogen protecting the woman against the effects of chemicals in the environment or foods that increase the loss or decrease the absorption of calcium. Estrogen may also help the body reabsorb and use calcium. It may be that estrogen was keeping something else in balance and when the estrogen declines then an excess of the other develops. The cause of osteoporosis could be something else that changes during menopause. Some older women may get more severe osteoporosis due to the use of certain drugs. For example, benzodiazepines (tranquilizers like Xanax® and Valium®) dramatically increase the risk of hip fracture.

Some doctors believe the secret to regaining lost bone strength is progesterone, not estrogen. But, like estrogen, it must be supplemented, because its normal production also decreases after menopause. The real answer may be as simple as the estrogen just doing what regular weight-bearing exercise would do. I believe that women who take estrogen to prevent osteoporosis are just treating an unbalanced condition that regular physical use (exercise) and a balanced diet of natural foods was intended to prevent. This is the most likely answer, because it is simple and natural and anyone can do it—like the millions of women who lived before the development of estrogen replacement therapy.

Men also get osteoporosis. Do they have a different reason for getting it than women? I do not think so. Men generally do not have high levels of female hormones. They have some estrogen (about one-fifth the amount a woman does) but less during their entire lives than most postmenopausal women. Why don't they get osteoporosis when they are young? Should we give estrogen replacement therapy to the men with this condition? I do not think many of them would be happy with the side effects. Some doctors believe that osteoporosis in men is caused by a decrease in testosterone. Why would it be a different cause in men than in women? That does not make sense. So, are men doomed to have weak bones? I do not believe so. They need the same things the women need—proper nutrition and weight-bearing exercise. If the testosterone level is the key to this disease, then exercise is still the answer, because heavy exercise stimulates the production of testosterone in both genders, helping to keep muscles and bones strong.

Fewer men than women get osteoporosis probably because they naturally have stronger muscles and generally do heavier work and exercise than women do. Who in the household usually carries the heavy things that need moving? Even if they do not do much physical work or exercise when they are older, many men will have built stronger bones in their youth. Therefore, it will take them much longer to lose enough bone mass to be a problem.

The parathyroid glands produce parathyroid hormone, which increases calcium absorption from the small intestine, decreases calcium loss through the kidneys and causes calcium to be removed from the bones—three things that increase calcium in the blood. The thyroid gland produces the hormone calcitonin, which decreases calcium in the blood by causing calcium to be deposited back into the bones. Women have lower levels of calcitonin than men do and postmenopausal women have less than younger women do. Most neck problems originate from vertebral misalignments at the base of the neck where the nerves go to and from the thyroid and parathyroid glands. Pressure on these nerves can affect the production and release of parathyroid hormone and calcitonin. If the nerve pressure stimulates excess parathyroid hormone, calcium will be lost from the bones. If calcitonin production and release is decreased, an insufficient amount of calcium will be replaced in the bones when appropriate. Therefore, abnormal function of the parathyroid and thyroid glands due to improper nerve flow, or for any other reason, may sometimes be a major factor in osteoporosis. Tightness in the neck and subsequent pressure on the nerves generally increase with age. Varying degrees of nerve pressure would also explain why some women have more bone loss than others of similar age and body type.

Most of my female patients have neck problems but my male patients usually have lower back conditions. There are reasons for this as there are reasons for everything. Women generally have weaker upper body muscles than men do. This makes their neck muscles more susceptible to overstress or traumatic injury. Most of them also carry heavy purses on their shoulders that put excessive stress on their neck muscles. Many of them also carry children in a way that stresses their neck muscles. This may be why women have lower calcitonin levels than men, and a part of why more women get osteoporosis. Men tend to do more heavy lifting and often carry their wallets in a back pocket. The wallet causes the hips to torque, and this can sometimes create pelvic and lower back misalignments and pain. Excessive sitting and improper lifting can cause similar problems.

I believe that an excess of sodium fluoride contributes to the fractures experienced by many of those with osteoporosis. This toxic chemical tends to accumulate in the system and causes bones to be abnormal and more fragile. Therefore, people who have used fluoride toothpaste and ingested water or other liquids containing fluoride will most likely experience more broken bones. Remember how important pure water is to good health.

Preventing osteoporosis should be a natural result of a healthy lifestyle that includes a balanced diet and regular strength-building exercises for the entire body. A good program has exercises that put compressive stress on the bones of the spine, thighs and wrists. I have read articles written by nutritional "experts" who recommend walking, dancing, tennis, climbing stairs and other similar activities to prevent osteoporosis. They call them "weight-bearing" exercises. Do not believe it. Those activities will do almost nothing to prevent losing bone strength and density. They are fine to do and usually enjoyable, but are minimally useful for keeping bones strong. Just think about it for a moment. Many older women walk around a considerable amount every day and some of them also climb stairs. So why do their bones get weak? Because the stress on the bones must be more than just the weight of their bodies in order to maintain enough strength to resist fractures.

Weight bearing means carrying something—something relatively heavy. Just walking around does not put weight-bearing stress on the thoracic vertebrae or wrists and hardly any on the thighbones. Do some hiking with a 25- to 90-pound pack on your back and you will get some weight-bearing exercise. Lifting it and holding on to the straps part of the time will even keep your wrists strong.

You will not find much osteoporosis in the countries where women still carry water, food or wood in their arms, on top of their heads or hanging from each end of a stick across the base of their necks. Keep in mind that these women eat natural diets devoid of calcium-depleting foods and drugs, and drink water without sodium fluoride. They do not stress their necks by carrying heavy purses on one shoulder. They do, however, have lower estrogen and progesterone levels when they get older. This is another reason why I believe that these hormones have little to do with causing osteoporosis.

I believe that the lack of stressful physical work is a primary component of osteoporosis and why the right strength-building exercise program is imperative. It is even more important if you already have osteoporosis. Inefficient or unsafe programs either produce minimal results or cause injury. Your program should include exercises that stress the wrists from different angles, but most importantly, a *full* squat exercise with added weight putting compressive pressure on the spine and upper thighbones. All exercises must be done properly to get the best results with maximum safety. A variety of exercise machines can be used to make the full squat exercise safe for the lower back and knees. Some of the other machines found in gyms and health clubs make exercising other muscles safer and simpler.

If your bones are already osteoporotic, you must proceed slowly and cautiously as you exercise to regain bone density and strength. Eating a pH balanced diet is also vital and you must avoid soft drinks and other calcium-depleting products. A calcium and magnesium supplement may be necessary in the beginning, but you should be tested for need so you do not disrupt your body's mineral balances. Once you stop depleting it, you should get all the calcium you need from a variety of natural foods and a daily multivitamin and mineral supplement.

Hypoglycemia

Hypoglycemia occurs when the blood sugar level drops below normal. It often happens suddenly and can cause a large number of unpleasant physical and emotional symptoms. A common cause of this condition is eating unbalanced foods that release high levels of sugar into the bloodstream at one time. Alcohol, sugar and most processed grain products are the main culprits. Frequent high blood sugar levels overstress the pancreas and sometimes cause it to overreact and secrete excess insulin. This causes the blood sugar level to drop abnormally low. It can easily occur in the 10 percent of the population who have inherited an overly sensitive pancreas, but can happen to people who stress the body's blood sugar balancing system enough.

The adrenal glands produce a number of vital hormones. One of them is cortisol, a glucocorticoid hormone that acts as an anti-inflammatory but also affects blood sugar levels by causing the body to convert protein to glucose. The adrenal glands can become overworked from stress, poor nutrition and excess salt. This may cause reduced production of cortisol and lead to hypoglycemia. Pressure on certain spinal nerves can inhibit the normal function of the pancreas and adrenal glands. A high-protein diet overstresses the pancreas, adrenal glands and other digestive organs and can cause, or contribute to, the development of hypoglycemia. This is another reason why a high-protein diet is not recommended.

A number of commonly used drugs have been shown to cause hypoglycemia. Normal blood sugar levels can be disrupted by anti-inflammatory drugs, analgesics, anticoagulants, diuretics, hormones, stimulants and tranquilizers, antibiotics, alcohol, nicotine, sugar (which acts like a drug) and numerous other chemicals. Other contributors to hypoglycemia include poor nutrition, lack of the trace minerals chromium and manganese, and abnormal liver or kidney function.

Here are some of the symptoms you could experience if you have hypoglycemia:

cold hands and feet	headaches
fatigue	muscle pains and cramps
fainting	numbness
nightmares	insomnia
crying spells	drowsiness
dizziness	strange breath odor
irritability	nausea
restlessness	excessive worry
nervous breakdown	itching or crawling sensations
depression	forgetfulness
allergies	excess anxiety
blurred vision	inner trembling
ringing in the ears	strange body odor
temper tantrums	sensitivity to noise and light
cold sweats	skin conditions
joint pains	loss of appetite
gastrointestinal upsets	dry or burning mouth
loss of sex drive	impotency
fast or pounding heartbeat	suicidal thoughts
inability to concentrate	illogical fears
tremors	blackouts
uncoordination	shortness of breath
hot flashes	

I told you there were a large number of possible symptoms. Do any of them sound familiar? This list should help you to see the importance of eating to maintain a normal blood sugar level and living a lifestyle that will not overstress your pancreas and adrenal glands. If you have inherited one or both of those organs as your weak link, you will be more vulnerable to developing hypoglycemia and experiencing some of these symptoms. There are other causes for these symptoms, but low blood sugar is a common one. Another frequent cause for most of them is nutritional deficiencies. If you regularly experience five or more of the above symptoms, you should seek advice from a doctor experienced in *properly* diagnosing and treating hypoglycemia and similar conditions.

Polio is uncommon in the United States these days but is still seen in underdeveloped countries. Evidence exists that hypoglycemia makes a person susceptible to polio.

As previously mentioned, the three main causes of hypoglycemia are alcohol, sugar and processed grain products. Almost every processed food contains processed flour and many contain sugar. These three things also lead to depletion of B-complex vitamins, vitamin A, zinc, calcium and magnesium. A deficiency of these nutrients can contribute to many of the symptoms seen in hypoglycemia. It is estimated that this condition affects Americans at the rate of 16,000 new cases every month.

Some of the problems in society that can be caused by hypoglycemia are violent crimes, accidents, juvenile delinquency, murder, suicide, marital difficulties and divorce, depression, mental illness, fatigue, excessive use of legal and illegal drugs, smoking, obesity and alcoholism. How many of these problems would be solved if more people got adequate nutrition? Does the fact that people of certain races seem more susceptible to this condition explain why more of them are in prison? The percentage of people suffering from low blood sugar problems is approximately the same as those with some type of mental illness. Do you think this is a coincidence? I don't. I am not sure of this, but I have heard that Adolf Hitler had hypoglycemia.

When I was in my mid-twenties, I developed hypoglycemia. It came on gradually and caused many of the symptoms previously listed. It became so severe that I lost my job and could barely function. I consulted numerous doctors, but got no help. Most of them wanted to treat particular symptoms or acted as if it was all in my head. One even suggested that I go to a psychiatrist for medication. This is a common response from doctors who do not know what is wrong, do not attempt to find out, or do not want to admit that they do not know how to resolve the problem. I did not think that psychotropic drugs would eliminate the cause of my condition. For many years, some doctors denied that hypoglycemia even existed. Finally, after much physical, mental and financial suffering, a six-hour glucose tolerance test was done to diagnose my condition. A mixed-meal tolerance test is generally used now to diagnose hypoglycemia, but I believe that the glucose tolerance test is better, because it is closer to the way many people eat.

Once I knew what was happening, I read four or five books on the subject of hypoglycemia. Several doctors and all but one of the books suggested eating a small high-protein meal every three to four hours to maintain a normal blood sugar level and control the symptoms. This approach made no sense to me, because that is what I had been doing and what I believe had overstressed my digestive system and caused the condition. Eating high-protein meals every three to four hours may cover up some symptoms for a while, but makes the condition worse by overstressing the weakened glands and organs. The goal should be to restore normal function, not just cover up symptoms.

Fortunately for me, I read the book *Hypoglycemia: A Better Approach*. The author, Paavo Airola, suggested doing the opposite of what the others were saying. He recommended a low-protein diet to give the digestive system a chance to rest and rejuvenate. I followed his advice and ate primarily *whole* complex carbohydrates (vegetables, whole grains and legumes) and healthful fats. These foods helped my body maintain a normal blood sugar level without stressing my system. I also did some internal cleansing and fasting occasionally to give my digestive system a complete rest. After four or five months, my condition was resolved and I was able to eat fruits and certain other foods again with no adverse reactions. I then became a vegetarian for almost two years. That almost killed me and then I began developing the program in this book. I have had no further hypoglycemic problems for more than twenty-eight years now.

A great deal of misleading information about hypoglycemia has been written in various publications and given to patients by doctors. This information is about diet plans that treat the symptoms while contributing to making the condition worse. Sadly, many doctors do not even attempt to discover and eliminate the cause of a patient's symptoms. They just prescribe drugs to treat individual symptoms, such as a headache, or refer the patient to a psychiatrist who often prescribes more drugs to treat other symptoms. Sometimes the drugs make the low-blood sugar condition worse. Unfortunately, many people just assume everyone else feels as badly as they do, so they do not even look for help. Those who do look usually go to a medical doctor who knows little, if anything, about correctly diagnosing or treating hypoglycemia. The people experiencing it or the doctors they go to for help most often blame the symptoms on stress. This is a common answer many doctors give to patients when they do not know what is wrong with them. Using anything (even herbs and foods) to cover up your symptoms is unhealthful, because the cause of the problem is not being dealt with and is usually getting worse.

In the year 2000 I attended a nutritional seminar. The instructor was a likeable person and had other good information, but recommended eating a high-protein diet. He knew that when complex carbohydrates are eaten, insulin is released to cause excess glucose to be stored as glycogen in either the liver or the muscles. For this reason, he believes that eating carbohydrates causes hypoglycemia. I agree that an excess of *processed* carbohydrates, which raise the blood sugar level excessively fast, contributes to the problem. The body can use some of the energy, but the excess causes a stress reaction and often the release of too much insulin. This causes low blood sugar and stress to the pancreas. It can gradually lead to further overreaction or a breakdown of the pancreas. He used the meat-eating Eskimo people as an example to justify his reasoning, but failed to mention the billions of other healthy people in the world who eat small amounts of complete protein. You already know Eskimo people need to eat that way to condition their bodies to their harsh environment and that all of these people start having health problems when sugar and processed grains are added to their diets. Also remember that my hypoglycemia was resolved by eating mostly complex-carbohydrate foods.

I was not convinced his high-protein diet was healthful, because he had a large belly and said he had suffered from hypoglycemia for a long time. He mentioned that he took herbs twice a day to strengthen his pancreas and other parts of his body. With all he was doing, why did he have excess fat and hypoglycemia? It makes no sense, because if people eat properly, they should be lean and have normal blood sugar response. Unfortunately, this doctor of chiropractic will eventually pay the price for just treating his symptoms.

What happens if you do not overeat and you eat whole foods like I have been suggesting throughout this book? The glucose from *whole* carbohydrate foods is released at a slow and constant rate. The brain and muscles can use it as it becomes available. Almost no insulin release is even needed. No crisis (threat of injury from excess sugar) is created so the pancreas does not overreact or get stressed. Let me give you some examples of whole food versus processed foods to make this more clear. The glycemic index of brown rice (a whole food) is 55, but instant white rice (a processed food) is 87. A grapefruit (a whole food) is rated 25, but grapefruit juice (a processed food) is 48. Even processed pumpernickel bread is only 51 compared to a highly processed French baguette (roll) having a glycemic index of 95.

Until hypoglycemia is treated correctly and eliminated, you will not be able to think straight and feel good about yourself and your life. You will never lose your excess body fat if you are depressed or experiencing some of the other symptoms this condition can cause. If the pancreas and other endocrine glands are constantly overreacting, a breakdown could occur that decreases their ability to produce enough of their vital secretions. Insufficient insulin or the body's inability to use it properly is what causes diabetes mellitus. I believe that hypoglycemia may lead to the development of this more serious condition.

Diabetes Mellitus

Diabetes mellitus is an extremely serious health condition that is usually just referred to as diabetes. In this condition, the blood sugar level gets excessively high because the body is unable to regulate it properly. The high sugar content in the blood causes a great deal of damage in the body, especially to the arteries carrying it. Damage to the small blood vessels of the eyes can cause many vision problems including blindness. In fact, diabetes is the leading cause of blindness in people ages twenty to seventy-four. As a side note, in *Health and Light*, John Ott relates a story of how indirect exposure to natural light was able to quickly stop the bleeding and improve the vision in a diabetic person's eyes after many conventional treatments had failed. High blood sugar levels also commonly damage the blood vessels and nerves of the feet and legs. This often leads to gangrene and is why many diabetics have had their legs amputated. About eight percent of diabetic men become impotent. Diabetics have increased risk for kidney failure, heart disease, strokes and infections. Their arteries are damaged by the sugar and this often leads to severe atherosclerosis and renal (kidney) vascular damage. Diabetes is currently the sixth leading cause of death in the United States. As you can see, this is an extremely serious condition you want to avoid if possible, and fortunately it can usually be easily prevented.

There are two forms of diabetes mellitus. Type I, insulin-dependent diabetes, often occurs at or before puberty and is usually caused by a genetic weakness or some permanent damage to the pancreas. Research suggests that during early development, cow's milk protein may trigger a reaction in the body that destroys the insulin-producing beta cells of the pancreas. This may be the primary reason why some people develop diabetes. Type I diabetes can be helped with exercise and proper nutrition but insulin injections must also be used.

Type II, non-insulin-dependent diabetes, used to appear after age forty and therefore was commonly called adult-onset diabetes. It accounts for 90 to 95 percent of all diabetes cases. According to the American Diabetes Association, about thirteen million Americans have been diagnosed with diabetes in 2004 and it is estimated that more than five million more have it but do not know that they do. Diabetes is increasing at a rate of about 800,000 new cases a year. Its incidence is much higher among African Americans, Mexican Americans and Native Americans. I believe this occurs because the diets they now eat are so different from the natural diets of their ancestors that it is easy for them to get fat and to not get adequate nutrition. Even those eating a diet like their ancestors will have problems if they also eat processed foods, especially sugar. Do not think using aspartame instead of sugar is going to save you. It has been shown to cause or worsen diabetes and many other serious diseases.

Because 85 to 90 percent of type II diabetes sufferers are labeled as overweight or obese, being fat increases your risk more than anything else. Every 20 percent increase in your body weight doubles your chances of getting this serious condition. A study done by a number of insurance companies compared three equally numbered groups of people over the age of forty-five. The group of very thin people had one case of diabetes, the normal weight group had five cases and the fat group had 227 cases. During the 1990s, the incidence of diabetes increased 33 percent and by 70 percent among people in their thirties. The term "adult-onset" is fast becoming obsolete. The frequency of diabetes is increasing right along with the incidence of obesity. The rate of type I diabetes does not seem to be increasing.

Why are people getting diabetes at such young ages? The answer is simple. If someone gets fat by age thirty and develops diabetes at age fifty, it took twenty years to create enough damage to manifest the condition. It is easy to see why a woman gets diabetes at age thirty-seven if she was fat at age seventeen, or why a man gets it at age twenty if he has been fat his entire life. Of course, how long it takes to create the problem varies based on diet, activity level, fat percentage, age, and function of the pancreas and other organs. If your pancreas is the weak link in your body, it is very important to avoid overstressing it and vital to give it the support it needs to function at its best.

Some of the symptoms of diabetes are lethargy, irritability, increased thirst, frequent urination, increased appetite, slow healing of cuts and bruises, numb or tingling extremities, failing strength and loss of weight. The weight loss is usually not noticeable in the majority of those who are obese. They may lose lean tissue and then gain even more fat due to an increased appetite. Skin infections or irritations and visual disturbances are also common. The excessive urination often leads to dehydration, a loss of electrolyte minerals and the symptoms they create. Diabetes also reduces your body's ability to heal properly, and degenerative changes often occur.

Excess body fat and overeating both put greater than normal stress on your pancreas and, like eating excess protein, can weaken it to the point where it can no longer produce enough insulin for your needs. Another important fact is that as your body fat increases you lose insulin receptors on your cells, so they are less able to use glucose. Your body reduces the number of receptors to compensate for the excess insulin created by overeating and eating processed foods. As your body fat decreases, your body increases the number of receptors. It is clear to see that achieving and maintaining normal body weight is extremely important in preventing or controlling diabetes. Physical exercise reduces your need for insulin and improves your insulin sensitivity so you need less. Therefore, regular exercise is also helpful for preventing or treating diabetes.

Living a balanced and happy life is important for us all, because it reduces stress and many other things detrimental to good health. Fear and anger stimulate the release of epinephrine, which increases the blood sugar level. This is especially harmful to diabetics. These two emotions are the origins of most of the others that have negative effects on our health and well-being. It is important to find positive ways to express and deal with these emotions.

Most doctors suggest exercising and eating a better diet to their diabetic patients. Sadly, the majority of them do not know how to eat well themselves or understand the best exercises to help people lose their excess weight. One drug currently being used stimulates the pancreas to make more insulin. This may stress the pancreas further and lead to more problems. Some drugs make the body's cells more sensitive to insulin and others slow the breakdown of carbohydrates in the digestive tract. These drugs do not help the person to learn what foods naturally break down slowly. They may prolong someone's life for a while but the condition will usually continue to worsen.

About one third of those affected with diabetes do not even know they have it, because it progresses slowly. Taking a long time to develop makes it easier to prevent but also easier to postpone doing anything about it. You must start exercising and eating well now. Do not wait until you have accumulated enough damage to start having symptoms. It is important to get a *thorough* physical exam about once a year. Be aware that many doctors do superficial physical exams and often will not find a problem until it has grown into something difficult to resolve. Find a doctor who cares about your health as much as (preferably more than) he does about money.

Alcoholism

Alcoholism is America's number-one drug addiction. It has been labeled a disease in the United States but the medical authorities of most countries do not share the same belief. Numerous theories attempt to explain why one person gets addicted to alcohol but another does not. Some people believe it is an attempt to run away from emotional problems or a result of being abused or neglected as a child. Certainly, psychological influences can play a part in why someone starts drinking, or contribute to the problem in some other way, but research and successful treatment of many alcoholics seem to indicate it to be primarily a physical disorder that can often be resolved by nutritional means.

Researchers have turned rats into alcoholics simply by feeding them a diet high in processed carbohydrates and low in protein, vitamins and minerals. (This is like the diet many people eat, especially young people.) Some of the rats did not develop the craving for alcohol until they were given sugar. These rats then became the heaviest drinkers of all. (Most people ingest excess amounts of refined sugar.) Another study fed the rats hot dogs, donuts, carbonated drinks, white bread, green beans, spaghetti and meatballs, salad, candy, cake and cookies. (That sounds like the diet of some of the people I know.) These rats drank a great deal of alcohol and even more when caffeine was added. Now, what happened when they were placed on a healthful diet? They gradually became ex-alcoholics. In these studies, none of the rats were psychologically stressed, physically abused or raised by uncaring parents.

Clearly, nutrient deficiencies can create a biological thirst for alcohol. A poor diet can cause the craving and a good diet can eliminate it. Another fact is that 70 to 90 percent of all alcoholics are hypoglycemic. You already know that caffeine, nicotine, sugar and many processed carbohydrate foods contribute to that problem. Many former alcoholics who no longer drink report craving alcohol, caffeine, nicotine or sweets when they experience low blood sugar. This explains why drinkers are not usually motivated to quit by dangers or losses they may face. Believe me, when your blood sugar drops dramatically, you do not care if you live or die, so the fear of losing your job, spouse, driver's license or anything else does not matter at that moment. The influence is extremely powerful, and because your brain is not functioning normally at that time, you can not see future consequences, nor would you care about them if you could. People in this hypoglycemic condition often turn to alcohol, because it is the fastest way to get glucose to the brain and relieve the discomfort.

When alcohol is ingested, the enzyme alcohol dehydrogenase breaks it down into acetaldehyde, which is a chemical similar to formaldehyde. Acetaldehyde acts as a free radical and damages the cells it contacts. It also makes people feel poorly. Drinking more alcohol temporarily makes someone feel better and a negative cycle is created that can lead to excessive alcohol consumption. When acetaldehyde is formed, the body then uses the enzyme aldehyde dehydrogenase to convert the acetaldehyde to acetic acid, which is similar to vinegar and not harmful. Some people's bodies do not break down acetaldehyde as well as others do, so it builds up to even more harmful levels. This could make a person more susceptible to becoming an alcoholic. Excess alcohol damages the liver so much that it cannot make enough aldehyde dehydrogenase and this also leads to a buildup of toxic acetaldehyde.

Alcoholics Anonymous (AA) has helped a large number of people with their Twelve Step program. Unfortunately, it has the potential to work only for someone willing to take the first step. This is very difficult for most alcoholics, because the physical effects of malnutrition and low blood sugar are extremely powerful. Most alcoholics never take the first step and the majority of those who do find the program too restrictive and end up dropping out. I believe that an important key is to get the body functioning normally again with proper diet and special nutritional supplements. Sometimes a social or psychological program may then be necessary to eliminate the person's emotional addiction. This is important to prevent the person from starting to drink again and re-creating the nutritional deficiencies and physical imbalances. Unfortunately, most alcoholic treatment programs do nothing to correct the nutritional deficiencies alcoholics have. Many alcoholics simply replace alcohol with nicotine, sugar, caffeine or processed carbohydrates. Attend an AA meeting sometime (I have gone as someone's guest) and watch most of them drink coffee, eat cookies and smoke cigarettes like there's no tomorrow. These substitutes perpetuate the hypoglycemic condition and cause the health of these people to further deteriorate. Physically they still crave alcohol so it would be easy to start drinking again.

Alcohol abuse (the person's body, family, friends and life are really what are being abused) is a vicious cycle that usually grows stronger as the person's life spirals ever downward. Here is basically how it starts and grows. First, alcohol is ingested and supplies calories that should be obtained from food. The calories from the alcohol are empty, because there is no protein, or vitamins or minerals. Just 20 ounces of 86-proof liquor contains 1,500 calories. That may be one half or more of someone's daily requirements. Second, the alcohol depletes the B vitamins, magnesium and other nutrients the person may be getting from foods or supplements. This can easily create a deficiency of these vital nutrients. Third, alcohol causes inflammation in the stomach, pancreas and intestine, causing these organs to function abnormally. This can lead to other problems like diabetes and can cause poor digestion and absorption of any healthful nutrients being ingested. Someone's body could easily get even less of the nutrients already being depleted by the alcohol as well as other vital nutrients. Fourth, alcohol and its byproduct acetaldehyde interfere with the activation of some vitamins by liver cells. This creates even more deficiencies. It is easy to see how all these deficiencies would reduce the digestive efficiency of a person's body more and more. This is a good reason to avoid drinking wine no matter how many people or "scientific studies" tell you it is good for you and your digestion. These nutritional deficiencies are what cause the many physical and mental problems normally seen in alcoholics. Sadly, many alcoholics attempt to treat the problems they experience by drinking more. This may make them oblivious to the problems for a while, but just makes everything worse.

Some of the problems common to alcoholics are abnormal carbohydrate metabolism, nutrient deficiencies, wheat allergy, hormone imbalances, liver dysfunction, and functional or metabolic disorders of the brain. If people do not get enough glucose for their brains to function normally, they may be stimulated to drink alcohol to supply the energy the brain needs, because it can use only glucose for energy. Alcohol supplies this need quickly, because about one-fifth of it is absorbed directly from the stomach. This may be the initial trigger for some alcoholics and what keeps many of them drinking.

Some doctors and health centers have had tremendous success helping alcoholics to recover using megavitamin therapy. The primary vitamin normally used is niacin (vitamin B_3). It may be that those susceptible to alcoholism need more of this nutrient, but I believe it is just the vitamin most depleted by alcohol and perhaps the initial cause of the alcoholic downward spiral. Meats, poultry and fish are the best sources of niacin but excess consumption of sugar and processed starches deplete niacin from the body.

A niacin deficiency causes many symptoms. In the beginning, muscular weakness, fatigue, poor appetite, indigestion and various skin eruptions occur. Another early sign of niacin deficiency is the loss of a sense of humor. Someone may also experience insomnia, bad breath, headaches, tender gums, nausea, vomiting, canker sores, irritability, tension and extreme depression. A severe niacin deficiency can result in rough and inflamed skin, tremors, nervous disorders and pellagra—a condition that causes dermatitis, dementia and diarrhea.

The symptoms of magnesium deficiency are also important to understand and eliminate in an alcoholic or anyone having a nervous disorder. Some of them are tremors, muscle twitches, apprehension, confusion and disorientation. Magnesium has helped neuromuscular disorders, nervousness, tantrums, diarrhea, vomiting, sensitivity to noise, and delirium tremens (DTs). Do you see some of the similarities with niacin deficiency? One study of patients with *mild* magnesium deficiencies found that 22 percent had convulsions; 44 percent experienced hallucinations; 78 percent were mentally confused; 83 percent were disoriented so badly they could not remember where they were, the year, the day, or the month; and all of them were easily startled and bothered by unexpected noise or movement. A more severe deficiency can cause someone to be extremely psychotic with tics, tremors, slurred speech and the inability to stand up. How many people living on the street or locked up in mental institutions are simply deficient in magnesium or niacin?

Magnesium is vital for nerve conduction and muscular contraction. It activates enzymes necessary for metabolizing carbohydrates and amino acids. It helps regulate the acid/alkaline balance in the body. Magnesium is necessary for proper absorption and metabolism of other minerals so without it you will most likely be deficient in others. It is needed in the conversion of blood sugar into energy and helps use the B-complex vitamins and vitamins C and E. With all of these vital functions, it is easy to see why a deficiency causes so many serious symptoms.

In *The Cure for All Diseases*, Dr. Hulda Clark states that besides the liver not functioning properly, two other things contribute to alcoholism. One is the chemical beryllium, found in coal products such as coal oil and kerosene. She believes that when the fumes are inhaled, the beryllium attaches to the receptor sites in the addiction center of the brain. The beryllium blocks the attachment of the amino acid glutamine that is supposed to stimulate joy and happiness. If the glutamine cannot attach, the result is chronic depression. When alcohol is ingested, placed on the skin, or made in the intestines by the *Candida albicans* fungus, a substance called salsol is formed. The salsol reacts with the beryllium and releases pleasure chemicals from the brain. This is why the alcohol stimulates a good feeling for a while.

Dr. Clark believes the other contributor to alcoholism is ergot mold. This mold is often found in nuts, grains and alcoholic beverages. Ergot and alcohol interact and make each other more toxic to the liver. Using a bit of vitamin C powder when eating nuts or cooking grains can neutralize the ergot.

Dr. Clark advises alcoholics to take a B-complex vitamin, niacinamide (a form of niacin), and glutamine with each meal. The vitamins help detoxify the ergot and the glutamine may help reduce the depression. She recommends that the person avoid inhaling the fumes from paints, automotive products, solvents and cleaners. Niacin has been successful at treating alcoholism but until now no one had an explanation for how it worked.

I believe that most alcohol and drug treatment centers are too generic. They attempt to treat everyone the same. Just like proper nutritional plans, programs must be designed specifically for each person if you hope to obtain permanent success. Alcoholics Anonymous works well for some people but may be completely wrong for others. I disagree with permanently labeling someone an alcoholic or with calling alcoholism a disease. It is a physical and emotional imbalance, which is true of all diseases, but labeling it as such gives many people the excuse of not taking responsibility for their own actions or their own healing. Constantly calling yourself an alcoholic reinforces this negative label and programs the subconscious to create an alcoholic. I believe that many people in alcoholic programs focus on their fear of drinking again and this sometimes creates what they fear, and that some become dependent on others to not drink. I believe it is possible to eliminate the physical *and* psychological addictions so dependency on others is unnecessary.

Drinking problems come in different degrees and for varying reasons, just like excess fat. Not everyone has to hit rock bottom before deciding to do something about the problem. Some people will be able to have an occasional drink after their bodies are balanced and they have eliminated their emotional reasons for drinking or learned healthy ways of dealing with them. Just like overeating, once the causes of excess drinking have been eliminated, it can be controlled and done in moderation if the person chooses to drink at all. On the other hand, some people will never be able to touch another drop of alcohol without starting to drink excessively again. These are people who have a genetic defect, or who will not or do not know how to eliminate the physical and emotional reasons why they drink to excess. If you have a problem with drinking too much alcohol, you may find your emotional reason for doing it in chapter twelve.

Most, if not all, of the problems found in alcoholics can be reversed and entirely resolved using natural methods. Because overeating, drinking to excess or using other harmful drugs are so similar, this book could have been titled *How to Cure Alcoholism* or *Ending Drug Addiction*. Some people overeat because of their physical and emotional imbalances and others drink excessively or use drugs. Some people do two or three of these destructive behaviors. I believe that many alcoholics, drug users, overeaters and other addicts are shy and lack confidence in their own abilities. They drink, use drugs, overeat or do other addictive behaviors to deaden their uncomfortable feelings or to fit in with the crowd. I believe that most of them are also extremely deficient in soul food and self-love. People with these problems need to learn to overcome their shyness, develop self-confidence, start loving themselves and get more soul food.

My method of treatment for alcoholics would be to do my PMBT therapy to make sure they have normal nerve flow to the liver, stomach, pancreas, adrenal glands and small intestines. Also, their nervous systems would be balanced if necessary and any abnormally functioning glands and organs treated to restore normal blood flow. Because alcoholics, like most fat people, are undernourished, they would be placed on a balanced diet of natural foods rich in the nutrients necessary to restore health. Those with hypoglycemia may need to avoid some natural foods until their bodies have recuperated enough to handle them. A few natural foods may have to be eliminated permanently by some people. A bit of extra protein may initially be necessary to strengthen and rebuild weakened and depleted tissues.

A special nutritional supplementation program would be used to reestablish normal levels of vitamins and minerals. This would be accomplished primarily by using the Super Spectrim multivitamin and mineral twice daily along with extra magnesium, zinc, calcium, glutamine and niacinamide. Supplements would include various herbs that calm and feed the nerves and others that help the liver to regenerate. Each person would be tested to determine the supplements and dosages needed. Vitamin C powder would be added to any nuts or grains. Caffeine and sugar would have to be completely avoided, because they impair recovery significantly. Nicotine would also have to be eliminated, because it causes a craving for caffeine and sugar. Doing this should not be difficult, because the foods, vitamins, minerals and herbs should help eliminate the physical desire for these harmful substances. Synthetic vitamin D, like the kind added to milk, and fluoride would have to be avoided, because they bind with magnesium and carry it out of the body.

During the start of treatment, an easy cardiovascular exercise program would be implemented to help normalize their blood sugar levels and reduce stress and nervous tension. A strength-building program would soon be added to stimulate the replacement of the protein and other nutrients stolen from their muscles when they were drinking. Both types of exercise would help alcoholics feel better by stimulating endorphin release and by improving their self-image and sense of accomplishment and self-worth.

I would have alcoholics get plenty of exposure to natural light and recommend that they install full-spectrum lights at home and in their workplaces. I believe that this "light" therapy would be extremely helpful because of its endocrine balancing effect. The next paragraph sheds more light (pun intended) on the importance of this.

When a group of rats was kept in total darkness for two weeks, they began drinking alcohol instead of water. When they were exposed to normal laboratory lighting, 75 percent of them went back to water. Chances are that this percentage would have been much higher if the lab had used full-spectrum lighting. Dr. Irving Geller states that when the rats were deprived of light, it stimulated their pineal glands to produce more melatonin and a melatonin-forming enzyme. He has made rats into alcoholics by injecting them with a melatonin solution. Based on this evidence, alcoholics should get an abundance of natural light and avoid taking a melatonin supplement for any reason.

Last, but certainly not least, any emotional causes for drinking would be determined and eliminated. New thought processes would have to be developed concerning how the people feel about alcohol and about themselves. In this book you will find many ways of changing your thoughts and feelings that can be applied to alcohol or drug addiction as easily as overeating or making poor food choices.

Alcoholics would be encouraged to feed their minds with uplifting and inspirational thoughts from books and tapes. This would be most important to do during the time of day they used to drink and just before going to sleep.

They would be taught how to see the positive side of everything instead of the negative and how to find ways to get an abundance of soul food to feed their starving spirits. Alcoholics, like fat people, must come to the realization that they have the power within themselves to overcome their problems. They just have to use it. Unfortunately, many of them do not know they have it, do not know how to use it, or do not feel worthy of using it. An important goal would be to help them realize that they can change as soon as they make the choice to change.

Mental Illness

Have you ever felt like you just can't take it anymore and are going to "crack up" at any moment? Haven't we all at one time or another? This is normal in extreme circumstances, but if this feeling occurs frequently or without an obvious reason, it is important to find and eliminate the cause.

Why you feel depressed and have little joy in your life most likely comes from a nutritional deficiency, not your job, the world's problems, your own real or imagined problems, your children or your spouse. These deficiencies can come from a physical disorder, but are most commonly caused by poor eating habits or the use of alcohol and various drugs that deplete the body of vital nutrients. In general, the greater the deficiency, the more severe the symptoms are, but many people experience severe symptoms from the combined effects of many small deficiencies, not from a large deficiency.

Every vital nutrient our bodies need to function normally affects and is dependent on others. It may be that one missing nutrient will prevent others from being assimilated or used. Frequently two or more nutrients work together to cause a certain reaction or produce a specific substance. Sometimes the ratio between nutrients is extremely important. A shortage of one vitamin, mineral, amino acid or fatty acid creates a snowball effect that can negatively influence every other nutrient. For these and other reasons, it is imperative to get adequate amounts of all vital nutrients.

An inadequate amount of calcium can cause an anxiety neurosis with symptoms including nervousness, exaggerated fears, loss of appetite, sleep disturbances and feelings of impending doom. You could also experience muscle cramps, stiff muscles, palpitations, sweating, a racing heart and anxiety. Infants and children may experience uncontrollable temper tantrums. If you are lacking in niacin, you will lose your sense of humor. Teenagers are often lacking in this vital nutrient. A zinc deficiency can lead to poor appetite, slow growth and a decreased sense of smell and taste. It can cause children to be lethargic and apathetic about their schoolwork. Students with the highest academic grades usually have substantial amounts of zinc and copper in their systems. A French scientist found suicide rates to be much higher where the soils were depleted of zinc.

The two main causes of nutritional deficiencies are poor eating habits and dieting. Both of these are completely within your control. The brain is extremely sensitive to nutritional deficiencies. This is why so many emotional problems can be caused by dietary deficiencies and why emotional complaints are common while dieting. Some of the symptoms often seen are insomnia, nervousness, irritability, confusion, depression, inability to tolerate stress, severe agitation, fatigue, neurosis, tension, inability to concentrate, anxiety, and manic or paranoid behavior. Do any of those sound familiar? Do not forget that the brain controls all other parts of your body. If it is not working properly, neither will anything else. A lack of essential nutrients to the brain creates a negative spiral. Even the good foods being eaten may not be digested well or used. This is why special measures must often be taken to stop the negative cycle and get things moving in a positive direction. Take a look at the symptoms you just read. Most of them are responsible for a lack of caring, poor food choices and overeating. This is another example of the intimate relationship among the body, mind and spirit and how each one affects the other two.

Not all nutritional deficiencies come from the lack of ingesting, absorbing or utilizing healthful nutrients. Many are caused or made worse by something else being ingested or inhaled. The five biggest culprits are caffeine, alcohol, refined sugar, refined flour and nicotine. You already know about many of their harmful effects. Nicotine impairs the absorption of vitamin C, which is used up protecting the body from the free radicals smoking produces. You know that nicotine creates a desire for caffeine and sugar. These five items not only deplete your body of vital nutrients and create the need for more nutrients to protect you from their negative effects, but can also lead to a hypoglycemic condition. Low blood sugar leads to a lack of fuel for the brain and can make you feel like you are going crazy. Hypoglycemia combined with deficiencies of certain nutrients can make otherwise normal people act extremely irrationally, even to the point of killing themselves or others. Many violent criminals are hypoglycemic and starved for good nutrition.

Numerous drugs can cause deficiencies of vital nutrients. Some having this effect are analgesics (pain medications), antacids, antibiotics, blood pressure and cholesterol lowering agents, diuretics, laxatives, and sedatives. Oral contraceptives are especially bad and the most common symptoms are mild to moderate depression, lethargy, fatigue, insomnia and restless sleep. When a woman is taking birth control pills, she needs about fifty to one hundred times more vitamin B_6 to normalize her tryptophan metabolism. Oral contraceptives also limit the absorption of folic acid from foods so supplementation is necessary to prevent a deficiency. Vitamin B_{12} supplementation is also necessary and as much as one to two grams of vitamin C may be needed every day. If you are a woman, you may now understand why you experience so many strange emotional symptoms when using the pill.

You can generally assume that any drug is going to cause a deficiency of something, because drugs are unbalanced products that create imbalances in our bodies. Particular nutrients are used in an attempt to reestablish balance and the liver is stressed detoxifying the drugs. When taking a medication for long periods of time, a competent, nutritionally oriented physician should test you to determine need and dosage of any nutritional supplements necessary to prevent deficiencies and unhealthy symptoms. I believe that many drug addicts could be restored to balance and health quickly with good food and proper nutritional supplementation.

Many people who thought they had serious mental conditions have been restored to normal simply by eating a diet high in essential nutrients. Some of them needed extra supplementation to resolve their problems. Even many schizophrenics have been helped tremendously with improved nutrition and the right supplements. Niacin is the most helpful nutrient for this condition.

There have been numerous cases of certain foods causing the symptoms of severe mental illness and of people being restored to normal when they avoided those foods. Some researchers believe that allergies may be a common cause of mental illness. Some allergic reactions are caused or made worse by hypoglycemia. Allergies are discussed much more in the next chapter.

A condition seemingly affecting more and more people is known as attention deficit hyperactivity disorder (ADHD). It is sometimes called attention deficit disorder (ADD), especially when hyperactivity is absent. You have learned that hydrogenated and partially hydrogenated oils are possible contributors to this condition. I believe that many people have it and do not even know it. It is generally more noticeable in young people, because their bodies are smaller and still growing, their diets are lacking in vital nutrients, their brains are being mentally challenged in school and their intellectual performances are being measured. I believe that most of those affected with this problem could be restored to normal with good nutrition. Some may need other natural treatments but few should need drugs. Many children with ADHD are probably hyperactive due to their consumption of caffeine and processed sugar. Many are prescribed a drug to calm them down. Their bodies are being stimulated and calmed at the same time. This is tremendously stressful and confusing for a brain that is most likely being deprived of the nutrients needed to concentrate, think straight and make wise decisions. It is quite easy to see why those with ADHD behave as they do. Chances are that most of them get a minimal amount of natural balanced light and a great deal of exposure to unbalanced light sources. A deficiency of sleep could also be a major factor in ADD, whether from a sleep disorder of some kind or from just not sleeping enough.

Before you rush off to a psychiatrist for the latest mood-altering or anti-depressant drug for you or for another drug to treat your child's ADD or ADHD, take a look at your nutritional habits. An extremely large percentage of emotional complaints can be resolved by supplying the brain the nutrients it needs to function normally. Sleep and natural light are two of the most important. Eliminate the nutrient vampires we have talked about and make sure you are getting an adequate supply of B vitamins and trace minerals. Some people may need St. John's Wort, valerian root or other herbs temporarily to help restore balanced nutrition to their brains and nervous systems.

Trace minerals are important for many vital processes. For example, if you are deficient in iodine, your thyroid gland is unable to produce enough of its hormones. This slows down your metabolism and causes numerous physical and emotional symptoms. Eliminate your nutritional deficiencies and physical imbalances before lying down on a therapist's couch and discussing what you do not like about your mother. Chances are that you will realize that your mother is a pretty neat lady who, like you, has always done her best, and that you have no need to discuss anything except how good you feel and what you want to accomplish with your life.

Besides the obvious, like noise and rush-hour traffic, other things in our environment can affect our mental state. Very low frequency sounds, known as infrasounds, are below twenty hertz and generally inaudible to the human ear. They can be generated by natural events such as earthquakes and major storms or by construction machinery, defective electric motors, aircraft and even from traveling in a car at certain speeds. These sounds can sometimes cause sane people to act crazy. Could infrasounds be a possible cause of road rage? The odorless fumes in our polluted atmosphere have been found to be responsible for a number of mental disturbances. Regular (not full spectrum) fluorescent lights, strobe lights and certain colored lights can also cause mental distress and bizarre behavior.

Now, guess what our two main defenses against these disruptive forces are. The answers are good nutrition and exercise. Are you surprised? You shouldn't be, after what you have learned so far.

Alzheimer's Disease

For more than thirty years, I have seen diseases that once seemed rare become commonplace. My belief has long been that the main reasons for this are what we ingest and the chemical toxins we are exposed to in our modern environments. People who eat simple diets of natural foods and who are not constantly exposed to numerous chemicals do not get these diseases. More than 100,000 man-made chemicals are in our environment and a large number of them can cause health problems. Many of them are added to our food or found in personal care and cleaning products. There seem to be two main interrelated causes of many diseases. The first is the accumulation of damage the toxic chemicals cause to our bodies. The second is that the nutrient-poor diets many of us eat reduce our bodies' ability to prevent some of the damage and detoxify and eliminate these chemicals. A lack of physical exertion and limited exposure to natural light also make us more susceptible to their destructive effects.

According to Dr. Hulda Clark, who has researched many diseases for their causes, toxic chemicals are part of the cause of almost all. She has determined the toxic chemical she believes is causing most of them. Frequently, the chemicals create an abnormal environment that attracts parasites to travel to and live in parts of our bodies where they would normally never go. Sometimes molds or fungi can overgrow because of the chemicals. Her research seems to have proved what I have suspected for many years. I believe her findings hold the answer to the cause of many diseases. I highly recommend her book, *The Cure for All Diseases*. Do not wait for mainstream medical researchers to come up with a miracle cure. Unfortunately, the companies with the funding to do the appropriate research only seem interested in developing a drug to treat your symptoms and make them millions of dollars. You will rarely hear anything except what they want you to hear.

Alzheimer's disease used to be unheard of but is now becoming more and more common. It has been known for a number of years that aluminum is somehow associated with the development of this tragic disease. I have been telling people for years to avoid products containing aluminum and to not use aluminum cookware. I have also told people to avoid sodium fluoride—a toxic byproduct of aluminum manufacturing. Almost all countries of the world have either not approved the addition of fluoride to their water supplies or have done it and abandoned the practice. I would like to see research done comparing the incidence of Alzheimer's disease in countries that fluoridate the water to those countries where the authorities are smart enough not to do it.

Dr. Clark has found aluminum in all Alzheimer's disease sufferers she has tested. Her research indicates that the chemical solvents xylene and toluene accumulate in the brain and attract parasites to travel there. These two pollutants are found in many popular beverages and carbonated drinks. Dr. Clark recommends avoiding commercial beverages, including water, because they are contaminated with these two solvents. Purify your own water and eat the whole foods that contain the juices. She also recommends avoiding aluminum in all forms. Baking powder sometimes contains aluminum, as do many antiperspirant products and commercial soaps and lotions. Aerosol antiperspirants are probably the worst because inhaled aluminum particles could be rapidly absorbed. To reduce body odor use a deodorant stone that contains natural mineral salts. These stones are available in most health-food stores. Avoid drinking anything from aluminum cans, cooking in aluminum cookware and using aluminum foil. Aluminum may be found in children's aspirin tablets and some white flour. Dr. Clark even recommends putting tape around aluminum tubing you may touch such as the handles of a walker or cane. Restaurant foods may be contaminated with aluminum and these other chemicals so if you eat out frequently I suggest asking them how your meal will be prepared and ordering foods you know are not cooked in aluminum.

Dr. Clark also finds mercury, Freon, thallium and cadmium polluting the brains of Alzheimer's disease sufferers.

The best thing to do with this tragic disease is to prevent it. Avoiding these contaminants seems the best way. It may be the interaction of these chemicals that causes the brain damage seen in Alzheimer's disease. If someone has the disease, cleansing the body of contaminants and parasites and avoiding additional contamination may halt its progression. Sadly, once damage is done it will most likely be permanent.

Various supplements seem to improve brain function. Niacin and ginkgo biloba increase blood flow to the brain and vitamin E decreases the need for oxygen in many tissues, leaving more available for the brain. A substance called vitamin T may also be helpful at improving memory. It is found in sesame seeds, raw sesame butter and egg yolks. Lecithin, which is also found in egg yolks, improves brain function, particularly memory. Turmeric (curcumin) seems to protect the brain from the damage that causes Alzheimer's disease. Many other nutrients are important for proper function of the brain, so balanced nutrition and a good vitamin and mineral supplement are imperative. Improved nutrition has reversed senility, which I believe is primarily caused by a lack of essential nutrients and oxygen to the brain. It is doubtful that Alzheimer's disease could be reversed, but stopping exposure to possible causes may slow its progression, and a possibility of some help for the symptoms exists. If the first vertebra of the spine is misaligned in a particular way, pressure is placed on the nerve that controls blood flow to the brain. Getting this bone aligned properly (and permanently) can greatly improve brain function. Some of my patients have experienced dramatic improvement in their memories after this bone was realigned.

Recent research indicates that melatonin inhibits the formation of the amyloid protein bundles seen in the brains of Alzheimer's disease patients. This is early research, so do not start taking a melatonin supplement, especially if you have a problem with alcohol. I believe that the best way to prevent this disease is to maintain your health in the ways described in this book. Whole, natural foods contain the nutrients necessary to make all the melatonin you need.

Rheumatoid Arthritis

Rheumatoid arthritis (RA) is an inflammatory condition generally affecting numerous joints, particularly the feet, hips, ankles, elbows, wrists and hands. It usually occurs between the ages of twenty-five and fifty and is often associated with physical or emotional stress. It is two to three times more common in women. Many believe it is an autoimmune disease that causes the body to attack and damage its own joints. The cartilage is destroyed first, and when none is left, the underlying bone is attacked. The body then heals the damaged joint with calcium deposits that may eventually fuse it and prevent movement. People with this disease often have liver problems.

Dr. Hulda Clark believes RA is caused by any of the four common types of roundworm parasites invading the joints. She believes that toxins, like mercury, thallium, cadmium, lead and chemical solvents, attract the worms to the joints. Because many people have roundworms, the type of toxin may be what determines whether someone gets RA. Ridding the body of these toxins may be the key to treating or perhaps even curing this debilitating disease. In *The Cure for All Diseases,* she describes how to make and use what she calls a zapper. This device can kill the worms in just seven minutes. Because we are easily reinfected, they should be eliminated every few weeks.

Foods of the *Solanaceae* (nightshade) family of plants (cape gooseberry, cayenne pepper, potato, tomato, eggplant and tobacco) cause joint pain in some people. Avoiding these foods for a few weeks can help determine if they are contributing to the symptoms of RA.

Completely eliminating rheumatoid arthritis may be possible using all of the healing techniques I use to reestablish balance in someone's body, but nutrition would play a large role and used alone can help the condition to varying degrees. I would first have a patient use a zapper to kill any roundworms and then complete a few cleansing programs to eliminate toxins and internal waste. Some people have improved dramatically by restoring a normal internal chemical environment. The main dietary problem seems to be an excess of acid-forming foods. A diet of mainly fruits, legumes, vegetables and fresh vegetable juices would be the most successful for getting rheumatoid arthritis under control. Almost forty years ago a relative of mine claimed to have cured her RA by drinking large quantities of fresh vegetable juices.

People with RA generally have low levels of zinc in their blood and high levels of copper. Some patients treated with zinc sulfate had moderate improvement. This supplementation probably helped because most patients have liver problems that cause low levels of zinc. A high intake of phytic acid, calcium and iron all interfere with the absorption of zinc. Alcohol consumption can lead to a zinc deficiency. When the body is low in zinc, the toxic mineral cadmium is stored in the body. Remember that cadmium levels generally increase with age and that it is found in refined flour, processed rice and white sugar. Coffee, tea and soft water also contain high levels of cadmium and it is often found in polluted air. Getting an adequate amount of zinc, cleansing the body of cadmium and then reducing intake of this toxin may be helpful in treating RA.

High intake of zinc interferes with the use of copper that in turn causes incomplete iron metabolism. Therefore, low zinc may increase the use of copper and influence iron metabolism in some way. This may be why many people with RA have hypochromic (iron-deficiency) anemia. Patients treated with iron supplements to help their anemia had a flare-up of their arthritis. This probably happened due to a decrease in zinc, because excess iron inhibits the absorption of zinc.

Numerous natural products have an anti-inflammatory effect. Bromelain, a pineapple enzyme, and the herb curcumin have anti-inflammatory properties if taken between meals. Chaparral herb and cayenne are also good for reducing inflammation. Fish oils containing omega-3 fatty acids have an anti-inflammatory effect and sometimes reduce the symptoms of RA. Flaxseed oil contains omega-3 fatty acids but is not helpful for treating RA. There must be something else in the fish oil that works with the fatty acids. I would have a woman with RA take milk thistle herb or an extract of it to help cleanse and strengthen her liver.

A nutritionist friend of mine has had great success helping people with rheumatoid arthritis. It has been resolved after they followed a program to cleanse their bodies of the yeast-like fungus *Candida albicans*. I do not believe that RA is an autoimmune disease. My theory is that something, probably a toxic chemical like mercury, accumulates in the joints. This chemical then causes the *Candida* to travel to and grow on the cartilage. By the way, *Candida* does have an affinity for mercury. As the body attempts to get rid of the yeast, it also eliminates a thin layer of the cartilage. Unfortunately, the yeast grows quickly on the newly exposed cartilage and the process repeats itself until no cartilage is left. The same process then starts on the bone. The body appears to be attacking and destroying itself for no reason, but there is always a reason. The chemical attracting the yeast may even be something created by mental stress. A person's negative thoughts or a powerful mental conflict may be creating the stress. This would explain why some people have spontaneous remission of this condition. Abnormal nerve flow to certain parts of the body could also be part of the cause of RA.

Some people have gotten some relief from RA using a supplement called MSM (methylsulfonylmethane). This product contains sulfur. I believe it helps either by killing off the *Candida* or perhaps by eliminating the chemical that is attracting the yeast to the joints. If someone is deficient in sulfur, it usually helps, but if a person is not deficient, I have seen MSM cause skin problems. I recommend being tested for need and dosage before using MSM or other specialized nutritional supplements.

There may be other nutritional imbalances working in conjunction with the yeast or toxic chemical. This would explain why some people improve dramatically with dietary changes but others improve only slightly. Other imbalances people have may be greatly reducing the nutrients they get from the same healing foods. I hope someday to be able to test and treat enough patients with RA so a common cause can be discovered and a successful natural treatment developed.

Degenerative Conditions and Aging

Numerous things can cause the human body to function inefficiently, age faster or just make us feel older than we are. Of all those associated with aging, nutrition and exercise are generally considered as the two with the greatest influence. Therefore, if you apply what you are learning about these two topics, chances are you will improve your body's efficiency, age more slowly and feel younger. You could add ten, fifteen, or even more *healthy* years to your life. My natural longevity book will be about the *other* contributors to aging. There are two that have perhaps as strong an influence as diet or exercise. I will explain many things that are rarely included in anti-aging books and programs.

There have been numerous instances where groups of primitive people were thriving and extremely healthy. They had strong immune systems, babies were delivered easily, they were strong and lean, no one had cavities and there were few degenerative conditions. They were then introduced to the refined foods of modern man. Not long after, cavities and many diseases became commonplace. Within one generation, structural changes were seen in the bones of these people. The face bones were smaller and affected breathing and chewing. There was less space for the teeth and this created the need for braces on them. It has been shown that the jaws of many people have been getting smaller with each generation. Is it any wonder why so many children need braces on their teeth? Changes were seen in the pelvic bones of the women and this led to more difficult and painful childbirth. Is this why many women can no longer deliver a baby the way Nature intended? Other signs of general deterioration of their bodies were observed. A decline in the mental and moral health and well-being of these people was also seen. Why did these changes occur? Because the natural chemical balances in their bodies were disrupted, the same degenerative changes and diseases plaguing modern man began to affect them.

Some of these people returned to their simple, whole food diets. This restored chemical balance to their bodies and along with it the good health they once enjoyed. This is just one more explanation of why modern man suffers from so many unnatural diseases and degenerative conditions. These problems can usually be avoided by eating a diet of balanced foods created by Nature instead of distorted foods created by mankind. If you eat distorted and unbalanced foods, you will create a distorted body and unbalanced health. It's that simple. The human body is an amazing creation but cannot create strength and health unless it is given the raw materials and a reason (exercise or physical work) to do it. Protecting your body from the high levels of free radicals found in modern environments is also important for preventing certain degenerative conditions.

If you ever plan to have children, you must realize that, whether you are male or female, what you eat now will be the foundation of the body of your child. Most women know how important it is to eat well and avoid alcohol, tobacco and other drugs during pregnancy, but for creating the strongest and healthiest offspring, a woman should follow those guidelines long before getting pregnant. She should continue a healthy lifestyle so her milk contains the best nutrition for her baby. It is important for the father to take care of his body so he will have healthy genetic material to pass on to his offspring. Both parents should be a good example for their child.

Osteoarthritis (OA) is the condition most often thought about when the word degeneration is mentioned. It is commonly called arthritis and is also known as degenerative joint disease (DJD). The root word "arthr" means joint and the suffix "itis" means inflammation, so the word "arthritis" means inflammation of a joint. According to the Centers for Disease Control and Prevention (CDC) an estimated 43 million people have arthritis and this number is expected to increase to 60 million by the year 2020. The symptoms of this crippling condition can be relieved somewhat with good nutrition, special supplements, stretching, moist heat, pain killing and anti-inflammatory drugs and certain exercises, but to truly resolve it the cause must be eliminated. Many people seem to believe that arthritis just naturally happens when someone gets "old." The truth is, with correct treatment, arthritis is preventable and usually curable.

Here is a story to illustrate. A man eighty-two years of age goes to see his doctor because his right knee is hurting. After the doctor takes X-rays and examines him, he informs the man that he has arthritis in his right knee. The man then asks the doctor what causes arthritis and gets the reply, "old age." The man then says, "But doctor, my left knee is also eighty-two years old and it's just fine." The point is that age has nothing to do with whether you get osteoarthritis or not. A man I know had one of his hips replaced at age thirty-three. It was the hip he had injured playing football ten or twelve years earlier. His injury created muscular scar tissue that caused a hip misalignment bad enough to completely wear away the cartilage in his hip socket in just over a decade. If the hip joints of a hundred-year-old woman have been fairly well aligned her entire life, the joints will not be painful and arthritic. Do not believe anyone who tells you osteoarthritis is inherited.

Here is an example to help you understand this concept. Start with an automobile with the front wheels properly aligned and new tires designed to last 50,000 miles. What will happen if the right wheel hits enough ruts and potholes to throw off its alignment to some degree? The right tire will start wearing out faster than normal, because the misalignment puts excessive stress on certain areas of the tire. The weight is no longer evenly distributed over the entire width of the tire. After 25,000 miles, the left tire will still have another 25,000 miles worth of tread but the right tire could be completely worn out. This is the same way arthritis of the spine, hip, knee or ankle develops.

Think of a woman who injures her right hip in an auto accident, from falls taken while learning to ice skate, or from the accumulated stress of carrying children on her right hip or sitting with one leg under the other for many years. Compensating for other structural misalignments (usually pelvic or lower back) is a common cause of overstress to the hip muscles. Any of these things can injure the muscles around her hip joint and lead to the development of fibrotic adhesions. A large enough build-up of these adhesions will make the muscles short enough to pull her pelvic bones, right thighbone, or both out of normal alignment. This creates a misalignment of her right hip joint. Now, just like on the tire, the weight is unevenly distributed on the cartilage of the hip socket. This puts more pressure on her right hip cartilage, causing it to wear out faster than normal. She may occasionally notice tightness in her right hip during certain activities, but will either think nothing of it or falsely label it an unavoidable part of aging. She may be puzzled, however, as to why it is only the right hip instead of both. By age fifty, her right hip will start to hurt and will get worse as the joint continues to wear out. By age sixty or sixty-five, an X-ray will show the left hip to be in good shape, but the right one will look worn out and ready for a hip replacement that could have easily been prevented. By the way, the right hip is usually the arthritic one and I know why.

Let's go back to our tire example. What if you noticed after driving 10,000 miles that the right front tire was wearing out abnormally fast? You would take the car in and have the wheel aligned. This would stop the excessive wear and tear, and the tire may now last for another 35,000 miles instead of only another 15,000 miles.

The hip joint is similar. If at age forty-five you notice that your right hip feels tighter than the left and occasionally hurts, what can you do? You can get your hip joint realigned with my PMBT therapy and stop the excessive wear and tear. Chances are that your right hip socket cartilage will now last for the rest of your life, instead of being completely worn out by age sixty.

Six primary variables determine the severity of osteoarthritis. The first is simply the degree of misalignment in the joint. Just like our tire example, if the structural imbalance is minor, there will not be much excess pressure, so hardly any inflammation and pain will be experienced. The worse the misalignment is, the more inflammation, pain and cartilage degeneration it will cause. If a man has a severe hip misalignment at age fifteen, he could have severe arthritic degeneration and intense pain by age twenty-five. About five years ago, I successfully treated a patient who already had a badly worn arthritic hip by age twenty-eight. His hip joint misalignment was caused by muscle injuries that had occurred when he was running track in college. He had no symptoms, however, until a new injury at twenty-eight made the misalignment bad enough to cause them. His other hip felt fine and looked perfectly normal on X-ray.

The second variable affecting the severity of arthritis is time. The longer a misalignment is present, the more wear and tear there will be on the cartilage. This is why arthritis gradually gets worse. This also explains why most people get arthritis in one place or another. As people live, work and play, they accumulate muscle damage leading to joint misalignments. As time passes, more damage accumulates. Because many of these imbalances are minor, most people do not notice a problem until they are fifty or sixty years old and have accumulated substantial cartilage damage. At that time, they start to have stiffness and pain in their knees, hips, fingers or whatever joints have been misaligned. Most people just assume it is a natural part of aging and are unaware that a successful treatment exists. They just live with the pain or use drugs or other treatments to cover up their symptoms. Unfortunately, as the condition gets worse, stronger drugs, more frequent treatments or surgical replacement are necessary to deal with the pain.

The third variable influencing the severity of arthritis is the amount of use the affected joint gets. If a man is physically active in his job, sports, exercising or other activities, his misaligned joint is going to wear out faster than if he is physically inactive. If you rarely drive a car with a misaligned wheel, the tire will last much longer.

The fourth variable is weight. It should be easy to understand why weight-bearing joints (those most commonly affected with arthritis) such as feet, ankles, knees, hips and spine are going to get more stress in a 250-pound person than in a 125-pound person. Losing excess fat and maintaining a more normal body weight not only reduces the pain of arthritis but also slows the progression of cartilage degeneration. Even non-weight-bearing joints have improved when sufferers have lost weight. This most likely occurred because the nutritional program used to lose the weight was more alkaline and helped to reduce the inflammation caused by the joint imbalances.

The fifth variable comes from the body's power of adaptation. When a joint is out of alignment, the body purposely creates other joint misalignments to compensate and reduce pressure on it. This can often relieve pain in the original misaligned joint and explains why many therapies seem to have resolved a problem when they really have not. They just treat someone's symptoms until the body has time to compensate. Unfortunately, the compensating muscles develop a problem of their own after a period of time due to the excessive stress they are getting. This creates a domino effect that leads to more and more misalignments.

The sixth variable affecting the severity of arthritis is how well the joint is lubricated. The joints are lubricated with synovial fluid. How well the body is functioning, and having the nutrients available to make this fluid are the primary factors. It is especially important to get enough essential fatty acids. Free radicals can oxidize the lipids in synovial fluid and reduce its lubricating ability. Therefore, getting enough of the nutrients that neutralize free radicals is also important for reducing the abnormal wear and tear on the cartilage of a joint.

Sunlight is an extremely influential nutrient that improves bodily balance and function. In his book *Health and Light*, John Ott tells the story of his own experience with arthritis. He was suffering with an arthritic hip and had spent many hours relaxing in the Florida sun with no relief. But he had always worn sunglasses. He noticed that his hip pain got worse after filming his weekly television program under artificial lights. His condition was getting more painful, even though he had tried many therapies and had used a cane for a few years. His elbow was starting to bother him due to using the cane.

Then one day he broke his eyeglasses. For a few days, he did some work outside without wearing them. He then noticed that his hip and elbow had stopped hurting. He started walking and went quite a distance with his hip feeling better than it had for years. He then began spending about six hours a day outside without glasses or sunglasses. His glasses were for distance vision, so he spent quite a bit of time reading in the shade of a tree. He avoided as much artificial light exposure as possible and limited his time behind glass. His frequent colds and sore throats stopped and friends who followed a similar regimen saw hay fever and other conditions improve dramatically or disappear entirely. After six months of wearing his glasses as little as possible, he began to notice eyestrain whenever he did. He had his eyes tested and was told that his prescription was too strong because his eyesight had improved. He then decided to have his hip checked and was told by his doctor that the X-ray showed something extremely unusual—improvement. His hip's range of motion was restored to normal from a 30 percent restriction.

The symptoms of arthritis can be treated in various ways. Some therapies relieve the excessive pressure on a joint temporarily and others help reduce the inflammation caused by the joint imbalance. None of these treatments eliminate the cause of arthritis as PMBT treatments do, but they are helpful to varying degrees.

Strengthening certain muscles can sometimes create a counterpull against the tight muscles that cause the problem. This can help realign the joint to some degree and this relieves some of the stress on the cartilage. But, if done improperly, it can cause increased pressure on the cartilage instead. What often happens when a person attempts to treat arthritis this way is that the opposing muscle eventually gets tight. This restricts the joint's movement and puts excess pressure on the cartilage or bursae of the joint and increased stress on related or nearby joints. This makes the arthritis worse and often causes bursitis in the tight joint and problems in related joints. Unfortunately, because most joint imbalances vary, a generic exercise program cannot be designed for arthritic conditions other than arthritis of the hands. This is possible only because the imbalances are usually the same for everyone. This exercise program is explained and demonstrated fully in my arthritic hands self-treatment video, titled *Treat Your Own Arthritic Hands*. It is designed to strengthen the muscles, making them less susceptible to new damage. This prevents the problem from coming back once the muscles have healed from the treatments.

Stretching is often helpful for relieving the symptoms of arthritis. It works best when the tight damaged muscles that are causing the misalignments are stretched. But stretching just relieves the pressure temporarily. If done a few times every day, it may help quite a bit. Unfortunately, this is time-consuming so most people do not do enough or stop altogether. Stretching is also demonstrated in my video to use after the cause of the arthritis has been eliminated. It helps to prevent the accumulation of any new muscle damage.

Most arthritis therapies use heat in some form. Applying moist heat to short, damaged muscles causes them to lengthen temporarily, thereby relieving some of the pressure on the joint. This gives some relief but heat also increases inflammation and makes the problem worse. Using heat to treat arthritis is a two-edged sword. It helps in one way but hurts in another. Massaging and stretching your tight muscles relieves the pressure and pain as much as moist heat does, but without the negative effect of increasing the inflammation. Whatever you do, never apply dry heat to your skeletal muscles. It also increases the inflammation, but because muscles are mostly water, the dry heat dehydrates them, causing them to get shorter. This creates a greater imbalance in the joint and makes your problem worse.

Painkillers, anti-inflammatory drugs, muscle relaxants and anti-depressant drugs just treat symptoms. They do nothing to eliminate the cause of chronic arthritic conditions. These drugs have negative side effects and some may even weaken tendons, muscles or ligaments, leading to more injury and even worse problems. The side effects are often caused by the nutritional deficiencies that the drugs create.

I have eliminated the pain of arthritis and stopped its progression in hundreds of patients. If you have an arthritic condition in your spine, hip, knee, hands or other location it can most likely be resolved by getting the PMBT treatments explained on my Web site. Even patients with no hip cartilage left have experienced some relief from my therapy. The arthritic joint is aligned properly and other joint imbalances that could stress the muscles that would re-create the problem are also aligned. Then we determine what caused the muscle damage leading to the joint imbalance. If it is caused by an activity being done using incorrect body movements or poor posture, the patient is taught how to do it correctly so as not to over-stress the muscles and re-create the problem.

If you are told that arthritis is caused by a nutritional deficiency, just ask the person why people usually get arthritis in one hip or knee and not the other. A nutritional deficiency would affect all weight-bearing joints equally so this idea makes no sense when discussing osteoarthritis.

Nutritional supplements cannot eliminate the cause of arthritis, but can be helpful in treating the inflammation and pain. You learned about this in the previous section on rheumatoid arthritis. Herbs are natural products and can often be used extensively without side effects, but it is still best to cycle their use.

Two supplements currently popular for treating osteoarthritis are glucosamine sulfate and chondroitin sulfate. Chondroitin sulfate supplies the nutrients that ligaments need to heal but glucosamine sulfate is the one creating the positive effect experienced by some people with arthritis. It is a much smaller molecule, so it is more easily absorbed and used by the body. It contains nutrients that improve the lubrication of the cartilage. This leads to less friction and slows down the cartilage degeneration. Less friction also means less inflammation and that translates to less pain. Therefore, this supplement can be helpful, but a lack of it is not the cause of osteoarthritis. I believe that it just makes up for the lack of essential fatty acids in most people's diets. You know now that antioxidant supplements also decrease the pain of arthritis because they reduce free-radical damage to the synovial fluid. These supplements along with plenty of natural sunlight and a pH balanced diet containing adequate essential fatty acids may give dramatic relief even if the arthritic joint is not realigned.

Feeding Infants and Children

This section is brief so please do not completely base how you feed your infants and young children on what you read here. Use this information as a foundation to make your own decisions. Read more about it, consult with your pediatrician, study the nutritional content of foods and use your instincts and good sense to determine what to feed your children. The responsibility of parenthood is great and feeding your children well is an important part of getting them started off right. Do not forget that what the parents eat before conception and the mother eats during pregnancy and nursing are vital for proper development and optimal health of the child.

Be mindful that your child's doctor is most likely extremely lacking in nutritional knowledge. Here is an example to illustrate. One of my patients had been feeding her daughter much like my upcoming recommendations. Her child had experienced far fewer health problems than the average child does. One day she took her daughter for a regular checkup. The pediatrician said the child was in the seventy-fifth percentile in height for her age but in only the twenty-fifth percentile in weight. Her daughter still had significant amounts of baby fat, yet the doctor recommended feeding her cheese and other fattening foods to increase her weight up to the seventy-fifth percentile. The doctor just blindly followed some chart rather than actually looking at the child. Luckily, the mother knew this suggestion was absurd and that it would just create excess fat and most likely constipation and other health problems for her child. Other patients of mine have had similar experiences. I believe that the weight recommendations for infants and children are excessively high, because they are based on groups of infants and children that have eaten improperly and have excess fat.

The formation rate of fat cells is rapid in the first few years of life. If more fat is stimulated to be stored than the existing fat cells can contain, the body will create more fat cells. Obese children often have three times more fat cells than children of normal weight do. Once the fat cells are formed, they stay forever and make it easier to get fat and more difficult to get and stay lean. Be especially careful not to fatten up your children when they are young. After adolescence, the number of fat cells normally stays almost the same throughout life. Getting fat in later years used to come primarily from filling up the existing fat cells. Now, however, many people eat so much that all their existing fat cells are filled to capacity. This forces their bodies to create more fat cells to store the excess calories that are being eaten. This is an abnormal condition.

Infants will thrive best drinking their mother's milk. I recommend using it for one to two years before completely weaning the child. Studies have shown that the longer a child is breast-fed the more intelligent that child becomes. When to start solid foods depends on the infant. Some have developed enough to handle solid foods after four months, but infants do not need solid foods before they are six months old. Breast-fed infants do not even need water during the first six months. If the mother is eating well, her breast-fed baby should get all the nutrition it needs for the first year without anything additional.

Breast-feeding has health benefits for the mother as well. Studies suggest that mothers who breast-feed have decreased risk for breast and ovarian cancer, osteoporosis and anemia. Breast-feeding improves the emotional bond with the baby and also stimulates hormones that help the uterus return to its normal size. A nice benefit for anyone around the breast-fed child is that, unlike those drinking cow's milk, the child's bowel movements do not have a bad odor.

If you have an infant who is not being breast-fed, I recommend feeding the child fresh, raw goat's milk. Powdered goat's milk can be used if fresh milk is unavailable. About one-fourth of this homemade formula could be soymilk when the child is young and after the child is six months old, grain milks, nut milks and a little blackstrap molasses may be added. I do not recommend any of the popular infant formulas, but there may be a healthful one developed someday. Use your nutritional knowledge to decide if a formula contains healthful ingredients and if you want to give it to your child.

I have a college textbook on nutrition stating that cow's milk is inappropriate for infants. I definitely agree with that. The same book, however, states that the diet of an infant needs fluoride supplementation. They base this on the fact that the fluoride concentration in mother's milk is the same in women who ingest small amounts of fluoride as it is in women who ingest large amounts. They are saying a woman's body does not know what it is doing when it filters out the excess fluoride being ingested by the mother. It seems to me that Nature is telling them loud and clear that the baby does not need that much fluoride. They say human milk is the best food for an infant but that it does not contain enough vitamin D or fluoride. Don't you think the mother's body knows more about the proper amounts needed by the baby? We already discussed the fluoride, and either the baby does not need as much vitamin D as scientists think or Nature intended the baby to get some sunlight exposure to stimulate the production of vitamin D.

I do not recommend commercial baby foods because many of them contain high amounts of sodium, or starches that are poorly digested by infants. Can you believe they sell desserts and cookies for babies? What does a baby know about eating dessert? Please do not condition your infant to be fat before it even knows what fat is. Some commercial baby foods do not taste good either and they may contain unsafe levels of pesticides.

Homemade baby foods are the best. Blended fruits can be added to an infant's diet after five to seven months and blended or mashed vegetables and legumes a month or two later. It is best if only one food is given at a time. Do not add salt, sugar or honey. Honey may contain the spores that cause botulism, and infants less than one year of age lack the immunity to resist these spores. Fruit juice and sugar-sweetened beverages are not recommended, because they can cause tooth decay. Infants should be given a variety of foods that have different textures and tastes. This helps them learn to like the taste of more foods. Often you can just blend or mash for your baby some of the same foods the rest of the family is eating.

When infants are about six months old, their bodies develop the ability to make pancreatic amylase, an enzyme that digests complex carbohydrates. Babies who are given breads, cereals, cakes, crackers, cookies and other grain products before then may develop a sensitivity or allergy to those products. Their bodies may create antibodies to the grain just like it would if exposed to germs from an inoculation or other source. Why are wheat, yeast and corn such common allergens? I believe it is because they are contained in the most common products given to infants before they are six months old. The early addition of cereal has caused diarrhea in some infants. Some people believe the body compensates for the lack of pancreatic amylase by increasing its production of salivary amylase. This may be true to some degree, but I believe most of the damage will already be done before the infant's body realizes it needs to produce more salivary amylase.

A big concern for many doctors and nutritionists is that infants get adequate amounts of iron. A baby is generally born with enough iron stores to last from four to six months. This is why many parents are advised to start feeding their children foods containing supplemental iron when they are about four months of age. My college textbook on nutrition suggests adding iron-fortified infant cereals to a baby's diet between four and six months of age. The authors must not have read the other section of their own book about babies being unable to digest grains until they are at least six months of age. The authors suggest waiting six to eight months before giving a baby strained fruits or vegetables—fruits that contain iron and need no digestion whatsoever. Their suggestions seem backward based on physiology and the digestive capabilities of infants. Commercial baby cereals are made from flour instead of something whole and natural. Many of them state on the package that the American Academy of Pediatrics recommends adding iron-fortified cereals to a baby's diet between four and six months of age. The people at the AAP must have read the same college textbook.

Why is iron deficiency so common in infants? A few possible reasons exist. If a mother is anemic during pregnancy, chances are her baby will be born with less than normal amounts of iron. Not being breast-fed can also lead to inadequate iron. Cow's milk given to a baby can cause bleeding in the intestines and lead to an iron deficiency. Also, if the umbilical cord is cut before pulsing has stopped, there may be decreased amounts of iron transferred from the mother to the child.

Feeding iron-fortified cereals to infants seems ridiculous to me. You already know that processed grains may cause an allergy to develop. To add insult to injury, the electrolytic form of iron that is generally used to fortify the cereal is poorly absorbed. Why use this type? It is used because it makes a more attractive product with a longer shelf life. It sticks to the cereal instead of settling and does not affect the flavor and appearance of the cereal like more absorbable forms of iron would. Unfortunately, this inferior source of iron increases the need for more of the cereal that is unhealthful for your baby. Why not give babies a natural food containing iron? That is what they got for thousands of years before iron supplements were developed.

Mother's milk is low in iron but what it does contain has a high bioavailability—babies can absorb up to 50 percent. To get the same amount of iron, far more would have to be ingested from other sources. For example, they would absorb only about four percent of the iron in a fortified formula. A baby drinking milk from a well-nourished mother should easily maintain normal iron status for the first year. Nevertheless, to be sure, I would feed the seven- to eight-month-old infant some natural foods containing iron. Eggplant is high in iron, tomatoes have a good amount and many legumes (lentils, kidney beans, lima beans, and soybeans) contain moderate amounts. Almost all vegetables (especially leafy greens like spinach and beet greens) contain some iron. Blackstrap molasses is a rich source of iron and many other nutrients. Fruits high in iron are peaches, apricots, dates, figs, prunes and raisins. I recommend going easy on the dried fruits until the infant is about a year old. Turkey, clams, oysters, sardines and shrimp contain high amounts of iron, as do walnuts, almonds, Brazil nuts, cashews, hazelnuts and pecans. The nuts would be best used as nut butters. Some powdered kelp or dulse could be added to your baby's food. These are two types of iron-rich seaweed. I do not see how an infant being fed as suggested here could develop an iron deficiency.

I do not recommend feeding an infant grain products, meats or eggs before the age of one. Fruits, vegetables, legumes, nuts, seeds, fish, fowl and eggs should supply great nutrition to an infant after age one. I believe it is best to wait until children are about eighteen months old before they eat red meats or moderate amounts of whole grains. Raw fruits and vegetables make great snacks for children age two and above. At about age three or four, children should be able to eat the way I have explained in this book. If you help your children discover that natural foods can taste great *and* make them feel good, they will eat better while growing up and this increases their chances of being healthy. This is a precious gift that will last a lifetime and may even be passed on to their children and to future generations.

Children and teenagers seem to be growing taller and larger with each generation. There are many possible reasons for this. I believe that it is caused by the consumption of something unnatural and unhealthful. It is not because they are eating nutritious meals, because that is certainly not the case. It may be from the fluoride in the water and the antibiotics, growth hormone and anabolic steroids found in the dairy products and meats they ingest. Other drugs and environmental toxins may also be involved. I believe these chemicals are major contributors to the increasing rates of obesity and certain other health problems we are seeing in children.

Some parents have mentioned to me that their children dislike most vegetables and some fruits. This is often true, but when I question the parents I find out they have not given their children many foods to try. How can children know if they like a food if they have never eaten it before? Parents need to give their children a chance to eat more varieties of fruits, vegetables, legumes and whole grains. They can also experiment with different ways of presenting the foods. A child may love a vegetable raw but dislike it when cooked. To this day, I am not crazy about cooked carrots but I love them raw.

Squash, parsnip or rutabaga steamed and mashed with some potatoes may strike a child's fancy or the same foods sliced and steamed may be preferred. The texture may be the key to a child liking a food. You may be able to put many different vegetables into an omelet your child will enjoy. Your children may prefer a slice of crunchy Jerusalem artichoke to an unhealthful cracker but you will never know if you never give it to them. The parents have not even eaten most of the foods I suggest they offer to their children. They also need to discover and eat these tasty and nutritious foods. Some nutritionists advise parents to pretend to like a food that they want their children to eat. Do not eat foods that you dislike, and be honest with your children as you help them discover healthful foods that they find appetizing.

Feeding your children nourishing, whole foods makes them better able to cope with the stresses of modern living. Chances are they will do better in school and be less disruptive at home. This has the added benefit of reducing your stress. You may find your children becoming less finicky eaters, because the healthful foods will make them feel satisfied. They will instinctively eat what makes them feel good physically and emotionally.

eleven

Lean for Life — Physical Causes of Excess Fat

his chapter and the next are dedicated to anyone with excess body fat. Even if you are not in this category, I highly recommend reading them anyway, because they contain many nutritional guidelines that apply to everyone. You will also find valuable health concepts applicable to your life, and ideas that may help you understand or assist a friend or family member. The physical and emotional obstacles to being lean that are included may not be influencing you to have excess fat but some of them could quite possibly be negatively affecting your behavior and health in other ways. Something you learn may help you to improve your life dramatically. Also, before you decide to skip these chapters, have your body fat percentage checked. You may be 5'3", weigh 110 pounds and believe you are in good shape, but I knew a woman once who had those statistics yet had 40 percent body fat. She was in terrible condition and considered obese, but going strictly by her height and weight you may have said she was a thin person. You must understand that being *thin* and being *lean* are often entirely different.

In this and the next few chapters you will be given numerous ideas to help you answer the question of why you have excess fat. I also teach you many methods for eliminating it permanently. I am going to reveal the truth about losing body fat and staying lean for the rest of your life. You should know by now it is not about losing "weight." The woman in the preceding example had been losing "weight" most of her life. She would starve herself all day and then eat a small meal in the evening. This had maintained her weight but was difficult and unhealthy. She lost lean body tissue during the day and her body stored most of the meal as fat because it felt the need to protect itself. Her body was malnourished and unhealthy, and she gradually lost lean tissue and gained fat. The loss of lean body mass lowered her metabolism, making it harder for her to keep from gaining even more fat. If you ever hope to accomplish your goal, you must supply your body with good nutrition so you will lose fat, not just weight. You should already understand the difference.

A belief shared by many is that it takes will power to lose fat. This may be what keeps most of them fat, because every time they cheat on their "diet," they criticize themselves and lament that they have no will power. This lowers their self-worth and usually leads to a defeatist attitude. They often give up, because they feel doomed to failure due to this lack. They are hypnotizing themselves into believing they will never succeed. The truth is, will power has *nothing* to do with it. It did not take will power to get fat and it does not take any to get lean. A good reason to lose excess fat is what is really needed and everyone should be able to find at least one. Also, will power can never win over hormone imbalances, certain nutritional deficiencies, subconscious motives, feelings of low self-worth, or certain other physical or emotional imbalances. The key is to eliminate these problems, not constantly attempt to defeat them with will power. Getting and staying lean should not be a battle. If it is, you are not doing it in a healthful and natural way.

Another erroneous idea is that food is the enemy. Nature has created a tremendous variety of foods to keep our bodies and minds healthy and strong. These nutritious and life-giving foods are friends you should get to know better and keep in your life always. It is possible to eat large quantities of great-tasting natural foods while losing unwanted fat and enjoying life. The real enemies are your poor habits, nutritional ignorance, low self-esteem, fear, guilt, shame, negative subconscious motivations and the health-robbing substances discussed in chapter four.

Find and Eliminate Your Root Cause(s) for Being Fat

Know the truth, and the truth will set you free. This statement applies to all aspects of life, including fat loss. There is one exception I will tell you about, but the truth is, if you do not find and eliminate the root cause of why you are fat, you will constantly struggle to lose weight, but will not succeed. It's that simple. You may lose some weight with each new diet program or "magic" pill, but you will gain it back if the cause is still there. There is a reason for everything and until your reason for being fat is discovered, faced, and eliminated, you will be stuck in a never-ending battle. Once you find and eliminate the cause of why you are fat, the struggle will end—then you can start being lean. Imagine how much more you will be able to accomplish and enjoy in life with the time you now spend struggling to lose body fat or to lose "weight."

Statistics tell us that about 95 percent of the people who go on diets fail to attain lasting results. Here is why. Most diets create "weight" loss, but much of the weight lost is lean muscle tissue, not fat. On some diet programs people actually gain fat when they are losing weight. Also, the body almost always lowers its metabolism (unless mostly alkaline foods are eaten) to compensate for a decreased intake of calories. As soon as people start eating the way they used to—the way that made them fat in the first place—they will gain back some of the lean tissue, and because of a slower metabolism, maybe even more body fat than they had before. This is why most people gain back as much, if not more weight than they lost and end up with a higher body fat percentage. The few people who do keep the weight off are usually those who gained it due to "creeping obesity." This is explained in an upcoming section.

You have one or more root causes for your excess fat and they can be primarily physical or emotional. Ultimately you will have both, because emotional and physical causes are linked—one always creates the other. For example, if a physical cause is making you fat, you will experience emotional stress, frustration and a poor self-image. These feelings often lead to overeating, not exercising and other self-debasing behaviors that make everything worse. As you gain more fat, your physical problems worsen making the emotional problems worse and the process continues to snowball. Likewise, if you have an emotional cause making you fat, the excess fat and internal waste create physical causes that make the condition worse and lead to the same downward spiral. Therefore, it is vital to determine and eliminate *all* of your reasons for being fat. One cause is often the primary key and once eliminated makes getting rid of the others easy.

You learned in chapter six how to develop the best eating program for your one-of-a-kind body. Soon I will explain how to find your truth—the unique physical or psychological reasons for your excess fat. This will give you a few more of the special pieces needed to complete your permanent fat-loss puzzle.

Determining the root cause, or causes, for being fat is not always easy. The most important characteristic you need is honesty with yourself. This is extremely difficult for many people, because they have never learned how to see themselves as they really are. Most of the causes are explained in this book, so you should find yours or at least learn how to discover it. If you are honest with yourself, you could find yours within the next few hours or the next few days. You may want to go over the various causes with a good friend (one who will be completely honest with you) to help you determine yours. I repeat—*discovering and eliminating your causes for being fat is the secret to permanent fat loss.* If you do not do this, you will continue to waste time and struggle as you have in the past. You may win a few battles occasionally, but will lose the war. Barring a truly uncorrectable physical problem, if you follow the nutritional program you develop from the guidelines in this book, your body weight should normalize quickly and naturally.

Please do not let anyone take away your hope of correcting a physical problem. Some rare conditions exist where nothing can be done, but remember that doctors (medical doctors usually) often tell people nothing can be done for them if the doctor does not know how to help them. This does not eliminate the possibility of someone else resolving the problem. I dislike seeing anyone's hope taken away. Remember that medical doctors primarily learn how to treat the symptoms of diseases, but few of them know much about health and how to restore, maintain or improve it. Many of my patients were told by more than one doctor that nothing could be done for them, but their problems were resolved after getting PMBT treatments. My PMBT therapy was developed (and resolved my many problems) after more than twenty years searching for pain relief. It has gotten rid of problems that patients had suffered with for more than forty years. Do not give up looking for something that, or someone who may be able to correct your condition.

If you have an emotional cause making you fat, you will not follow the nutritional and other guidelines recommended in this book. If you follow the program, it will work for you unless you have an extreme and uncorrectable physical cause. If you do not follow the program, an emotional reason is preventing you from doing so. And, if you do not do it, it cannot work for you.

I will be using the term "fat" instead of "overweight," because "overweight" fails to differentiate between fat and muscle. I am going to be unusually honest and open in talking about fat loss, just as you must be with yourself if you ever want to be free from the bondage of excess body fat. Sugar coating the subject (pun intended) is not going to help you accomplish your goals. Let's first discuss physical causes and then take a look at the most common physical reasons why people have excess body fat.

Physical Causes of Excess Fat

Some people get fat because of a physical reason. They often spend their lives struggling to lose the excess fat. The battle is frequently expensive, time consuming and usually creates a great deal of emotional stress and frustration that can easily lead to a defeatist attitude and overeating. The excess fat causes physical stress that drains their energy and makes them more susceptible to almost all diseases. People with excess fat usually have more physical problems, because, whether dieting or overeating, they are almost always undernourished. They are also more likely to develop structural problems due to the excess stress the additional body fat puts on their muscles and joints.

Unfortunately, most dietary programs, weight-loss centers, support groups and others do not know how to determine or eliminate the root cause for being fat. Some of them teach people how to eat a bit better but rarely are the recommendations truly balanced and in harmony with Nature. Sometimes the advice is sound, but as you have learned, if there is an emotional cause, people will not eat as they know they should. Many of the people in these groups attempt to help each other, but their help is usually based on misinformation. They often see fat loss as a war where they need to support each other as they fight. Losing body fat is not a struggle if done properly. It should be simple and easy, because the natural state your body wants is to have only enough body fat for good health. Once you truly understand this, you can see why most weight-loss programs fail.

Just because something is low in calories does not mean it is good for you. It may do nothing to build health and it may not help you lose body fat. In my opinion, the majority of weight-loss foods marketed to desperate people are total garbage. They are lifeless, unbalanced and misleading. People are told they will lose fat if they eat these low-calorie, so-called "healthful" meals. Your goal is fat loss, not weight loss—building health and learning to eat healthfully—not just dieting. Good health comes from eating a variety of whole, natural foods, not from expensive diet shakes, protein bars and processed TV-dinner meals. I hope that after reading this book, you will understand and embrace the truth about fat loss and be honest enough with yourself to discover your underlying causes, eliminate them, and spend the rest of your life lean, healthy and happy.

As you learn about the physical and emotional reasons for being fat, be aware that many of them can be caused by imbalances created by legal and illegal drugs and from most of the enemies you learned about in chapter four. Now, pay attention, because the cause of *your* excess fat may be the next topic.

Not Knowing How to Eat Healthfully

The saying, "What you don't know won't hurt you" may be true in some situations but when related to eating well and staying healthy, a lack of knowledge can make your life miserable and shorten it by many years.

Most people rarely think about how they are affecting themselves (body, mind and spirit) by how they eat. They have little or no awareness of the consequences of their nutritional habits. Some make an effort to eat more nutritious foods but do not know what is good for them nor do they know that how and when they eat and drink has profound effects on the results they get. Most people do not know that this knowledge can give them the power to control to a large degree what their bodies look like, so they do not attempt to learn how to eat properly.

Everyone knows something about eating well—everyone has a few pieces of the puzzle. Most people, however, are missing too many of the pieces to make any sense out of the ones they do have. They have heard they should eat more fiber, less fat, and reduce consumption of certain foods and those containing harmful chemicals. Unfortunately, few people know why certain foods are bad, how bad they are, or what they should eat instead. If you knew how bad it was to eat certain processed foods, you would never put another bite in your mouth as long as you live (and you would live longer). We now hear that we should eat more fruits and vegetables, but most people do not know the right time to eat them or how to incorporate them into meals that are healthful and easy to make.

A great deal of the nutritional information made available to the general public is false and publicized simply to market a product. Bread manufacturers tell you that processed white (lifeless) bread will build some form of health and they are right. It will build poor health. It will also make your body more susceptible to diseases and much of it will be stored as excess body fat. When health research organizations "discover" what they consider great new dietary revelations—like eating fiber to reduce your chances of colon cancer—food companies jump on these "new" health breakthroughs. Suddenly everything processed and lifeless has bran added to it in an attempt to sell more products to unknowing consumers. The bran has a few beneficial effects but the food is still unbalanced, essentially worthless and nothing like a wholesome natural food.

Most of these nutritional "breakthroughs" are so ridiculously obvious that anyone with even a little good sense and awareness could come up with most of them in a few minutes of thinking. Books on nutrition written more than a hundred years ago stressed the importance of eating some whole grains and plenty of fruits, vegetables and legumes to get the different types of fiber necessary to keep your colon clean and healthy and your bowels moving easily and regularly. They had the same good reasons for recommending these foods that you have been reading about in this book. Because so many people are afraid of osteoporosis, you now see numerous products with added calcium. Do you think they care about your bones being stronger or about selling more of their products?

Another thing that sells non-nutritious foods to unaware consumers is the labeling. You often see large letters across a product's package spelling out "LOW IN SUGAR" or "NO SUGAR ADDED." You are not told it is loaded with unhealthful forms of fat. On the other hand, the product with little or no fat but large amounts of sugar is often labeled "LOW IN FAT," or "NO FAT," leading some people to believe it is a healthful product. How much of the product do you think they would sell if they were honest and labeled it "LOADED WITH SUGAR" or "HIGH IN SATURATED FAT?"

The terms "natural" or "from natural sources" trick some people into believing they are eating something healthful. Everything on earth comes from natural sources but that does not mean it is good for you. Would you drink a toxic toilet bowl cleaner and consider it to be good for you? It came from natural sources. All "food" products on the market come from natural sources. The problem is they are so distorted, denatured and lifeless by the time the processing is done that they have very few, if any, of the nutrients the natural product originally contained. It amazes me that a multitude of vitamins, minerals and enzymes can be processed out of a food until absolutely nothing worthwhile is left and after a few nutrients are artificially added it is labeled "enriched." For example, during the processing of wheat to make flour, twenty vitamins and minerals, all the bran, all the wheat germ, and all of its other vital nutrients are eliminated. It is completely worthless at that point except perhaps for making glue. Various chemicals that are not conducive to building good health are added to age and bleach the flour. Then, usually three vitamins and one or two minerals are added and it is now "enriched." If some people burned your house down, stole your car, took all your money and clothes, and then gave you a torn shirt, one shoe, five dollars and an umbrella with holes in it, would you feel like they enriched your life?

Another marketing gimmick you may be unaware of is fat percentage labeling. If you saw a label on some lunchmeat that read "93 percent fat-free," you might assume that it contains only seven percent fat. That is what most people think and what the food processors want you to think. You would be correct in one way and this would seem to be healthful to most people, but let's look closer and find the truth.

The law allows the fat content of foods to be labeled by weight, not calories, but the calories are what can make you fat. Let's calculate the calories in our lunchmeat example and see how many calories you are getting from fat. One serving has 60 calories and contains three grams of fat. Three grams multiplied by nine calories per gram equals 27 calories or 45 percent of the total calories. That's much different than seven percent. Let's take a look at two-percent milk. The nutritional information on the back of the carton lists 120 calories per cup with 45 calories from fat and 27 of those from saturated fat. Divide 45 calories by the total of 120 to calculate the percentage of fat and you will see that two-percent milk is really 38 percent fat. Divide 27 by 120 and you will see that it is 22.5 percent saturated fat—the form of fat you should minimize in your diet. Thirty-eight percent fat and the milk is labeled "low fat." It is lower than whole milk that gets 48 percent of its calories from fat. I calculated the fat content of an "80 percent fat-free" product that was labeled "Lite." This one gets 77 percent of its calories from fat, not 20 percent as many people might assume. Would you buy a product labeled "77 percent fat"? I doubt it. That is why food processors fought hard to be able to label fat content by weight. The government advises you to eat less fat but at the same time allows this deceptive labeling. The label on the back tells you the facts but few people look at it or know how to interpret it correctly. To calculate the fat percentage by calories, divide the number of fat calories by the total number of calories and multiply the answer by 100. I think that you will be shocked by what you learn.

The term "low fat" is relative and rarely has anything to do with whether a food is healthful or will keep you lean. You should also be aware that nutritional labels may be inaccurate. I saw one recently that listed 140 calories per serving with five calories from fat. Below, it listed one gram of fat, which is equal to nine calories, not five. The fat calories were listed 45 percent lower than what they really were. Another trick used on food labels is to list the nutritional contents by the slice (very small slice) instead of per serving. This makes it look lower in harmful ingredients than it is per serving.

If you are interested in knowing more about the true fat content of foods, buy a book that lists the number of calories and fat grams of numerous foods. Multiply the fat grams by nine, divide by the total calories and multiply by 100. This gives you the percentage of calories from fat. Checking out some of your favorite foods will most likely prove enlightening and give you some valuable guidance as you develop your personalized nutritional program. Keep in mind, however, that some natural foods are high in fat—healthful fat. Do not avoid these foods; just eat them in the morning or early afternoon so the calories will be burned for energy. Also, think about how food is cooked and packaged. For example, tuna in water has less fat than tuna in oil, and boiled or baked chicken is lower in fat than fried chicken.

Advertising firms are paid tremendous sums of money to come up with ways to convince you that worthless products are good for you. For a while, pay attention to the commercials and advertisements you see. If you disregard the automotive ads, you will see that most of them are for fast foods, beer, soft drinks, processed foods and drinks, or drugs. It is not hard to see why the rate of obesity is rising so fast in the United States. The drug companies saw how well advertising worked for fast foods so they decided to do the same. Now people diagnose themselves from a television commercial and then go to a doctor and ask for a particular drug. Many of these prescription drugs are also advertised in "health" magazines. I was recently offered a free one-year subscription to one of these magazines if I filled out a questionnaire primarily made up of questions about what diseases the people in my household had and what drugs they currently used. According to the National Institute for Health Care Management Foundation, prescription drug spending increased 19 percent in the year 2000, nearly half of that was from sales of the fifty most advertised drugs. Remember that these ads are trying to sell you something and there are more of them now. Most of them do not provide adequate and easy to understand information about the risks, some make false, misleading or unsupported claims, and many doctors feel pressured to prescribe the drug their patients say they want. Do not let a television commercial convince you that you need a drug to cover up the symptoms of a poor diet and lack of exercise. Many prescription drugs can be obtained now over the Internet without even seeing a doctor. This is an extremely dangerous situation.

Do you believe the government cares anything about your health? They tell you mostly what they are told by food producers and drug companies or nothing at all. Never forget that your health and well-being are *your* responsibility. This is why you must learn to see through the facade of advertising and marketing campaigns to find the truth about healthful eating. Following the suggestions in this book eliminates most of the threats from these deceptions, and now that you are armed with the truth you should not fall victim to these advertising gimmicks.

Sadly, those most easily influenced by misinformation and advertising are our youth. Cartoon characters easily control what young children want to eat and famous multimillionaire athletes are paid more millions to sell junk food to our adolescents. Most schools do not teach healthful eating or offer nutritious lunches. According to the CDC in Atlanta, children can purchase soft drinks and junk food at 43 percent of all elementary schools, 74 percent of middle schools, and 98 percent of high schools. The CDC also reported that only 42 percent of U.S. schoolchildren attended a daily physical education class in 1991 and that by 1999 the percentage had dropped to 29. You have learned that your children will be healthier, happier and learn better if they get adequate nutrition and exercise but few are getting it at school. Therefore, it is up to you to teach your children and to be a good example.

I hope that someday schools will have safe and effective strength-training classes (two to three times a week) for children over age thirteen, and offer fun and challenging strength games for younger children. Strength training is the most beneficial type of exercise and can be done for as long as they live. They would have much better bodies when they graduated and hopefully be inspired to continue exercising. Many of the boys would make excellent progress because of their high levels of testosterone. This could possibly prevent some of them from using illegal and dangerous anabolic steroids. On the alternate days I would like to see school children have the option to participate in sports or other physical activities they enjoy. Tennis, golf, archery, running, cycling, self-defense and other activities that they can continue doing as adults would be the best for most of them.

I believe that many children are doing less walking, hiking, biking and playing outside. The main reasons are the fear of abduction, the lure of computer video games, television and the Internet, and a lack of energy due to being fat, undernourished or both.

Many people eat large amounts of processed, denatured, chemical-laden foods that are incapable of sustaining normal health. They may barely sustain your life, but hardly supply your immune and other systems of your body with anything they need to function effectively. Most of these foods are like vampires, depleting you of nutrients you already have in an attempt to burn their empty calories. Many people would easily lose their excess fat if they just ate whole, natural foods instead of processed foods. Choose your foods as recommended in this book and eat them as close to their natural states as possible. This is the foundation on which you will build your body, but far from the total. Whatever other variables may apply in your case, remember that you cannot build a brick house out of straw. You must supply the raw materials your body needs or it cannot create the results you want.

Another part of proper eating that is unknown to most people is how inefficient it is to eat an excessive number of foods at one time. Good examples of this can be seen in smorgasbords and restaurants with salad bars where many people think they need to have some of everything. Doing this creates difficult-to-digest combinations and leads to overeating, both of which make digestion more complex and time-consuming. It forces your body to work harder and can lead to incomplete digestion, absorption and use of some of the foods.

Some people have some good complex carbohydrates and a salad for lunch. This would be fine, but they often think they need some dessert. Some eat the sugar and bleached flour desserts but others eat fruit, thinking it is much better. It is certainly a better food than the dessert, but eating fruit with or after the other foods makes digestion of the meal more complicated and less efficient. Eating fruit at the end is an easy way to add extra calories to the meal, something you do not want to do. For example, the fruit would have been excellent if a woman had eaten it 15 to 20 minutes before she ate the meal, because the fruit would have been out of her stomach by the time the other food was eaten. Also, her appetite would have been partially satisfied so she would eat less at the main meal. You should understand this concept fairly well by now because of what you learned about food combining in chapter five. Your meals should be relatively simple, yet great tasting and satisfying. You should eat the whole, natural foods you enjoy, but at the proper time.

Eating proper food combinations is a good idea for anyone, but is most important for those who desire to lose excess body fat and improve the efficiency of their internal systems. For example, eating one type of fruit for breakfast is a fine way to start the day. You can also eat more than one fruit if they combine well. Then, a good lunch would be a baked potato, some steamed vegetables and a salad with olive oil as dressing. For dinner, fish or chicken along with some string beans and a salad would be great. Remember, no oil in the dressing when eating meat. A raw vegetable or fruit is a good between-meal snack if you feel hungry. This is an ideal eating pattern to normalize someone's system quickly. Following some cleansing programs for a few weekends would restore the person's system to peak efficiency even faster.

Eating just one food at a time (a mono-diet) is an excellent eating plan for grossly obese people or anyone wanting the fastest results. A mono-diet allows the digestive system, which is most likely weak and inefficient, to break down only one type of food at a time. This simplifies its work, giving the overworked pancreas, liver, stomach and adrenal glands time to rejuvenate. This can return big health dividends and may eliminate hypoglycemia or other physical causes for being fat. The removal of internal waste helps normalize and improve the body's elimination system. Eating in this way simplifies the identification of any foods that cause allergic reactions. I will soon explain why this is important. Many wild animals eat a mono-diet. Did Nature intend us to do the same?

Timing is another component of proper eating where many people lack the knowledge of how it effects the results they get. The longer I live, the more I believe that timing is everything. For example, if you are not ready to let go of your fat and the reasons for it, you will read this book, find the answers you need, but do nothing. But when the timing is right, you will reread it, take action and be lean for life. I hope you are ready now or will find in the upcoming pages what you need to get ready. The principle of timing applies to eating just as it does to everything else in life. There is a time for everything.

Some people eat the right foods but at the wrong time. For example, we have discussed providing your body with essential fatty acids from whole foods or good vegetable or seed oils. It was recommended that you ingest these in the morning or at lunchtime to supply your daily needs. If you were to ingest these good fats in the late afternoon or evening, they may be stored as body fat. By ingesting them at the proper time, the fat will satisfy your appetite, eliminate cravings for bad fats, give you long-lasting energy and supply your body the essential fatty acids it needs. Another example of poor timing would be eating complete protein foods in the morning or at lunch and eating complex carbohydrates in the evening. The protein would make you tired during the day, and because your body does not normally need high-energy foods before bed, chances are the carbohydrate foods would be stored as fat. They would also inhibit the release of growth hormone, which stimulates fat burning. You already know the benefits of drinking water at the right time.

If you give your body what it needs, when it needs it, it will function well and maintain a healthy body fat level. Even good foods, if eaten at the wrong time, can produce the opposite results of what you want. Eating the same quantities of the same foods will produce radically different results if you eat them at different times. If you ate all of the foods in the morning in one or two meals, you would have energy and lose body weight—some fat and some muscle. If you were to eat the same types and amounts of food in one or two meals after six in the evening, you would not have much energy during the day and would gain body fat and lose muscle. Your body would cannibalize muscle tissue during the day to function and then store most of the food you eat in the evening as fat. This is an extreme example, but illustrates the importance of eating the right foods at the right time. Unfortunately, this example is common. I have talked with many people who, in an attempt to lose "weight" or keep their weight at a certain level, starve themselves all day and eat one meal in the evening. Remember our 110-pound obese woman? This is the absolute worst way to attempt to regulate your body fat level. It may control your weight, but your body fat will increase as your lean mass is eaten away.

Most people do not eat healthful foods because they have never eaten them. They have never experienced how delicious they taste and how good these foods can make them feel mentally and physically.

Do not feel badly and put yourself down if a lack of knowledge is the cause of why you have excess fat. You were not taught how to eat healthfully in school and chances are your parents did not know how. The past cannot be changed, but the future can be if you live in the present moment and apply the knowledge of proper eating that you now have.

The Negative Cycle of Overeating

The negative cycle of overeating leads to increased body fat because it decreases body efficiency. The less efficient your body is at digesting and using the foods you eat, the more food it will ask for in its attempt to fill its needs. This creates a negative cycle, because your body will keep telling you it is hungry until it gets the nutrition it needs. This is why people can sit all day long eating foods containing little, if any, nutritional value and still be hungry. Their bodies are actually starving and will never be satisfied until they get the vital nutrients that are needed.

My nutritional program can help you achieve and maintain healthy body weight, because it accomplishes the primary goal of eating—supplying your body and mind with the nutrients they need to function normally. Once this is done, your body stops craving food. Your hunger is satisfied and that gnawing, empty feeling goes away. You should feel a normal, natural satisfaction and not have to struggle against overeating. A big difference exists between how you feel when your body is truly satisfied and when your stomach is just full. You may even stop eating before you feel full, because your body is satisfied. Eating nutritionally deficient food, or even good food in a way that your body cannot use it, creates an ongoing struggle against overeating, because your body is always hungry. You now know how easy it is to end this struggle.

Overeating makes our bodies less efficient and as the problem worsens we need to eat more to get the same amount of nutrition. The excess food accumulates as fat and internal waste and makes our bodies even less efficient. This increases the *need* to eat even more as the negative cycle progresses at an ever-increasing rate. As people struggle against this constant craving for food, they develop emotional problems. Some believe they are worthless. Others believe they have no will power or self-control. Some eat more to punish themselves for being so weak willed. Many of them stress their bodies with diet programs or pills that cause a loss of lean body mass. This leads to more fat and even greater feelings of failure and hopelessness. These negative feelings and the stress they create make the overeating problem worse, because now people often stop caring if they gain more body fat. They feel powerless. Many give up and sink deeper and deeper into the negative cycle of despair and fat gain. The powerful forces of Nature, habit, inertia, momentum, the subconscious mind, and love are all working against them.

Fortunately, you now understand what is happening and have the knowledge to reverse the process by creating a positive cycle. It's simple. When you supply your body with nutritious foods in a way that it can get maximum benefits from them, you fill your nutritional needs with less food. Your body then has the chance to burn stored fat and start cleansing out internal waste. As this happens, your entire system gets more efficient and you supply your body's needs with even less food. The power of this positive cycle increases as your body gets more efficient and requires smaller amounts of food to get the nutrition it needs.

As you lose stored fat and internal waste, your negative emotional feelings will start to diminish. You will no longer feel powerless, because you now know how to reverse the negative cycle and lose your excess fat. As time goes by, the physical and emotional components help each other to progress. Your improved attitude makes it easier for you to keep eating properly and this helps your body become more efficient. Looking and feeling better physically boosts your emotional outlook even more. You will have created a positive physical and emotional cycle and harnessed the six powerful forces that were working against you to constantly work for you. Another important emotional benefit is your understanding of why you had the excess fat. This makes it easy to keep it gone for good.

Learned Bad Habits

Many of us grow up eating in the same way as our parents. Just look around. When you see a fat child, you usually see fat parents. There may be some hereditary predisposition for being fat, but they are most likely all fat because they are eating the same foods with the same poor habits. The attitudes and behaviors that made the parents fat made their children fat. I have known quite a few people who are the only lean ones in their families and the only difference is an active lifestyle and better eating habits. Even if someone has an inherited problem, it can usually be compensated for or overcome entirely. Take a moment to think about your parents. Are or were they fat? If so, you need to change the eating habits you learned while growing up. These habits may have caused you to develop excess fat cells as a child. This may make it a bit more difficult for you, but should not prevent your success. Poor eating habits will keep you fat until you develop healthier habits.

Parents usually want the best for their children so please do not blame yours if you have excess fat. They taught you what they knew; they just did not know how to eat healthfully. What's done is done. Your life is your responsibility, not your parents'. You can change what you do not like at any time, and you now have the knowledge and power to achieve permanent victory over your fat if you so choose. Do not waste any precious time blaming or condemning. Use it to improve your life and the lives of others. If one of your parents is fat, share this book with them and work through it together if you can. It will supply soul food for both of you and may improve your relationship.

Overeating is often nothing more than a bad habit. It can be caused by eating foods that are lacking in nutritional value or by eating too fast and putting in more food than your body needs before it has a chance to tell you that it has had enough. This habit is simple to change. Just eat foods high in nutritional value (natural, not artificially added) and eat more slowly. This gives your body the chance to tell you it is satisfied. Relax and enjoy your meals. It is easy if you eat whole, natural foods, because most of them are difficult to eat fast.

Eating large meals late at night and eating unhealthful nighttime snacks are two bad habits. Eating ice cream late every night or eating greasy and salty snacks in the evening when watching television or a movie are common examples of this. Eating candies, desserts and other foods lacking nutritional value is another bad habit you can easily change once you choose to have the benefits that changing will give you. Some people condition their children into believing that they need to eat an unhealthful dessert after they eat dinner. A rapidly growing child is not going to grow up strong and healthy eating sugar and fat-filled desserts.

It is a bad habit to have nutritionally void foods in the house as temptations. If people have cupboards full of chips, cookies and other junk foods, what are they and their families going to eat? People, especially children, generally eat what is available. Do not expect your young children to assume responsibility for their own health and say, "I'd rather eat an apple than a candy bar." It will never happen. They are influenced too much by advertisements, their peers, and by your example. If they are hungry and want a snack between meals, give them a bowl of blueberries or an apple. Let them learn how delicious these natural fruits are and how good they make them feel. It is your responsibility to help them develop healthy eating habits.

Forcing children to eat everything on their plates is another bad habit that parents often instill in their children. Some do it by telling their children that if they do not "clean up the plate" they will not get any dessert. The children overeat and then eat an unhealthful and fattening dessert. Other parents say that it wastes money or that food cannot be wasted because children are starving in Africa. If the parents really want to help, they should give their children less food and donate the money they save to help the starving children of the world. Some children will eat more than they want just to please their parents. Others will do it because of a fear of punishment or the fear of losing love from their parents.

Forcing children to eat everything on their plates can create excess fat, and not eating it all usually causes guilt feelings and a lower sense of self-worth. You have no idea how hungry your children are at any moment. If you fill their plates with more than they need, you are teaching them to overeat. They will soon need the quantity you are giving them and then even more. You will create the negative cycle of overeating for them. If this habit was instilled in you as a child, realize that you are an adult now and can easily change it with the knowledge you are acquiring from this book. Avoid creating this habit for your children by having them eat a small amount of most, if not all, of the foods of the meal and if they want more, give them some of each different food until they feel satisfied. Let them experience and learn to enjoy a wide variety of natural foods.

An especially bad habit is rewarding children with candy or other unhealthful "treats." Punishing them by not feeding them is another bad habit. These two habits often create a desire to overeat or to eat an unhealthful food if people feel like they have been good on a particular day. These habits plague millions who have carried them into adulthood. If you are one of them, you need to learn to treat yourself with positive things like a vacation, new clothes, feeling and looking terrific, or gifts, instead of eating foods that rot your teeth, make you fat, depress you and cause numerous other health problems. Foods that make you fat and undermine your health are not treats. Treat yourself to a vibrant, active life instead. It is much less expensive in numerous ways. If fat people figured out how much money they spend on junk food it would boggle their minds. Some could buy a new car with the money they now spend on lifeless foods and on the diets and programs used in an attempt to get rid of the fat created by those foods. "Weight loss" is a billion-dollar industry. How much of it is your money? Billions more are spent each year treating the diseases caused by unhealthful foods and excess fat. Do not forget about the costly negative effects to your self-image and sense of self-worth.

Other bad habits include adding salt to meals, eating large meals, frequently eating dessert, and numerous others I will be describing soon. These bad habits lead to the negative cycle of overeating. Most of them come simply from a lack of knowledge about what to eat, how and when to eat it, and what negative effects these habits have.

To eliminate a bad habit, you must be self-observant and aware enough to realize you have one. Then you must be honest enough to admit it. You cannot eliminate a bad habit if you do not acknowledge that it exists. You must learn to be objective and see yourself as others do. You have to see yourself shoveling spoonful after spoonful of sugar on your sugarcoated cold cereal before you can stop doing it. A simple way to get rid of a bad habit is to replace it with a good one. This can be as easy as eating popcorn without butter and salt or having a piece of fruit and some water instead of coffee and a donut. I will explain more ways to eliminate bad habits in upcoming chapters.

If you have children, you already know that they learn many of their behaviors by imitating their parents, friends and siblings. But you are the one who generally has the most influence. Be aware that your bad habits are going to affect more people than just you. If you head for the refrigerator or cookie jar every time you feel stressed or frustrated, what do you think your children will do when they get angry, upset or frustrated? If you use alcohol or drugs, what do you think they are going to do? Refer back to the "reduce stress" section in chapter nine for positive and constructive ways to deal with stress. Then let your children learn how to do it by observing you.

We are not our bodies, but unfortunately people often react to us based largely on our physical appearance. Please spare your children the anguish and despair you may have experienced. As you develop better eating habits and other ways of being healthier, pass this knowledge on to your children.

Let them grow up with the chance of being lean and healthy for their entire lives and the chance that their lives will be longer and filled with health and happiness instead of disease and suffering. If any of your children are already fat, share this book with them and work together to help each other shed excess fat. Children who get fat are often victims of ridicule from childhood onward. Unfortunately, most of the ridicule comes from within, undermining their self-image, confidence, success and happiness, and making it easier to develop negative and destructive behaviors. Your time, unconditional love and help in developing a good self-image are the three most important gifts you can give your children. Keeping them lean and well nourished is a big key to the development of a good self-image.

Keep in mind that your children will probably pass on the good eating habits to their children and so it will go from generation to generation. Always remember that your example has the greatest influence on them—what you *do*, not what you say. They may rebel and eat junk food in their teenage years, but chances are they will eat just like you when you are not looking and when they get a few years older. When it is their choice, they will often choose what they have learned is best for them.

Bodily Malfunction

A number of malfunctions (dysfunctions) can occur in your body, causing it to store more fat or inhibit the loss of excess you already have. Most of these can be corrected so you can achieve the lean, healthy body you want. These dysfunctions can affect you emotionally and physically. Many areas of your life will be improved by discovering and correcting these imbalances. You have already learned about the inefficiency of your digestive system due to an accumulation of excess fat and internal waste. An excuse given by some fat people is that they have a glandular problem. This is often true, but the glandular problem was usually created by excess waste and body fat overstressing the liver, pancreas, adrenal glands, and other glands and organs. You have learned that it is usually possible to reverse this with cleansing and dietary changes that give the overstressed glands and organs the chance to repair and rejuvenate.

You have learned that if the spinal nerve supplying a particular gland, organ or other structure has pressure on it that normal function is affected. One important area of the spine is where the nerves go to and from the thyroid gland—a gland that plays a major role in regulating your metabolism. If your metabolism is slowed down due to pressure on these nerves, it is easier to gain body fat and harder to lose it. If nerve flow is restored, your thyroid gland should function properly again and increase your metabolism back to its normal level—provided the thyroid gland is getting adequate blood flow and enough iodine to make the necessary amount of thyroid hormones.

About twelve years ago one of my patients had a misalignment of the vertebra at the base of her neck where the nerves supply the thyroid gland.

After the vertebra was stabilized in its proper position, she began losing excess body fat. After three weeks she had lost 15 pounds and told me that her eating and exercise habits had not changed. Normal communication between her brain and thyroid gland had been restored thereby normalizing her metabolism. Since then, many of my patients have lost excess fat after having misalignment of the same vertebra corrected. If fat loss is your goal, it is extremely important to have proper nerve flow to and from the internal organs of your body—especially those dealing with digestion, elimination and control of your metabolic rate.

Unfortunately, only one therapy I know of is capable of balancing the spine and restoring normal nerve flow permanently. The aforementioned patient had been treated over a thirty-year period for her chronic neck pain and severe headaches with many different conventional therapies (chiropractic, physical therapy, acupuncture, stretching, exercise, massage, ultrasound, heat therapy, Hellerwork and more). Her problems continued to worsen until she got my PMBT treatments. Her chronic headaches were resolved and her severe dowager's hump (excessive upper back curve) was restored to a normal curve. We achieved success, because I eliminated the *cause* of her vertebrae and certain other bones being out of alignment. Most conventional therapies simply manipulate or force the vertebrae back in place and hope they stay. Rarely do the bones stay in place long enough for the body to reestablish normal function. Some problems may seem to improve if the body compensates with another area. Unfortunately this leads to the eventual development of a new problem. Two wrongs don't make a right even though someone's original symptoms may be improved. PMBT therapy not only eliminates the cause of the vertebral misalignments, thereby giving lasting results, but I seek to determine the "cause of the cause" and eliminate this as well. This is the true root of the problem, and if not eliminated, will one day re-create the problem. You must use the same concept to obtain permanent fat loss. The cause must be discovered, eliminated and then not re-created.

The most common area of injury or overstress to the neck is at the junction of the neck and the rib cage. This is where it gets the most stress so this is where misalignments are most common. As people live their lives they accumulate problems there and nerve flow to the thyroid gland is diminished. Is this why low thyroid conditions are so prevalent? I believe it is, based on the success of my therapy in resolving this and many other dysfunctions by realigning the spinal vertebrae and restoring normal nerve flow to the affected area.

You already know about the autonomic nervous system and its two parts, the sympathetic and parasympathetic. This system functions through the nerves coming from your brain, down the spinal cord and exiting between the vertebrae of your spine. It is the system affected when vertebrae are out of alignment causing inflammation that puts pressure on the nerves. You also know that the two parts of this system can become unbalanced by a physical or emotional trauma. If they are out of synchronization, it can wreak havoc on proper digestion, assimilation and utilization of foods. Improperly timed blood flow can influence your fat-loss program by decreasing blood flow to the thyroid gland, thereby slowing your metabolism. This is another example of the principle of timing.

A hormone from the pituitary gland stimulates the thyroid gland to do its job, and the pituitary gland is controlled by the hypothalamus of the brain. All of these can be negatively affected by a nervous system imbalance. To restore balance to the autonomic nervous system and then treat any affected organs and glands, I use the Neurovascular Dynamics (NVD) technique. This technique has reestablished normal blood flow to parts of the body when normal nerve flow was being restored to the same areas using PMBT therapy. NVD is not widely available, but is practiced by some chiropractors and other therapists.

A nervous system imbalance may be why you have excess body fat or why you have been unable to lose it even if you are following my nutritional recommendations. Even if you have nervous system imbalances, you should still experience great results. They will just be slower and you may have to be stricter in some areas of your program to stay lean. You may already be taking medication to compensate for a dysfunctional thyroid gland. The best course of action would be to reestablish normal nerve and blood flow by getting the spine aligned, the two nervous systems balanced and all affected glands or organs treated and restored to normal function. Most people would be able to stop using the medication, but this should be done only under a doctor's recommendation and supervision.

For its size, the thyroid gland normally has more blood flow than any other gland or organ in your body, and the arteries supplying it pass through muscles in the front of your neck. If these muscles are excessively tight (as they are in most people), they constrict the arteries and reduce blood flow to the thyroid gland. If your thyroid gland does not have adequate blood flow, it cannot do its job properly and consequently your metabolism is slowed. Treatments with my PMBT therapy can eliminate the tightness in the neck muscles and restore normal blood flow to the thyroid gland.

I believe that spinal nerve pressure at the base of the neck and tight muscles in the front of the neck are part of the reason why people tend to gain body fat as they age. It makes sense, because these areas generally get tighter over time and both can slow the metabolism. This, along with poor nutrition and a lack of strength-building exercise to maintain lean body mass makes it easy to see why so many people lose muscle and gain fat as time passes. They grow weaker, fatter and older even though their activity levels stay the same. Low thyroid function and loss of lean body mass are the two primary causes for the now obsolete expression "middle-age spread." Excess fat and loss of strength contribute to many of the symptoms of "old age." With proper exercise and nutrition, you could be physiologically younger five years from now than you were ten years ago.

A simple way to determine if the muscles in the front of your neck are tight is to stand normally and have someone look at you from the side. Have the person visualize an imaginary line upward from the center of your shoulder or hold a ruler or other straightedge in the same location. The muscles are tight if the center of your ear is forward of the shoulder centerline. Even if your ear and shoulder are aligned, the muscles may still be tight if the muscles in the back of your neck are equally tight or if other shortened muscles are causing your shoulders to round forward. This latter scenario is another extremely common problem. Stretching can give some temporary relief, but cannot restore these muscles to their normal lengths. The cause of why they are short must be eliminated before permanent results can be obtained. My PMBT therapy eliminates the cause, allowing the muscles to heal back to normal. Restoring certain neck and shoulder muscles to their normal lengths also improves your posture and reduces neck stress. If the muscles in the front are tight, you will feel stress in the back muscles between your neck and shoulders, because they have to work harder than normal to create a counterpull against the front muscles. This is why most people "hold their stress" in the muscles at the back of their necks.

You can easily test your thyroid function at home. Women should not do it during menstruation. Just put a regular thermometer in your armpit for 10 minutes after awakening in the morning. Do not get out of bed or move about. Just reach for and position the thermometer and then lie quietly for 10 minutes. Do this on two or three different mornings and figure the average temperature. The temperature should be between 97.8 and 98.2 degrees. If it is low, you may want to have a blood test done to check your thyroid hormone levels. Even if your blood test results are normal, a low temperature may indicate that your body is not using the hormones properly. Your metabolism could still be low. This may be caused by a nutritional deficiency, a lack of strength-building exercise or from other imbalances.

Most parts of your body need three things to function normally. They need good communication with the brain (this is like the foreman who knows how to build a brick wall). They also need adequate blood flow (this is like the workmen who build the wall) and they need the raw materials to do the job (this is like the bricks and mortar). Without an adequate amount of all three of these components there will be less than normal function in that part of the body.

You have learned that the vagus nerves and chemical ligands link the emotional centers of your brain to many parts of your body. Therefore, your emotional state and thinking patterns can be another source of bodily dysfunction. I will teach you how to improve your thinking habits in the next few chapters.

Unhealthy dietary habits can cause your glands and organs to malfunction. For example, eating excess sugar can lead to a pancreas problem and decreased or increased blood sugar levels. You already know that most people who develop diabetes are fat and that hypoglycemia can create a mental and physical roller coaster that leads to fat gain. Excess salt intake can cause increased blood pressure, water retention, adrenal gland dysfunction and numerous other problems. Some of the symptoms of adrenal gland dysfunction are light sensitivity, dizziness when getting up from sitting or lying down, fatigue, feeling stressed out and craving salt. Remember that salt has a stimulating effect on the adrenal glands, so if you give in to the craving, you will make the condition worse. Resolving adrenal problems is sometimes as simple as reducing salt intake.

Ingesting excess fats, the wrong kinds of fats or eating fats at the wrong time leads to body fat being stored and stresses the entire body, making it sluggish and inefficient. Not eating enough fat may cause your body to manufacture excess cholesterol and raise the amount in your blood to unhealthy levels. A deficiency and sometimes an excess of a nutrient can create chemical imbalances and related health problems. Following a low-calorie diet or going hungry all day and then eating one small meal causes your body to lower your metabolism as a protective response. It will take a while to get your body and metabolism normalized again once you start eating healthfully. If you have been starving yourself, be especially careful in the beginning. Eat small, light meals and gradually increase as your metabolism normalizes.

Many people experience abnormal food cravings. There are numerous reasons for this. You have learned why you may crave alcohol and foods that contain bad fats, sugar, salt and processed carbohydrates, and why you may crave more food. Some cravings are stimulated by bodily dysfunctions caused by poor nutrition or abnormal nerve or blood flow. Chapter twelve contains numerous emotional reasons for abnormal food cravings, but here are a few more physical ones.

If you have an overgrowth of *Candida albicans* in your system, it can cause a craving for sugar, processed carbohydrates and alcohol. The obvious solution is to kill off the *Candida*. This is best done with specific nutritional supplements and by temporarily eliminating certain foods from the diet. I have taught numerous people how to eliminate this stubborn yeast.

The ability to convert the linoleic acid found in some good fats into its usable form, gamma-linoleic acid (GLA), is often reduced as people age. When this happens, they may start eating more fried foods, pastries and other foods that contain bad fats. This problem can be resolved by ingesting GLA supplements. Borage oil is an excellent source and can be found in capsule form in most health-food stores. If you crave bad fats, get tested for need or take one capsule a day for a week or two and see what happens. If you still have the craving, take two a day for a week or two. Increase the number of capsules in a similar manner until the craving is gone. One to four capsules a day should be adequate for most people. In the winter you will be getting more good fats from whole grains, nuts, seeds and avocados, but you may still need more oil due to the body's increased need for good fats during cold weather. I suggest using a combination of flaxseed oil and borage oil capsules. Determining how much you need is usually quite easy. If your skin is dry and your heels dry and cracked, you need more oil and if your face feels oily, you need less.

Some people continually crave food. For them, the first step is to make sure their bodies are getting good food that is eaten at the right time and digested well. This will resolve the problem for many of them. If someone still wants to eat all the time, there may be another internal imbalance triggering it. An inadequate amount of serotonin decreases our sense of well being, happiness and contentment. This can cause us to eat excessively but never feel satisfied. L-5-hydroxytryptophan (5-HTP) is the precursor to serotonin and is normally made in the body from the amino acid tryptophan. It is available as a supplement and has reduced the appetites of many people who do not get enough tryptophan or who are unable to produce enough 5-HTP from the normal amount they do get.

Eating foods that are lacking in nutritional value is another reason your body's systems may function poorly. It is a common cause of people who have excess fat and the primary reason why most of them are severely malnourished. Prolonged malnutrition slows your metabolism by 20 to 30 percent, because when your body does not get what it needs, it must slow or curtail certain functions. The body also does not get the nutrients needed to complete all necessary chemical reactions. Many people assume that eating all day is all they need to do, but are unaware of the effects of what they are eating and when they are eating it. I cannot overemphasize the point that the food you eat must contain nutritional value if it is going to build health and keep your body looking good. Think about it when you make your food choices and please never forget it. Also don't forget the other three vital steps necessary to reach the bottom line of supplying your body with the nutrients it needs.

If you do not get enough UV light through the pupils of your eyes (*never* look directly at the sun), you can become undernourished and develop the winter blues. This condition affects millions of people and has numerous symptoms—moodiness, fatigue, excessive sleeping, feeling down, lethargy, difficulty getting up, loss of sex drive, social withdrawal, weight gain and a craving for processed carbohydrates. It is similar to, but less severe than, seasonal affective disorder that was discussed in chapter three. The cure is to get enough of the full-spectrum light you need.

Digestion, absorption, and utilization of foods can be affected by various inborn capabilities of your unique body. Some people have strong digestive systems and others have weak ones. If the nerve and blood flow are normal, you are left with your inherited capabilities. This is just the way your body is. It does not mean something is wrong. You just have to be aware that parts of your system may be less efficient than those parts in someone else. You must experiment and learn about your body and its capabilities, and then give it special support when necessary.

If a woman has had her thyroid gland surgically removed, she will need artificial thyroxine to keep her metabolism normal. Fortunately, most genetic weaknesses or cases where certain glands have been taken out can usually be dealt with using herbs, other natural substances or artificial hormones. For example, if your natural production of digestive enzymes is low, taking supplemental enzymes with large meals or particular foods can help your body to digest them effectively. A bile supplement taken when ingesting fats will help someone who has a dysfunctional gallbladder. Gallbladder problems have resolved after normal nerve flow was restored, and eliminating gallstones can be done with a relatively simple nutritional procedure. It should rarely be necessary for a gallbladder to be surgically removed. Some doctors tell people that removing the gallbladder has no effect, but it does. The liver still makes bile but the quantity is insufficient to handle most fatty meals. This is the reason people who have had their gallbladders removed should take a bile supplement with every fatty meal.

Apple cider vinegar or betaine hydrochloride tablets can be taken with protein meals if your natural production of hydrochloric acid (HCl) is low. Inadequate HCl may be causing a deficiency of the minerals necessary for the fat-burning process. Something as simple as that could be why you have excess fat, even though your nutritional intake is relatively good. No matter what problem you may have, the dietary guidelines in this book should make it easier to supply the nutrition your body needs to be lean and function at peak efficiency. Do your best to deal with inherited problems using herbs, special supplements or various natural treatments. Resort to drugs only as a final alternative and preferably just to replace a natural substance your body is not producing.

Keep in mind that you may have more than one cause reducing your body's normal function. Eliminate them all and you should easily lose your excess fat. Remember that the enemies discussed in chapter four stress your body and cause hypoglycemia, hypothyroidism, and other dysfunctions that can make you feel lousy and gain fat. Eliminating these harmful substances may be the most important thing you can do to accomplish your fat-loss goal. Attempting to treat their negative influences is difficult and usually only partially successful.

Damage to the hypothalamus (a part of the brain) can stimulate excessive eating. People may also have a genetic abnormality affecting the chemistry of fat storage in their bodies. Both of these conditions and possibly other inborn imbalances could cause obesity. Some affect the quantity of food eaten and others may affect the type of foods eaten. I believe that these conditions are extremely rare and with good eating and exercise habits can be compensated for to a large degree.

Why do so many children suffer with allergies, ADHD, other health problems and excess fat? I believe many of them got off to a bad start, because they were born of poorly nourished parents. Then they were fed dairy products, sugar, hydrogenated oils and other harmful "foods" while growing up. Chances are most of them are still eating mainly lifeless junk. They have weak bodies because they never got the nutrients necessary to grow strong, and some formed abnormally high numbers of fat cells. Many of them were given drugs whenever they had even a slight sniffle so their immune systems never had a chance to develop properly. Some children become addicted to the drugs their parents use (caffeine, alcohol and nicotine, most often). If this is how you started out, you may be experiencing extensive abnormal function. You now know how to eliminate most, if not all, of your problems.

Numerous drugs have side effects that affect your body's function and nutritional status. They can increase your appetite, cause high or low blood sugar, malabsorption, high or low levels of cholesterol and triglycerides, and decreased protein metabolism. I suggest finding out the possible side effects and health consequences of any drug prior to taking it. You should also be aware of possible interactions with other drugs you may be taking. The best thing to do is build health with proper nutrition and regular exercise so drugs are not needed.

Electroacupuncture can test for numerous physical problems such as allergies, heavy metals, nutritional deficiencies, viruses, bacteria, hormone imbalances and dysfunctional glands and organs. The search for your physical problems will be simplified if you can find a holistic practitioner who does this. Otherwise, look for another holistic practitioner who can help you track down and eliminate your particular physical causes for being fat.

Fatigue

"I'm so tired." Scores of reasons exist for this common complaint, and most of them contribute to gaining excess body fat either directly or indirectly. Some of them make you fat and this causes the fatigue. Others decrease energy production or deplete your energy. Anything making you tired reduces your motivation to exercise or be physically active and at the same time increases your desire to eat in an attempt to get more energy. Fatigue also reduces your interest in mentally stimulating activities that keep you from thinking about eating all the time. A lack of energy often creates an "I don't care" attitude that frequently leads to overeating or making poor food choices.

Injuries and diseases cause fatigue because your body channels energy internally to repair damage or to fight an unwanted invader. Remember why internal cleansing causes fatigue? Many diseases cause fatigue for the same reason and there is usually repair work being done and the immune system is working harder. Chronic back, neck or other joint pains use up a great deal of energy. Even something as simple as poor posture can rob you of energy, because of the increased workload on your postural muscles.

Muscles that are tight from an accumulation of fibrotic adhesions can make you feel tired and old. Because of postural habits and lack of exercise, most people develop tightness in their lower back muscles, calves, hamstrings and upper back and neck muscles. The tighter these muscles are, the more energy it takes to move, and because the opposing muscles are attempting to establish balance, they use energy even when at rest. This and excess internal waste are the two primary reasons why older people generally have less energy for physical activities than younger people do. My PMBT therapy can eliminate the adhesions and restore the muscles to their original lengths. More energy would then be available for productive pursuits.

The causes of fatigue are many, including anemia, hypoglycemia, low thyroid function, adrenal gland exhaustion, allergies, internal imbalances, constipation, over-breathing, dehydration, *Candida albicans*, and the use of drugs, tobacco and caffeine. The list goes on and on: poor circulation, Epstein-Barr virus, vitamin B_1 or B_{12} deficiency, stress, poor absorption of nutrients, acute and chronic illness, heavy drinking, depression, anxiety, other psychological disorders, and negative emotions. Exposure to positive ions and emf (electromotive force) radiation from many types of electrical and electronic equipment can also cause fatigue. And, do not forget about eating foods lacking in the nutrients necessary for energy production. Many of these causes make some of the others worse so a negative health cycle is created. For example, low thyroid function causes a decrease in blood sugar and can contribute to constipation, poor circulation, poor absorption, illness, depression and other health problems. The goal when dealing with these conditions should be to find and eliminate the primary cause instead of just treating the symptoms. Treating the symptoms may be helpful in the beginning, but should not be necessary after the root cause is gone. Over-breathing will affect almost all of the other causes, because your cells will not be getting enough oxygen to function normally.

Eating an excess of energy foods at night (even healthful ones) can lead to fat storage and also restless sleep. The lack of restful sleep makes people wake up in the morning feeling tired. Many of them reach for a stimulant of some kind. This can create a negative cycle of eating and stimulant ingestion that starts their blood sugar levels on a roller coaster ride that may last all day. This is another example of why it is important to eat foods at the right time.

Lack of exercise can lead to fatigue and conversely, correct exercise can increase energy. Training to make muscles stronger allows them to work less during all activities and being in good cardiovascular condition increases oxygen to your body, so it can work longer and harder without getting tired. Endorphin release, improved self-image and other benefits of exercise you have previously learned, all give you more energy.

Many people experience fatigue simply because they have *minor* nutritional deficiencies. Lack of certain trace minerals and not enough water are the most common. Many other people create their own fatigue by constantly stressing their bodies with stimulants such as sugar, caffeine, nicotine, alcohol and certain drugs. They overstress their adrenal glands and other organs and block the message from the body when it is truly tired and asking for rest. Sometimes they get the message but do not rest.

Not getting enough of the electrolyte minerals potassium, magnesium and sodium can cause fatigue. Taking a supplement of these minerals could give you the energy to go to the gym and complete an exercise program. I use the electrolyte product available from Super Spectrim [(888) 772-6398] because it is much less expensive than similar products sold in health-food stores. Taking the electrolytes prior to working out "supercharges" my energy to greater than 100 percent so after the workout my energy level is at 100 percent instead of being depleted and then needing time to build back up to normal. I do not recommend the numerous sports drinks that contain electrolytes because they are expensive and many contain sugar and excess salt in order to cater to the sugar and salt addiction and distorted taste buds of most Americans.

Overeating causes fatigue in three primary ways. First, it uses more energy to digest and eliminate the excess food being eaten. Second, it increases your weight, requiring your muscles to use more energy for everything you do. Third, excess fat and internal waste create internal friction that robs you of energy and makes your body less efficient at everything it does.

If the first cervical vertebra in your neck is misaligned, it affects the nerve that controls blood flow to your brain. If blood flow is reduced, the resultant lack of oxygen and nutrients to the brain causes fatigue and lethargy. A number of symptoms can be created. Correcting this misalignment has resolved chronic tiredness, migraine headaches, high blood pressure, nervousness and insomnia for many of my patients. Remember that the cause of the vertebra being misaligned must be eliminated to obtain permanent relief. Snoring and sleep apnea have been resolved for patients by realigning other vertebrae in the neck.

If a misalignment of the first cervical vertebra is causing decreased blood flow to the brain, the brain will send a message to the body to increase the blood pressure. The brain will then get adequate blood flow to function normally. If someone has high blood pressure for this reason and takes medication to reduce the pressure, then the brain will not get adequate blood flow and the person will experience fatigue.

The stress and tension of a noisy, fast-paced life can cause fatigue. Working odd hours or worrying about and dealing with money problems, relationships, work and children can also cause fatigue. If a man wants to avoid doing something, he may create fatigue as an excuse. Fear can also lead to fatigue.

Adolescents commonly experience fatigue for numerous reasons. They are living in rapidly growing bodies and experiencing powerful hormonal changes. This takes energy, as does learning many new things in school. The excitement and anxiety about self, sex, career, God and the world can be extremely draining. Late nights, self-consciousness leading to isolation and boredom, not enough sleep, poor nutrition, lack of exercise and worrying about appearance and performance can also contribute to their fatigue. Some fatigue is a rebellion against authority and a way to exert their independence.

Some of the most common emotional causes of fatigue and overeating are boredom, loneliness and frustration. Your brain needs good nutrition to function normally but you must also feed your mind by learning new things, thinking uplifting thoughts, seeing the positive side of your experiences and expressing your creativity in some way. When their minds are starving, some people attempt to fill the void it creates with food and others just sit around with nothing to do but eat. Do not just sit and feed your face; get involved in living your life. Read a good book (or write one), talk with informed, enlightening and inspirational people, take a class to learn something you enjoy, start a business, learn to play a musical instrument or get involved in a worthwhile cause. The choices are endless.

Another common cause of fatigue and overeating is a lack of soul food. Remember that you are a spirit inhabiting a physical body, not a body with a spirit. If your spirit (the real you) is starving, the emptiness you feel inside will make life seem dull, boring and pointless. This often leads to depression. Some people use drugs in an attempt to find what is missing in their lives or to deaden the pain and loneliness they feel. Other people shovel food in as fast as they can in an attempt to fill up this seemingly bottomless pit of emptiness. Some people overeat, drink alcohol *and* use other drugs. Alcohol and drugs only make the situation worse and food will never help, because the spirit is not nourished with physical nutrients. You must supply it the spiritual food it needs for good health. Your spirit thrives on love, a sense of worthwhile purpose and the feelings you get from a job well done, when you see a lovely sight, hear beautiful music, hug a loved one, or give of yourself to others. Get into life and start nourishing your spirit (you) with positive and loving actions toward yourself and others. The benefits you will get from the feelings you experience are worth far more than the time and effort it takes. Old age is a common reason given to people as the cause of their fatigue. You now know age has very little to do with it and that most of the causes can be eliminated.

Probably the most common cause of fatigue is a deficiency of the vital nutrient sleep. This deficiency is almost universal in this day and age. We get much less sleep than people did fifty to one hundred years ago because of electric lights, around-the-clock television, the Internet, many more activities we can do, less physical labor or exercise and for a variety of other reasons. I believe that a lack of sleep is a major contributor to the obesity epidemic in America because being tired dramatically reduces our judgement and decision making about what foods to eat and how much. Fatigue also decreases our daytime alertness, so people constantly reach for drugs or unhealthful and fattening pick-me-up foods. One of the best ways to help keep your children from using drugs may be to make sure they get enough sleep. Sadly, many traffic fatalities are blamed on a lack of sleep, and people eating while driving probably cause others.

Here are a few tips on how to sleep longer and get more restful sleep. Do not have a television in your bedroom. If you want to watch late night television programs, record them and watch them the next day at an earlier hour. Determine a reasonable time to stop working or playing on your computer. Do not watch the late-night news or disturbing or action-packed television programs or movies prior to going to bed. Do not ingest high-energy snack foods or drinks in the evening after dinner. Go to sleep and wake up at the same times on most days. Do not exercise late in the evening. Use only a dim night light when you get up during the night. Take a 20 to 30 minute nap during the day whenever possible, but do not sleep more than 30 minutes or it will be difficult to wake up. This is especially important for teenagers because the change in the circadian rhythm (the 24-hour biological sleep cycle) that occurs at this time in their lives makes them stay up late. They have to get up early to go to school so they rarely get the nine hours or more of sleep they need. It will be challenging to get most teenagers to take a nap after school but once they experience how much better they feel, chances are they will continue this healthy habit.

Sleep in a comfortable position. The best position is to sleep on your back with a cervical pillow that maintains the normal curve of your neck. Visit my Web site, DrAlexander.com, to see the type of pillow I recommend. Using a regular pillow under your head will strain your neck muscles and create an abnormal forward curvature of your neck and upper back. Do not use a pillow under your knees when sleeping on your back or you will flatten out the normal curve of your lower back and create problems. The next best sleeping position is on your side. The pillow used should be thick enough and firm enough to keep your neck in alignment with the rest of your spine. When sleeping on your side, put a pillow between your knees to keep your lower back from twisting. Do not sleep on your stomach. In addition to these tips on sleeping, follow the guidelines in this book to exercise regularly, eat good foods at the right times, reduce stress, get organized and so on. If you are well rested, you will be more productive, feel better about yourself and your life, and you will make better choices for the health of your body, mind and spirit.

The Wrong "Good" Food for You

Just because a food is healthful and nutritious does not necessarily mean it is right for you. As you have already learned, you must find the proper ratio of complete proteins, carbohydrates and fats that supply the nutrients needed for your body to function efficiently. If your body would do best eating primarily vegetarian foods, you will make your body fat if you eat quite a bit of red meat. If your body needs red meat but does not get enough, it will function poorly and in an attempt to get the complete protein it needs, may cause you to overeat vegetarian foods (particularly dairy and processed grain products) and get fat. I have counseled a number of vegetarians. Many were fat and most of the others were thin, pale and sick all the time. Even though it makes a great deal of sense on paper, in practical application a strict vegetarian diet does not work for most people. You have already learned that it did not work for me. On the other hand, I have known people who have been vegetarians for many years and have done fine. Clearly, it is right for their bodies. As you know, I recommend primarily vegetarian foods with just the right amount of meats for your unique body.

Many people have read that they should eat a low-fat diet if they want to be healthy. But, if they limit the healthful fat in their diet, they may become deficient in essential fatty acids. This can lead to deficiencies of other vital nutrients. A low-fat diet can cause other problems. For example, if a woman's body does not get enough healthful fat, it will usually store some of the carbohydrate and protein foods she eats as fat. This is a protective mechanism our bodies use when they do not get enough of something. Many people think that the cause of water retention is drinking too much water and that the excess will be eliminated by not drinking. This could not be further from the truth. There are other causes for water retention but a frequent cause is not drinking enough. The body stores it for self-preservation. Not getting enough water creates other problems. Similarly, not eating enough healthful fats often causes fat to be stored and leads to other problems.

Another example of the wrong good foods is eating the foods your body just cannot handle well. Dairy products can easily make you fat. The nightshade family of plants may cause inflammation, making it difficult for you to exercise. You may be allergic to certain foods, because you were exposed to them before your body was able to digest them, because you have eaten an excess of them or because your body cannot handle them for some other reason. If you are in a rut and eating a limited variety of foods, you can easily overload your system with something. Also remember that if your variety of foods is limited, your body will crave the nutrients it is not getting. This may cause overeating in an attempt to get those nutrients. Never forget that even nutritious whole foods can be stored as fat if you eat them to excess.

As you can see, even nutritious natural foods can sometimes be detrimental to your health and your fat-loss program. This is why it is imperative to determine the right eating program for you. Once determined, it simplifies your eating and helps put an end to your struggle against excess body fat and perhaps one or more mysterious health problems. Determining the right program takes some time, but once it is done you will be extremely happy you took the time to do it. You may feel like you have been freed from a prison. From then on you will have more time to accomplish other goals and to enjoy life more fully with a lean and healthy body.

Creeping Obesity

Creeping obesity is what has happened to people who step on the scales one morning and find themselves 20 pounds heavier than they thought they were, and the extra 20 pounds is fat and internal waste. To understand how this happens, let's look at a few different scenarios. Our first person is a man who gets up and eats a large high-protein breakfast, because he has heard from the meat and milk producers and other advertisers that this is a good way to start the day. In reality it is a bad way, because a high-protein meal takes a great deal of energy to digest. You have learned that if more energy goes to your digestive system, your brain and muscles get less. This man will feel tired and lethargic, so will often stop and buy a cup of coffee and a donut or get an unhealthful pick-me-up from the catering truck when he gets to work. This is how the negative cycle starts. Does this sound familiar?

Our second person is a woman who eats a healthier breakfast but goes out five days a week and has a high-protein lunch. By the time she gets back to work, she will usually be ready for the proverbial siesta. To stay awake she drinks a cup of coffee with a few scoops of sugar or goes down the hall to the candy or soft drink machine. She will most likely need another sugar or caffeine energy boost about four o'clock in the afternoon, because her lunch had hardly any fats or complex carbohydrates for long-lasting energy. Some people add other unhealthful energy boosts by smoking cigarettes.

Our third person is a man who eats well all day but goes home and eats a large (and perhaps late) dinner of complex carbohydrates and protein. Now there is an abundance of energy foods (the carbohydrates) in his system that are digested and available for use just in time to go to sleep. Because he does not need much energy, his body will store most of it as fat. This can happen even if the foods being eaten are healthful and nutritious. The available energy may make it difficult for him to sleep well so he will be more tired the next day and possibly seek out a stimulant. And, as you have learned, eating carbohydrates prior to bedtime decreases the output of growth hormone, which stimulates fat burning and the body's rebuilding processes.

These common scenarios not only add 15 to 20 pounds of fat to someone's body in six months to a year but also cause other negative effects. The first two scenarios have the most harmful effects. First of all, the excess protein overstresses the digestive system. Second, not supplying the body with good energy foods during the day forces it to work harder to meet its energy needs, and some internal functions get shortchanged because not enough energy is available to do everything efficiently. Third, the protein and lack of energy foods causes many people to use harmful stimulants like caffeine, nicotine and sugar. Forcing the body with stimulants causes stress and is like whipping a tired, undernourished horse to make it run. Instead of feeding it so it will be strong and able to do what you want, it is forced to work harder when it is already in a depleted condition. This will eventually break your body's weakest link and create a serious health problem. Last but not least, protein and the complex-carbohydrate foods most people eat (processed grains) are acid-forming and you know the results of an acidic bloodstream.

Creeping obesity comes on so gradually that many people are unaware of it until they have gained about 20 pounds. You must develop an awareness of your body and what it is doing—rather, what you are doing to it—if you want to be healthy and lean for life. Besides a gain of excess fat, there is often a loss of lean body mass caused by a lack of correct strength-training exercise. This compounds the problem and can mask what is really happening if people only weigh themselves. If they lose 10 pounds of muscle and gain 20 pounds of fat, they will most likely think they only gained 10 pounds of fat.

Obesity can creep up on people if they eat a few more calories every day than they need, eat the wrong foods, or eat inefficiently or with poor timing. An extra slice of toast, a donut or a glass of wine each day will add about a pound of fat every month. Sooner or later, people notice their clothes feeling tighter and are often shocked when the scales register 10 to 15 pounds more than expected.

Creeping obesity can easily happen to parents who eat the leftover food of their children. This is seen less frequently in women, because many of them are always dieting in an attempt to maintain or regain their girlish figure. Unfortunately, most of them do not worry about overfeeding their husbands, even though he is gaining excess fat and getting closer to a heart attack, stroke or diabetes every day. Stop giving your children so much food and the problem is solved. As an added bonus, it saves money.

Why do about five percent of the people who follow one of the many diet plans lose weight and keep it off? This happens because creeping obesity was the reason they had excess fat. Once they lose the weight and stop drinking the special diet shake or whatever else they are using, they keep it off, because they finally understand that the weight will creep back again if they do not increase their awareness of what they are eating. They pay more attention to what they eat, they stop eating the children's leftovers, they stop the wine every night or they just cut back slightly on everything. They have eliminated their cause for having excess fat—simply not paying attention.

Excessive Dieting

Another common cause for being fat is frequent dieting. This may seem like a contradiction but makes perfect sense when you understand what is really happening. Unhealthful diets are followed because the average person does not know how and why the body burns fat. Many people believe a low-calorie diet will help them lose weight. Unfortunately, most of them end up eating a low-calorie diet that supplies their bodies with hardly any of the nutrition they need. They may lose weight, but most of it is usually lean body tissue, not fat. Then they start eating "normally" again—the way that made them fat in the first place. Their weight usually goes back up quickly as some of the lean tissue is replaced and they gain back even more fat than they had before. People see this as failure and you know what that can cause. It is a good thing some of the lean tissue comes back, otherwise they would be in much worse shape than before.

The human body is extremely adaptive to different conditions and circumstances. If people diet frequently by limiting their calories, their bodies simply adapt by slowing down internal metabolic processes. Now, however, it is much easier to gain body fat because their metabolisms are slowed down. Because their bodies have adapted to the 1,000 or 1,200 calories a day, every extra bite will be stored as fat. If they eat 1,700 calories, they will gain body fat quickly.

Many fat people do not eat very much so they cannot understand why they are fat. Most have slowed the metabolism of their bodies to such a degree that they do not need much food to maintain their lean body weights. This makes it easy to gain more fat. The majority of them have also lost lean body weight, because they have not exercised to maintain it. To make matters worse, they usually eat high-calorie foods with little nutritional value and eat at the wrong times. Keep in mind that food is primarily needed only for your lean body mass. For example, let's say that two women have the same activity level, the same metabolism, and 90 pounds of lean body mass. One could weigh 110 pounds, the other 190 pounds and they would maintain their weights with the same number of calories. One of them just has 80 more pounds of fat. The fat burns hardly any calories so essentially just goes along for the ride. You have been taught that it is possible to lose more body fat by eating large quantities of food (the right kind at the right time) than by not eating anything.

By following the program in this book, you will not waste your time counting calories or points, replacing one worthless food with another, or following other negative and futile pursuits. Your body will naturally tell you when it has gotten adequate nutrition and it will be easy to stop eating, because you will feel satisfied. When you start listening to your body, you gradually learn to hear what it is telling you. It will help you achieve your goal of getting and staying lean and healthy, because that is what it is programmed to do. If you are extremely active one day, your body will stimulate you to eat more. If you are inactive another day, your appetite will adjust and you will eat less. You will start living in harmony with the natural way of your body and mind, instead of attempting to trick it, stimulate it, manipulate hormone levels or fool it in some way with an unbalanced dietary program.

Muscles help maintain a normal metabolism because they use energy. Body fat uses few calories so does almost nothing to stimulate your metabolism. The larger your muscles, the more energy they use and the more calories you can consume without gaining fat. This is why gaining, or at least maintaining, lean body mass helps you move faster toward your goal of losing excess body fat. Correct strength training also shapes and tones your muscles, giving your body a more natural and attractive shape. If you are losing fat and gaining muscle at the same rate, you can shape and tighten your body even though your weight stays the same. You will lose inches, because muscle is far more dense than fat. Compare one pound of lean muscle meat to one pound of fat sometime. You may end up weighing close to what you did before you started your program but be much smaller, firmer and leaner.

Remember the 110-pound woman at the beginning of the chapter who thought she was in good shape but was actually obese and terribly unhealthy? Because of her small amount of lean body mass and her lowered metabolism, it was an ongoing struggle to maintain her weight. She was constantly starving herself as she had done to get herself into such terrible shape. Maintaining her weight became increasingly difficult as she lost more lean tissue and her metabolism slowed even more. Even though her efforts were increasing, she was unknowingly making the negative cycle worse. This is a clear example of not understanding what is happening. With proper knowledge, she can start a positive cycle and create and maintain a normal lean body easily and naturally.

Environment

This cause has emotional aspects, but I chose to put it here because of its physical components. Your environment consists primarily of four parts: where you live, where you work, the people you associate with in social activities, and your internal thought processes and programming.

Where you live

Where you live can affect your amount of body fat in part based on the culture and customs of the area. For example, if your community often has sales of baked goods and other get-togethers where food is a major reason for being there, you will constantly be tempted to overeat or eat unhealthful foods. Generally, people who live in the country eat more whole foods than city dwellers because they or their neighbors grow the foods. If you live where it is cold four or five months every year, you may accumulate excess body fat to keep you warmer, but it is easy to stay lean if you eat the right winter foods. If you live in a tropical climate, you may instinctively eat more fruits and lighter vegetables that keep you cooler and make it easier to stay lean. But you have to eat whole foods, not processed. Before refrigerators and supermarkets, the choices were easy. People ate what they could find or grow in their environments at a particular time. The availability of numerous foods (especially processed foods) throughout most of the year has many people confused about when to eat what. Nevertheless, with the knowledge you now have and a little desire you can be lean no matter where you live.

People who immigrate to the United States often gain quite a bit of weight for three primary reasons. They are exposed to much larger portion sizes when they eat in restaurants and when they buy processed foods, they generally eat more processed foods and fewer whole foods, and they usually walk or ride a bicycle much less than they did in their native countries. Many of them also do less physical activity because they have access to garage door openers, television remote controls, escalators and elevators, leaf blowers, riding lawnmowers, automatic clothes washers and dryers and other labor-saving devices and products.

In the early 1960s only 13 percent of Americans were considered obese compared to today's figure of almost 31 percent. Americans have gotten fatter for the same reasons that so many immigrants gain excess fat—larger portion sizes, eating more processed foods and fewer whole foods, and less physical work due to automation in more jobs and the abundance of labor-saving devices.

At work and home

Our home and work environments are extremely influential because we generally spend most of our time at these two locations. It is easy to eat well at home. Have a meal schedule, keep only good food in the house and do not have junk food delivered. If you have potato chips, soda pop, candy and cookies around, it is not going to just sit there. The members of your household (maybe you) are going to eat it and it is not going to do anything good for them. Always keep your home stocked with a variety of great-tasting, nutritious foods for meals and snacks. This is the easiest place to control how well you and your family eat. Take full advantage of it.

Eating well at work is a problem for many people. If someone works at a fast-food or conventional restaurant, bakery, donut shop or similar place, the sights and smells of unhealthful foods will be a constant temptation. But eating well even in these environments is really not difficult. The key is to eat healthfully before and after work, and to take good foods for lunch and snacks. Just because people work as pharmacists or clerks in drug stores does not mean they have to use drugs. You may work where a snack truck comes two or three times a day and people buy coffee, donuts, soft drinks, potato chips and other fattening foods. There may be vending machines with the same junk foods. It can be a big temptation when you see everyone else eating so often, but there is an easy way around this dilemma. You know these foods are unhealthful and expensive, so all you have to do is have a healthful lunch and snacks with you. Do not feel like you are missing out on something good. The only things you will miss are poor health and excess body fat.

I spent many years working for large corporations and never had a problem taking nutritious meals and snacks with me. Unlike processed foods, my meals needed refrigeration to stay fresh. Some employers had a refrigerator available, but if not, I just took my foods in a small ice chest. I also did this for years while studying to be a doctor. I observed some of the other students spending substantial amounts of money on junk food from the cafeteria. What did they get? Poor health and extra body fat. Are these what you want for your money?

The people in your life

The people you associate with can greatly influence how and what you eat. Is your mother or grandmother always telling you to eat more, because you look so thin? Your ethnic background and religion may be major influences for you. If you travel frequently, you will be eating out often. You already know how to deal with this. If your job involves "wining and dining" clients, you will be eating out more or having them come to your home. Many of your clients will not be used to eating the wholesome, nutritious meals you normally eat. If their taste buds are desensitized from eating salty and processed foods, your meals will taste bland to them. Nevertheless, with some spices and a little imagination you can make many healthful dishes that appeal to your clients' taste buds. Your example may inspire them to eat healthier themselves and no matter how they may tease you, in reality they respect you and your healthy lifestyle. This added respect might even be beneficial for your business relationships. If you are having a business dinner, you may want to pick up some foods for your clients that evening that you do not normally eat. You can eat the healthful foods and let them eat whatever they want of the healthful and unhealthful foods. Give away any unhealthful foods that are left over or store them for future business dinners only.

Some people do a great deal of socializing with friends or belong to clubs, bowling leagues or other groups. Many of these social activities include or revolve around eating. Studies have shown that people eat more when they go out with friends than when they are alone. There seems to be an unconscious contest about who can eat the most. Chances are also higher that dessert will be eaten or that each person will get a different dessert and everyone will eat some of each. When going out to dinner, being aware of the trap people often fall into can save you, if you let it. You can eat before you go to some social events and perhaps take along a small snack. At other times, you may be able to take a healthful meal with you. When others are eating hot dogs and greasy, salty potato chips, you can enjoy a great-tasting healthful meal or snack. As I have already said, you will be teased (and envied), but remember that you can be a positive role model for your friends. Be a leader, not a follower. Even if you are in junior high school, do not let peer pressure dictate your appearance, health and future.

Studies have shown that a woman will eat far less if she eats dinner with a man she is attracted to than if she eats with a male friend. Again, awareness is the operative word for women when eating with a male who is only a friend.

Another part of socializing is eating at other people's homes. I hope some of the friends you associate with eat well or at least understand your lifestyle and will prepare healthful foods for you. You may sometimes socialize with people who eat processed foods and other foods low in nutritional value. If asked, just tell your host you can eat only the healthful foods, because your doctor has you on a special diet for your allergies. Because the unhealthful foods would affect your sinuses and health, and because I am a doctor, your story would be true. Some people, when invited to someone's home for dinner, think it is rude not to eat portions of all the foods being served. I believe, however, that if I eat the healthful foods, it is fine to just say no thanks if offered other foods. If the people you socialize with are offended by your desire to be healthy and stay lean, you should find some different people to share your life with—people who at least respect your lifestyle, if not share it.

When you are out, choose the nutritious foods available or if there are none, take your own food, or eat before you go. Just be prepared. If you have healthful foods with you, there will not be a reason to eat expensive and fattening junk foods. With some good sense, creativity and planning, you can easily maintain your healthy and lean lifestyle wherever you go. Even all day at the amusement park or zoo can be easily dealt with by taking some water and a few healthful snacks along. Take some apples, bananas, grapes, figs, dates, prunes, raisins or other dried fruits. Nuts and seeds contain protein and fat, which satisfies your hunger for a long time. Dried figs, dates and raisins combine well with nuts and seeds. Be prepared when you go shopping. You know it always takes longer than planned and few foods available at the mall will help you stay lean and healthy. When you go to a movie prior to dinner, take along some water and a bag of grapes, apple slices or other fruit. It would be best not to eat anything during a movie after dinner, although a bag of plain popcorn may be all right if your body handles corn effectively. If you go to a matinee, you can eat more substantial snacks like seeds or nuts.

Do not forget about the money-saving side of this healthy habit. For example, if you go to a movie once a week and spend six dollars on buttered and salted popcorn, soft drinks and candies, you are spending about three hundred dollars each year. That would buy a new television, camera, stereo system or some new clothes. Wouldn't having one of those presents be better than having excess body fat?

Your internal programming

Your internal programming creates most of your self-talk—your thoughts and ideas. If people are in tune with their inner spirits, some self-talk comes from the truth within. This is the angel on one shoulder you may have seen in cartoons. Unfortunately, for most of us, our false worldly programming does most of the talking and talks much louder, this being the cartoon devil on your other shoulder. This internal environment is always with you and controls how you act or react. Your self-talk has the greatest influence on you and your life. To achieve permanent fat loss, you must get rid of your false programming and feelings about food, eating and yourself. Do not let advertising agencies control your thinking and your life. I will soon be explaining more about false programming and various ways to eliminate it. You will also be taught how to live in the moment and develop the awareness necessary to hear the wisdom of your true inner spirit—thoughts of unconditional love that will keep you lean, healthy and happy.

An Excess of One Type of Food

People can get fat from eating an excess of certain foods. Theoretically, the fat vegetarians I have counseled should have been lean. The two major reasons they were not were the excess of dairy products and processed "whole" wheat they ate. Look around a health-food store and you will see what many people think are healthful foods. Things like whole-wheat cookies, whole-wheat crackers, whole-wheat bread, whole-wheat flour and whole-wheat pasta. You will see numerous products made from whole wheat, corn and other processed grains. Those who do not understand what good nutrition is think these are nutritious foods. The truth is, most of the foods found in health-food stores will not build health or keep you lean. The processed convenience foods are the main offenders. They start as a better (organic) food initially and sometimes have less done to them, but the processing still destroys the balance and most of the nutritional value.

Let me explain why an excess of certain foods can be a problem. Your body can use only a certain amount of something at one time. Once your body reaches the limit of what it needs of a particular nutrient, it has to do something with the extra. Sometimes it can be eliminated, but it is often stored as fat or internal waste. Excessive amounts of one food can also create an overload in your system, causing you to develop sensitivity (an allergy) to it. And if you are bombarding your body with the nutrients from one particular food, chances are it is being starved for the different nutrients other foods contain. It would be difficult to create an allergy or internal imbalance by eating an excess of lettuce or apples, but meat, milk and grain products can easily create problems, because they are all concentrated foods. Most fat people have overdosed on those three.

Years ago one of my nutritional clients was sneezing and coughing throughout his entire consultation. He told me that he had hay fever. I asked him if he ate many whole-wheat products. He answered that he did, because he was attempting to eat healthfully. I suggested that he avoid wheat products for three months and gave him some ideas about what to eat instead. I told him that after his body cleansed out the excess processed wheat that he may be able to eat *whole* wheat occasionally without any negative effects. He would need to be tested by me or experiment on his own to see if this would be possible. Two weeks later I saw him at the gym and asked how his hay fever was doing. He said it was completely gone. His hay fever was actually a wheat allergy that had been created by overconsumption.

You have been taught to cycle your meats and grains and to avoid dairy products and processed flour products. If processed grains and dairy products were eliminated from the American people's diet, billions of pounds would soon be lost. Of course, this is not going to happen, but it can happen on a smaller scale for you. These products are the two worst offenders when it comes to gaining excess fat and causing colds, allergies and many other health problems. If you have been eating an excess of a particular meat or grain, eliminate using it for one to three months. You may be able to eat it again, just less often. Eating a wide variety of whole foods is an easy way to avoid excesses and the imbalances they create.

Food Allergies

I have briefly discussed food allergies, but because they are so common I want to give you more information about them. If you read the label of most nutritional supplements, you will see something like, "Contains no corn, soy, yeast, rice, wheat, barley, lactose, and all milk, citrus, fish and egg products." These products are listed because they are common causes of allergic reactions. Many people are allergic to at least one of them and fat people are usually allergic to quite a few. Be aware that products with other names could be derived from these common allergens. For example, sorbitol is a sweetener that is obtained from corn.

You now know that some people are allergic to certain foods because they have overloaded their systems with excessive amounts, and that this is easily resolved by avoiding the food for a while and giving the body time to restore balance. After that, the food can usually be eaten again in moderation without any problems developing. Some allergic reactions occur because the food is incomplete and the person's body is unable to use the part of the food being eaten because the other parts are missing. This problem is easily resolved by eating whole foods.

I believe allergies can be created if people eat certain concentrated foods before their bodies have developed the ability to properly digest them. You have learned that this can happen to babies who are fed grain products before they are six months old. Sometimes even the whole food may have to be avoided permanently. Casein seems to cause certain forms of allergies in infants and children. It may also cause autoimmune reactions.

Processed foods almost always contain artificial colorings, artificial flavorings and other chemicals that are sometimes the true allergen. Once again, this problem is resolved by eating whole foods. Numerous foods (spoiled fruits or vegetables, grains, nuts) can be moldy or contain other toxins that may cause allergic reactions. Avoid spoiled foods and add a quarter teaspoon of vitamin C powder to nut butters and grains to detoxify any mold and make the food safer to eat. Fat people tend to have more allergies, because excess fat and internal waste decreases the body's ability to use foods normally or eliminate excesses.

The alcohol in wine and other drinks increases your chance of developing food allergies. Wine may contain molds and yeasts that trigger allergic reactions. Most wines contain sulfites that can cause uncomfortable symptoms, especially for asthmatics, and particularly red wine contains histamine, the main chemical responsible for the symptoms of allergies. Wine also contains the chemical tyramine, which has effects in the body similar to caffeine.

Many behavioral, psychological and neurological symptoms are caused by food allergies. Those with the most documentation affect the gastrointestinal tract, respiratory tract or skin. Because the symptoms are often caused by your body's attempt to rid itself of the allergen, these three make sense, because they are all avenues of elimination. It is easy to see how numerous other symptoms can be caused by the systemic disruptions and imbalances created by an allergic reaction. Some of the most common confirmed symptoms are abdominal pain, asthma, diarrhea, dermatitis, urticaria (hives), vomiting, itching, rash, malabsorption, and rhinitis (inflammation of the nose). Other possible manifestations of food allergies include arthritis, arthralgia (joint pain), canker sores, colic, deafness, epilepsy, fever, menstrual irregularity, migraine headache, neuralgia (nerve pain), vertigo, personality changes, cheilitis (inflammation and cracking of the lips), incontinence, ear ache, and amblyopia (dimness of vision). I believe that allergies are the cause of many other diseases that medical science currently labels as "cause unknown."

Can an allergy make you fat? It most certainly can. Besides eliminating an allergen, your body can store it as fat to get it out of your bloodstream. And, because allergies almost always affect the gastrointestinal tract, the digestion and absorption of various nutrients will be adversely affected. Many people with "mental" conditions express their problems when they eat a food they are allergic to and some allergic reactions are either caused or intensified by hypoglycemia. The "mental" condition and hypoglycemia can both lead to overeating and poor food choices.

Some people become addicted to the food they are allergic to and end up eating an excess of the very thing causing their problems. Food addiction is like drug addiction. Food addicts experience unpleasant withdrawal symptoms when their bodies start cleansing out the stored residue of the food. They learn that the uncomfortable symptoms stop if they eat more of the food. This occurs because the food "fix" forces the residue back into the cells and stops the cleansing process. Now, however, even more residue gets stored and this accelerates the negative cycle by causing the body to start cleansing itself in ever-shortening intervals. The food addict eats more chocolate, sugar, bread, milk or whatever the culprit is. This is what happens to alcoholics, cigarette smokers or other drug users. They have to use the drug more and more frequently to prevent the withdrawal symptoms.

If the second vertebra of the neck is out of alignment (which it commonly is), the nerve pressure it causes can make the sinuses hypersensitive to pollens and other allergens in the air, but may also be a component of food allergies. A misalignment of the ninth thoracic vertebra affects the nerves to and from the adrenal glands and this vertebra is the one associated with causing food allergies. Other vertebrae may be misaligned, affecting normal nerve flow to the stomach, liver, intestines, pancreas and other organs. This can cause abnormal function of the digestive system and make someone susceptible to numerous food allergies. Remember that low hydrochloric acid production can cause numerous allergies, especially to complete protein foods. This is one of the first things to check for if you seem to be allergic to many foods. Inadequate amounts of digestive enzymes can cause similar problems. Restoring normal nerve flow to the stomach and other digestive organs may correct the problem or supplementation with betaine hydrochloride or digestive enzymes may be necessary.

Various tests for food allergies exist. The two I prefer are electroacupuncture and applied kinesiology. Both are fast and based on direct biofeedback from the body. After one of these tests, or if you just suspect a certain food, stop eating the food for at least fourteen days. After that time, eat a moderate portion of only the suspect food so no other foods or additives can interfere with the test, and see what reaction you get. After you determine an allergen, stop eating it for two to three months. Cleansing the body helps rid you of the residue of the allergen faster, but the withdrawal symptoms will be more intense. The physical reaction to that food may not happen again once its residue has been eliminated. You may be able to occasionally eat the food again without problems. The best thing to do is to get retested to see if your body is still sensitive to it. I think you will be pleasantly surprised at how good you feel after you cleanse your body of wheat, dairy, yeast and other products to which you are allergic. Be aware that there is often an emotional addiction to certain foods that can lead you right back into the physical reaction/addiction cycle if it is not also eliminated.

I rarely eat whole wheat, because mankind has modified it to contain more gluten. This was done so that numerous products can be made from the flour, because it is the gluten that makes the products stick together (like glue) instead of crumble. Try baking a loaf of bread with only rye flour and see what happens. Billions of baked goods are made (and consumed) from this processed wheat flour every day. I believe that eating an excess of gluten is the reason so many people are sensitive to it. This is another example of why refined flour products are not good for you.

Besides allergy problems, someone may experience intolerance to certain foods. Various chemicals, contaminants, gastrointestinal difficulties, unnatural foods, enzyme deficiencies or psychological influences can cause this. Food intolerance can cause abdominal pain, diarrhea, flatulence, dizziness, increased or decreased blood pressure, asthma, hives and headaches. These are similar to allergy symptoms and why lactose intolerance can easily be confused with cow's milk protein allergy. Certain toxins can cause severe symptoms and even death.

Some "health" drinks and nutritional supplements contain a large number of ingredients that are supposed to give you energy or have other positive effects. Sometimes these products are fine, but if you have an allergy or intolerance to just one of the ingredients, you will have problems. This is why it is important to keep your meals simple and to be tested for need and sensitivity before using nutritional supplements.

Loss of Lean Body Mass

You already know some of the negative effects of losing lean body mass but here are more. Have you ever heard a man say "I'm fifty years old and I weigh the same as I did in college"? Because of this he may believe he is almost as healthy at age fifty as he was at age twenty. Most of the time, this is untrue. He may weigh the same but chances are his fat-to-lean ratio has changed drastically. In college he may have had 15 percent body fat and now it is 28 percent. This is a dramatic change and a good example of why your weight is not an accurate indicator of your health.

Most people lose muscle tissue and gain fat as they age. As lean body mass decreases, their metabolisms slow down, making it easier to gain fat. People with fast metabolisms eat anything and everything in an attempt to maintain their "normal" weights. Even for them, as muscle is lost, fat is gained. For these people, however, the fat gain is difficult to detect, because they may not look fat and are able to pinch about the same amount of fat they always have. So where is the extra fat going? It is accumulating inside the muscles like the fat you see marbled throughout a steak. This is why the charts used with fat calipers list a higher percentage of body fat if you are older even if the same amount is measured subcutaneously (under the skin).

Why does the average adult lose five to seven pounds of lean body mass every decade? It is simply the lack of regular strength-building (or maintaining) exercise. Hormone production does gradually decrease, limiting the amount of muscle you can maintain, but correct exercise stimulates hormone production—testosterone and growth hormone primarily. You know that these both have anti-aging effects and that testosterone levels affect sexual drive and performance. Time marches on, but regardless of the inevitable, a great deal of muscle size and strength can be maintained into advanced age. This is why it is extremely important to consistently exercise intensely enough to at least maintain your muscle strength and size.

I have talked with many people who believe all they have to do is walk, go bowling, play golf or do other similar activities to stay healthy and strong as they age. Nothing could be further from the truth. These types of activities are not intense enough to maintain normal muscle (or bone) strength and mass. Many people even lose the strength to walk normally, because they spend most of their days sitting and never do anything to strengthen the muscles used for walking. Look at the average older man and you will see that his gluteus maximus muscles (the ones you sit on) have atrophied (gotten smaller) due to lack of use. It is less noticeable in older women because of the excess fat normally stored in that area but it also happens to most of them. The gluteus maximus muscles are the largest and strongest muscles in the entire body but ironically (and sadly) the first ones to shrivel up from lack of use.

They are the most important muscles to keep strong, because they are the foundation of your physical and sexual powers. Lack of strength is why you see more and more people using walkers, canes and other supports just to walk. Sometimes joint or balance problems are involved, but many of them are simply too weak to hold themselves up or take a normal stride. If these people were put on an *effective* exercise routine (and good nutrition, of course), within three to six weeks most of them could throw away their canes and walkers for the rest of their lives.

The benefits of regular exercise to build or maintain strength and muscle size are numerous. First of all, barring injuries, you should be able to do most of the things when you are sixty or seventy that you did when you were twenty if you have the same strength as you did then. If you keep your buttock, thigh and leg muscles strong, fluids will not pool in your ankles and feet causing edema, and the veins in your legs will not distort and become varicose. Your heart will have less stress, because the lower body muscles act like pumping stations to squeeze blood back up to the heart. These problems may occur if you have abnormal nerve flow to your lower extremities, but stronger muscles usually help. Maintaining your lean body mass reduces cellulite and keeps your skin tighter and your body more attractive. Exercising for strength (and endurance) improves circulation and can stimulate the creation of more blood vessels. This helps your body get the nutrients and oxygen necessary for good health.

Maintaining normal lean body mass is simple if you know how to exercise correctly. When I was attending chiropractic school, I maintained my physique and perhaps even built more muscle tissue while exercising for only 60 to 90 minutes twice a week. The key was knowing how to get maximum results from the time spent. Countless people have given up on strength training because they got little, if any, results. Because their training was inefficient or the program being used was ineffective for accomplishing their goals, they got discouraged and quit when nothing happened. I am currently in the process of writing a book about how to exercise safely to get maximum results in a minimum amount of time.

For more than thirty years, I have observed people using unsafe exercise form, doing exercises that will do nothing to help them reach their goals, or exercising so inefficiently it is almost a total waste of time. Many of the exercises that people commonly do actually hinder their progress instead of helping it. Anyone can "lift weights" for years and accomplish nothing. I have observed the training sessions of many professional bodybuilders and the majority of them used inefficient and often unsafe exercise techniques. Most of them achieve incredible (but unnatural) results because of growth-enhancing drugs, not correct training methods.

If you want to get lean and healthy and stay that way, an exercise program to strengthen and tone your skeletal muscles is essential. This can be done with exercises that use your body weight (push-ups, pull-ups and others) but this is inefficient and the results are quite limited. It is far more productive to use exercise machines and free weights, because the resistance can be adjusted in small increments to be less or more than your body weight. How to build strength and lean body mass is explained in chapter fifteen.

Do not use the excuses that you are too old to exercise or it is just not your "thing." First of all, the older you are, the more important it is. Second, you are never too old to start exercising and building strength. (A hundred year-old woman could experience noticeable changes in just a few weeks.) Third, anyone who wants to be as healthy, active and attractive as possible must exercise regularly. There are no exceptions. Finally, our bodies were designed for physical activity, so exercise is everyone's "thing."

Hormones

Hormones are extremely powerful chemicals that are tremendously difficult, if not impossible, to fight against. If you are a woman who has ever experienced premenstrual syndrome (PMS), you know what I am talking about. The pancreas and adrenal glands secrete hormones that control blood sugar levels. You already know the numerous negative effects hypoglycemia can have on how you feel physically and emotionally and what a strong eating stimulus this can be. Therefore, the proper function of these glands is crucial. Inadequate amounts of thyroid hormones (primarily thyroxine) can also lead to hypoglycemia and a lower metabolic rate.

The hormones testosterone, thyroxine and growth hormone increase protein synthesis and stimulate fat burning. Strength training stimulates the production and release of these hormones that are so helpful for getting and staying lean. Other hormones are produced that cause the release of these hormones. Some hormones appear to signal us to stop eating and others may make us eat less. Epinephrine and other adrenal hormones increase the release of fat from fat cells. Therefore, it is important to have normal levels of all hormones if we are going to be lean and healthy. Hormonal effects may also come from endorphins and other substances. Proper nerve and blood flow to the glands and organs that produce hormones is important, as is providing the precursor nutrients. I believe that an adequate amount of balanced light is also vital to the proper function of the endocrine glands and for normal hormone production.

Hormones are made from proteins, peptides (two or more linked amino acids), cholesterol or the amino acid tyrosine. Enzymes and other nutrients are needed for hormone production and use. If you fail to supply your body with the raw materials to make the hormones, you will not have enough produced to get or stay lean. Your thyroid gland may be functioning perfectly, but without enough iodine it will be unable to produce the amount of thyroxine necessary for normal metabolism.

Fat people generally have an imbalance of hormones, because they are malnourished and because fat cells produce estrogen. The excess estrogen may create an increased need for certain nutrients and cause overeating in an attempt to get them. Have you ever seen a man or boy with breasts? I am sure you have, because 12 percent of breast reduction surgeries are performed on men. Male breasts are partially caused by excess fat but the breast tissue itself is often stimulated to grow by the estrogen the fat cells produce. An excess of estrogen will also decrease your sexual desire and function, whether you are male or female.

Why do women often crave sugar, processed carbohydrates and fats during menstruation? I believe it is due to their bodies asking for the nutrients necessary to make the hormones and other chemicals that they need. Why do women get PMS? Often simply because they are lacking certain nutrients their bodies need at that time. The wife of one of my patients was obviously lacking in certain nutrients, because after she started taking the Super Spectrim multivitamin and mineral supplement she no longer got PMS. Why do many women gain fat as they go through menopause? Most likely because they no longer have the same balance of hormones that used to keep them leaner. I believe that this problem, like osteoporosis, can be prevented with proper nutrition and strength-building exercise.

Pregnancy

Many women gain excess fat during pregnancy. They often say that they are eating for two. The question is, "How much food does a one or two pound baby need?" Certainly not the same as an adult but some women seem to think they need to eat that much. Their bodies do need some additional energy during pregnancy, but the main concern should be on supplying good nutrition to the mother and the growing baby. The total weight gained during pregnancy should be between 20 and 25 pounds. If you eat well during pregnancy, you should gain hardly any fat and be back to your pre-pregnancy weight soon after the baby arrives.

One of my patients had a child when she was fifty-six years old. Six months into her pregnancy, she had gained only five pounds. She had an obstetrician and a high-risk pregnancy doctor. They both were worried that she had not gained enough weight, but neither one bothered to ask what she was eating. One of them told her to go home and eat some cheesecake. (Not a "food" I would recommend for mother or baby.) She had begun to follow my nutritional program and was losing excess fat while gaining for the baby. She and the baby were getting all the vital nutrients needed for excellent health. She had no morning sickness, no back pain and continued working more than 40 hours a week until she had a healthy baby girl. She gained only 14 pounds during the pregnancy, but lost almost 20 pounds within a few days of having the baby. This same patient gave birth to twin boys about thirteen months later when she was within a few months of her fifty-eighth birthday. We believe she may be the oldest woman to do this. She gained only 29 pounds with the twins and lost all of it within five days of giving birth. She then lost 20 more pounds in the next two months.

You now have at least a basic understanding of numerous physical causes for having excess fat. If you have excess fat to lose and your cause is primarily physical, chances are that it was discussed in this chapter and you now know what you may be dealing with and can get tested for the condition and properly treated. If the root cause of your excess fat is not physical, you will most likely find your cause among the emotional causes you will learn about in the next chapter.

twelve

Now you are going to learn about the most common emotional causes of excess fat. They are all usually made worse by overeating, because it causes more fat gain and increased feelings of hopelessness and lack of control. As you already know, physical and emotional causes create and amplify each other so everything gets worse as one negatively influences the other. Many people lose the desire to do anything about their excess body fat and feel more helpless and hopeless as they spiral downward emotionally and physically. This creates lower self-esteem, deeper depression, other destructive emotions and leads to more overeating and less interest in exercise and other activities that would help them. It is understandable why people get discouraged when they are doing all they know how to do and it is not working. The key in this, or similar situations, is to learn what does work. My hope for you is that you will soon learn and then find a reason to apply what works for you.

Emotional Causes of Excess Fat

Read the upcoming emotional causes carefully. If you are extremely honest with yourself, you should be able to determine which ones may be affecting you. Eliminating these destructive emotional patterns can improve your relationships, career, other areas of your life, and lead to more happiness and fulfillment. Even if you have a healthy body fat percentage, chances are your life will dramatically improve by eliminating certain problems or learning to deal with them in positive ways. As you read the upcoming causes, keep in mind that many of them overlap and cause a negative cycle as they feed on each other. Also, be aware that many of these different causes may be affecting you to some degree. Most people with excess body fat will find their primary or secondary causes in this chapter. If you do not, you will learn ways to discover your unique and uncommon causes.

Low Self-Worth

Feeling unworthy may be the most common reason why people have excess fat and is a part of all emotional causes. Most, if not all, of our problems stem from not feeling good enough. We are often programmed to believe that we are not good enough and never will be no matter what we do. These feelings send out vibrations that attract what we feel we deserve. Some people may starve themselves to death because they do not believe they are thin enough. Other people may be workaholics and misers if they do not feel they are rich enough. They may live lonely, unhappy lives and die with millions of dollars that did nothing good for them or anyone else. The absolute truth is—*you have always been, are now, and always will be good enough just as you are.*

If you do not feel worthy of the healthier and better-looking body that comes with losing excess fat, you will not do what it takes to have it. You will create and maintain the excess fat with your own subconscious thinking, and sabotage any efforts you make to lose it. You may also create illness, poverty or other hardships for yourself.

The secret to increasing your self-worth is to learn to love yourself. This is the topic of another entire book I have planned, but I will explain it briefly here.

Before you can learn to love yourself, you must first understand what real love is and that loving yourself is completely different from liking yourself. Love is simply accepting yourself 100 percent unconditionally as you are right now with no desire whatsoever to change yourself. This is true divine love that never has conditions or strings attached.

Loving yourself is easy and natural once you start to realize who you really are. As you eliminate your false programming, labels and phony facades, you will realize it is your true nature to completely accept yourself. Like a mother loving her newborn infant, no effort is necessary. An excellent way to see your true self in action is to do selfless service for others. It helps you to see what a beautiful being you truly are.

You are a beautiful spiritual being, not a collection of your past thoughts and actions. A bullterrier (pit bull) may be born with a particular inborn nature but can be conditioned to be a vicious attack dog or a gentle and playful pet. The inborn nature of human beings is to love. Some people are able to express much love in their lives but others have been conditioned to cheat, steal and even kill. These harmful actions do not come from the true self, but from false programming and conditioning.

Loving yourself has nothing to do with liking who you think you are—your false self. You can love yourself 100 percent unconditionally yet dislike everything you have ever done, every thought you have ever had, everything you have ever wanted to do but didn't, and everything about your body, occupation and life circumstances. You may hate everything about yourself and your entire life. It doesn't matter. Once you start loving yourself, however, you will notice that you have freed yourself to change your life. You do not have to change anything, but when you truly love yourself, you just naturally start changing the things about your false self that you dislike. It will be easy to see yourself as others do and develop clear courses of action to eliminate your unwanted behaviors. The changes happen easily and naturally because you are moving toward expressing the real you. No pressure exists, no one is forcing you and no parental programming is pushing you to change. A positive cycle is created when your physical body and mind start expressing your true inner self more accurately as each bit of worldly programming is stripped away. You will realize that you are a beautiful, loving being who deserves better than what you have given yourself up to this point. You will start creating the life you now feel you deserve—the one you truly do deserve. The only way to create this new life full of health, happiness and satisfaction is to change your programmed thoughts and actions. One by one, the habits, thinking patterns and behaviors you dislike will be eliminated. Soon you will not only love yourself, but truly like who you are as well. This will increase your feeling of self-worth, improve your self-image and give you the reason to purge the conditioned thinking that has been keeping you trapped in a fat body.

Another positive result of loving yourself is the elimination of judgments that create labels. You are a beautiful, loving being with tremendous potential for change and creative expression. Labels limit or stop your actions and progress. Some of the labels fat people burden themselves with are heavy, plump, chubby, overweight, obese, big, heavyset, beefy, pudgy, big-boned, stout, portly, full-figured, chunky, stocky and ugly. Your fat labels will soon be gone if you love yourself. Another label you must get rid of is the one that defines you as unworthy to live a happy and healthy life. Forgiving your parents and yourself for creating this belief helps eliminate it. As your self-image improves, you will see being fat as unhealthy and disabling not jolly or prosperous. You will also realize that your body is fat, not the real you. You are a spiritual being who was given a vehicle that allows you to function in a physical world. You were also given a great deal of power over your vehicle.

Let's say that you are given a car for your twenty-first birthday and it is up to you to take care of it. You can dent it, abuse it, ignore necessary upkeep and it will look terrible and run badly within six months. On the other hand, you can keep it clean inside and out by washing it, and running well by using clean-burning fuel and giving it regular tune-ups and maintenance. Do this and your car will serve you well and look great for many years. Your body is essentially fully developed by age twenty-one but then starts to deteriorate if not given regular maintenance (exercise) and good fuel (nutrition). Take care of the vehicle you call your body and it will look great for many years and serve you well on the journey called life. Its care is entirely up to you.

Some people get fat after they get out of college. This occurs primarily because they are not learning much so their brains use less energy, their bodies have finished their natural growth and they are usually less physically active. Of course, others get fat during college if they eat mostly junk food, drink alcohol and eat to reduce the stress of school.

If you are a parent and you feed your children well and are a good example for them, when they are twenty-one, chances are they will have strong, healthy bodies. That is like giving each of them a brand new car for graduation. If your children grow up eating mostly fast food and processed junk foods, their bodies will not be able to build a healthy vehicle for them. This is like giving them each an old, rundown car for graduation. Make the choice to take care of your own vehicle and to help your children build a strong and healthy one to get them started in life. Also teach them how to keep it that way.

If you feel unworthy of being loved, you may sabotage a healthy, loving relationship. You may use alcohol, drugs or excess fat to drive the other person away. This destroys a valuable source of soul food and creates a negative cycle of lower self-worth, self-destructive behaviors and perhaps the loss of other healthy relationships. It also reduces your opportunities to do loving things that will help you to discover the beautiful being that you are.

When you stop judging yourself as bad, weak-willed, fat, ugly, or whatever you believe yourself to be, you become free to see and express more of your true self. When you stop blocking what you truly deserve, the truth within you can create more of the love, health and happiness your heart desires. If you look in the mirror and notice your hair is longer than you want it to be, you get a haircut. If you look in the mirror and see excess fat you no longer feel you deserve, you simply eat healthier and exercise regularly. The excess fat will soon be gone and will stay gone forever, because you have eliminated the reason it was created in the first place. If the cause stays gone, so will the excess fat.

Think about it for a moment. You are essentially the same person you were as a child, teenager or middle-aged and you will be the same when you are older. Your body is different and you have had numerous experiences but it is the same "you" inside. As you continue to love yourself and get more in touch with who you are, your behaviors will change for the better and there will be more reasons to like who you are. As your self-image and self-worth improve, losing body fat or staying lean will get easier and feel, as it should, completely natural. You will also enjoy positive changes in other areas of your life as you create more of the good things you feel you deserve.

An exercise that may help you to decide what behaviors you want to change is to write down what people who know you would say about you at your funeral if it was held today. Then write down what you would like them to say and how you would like to be remembered. This can help you to become the person you want to be.

Some people feel unworthy if they are not doing something they believe is "great" to change the world. This is an unhealthy judgment that can depress you and prevent you from doing anything good for anyone. You are a unique person and have a purpose for being here. If you did not, I do not think you would be here. I also believe that if you love yourself, you will be guided to use your special talents in the best possible way. Your job is to be happy, and if you do this, you may significantly influence the lives of thousands of people and will brighten a few moments of a day for millions. If you do nothing more than give others a smile, a friendly hello and an honest compliment, you may leave a legacy greater than any king or celebrity. Always remember how special you are and what joy and goodness you can bring to your own life and the lives of others. Also remember that happiness will *never* be found in drugs, alcohol, junk food or excessive eating.

Role Models

Who you think you are or who you think you want to be often comes from past or present role models. You may gain excess fat in an attempt to be more like an important role model. You must realize that emulating that person or their achievements comes from within. Your thoughts, feelings and behaviors are what count, not if your body is fat.

Here is an example to help make this role model idea more clear. Let's say you want to be a good mother and that all the women you felt were "good" mothers are fat. You may have known some thin women you believed were bad mothers. You have created the false belief that in order to be a good mother you must be fat. You need to stop for a moment and consider the basis of your belief. It should not be difficult to understand that being fat has nothing to do with being a good mother. If you are constantly baking (and eating) cakes, pies and cookies for your family to eat, is that a good thing? Do you think that you being obese may be an embarrassment to your children? Is dying fifteen to twenty years before your time a good thing for your children and grandchildren? On the contrary, if you are a lean and healthy role model and feed your children nutritious meals so they do not get fat, you can be a better mother than the fat ones you admire.

Remember that you may be the most influential role model your child will ever have. If a child's parents are fat, the child's mind sees this as normal and not something to avoid. If children never see their parents exercise or eat well, what training do they have to exercise and eat well? Your children learn your thinking and behavioral patterns toward food—patterns they will most likely pass on to your grandchildren. Would you rather see your children and grandchildren fat and unhealthy or lean and healthy? The things your children see you do for yourself have a tremendous influence on them. Being fat is a great disservice to your children and anyone else who sees you as a role model. You may be condemning your children and others to a lifetime of being fat.

If you want to be a jolly, happy-go-lucky person and you equate it with being fat, this idea may be causing you to maintain your fat. You may believe that if you lose the fat, you will also lose your happy-go-lucky attitude. You will not become mean if you get lean. In reality you will have much more to be happy about. Do you think Santa Claus would stop saying "Ho, Ho, Ho" and become a miserly old man if he lost some of his excess body fat? Some fat people may seem jolly on the outside, but if you get to know them, you will find that they are often depressed, have a low self-image and feel helpless because of their excess fat.

Take some time now—right now—to write down who you think you are. You may be a woman, daughter, granddaughter, wife, mother, brain surgeon, great cook, animal lover, and so forth. We all play many roles but are actually much more than the total of them all. Next, write down the names of your past and present role models and what you admire about them. Now, read your lists and consider this—are any of the images of who you think you are or any of your role models fat? If so, you need to do some serious thinking about the influence this is having on you.

Advertisers know the power of role models. Why do you think they pay millions of dollars to celebrities and famous athletes to endorse their products? They use lean people to sell foods that will make you fat, because you would not buy it if a fat person advertised it. Doesn't that seem a bit deceptive? Children are the most easily influenced, so if you have children, you need to help them realize that the sports superstars do not eat candy bars all the time, if ever, or at the fast-food franchise on a regular basis. They would not be superstars for long if they did.

To eliminate this cause you must admit that your role model was less than perfect or did not have all the answers—at least about being lean and healthy. You must realize that your role models are humans who make mistakes, have limited knowledge of eating well or have physical and emotional reasons for being fat. This is difficult for some people to do but your new knowledge should make it easy. Do not condemn and punish yourself for choosing some fat role models. Reevaluate these people based on the spiritual beings they are, not the appearance of their bodies. Their positive actions are what you want to learn from and emulate. Doing similar positive works in the world or even surpassing their accomplishments is a great way to honor them or their memories.

Think about your friends and the other people who know you and look up to you and your accomplishments. What good would you do for others by losing your excess fat and keeping it off? You may be instrumental in helping other people lose their excess body fat. Your success may even inspire one of your role models to get leaner and healthier. Tell others about this book so they can learn how to do it, but most important of all, prove to yourself and others that it can be done. Being a good example is an excellent way to help others and that, in turn, helps you to know and love more of the person you really are. This is another one of the many positive cycles you can create to improve your life.

Punishment

Some people get fat to punish themselves for past or current actions, thoughts or lack of action. They feel guilt, shame, anger and other negative emotions created by self-judgment. These feelings usually lead to more and harsher self-judgment, lowered sense of self-worth and a greater need to punish themselves. The punishment creates something new to judge, creating a negative cycle of judgment and punishment that is extremely detrimental to the self-image and sense of self-worth. By loving yourself, you can create a positive cycle to replace this negative one.

We are not qualified, nor meant, to judge anyone. When we judge ourselves, we create negative emotions that are destructive to our lives and the lives of others. You may have learned that we are usually most critical of ourselves. When friends do something we consider "bad," we can usually find excuses for them and then forgive them. Sadly, it is rare if we can find the same excuses and forgive ourselves for doing the same thing. When we are judgmental, we become our own judge, jury and executioner. The most common punishments we impose are poverty, poor health, loneliness and a lack of joy and love. Being fat and less attractive is part of most of these punishments, especially poor health.

Ironically, the form of punishment we usually choose is the part of life most important to us. If financial success is your greatest goal, chances are that you will punish yourself by creating poverty, business failures or financial hardships. I believe that many people choose poor health as their punishment. They know that an easy way to create health problems is to gain excess fat and they often continue to gain until they get what they feel they deserve. If being loved is what you want the most, being fat can decrease your attractiveness and your chance of experiencing it. Being fat can also make you depressed to the point where nothing (even being loved) brings you any happiness. You may punish yourself with excess fat if you are angry at or disappointed in yourself for not yet accomplishing certain goals. This problem often worsens with age. Let your true self choose your goals, not your worldly programmed ego. Understand and be content with the success your spirit creates for you, because it (the real you) knows what will make you truly happy. Remember that just because a goal has not been reached does not mean it never will be.

I once saw a television program about some former prostitutes who lived at a halfway house. The kind woman who ran it was helping these women start new lives. I was not surprised, however, to see that they were all extremely fat. They were not fat before, so they must have gotten fat for psychological reasons. Perhaps it was punishment for what they had previously done or a protective mechanism to keep them from returning to their previous occupation. It may have been because they saw the woman who was helping them as a role model. You may have already guessed that she was fat.

I know someone who used to cut and burn her skin when she was a young girl. When she was a teenager she stopped the self-mutilation, but became addicted to illegal drugs. In her early twenties she stopped using drugs and then she became obese. It is easy to see that she was just using different ways to punish herself. By being fat, she can punish herself without others knowing and without losing her job. She told me that she knew what she was doing and had no intention of improving her diet in any way. She will stay fat until she eliminates her reason to punish herself or starts using an alternative form.

You may have gained excess fat in an attempt to punish other people—perhaps your parents. If what you do never seems good enough for them, you may get fat if you think it will embarrass them or prove to them that they are right. You must realize that your life belongs to you, not your parents. Love yourself and live from your own spirit and chances are your relationship with your parents will be much more gratifying and harmonious for all of you. If you are unhappy with your significant other, you may get fat to make yourself less attractive or perhaps even to get the person to leave you. This will punish you and perhaps your mate as well. Unfortunately, getting fat usually backfires and creates more problems between you. Resolve your conflicts in positive ways so you can achieve your goal of a lean and attractive body and perhaps save a loving and satisfying relationship. Think about how your being fat may possibly be affecting the other people in your life but remember that whatever your reason for being fat is, it has its greatest negative impact on you. If punishing yourself or someone else is your reason for being fat, make sure you eliminate the true cause. Do not just replace being fat with another form of punishment.

Excuse

Being fat can be a powerful excuse to avoid doing something. For example, if you have a fear of developing an intimate relationship, a fat and less attractive body creates a great excuse to avoid opportunities for intimacy. It gives your friends and family a reason why you are not in a loving relationship. You must understand that you have the choice, fat or lean, of having a relationship or not.

If you are an attractive woman who does not want an intimate relationship, gaining excess fat will stop many men from asking you out. It reduces or eliminates your need to constantly say no. This is a welcome relief if saying no is uncomfortable for you, as it is for most of us. Better ways to deal with the situation are to either avoid locations where men would see you or to learn how to say no with grace and charm. You could wear a wedding band or tell them you already have a boyfriend. This would at least deter the gentlemen.

Sometimes people get fat to avoid doing a physical activity they do not want to do. This often occurs when people are afraid of losing something if they fail to live up to another person's expectations. For example, a father may want his son to become a professional baseball player. If the son lacks the talent or does not share that goal, it puts him in a stressful predicament. He is afraid if he works hard to be a great baseball player but fails, that he will lose his father's love. He has the same fear if he does not attempt it at all. Getting fat gives him an excuse to not play. This lets him off the hook and gives him hope that he will not lose his father's love.

Of course, the son should simply explain to his father that he does not believe he can be successful at it or that he does not want to play professional baseball. He should express that he wants to make his father proud of him by excelling at something he does have a high aptitude for and a strong interest in pursuing. Sadly, not many young people are able to say this to one of their parents. Because children always want to please them, it is the parents' responsibility to avoid putting these kinds of demands and pressures on their children. It may be the parent's idea of a wonderful life but the child may have no interest. Parents should not attempt to live their own dreams vicariously through their children. They must accept them as they are and let their children find their own paths and live their own lives.

A child may want to become a tennis professional and make her parents proud, but if she is afraid of failing, she may create a fat body as the excuse to not even attempt to reach that goal. The love (total acceptance) of their parents is the most important thing children want while growing up *and* throughout life. Children will do almost anything to prevent losing it. A parent's love has extreme value, because it is usually unconditional. This is the love we all constantly seek and the kind we must get from ourselves if we are to enjoy happiness and peace of mind. It must come from you, because you are the only one who will always be with you.

If a woman does not want to have sex with her partner, getting fat may reduce the frequency that they have sex. Being fat can give her the excuse that she is too tired or provide an excuse for her partner because she is less attractive and sexually stimulating. What if a woman's partner is not having sex with her for an emotional reason she does not want to face? Getting fat creates an excuse for her partner not to have sex with her and by believing this reason, she can avoid facing the real reason.

Some people get fat as an excuse to limit their success in life. For example, if a man works in a business where the next step in his advancement requires meeting new customers and presenting a sharp, pleasing physical appearance, he may sabotage his promotion by getting fat. If he does not want the responsibility of the new position or is afraid he will fail in it, getting fat will ensure that he will not get it. He may have the skills necessary to advance but if he feels unworthy of the rewards the new position would bring, he can punish himself by not getting it. Being fat may be a result of low self-worth, fear, a form of punishment or an excuse.

These are just a few examples of excuses people create by being fat. As you search for the cause of your excess fat, look for any excuses it is giving you. If you find that being fat is creating excuses, you must learn how to face the real issues and deal with them openly and honestly. This is the only way you will eliminate your abnormal need for excess body fat.

Attention

We all want to feel loved. It is the underlying force behind almost everything we do. People often join clubs, gangs, cults and other groups just for this reason. Sadly, many of us look for love in all the wrong places because we believe attention is the same as love. Some of us learn this as children and determine that even negative attention is better than no attention. Because love is total acceptance, its opposite is not hate but total indifference. Think about how you feel when people act as if you are not even there. You often want to do something (even if it is negative) to get them to acknowledge your existence. If a child does not get enough positive attention or does not believe he is capable of doing anything good enough to deserve positive attention, he will develop negative behaviors to get attention from his parents and others. This is a painful and unhealthy attempt to get the love he desperately seeks. His actions lower his self-worth and lead to other problems for himself, his family and society. These negative behaviors and low self-worth are often carried into adulthood, sometimes with extremely destructive consequences. Many career criminals may be committing crimes purely as an attempt to feel loved. Even negative attention from the police, prison guards, news media or other criminals is better than no attention. Think about how famous some criminals have become.

Some children may get attention from being able to eat large amounts. Grandma may say something like, "Johnny can eat more than his father" or "Little Johnny sure has a good appetite." This may keep little Johnny eating excessively until he becomes big (fat) Johnny. Getting attention for how much he can eat could easily continue for the rest of his life.

Being fat is an unhealthy approach some children and adults use to get attention. As a child you will attract ridicule, jeers and criticism from your peers. This will have detrimental effects on you, but you will do it anyway, because the negative attention is better than being ignored. You may also get attention from your parents through their attempts to help you lose your excess fat. When you are older, your friends and family may give you attention by teasing you or in their efforts to help you. If you are obese, everywhere you go you will draw stares from others. You may go to nutritionists, support groups, doctors and therapists seeking help at losing your excess body fat, but these attempts will fail if attention is what you want. If you lose your excess body fat, you will also lose the attention (false love) you have been getting. Unfortunately, false love (like drugs and unbalanced foods) can never create lasting satisfaction. You must constantly get attention from one source or another. This wastes a tremendous amount of time and energy in negative, non-productive activities and therefore limits your success and happiness. If you are fat for this or another reason, the negative attention you get may have extremely detrimental consequences. Some fat teenagers have dropped out of school or out of life by committing suicide, because of the negative attention they received.

Some fat people get the attention they seek through sympathy. They constantly tell others how hard they are trying (a negative word giving you an excuse to fail) to lose weight and how many sacrifices they have made. They usually get attention for their aching joints, diabetes or other health problems the excess fat has created. They also get attention when they occasionally lose a few pounds. Curiously, no one is ever notified when they gain it back the following week. Some fat people have a great sympathy and praise system going so why would they want to lose weight permanently? It would be like a child losing the attention of a parent or the comfort of a security blanket.

Another way to get attention is by joining a particular group. This may be why some people use alcohol or other drugs when they are with others and why they later join AA or another alcohol or drug abuse treatment group. If you belong to a fat loss group or a club where most of the members are fat, you may get a great deal of attention and develop many friendships. If you lose your excess body fat, you will no longer feel like you belong to the group— you will not fit in anymore. Wanting to belong and get attention can keep you desperately hanging on to the body fat you think and say you want to lose. Belonging to clubs and groups can be rewarding, but always understand your motivation for being there. If you can give and receive love (total acceptance), it should help you reach your goals; otherwise it will hinder your progress. Enrich your life and the lives of others by joining the right group.

Negative and destructive attention-getting behaviors will continue until you learn positive ways to find the love you need. The best way to do this is to find divine unconditional love. The first place to look for this is within. Loving yourself will turn your life into the joyous adventure it is meant to be. Self-love is the only love you really need but you will notice amazing things happening after you start loving yourself. Others will see you as more lovable, you will believe others can love you and you will accept (instead of reject) more of the love they offer. Have you ever noticed that when you are seeking companionship it is difficult to find? Now, what happens when you find someone you like? Suddenly you become very popular. This happens because, when you are in love, the chemicals your body releases and the loving thoughts you project attract others like a magnet. By loving yourself, you can create the vibrations and aura that attract the love of others.

If you cannot or do not want to find unconditional love (remember, all you need is your own), at least find positive ways to get attention. Get it from doing things that improve your self-image and create another positive cycle in your life. This may help you find the love you seek. An important accomplishment can be losing your excess fat and getting your body looking great. Now you will get noticed because you look good, and you will also attract attention by eating healthfully. Remember that others may tease you but in reality will either envy or respect you.

Do not be eccentric or fanatical with your nutritional or exercise programs. Examples of this are eating healthful foods but with hardly any variety, being extremely strict or becoming an exercise junkie who gets upset if a planned three-hour (much too long) workout has to be cut short by 10 minutes. These are ways of getting negative attention. Some people become workaholics to make large amounts of money to get attention from their positions in life or their worldly possessions but lose the love of their families and themselves in the process. Do not just channel your abnormal behaviors into healthier outlets. Eliminate your abnormal thinking and behaviors and live a balanced, happy life.

Stress Release

Some people make poor food choices or overeat when under excessive stress. This may sometimes be a physical attempt to get the nutrients needed to handle the stress. Vitamin C and B vitamins can help someone deal with physical and emotional stresses. Unfortunately, many people turn to the stress-causing foods that also reduce the ability to deal with it. These are the enemies we discussed in chapter four.

For many people, eating to relieve stress is a conditioned behavior developed as a child. When they were upset or crying, their parents gave them candy, ice cream or a cookie to soothe them. If you are a parent, please do not create this behavior in your children. Determine and deal with the cause of the problem instead of attempting to distract or comfort them with unhealthful foods. Teach your children how to deal effectively with their problems instead of distracting themselves by eating. If you do not know how to do this, you need to learn for the sake of your children and yourself. The parasympathetic nervous system is activated when we eat, channeling blood away from our brains and muscles. This is why eating calms most people down. Learn to relax and reduce stress using healthy methods.

Stress can lower your self-worth and cause you to think things like, "I don't care if I gain five pounds," or "I don't care if I eat this pizza and ice cream." These temporary lapses often become more frequent, because the fat gain they cause leads to more stress, guilt feelings and a lower sense of self-worth. A negative cycle is created generating more fat, more guilt and more stress. As your self-worth decreases further, it creates other problems in your life and lets your other causes for excess fat, as well as other negative influences, affect you to a greater degree.

Many techniques can help you deal with stress. Meditation, biofeedback, correct breathing and progressive relaxation are just a few of them. Proper breathing is excellent, because it takes no extra time and can be done by anyone. If you eat when you get stressed, it is time to learn healthy ways of reducing or dealing with it. These new ways will gradually replace the old, ineffective methods you are currently using. Physical stress from work or exercise reduces a great deal of the mental and emotional stresses people have. You may think this would create more stress and increase the problem, but instead it uses up the epinephrine stimulated by mental and emotional stresses and this allows the muscles to relax. Physical work or exercise also conditions and strengthens your body, making it better able to withstand stress. It improves the balance between each of the four aspects of your being. While attending chiropractic college, I noticed that the few people who exercised regularly handled the intense mental and emotional stresses of school far better than the ones who did no physical exercise. Many of the non-exercisers ate to reduce their stress and got fat because of it. I was called "Mr. Cool" by some of my classmates, primarily because regular exercise and a nutritious diet kept me in balance and minimally affected by the stress.

Some people are extra sensitive to environmental stresses and the negative vibrations of others. It is especially important for these people to supply their bodies with good nutrition and to learn ways of eliminating or reducing their stress.

Most of the stress in your life can be eliminated, because you are the one creating it. It is then relatively easy to deal healthfully with whatever stresses remain. Eliminating and dealing with stress is the topic of another book I have planned.

Fear

Fear can sometimes be an extremely powerful motivator but is never a healthy one. Use love, joy, appreciation and other positive feelings to motivate you. If fear is keeping you fat, it will be difficult, if not impossible, to get lean until you find and eliminate your fear. This section includes some of the common fears that can make and keep someone fat. If your fear is not mentioned, you should still be able to discover what yours is and eliminate its control over you. Think about it and you will see that the other emotional causes are just different forms of fear.

Our greatest fear is the fear of rejection, because this makes us feel ignored and unloved. It is the opposite of our greatest need—acceptance (love). I believe that fear is our greatest obstacle to happiness and creating the life we want. Whenever you feel uneasy or unhappy just determine what it is that you fear. Most fears are based on incorrect facts, failure to think about current circumstances or a lack of faith in your right to be happy. Most fears are just (F)alse (E)vidence (A)ppearing (R)eal. After determining why you are unhappy, stop thinking about what you are afraid may happen and think about what you want to happen. Imagine and feel the joy you will experience when what you want happens, and expect it to occur when the time is right. Do not generate negative energy by worrying about when it will happen, just be happy and know that your positive energy will attract it. If you focus your attention on what you fear, your thoughts and subsequent feelings will attract it. You will create a self-fulfilling prophecy. Always focus on what you want, not what you don't want.

Part of our fear of rejection is the fear of losing friendship or love from others who are fat. If your parents are fat, you may fear losing some of their love and attention if you lose your excess fat. If you have some fat friends, you could fear losing them as friends if you get too lean. You may be afraid of them getting jealous or not wanting to associate with you anymore, because you make them look bad or feel guilty about not following your example. As long as you maintain a certain level of body fat, you may feel like the friendship will not be threatened.

Let me tell you the story of one of my former nutritional clients. She had about 30 pounds of excess fat when she started my program. She lost 20 pounds in the first month and we determined that she would have a healthy body fat percentage if she lost 10 to 15 more pounds of fat and internal waste. This should have been easy but another month went by and she had not lost one pound more. I suggested some minor changes that should have sped up the fat burning. She told me she had made the changes, yet the fat loss still did not come. This was puzzling, because she should have kept losing fat even with her initial program. Eventually, under hypnosis, she revealed the cause of this mystery. She subconsciously believed that if she lost any more fat she would also lose the friendship of her two best friends. I am sure you have already guessed that both of them were fat. To prevent the imagined loss of love, she had sabotaged her nutritional program by eating candy, cookies, pies and other fattening foods she had rarely even eaten in the past. I explained to her subconscious mind that if her friends did not like and accept her for who she was that they were not true friends. Her body weight should have nothing to do with their friendship if they truly liked her as the beautiful being she was. Once she realized the truth, she stopped sabotaging her program and quickly achieved her fat-loss goal. She also kept her friends.

If your friendship with someone will be affected negatively by you losing your excess fat, you should find some new friends. True friends will be happy for you, and if they feel worthy will lose along with you or have you help them do the same. The "social" eating of unhealthful foods often comes from the fear of not fitting in or being accepted by others. It is like the peer pressures many teenagers experience. Dare to be a healthy, loving person and then find people who accept and love you as you are.

Famous fat people may keep themselves fat if they fear losing work or the acceptance and attention of their fans. People who have an influence on many others may stay fat if they fear that their followers will no longer trust or be able to identify with them if they get and stay lean.

Some people make and keep themselves fat to eliminate the temptation to cheat on a spouse who mistreats them. For example, if a lean and attractive woman is unhappy in her relationship with her husband, there may be a strong temptation to cheat on him. If she wants to be faithful, she can reduce, or eliminate, the fear and temptation by getting fat and being less attractive to other men. Of course, the healthy thing to do would be to get help for their relationship and make it loving and happy again or to leave and find happiness elsewhere. Then she can feel confident being her lean, attractive self again. She would either be happy with her husband or would look good as she worked toward finding and developing a new relationship.

Some people get fat because they are afraid of never finding the unconditional love we all want. Their fat bodies give them a reason for not being loved. They dislike it, but it is less painful than facing the realization that no one loves them. These people have to understand that the only love that truly matters and cannot be taken away is their own. They also have to remember that loving themselves is the key to attracting and accepting the love of others.

The fear of starving is another possible cause for being fat. This fear can come from childhood or subconscious memories. The upcoming idea is for information only. I am not attempting to change your spiritual beliefs in any way. No one knows for sure if our spirits live multiple lifetimes and inhabit many different bodies as they learn and progress, but a great deal of evidence suggests it. Living multiple lives explains most of the mysteries of life. Using hypnosis, I have tapped into what "seemed" to be someone's past life memories and eliminated physical and emotional problems that appeared to have originated in a previous lifetime. No, no one ever claimed to have been Cleopatra. I have read numerous cases where migraine headaches in this lifetime seemed to have been caused from a head injury in a past lifetime and after the people's subconscious minds were made aware of this, the migraine headaches stopped. Some people believe these subconscious memories are actually memories of our ancestors that were passed on to us genetically. No matter what the truth is about where these memories come from, the fact is that they exist and can affect you in the here and now.

No matter what the explanation, it is still possible to eliminate the negative influences of subconscious memories. If a man starved to death in a "past" lifetime, the memory of it, if strong enough, could be affecting him. His mind may be unconsciously causing him to eat excessively to store body fat to prepare for another famine and protect him from experiencing the starvation it remembers from the past. A qualified hypnotherapist should be able to help you discover if you have subconscious memories of extreme hunger or starvation. Hypnosis can be a valuable tool for determining other emotional causes of why you are fat. Some people have a fear of hypnosis, but it is nothing more than a tool we can use to help us. It is not some evil mind-control technique. On the contrary, it is perhaps the best way to eliminate the hypnotic programming we have created and give us back the freedom to express our true selves without the distortion caused by false and irrational conditioning.

Some people are afraid of being seen (who they are, not their bodies) by others or even by themselves. Being fat is a way of hiding. For example, this may be done if a man feels ashamed of who he thinks he is, but is frequently done because he is afraid that no one loves him. This fear is often expressed by using drugs and alcohol, overeating or isolation. Never forget that the only love and acceptance you really need is your own and that without it you will not feel worthy to accept the love of anyone else.

Some people hold on to their excess fat because they are afraid that their personalities will change when their bodies change. The funny thing is, they are right. The changes, however, should all be positive and toward a more perfect expression of their spirits. Some people are afraid that if they start looking like someone they know who has a poor sense of humor or is cold and uncaring that they will become like that person. Nothing could be further from the truth. If you have a good sense of humor when you are fat, it should be even better when you are thinner, because you will feel better about yourself and be more able to truly laugh at yourself. You will not just be laughing on the outside and hating and condemning yourself on the inside. Losing excess fat should help you to be a better and more likeable person than you are now. Remember that you are the spirit in your body, not the body itself.

Many of us are afraid to be different because we want to fit in and be accepted by others. Remember that your life and goals are yours and that you are free to act in ways to achieve your goals and make your life happy. Just because others are using drugs, drinking alcohol or eating poorly does not mean you have to do the same. You do not want your children to smoke or take drugs just because their friends do, so you should not eat unhealthful foods just because your friends do. Instead, be a good example for your friends and family. If you cannot embrace your uniqueness and not let your friends' unhealthy behaviors influence you then you should consider finding some friends with healthier habits.

Two of the strongest fears you must eliminate are both part of the fear of change. They are fear of the unknown and fear of what will be lost in the change. Both are easy to eliminate after you understand that life is change and that everything is constantly changing. Those who fear and resist change lead boring, unhappy lives and make minimal personal progress. People who look forward to and embrace change grow and improve rapidly and experience life as the exciting adventure it is meant to be. Look forward to and rejoice in the new and exciting changes occurring each day in yourself and your life. This is one reason why most children have so much energy and enthusiasm. Remember that what you are doing now is a change from something you used to do. If you change something and dislike it, you are usually free to change back to what you were doing or to something new. You are not going to lose anything positive and beneficial when you lose your excess fat. Instead, there will be numerous healthy and positive changes to enjoy.

The fear of failure stops most of us from doing many activities where we could be successful. It can prevent you from starting a healthful eating program. This fear can have many variations. Think for a while and write down what you may be afraid of failing at that would prevent you from reaching your permanent fat loss goal. It may be an emotional reason covered in this chapter or something entirely different. Many ex-convicts commit crimes so they can go back to prison, because they are afraid of failing on the outside. Do not let a fear of failure keep you in your "fat" prison now that you have the keys to unlock all of the doors.

The fear of success is like the fear of failure and can be just as powerful. Also write down what you may be afraid of succeeding at that may be preventing you from reaching your permanent fat loss goal. This could be the key you need to free you from the bondage of excess fat.

Encouragement from Someone

If someone has an interest in keeping you fat, that person will encourage you to overeat and make poor food choices and discourage you from developing healthful exercise and eating habits. Surprisingly, the people who want to see you stay fat are usually your spouse, friends or family. It may seem strange that the people you think would be your greatest supporters are often the ones who least want you to lose your excess fat.

Some of your friends or family who are fat do not want to see you lose your excess fat because it makes them look bad. Many of them would feel guilty if they did not lose their excess fat. The better you look, the more guilt feelings they may have about not doing the same for themselves. You are a constant reminder that it is possible and they are either unable to face the reason for their excess fat, unwilling to accept responsibility for what they look like, or simply too lazy to do anything about it. They will encourage you to have a "small" piece of pie or tell you things like "Gee, I think you've lost enough weight" or "You're getting too thin" or "You should eat a little more, I think you're starving yourself." If you know what is happening, you can easily see that their comments are designed to make you regain some fat. Be aware of what they are doing and take responsibility for your own actions and the healthy consequences. You now have the knowledge that gives you the power to lose excess fat permanently. All you have to do is use it.

Your friends and family generally say the things they do out of ignorance or a subconscious motivation. Some may be afraid that if you get lean that you will get mean and they will not like you anymore. Others may have the fear that you will reject them if you get lean. Just politely decline their offers for the foods you know would fatten you up. Do not get angry with them; simply understand that it is their problem, not yours. Their comments are often humorous so enjoy a little internal chuckle, but do not be cruel with comments directed at friends or loved ones. If you respond lovingly, your example may help some of them improve their health and appearance. Keep in mind that helping others is extremely rewarding. Never attempt, however, to make people do something they do not want to do. It is not going to happen and they may resent you.

Your greatest encouragement to get and stay fat may come from your spouse. If he is fat, his reasoning may be the same as that of your friends and family. If he is not, his reasoning will be different. Here is an example. Think about a man who marries a lean, attractive woman. If he does not do things to keep his attractive wife happy, he may be fearful that she will be tempted to cheat on him or end the relationship. Chances are high that other men will be attempting to get to know her when she is away from him. If he is afraid another man may tempt her, fattening her up and keeping her that way makes her less attractive and reduces his fear of losing her.

His fear may be justified if he lacks the self-confidence or initiative to maintain a good relationship and keep his special lady happy and satisfied. His fear may cause him to get jealous and falsely accuse her of doing certain things. This could possibly drive her away or cause her to do them. It would most likely create a great deal of stress that may cause her to overeat. This fear is a common reason why many men do not want their wives to succeed in the fat-losing quest. A man will say something like "Sure honey, try the new diet," and give her some mild encouragement once in a while. Then he will take her out to a late dinner and tempt her to eat a fattening meal. He will subtly sabotage her fat-losing efforts. He may use comments that reduce her self-worth and make her believe she deserves to be fat, or imply that she will never be successful, so why keep making an effort. He may say he still loves her even though her body is fat, but if he truly loves her, he will want to see her lose her excess fat and be as healthy and happy as possible.

If a man prepares a dinner of fattening foods, his wife may eat more than she wants because she does not want to imply that she does not like his cooking or appreciate the work involved to prepare the meal. Similarly, a woman may get upset if her husband does not eat much at a meal she prepared or says no thanks to fattening foods. He may then eat more to avoid feeling guilty for hurting her feelings. Children sometimes overeat to avoid offending their parents. This occurs both when the children are living at home and later when visiting their parents after they are grown up. These problems can be avoided simply by preparing healthful meals.

Some of your behaviors will be different from those of the fat and unhealthy people around you. Your actions will go unnoticed by most people, but your improved appearance will be a constant reminder to the ones who know you. You will get teased and prodded in an attempt to make you eat something fattening. Do not be like a young person who gives in to a friend's dare to take drugs. By the way, if you and your children are eating well, it will be much easier to say no to drugs and other harmful activities. For most of my life, some of my friends and family have attempted to get me to eat foods that would make me fat like they were. I never gave in to their remarks. They would sometimes say, "Why eat so healthfully? You will probably just be hit and killed by a truck." That is the excuse they use to justify their own lack of action. What they are really saying is "Why don't you get fat and die young of cancer or heart disease like me." My response was always, "What if I *don't* get hit by a truck?" Another thing I used to hear from the older ones is, "Wait until you get older and you'll be fat like me." I am older now, but still not fat. Now I get to hear about their diabetes, aching feet and other ailments. They no longer mention anything about me. Please do not let people talk you into limiting your life by eating unhealthful foods like they do. Do not let *anyone* make such an important decision for you.

Most of us want to fit in somewhere or belong to something greater than ourselves. If you are a balanced and whole person, you should feel like an important part of Nature's plan. Belonging to a group that gives you constant attention or support may be based on an unhealthy need. We are social beings so you may want to belong to a group where you can share enjoyable experiences, express your creativity and spirituality, or give of yourself to others. It is healthy if your attendance is not based on an abnormal need. Take a look at your membership in clubs or groups. If you are there because everyone else is fat, you should leave, because after you lose your excess fat you will no longer belong there. You will now be an outsider who behaves differently and has removed the cause of your condition. Most of the members of your group will not be ready or willing to face their own truths and you will be a constant reminder of that. Therefore, like fat friends or family members, these people can sabotage your success.

Maintain awareness that you are almost constantly being encouraged by numerous advertisers to eat fast foods, processed foods and other products that create excess fat and poor health. This is the primary reason why the obesity rate is increasing so quickly and the health of our people deteriorating so rapidly. Going on a fast-food sandwich diet or eating a particular breakfast cereal and not exercising are not the answers to your problem. Please do not let this endless attempt to make money undermine your health and happiness. I have nothing against people making money, but I would like to see them do it by providing healthful foods instead of preying on the lack of knowledge, addictions and gluttony of their customers.

Power

Some people gain excess body fat in an attempt to feel more powerful. For example, if a man physically or emotionally abuses his wife, she can balance the power to some degree by being fat. The fat cushions the blows and the extra weight gives her more power to defend herself against physical abuse.

If her husband berates her verbally, the excess fat literally acts like a thick skin to shield against his psychological attack.

Most women are extremely protective of their children and may get and stay fat if they feel it gives them more power to protect their children from harm. Sadly, the majority of them do not realize that being a lean role model and teaching good eating and exercise habits will protect their children from most of the physical (disease) and emotional (ridicule from self and others) threats they will encounter.

Excess body fat may make some people feel more powerful at disciplining their children. Other people may gain fat to look more capable for a physically demanding job. Others may be fat if they believe they will get advancements because an employer feels sorry for them. It may get them out of doing certain tasks they dislike.

Some people gain body fat in an attempt to balance out the power between themselves and a strong and intimidating parent. The smaller they are, the more intimidated they often feel. Being physically larger can have a powerful psychological effect. This may happen more frequently when the parent is fat, because the child sees the fat as part of the parent's power. Some children get fat if other children bully them. Others use being fat as a way to manipulate one or both of their parents. Some children get fat as a rebellion against their parent's rules and guidelines. What they put in their mouths may be the only thing they feel they have control over. Some children use food and others use alcohol, drugs or cigarettes. Give your children (especially teenagers) positive and significant things to have control over. It may be the rewards they get for good grades, doing various chores or for other positive behaviors. You could give them a vote or say in the house rules. Young children can frequently be given a choice between two acceptable activities. Let your children choose between two healthful foods, not between a hamburger and pizza. An important thing is to give them control over their health and appearance by teaching them how to eat healthfully and exercise effectively.

Keep in mind that you may still be rebelling against your parents even if you are fifty years old. You may feel powerless against society or your boss. This could be your cause for being fat, if eating is about the only thing you feel you have much control (power) over.

The secret to eliminating this cause is to realize that true power does not come from excess fat. In fact, being fat makes you feel weak-willed and less capable. It supplies you with more verbal ammunition to put yourself down. If you want greater physical strength, you must exercise against increasing resistance. If you need psychological strength, you have to learn where your weaknesses are and determine how other people (and you) play on those weaknesses. This requires soul-searching and learning about yourself, why you do certain things, and what you truly want to do in life. If you accept yourself as you are, it will be easy to make these changes, because you will start finding books and people to help you learn how to develop more psychological strength and eliminate your weaknesses. Remember that when you truly love yourself, solving your problems and changing the things you dislike about yourself happen easily and naturally. A friend may tell you about a book or you may walk into a bookstore and a book may "jump out at you," providing what you need at the time.

Learning more about yourself and what you truly want from life can help you get away from someone who is physically or mentally abusing you. You will develop the physical or emotional strength needed to get yourself out of almost any unhealthy situation.

How we eat and what our bodies look like are among the few things in life all of us have a great deal of control over. Accepting responsibility for looking and feeling your best gives you a sense of power and confidence that often motivates you to improve other areas of your life.

Depression

People often stop caring about themselves when they are depressed. They develop an "I don't care" attitude that can be expressed in many negative ways but is frequently seen in eating patterns. People overeat or ingest foods and drinks they know are unhealthful and fattening. They know what they are doing, but the depression prevents them from feeling good enough to not do it. Some people go to the other extreme and starve themselves. Sadly, some people believe their depression is a weakness or sin for which they must be punished. Overeating and getting fat is often part, if not all, of that punishment, and another negative cycle is started.

We all get depressed occasionally. Sometimes it is a natural and appropriate response. If a loved one dies, or you lose your job or experience other losses or problems, it is normal to mourn or be depressed for a certain period of time. But the depression should not last long. Your thinking (if your mind and soul are well fed) should lead you to positive action and soon have your life back on track and moving forward. For example, after you lose a job you should be looking for a new one or educating yourself for a better one instead of sitting at home feeling sorry for yourself and overeating. Losing a job is often how life gets you out of a rut and moves you on to something better. You should view it as a great opportunity. I have never lost a job where I did not end up finding a better one. Eventually I started my own business and later went back to school and then started a more lucrative business.

If you are frequently depressed, you need to determine and eliminate the cause. I am talking about getting rid of the true cause, not just taking a pill to cover up the symptoms and then pretending everything is fine. Unfortunately, this is the course of action taken by millions who think it will magically resolve their problems. Like most magic, however, it is only an illusion. The drug companies certainly love these people but I doubt if the people love themselves. The real magic is found within us when we look honestly at ourselves with love and understanding. If obese people were truly honest with themselves, I believe that the vast majority of them would admit to frequent bouts of depression. Sometimes medication can be helpful for a short time as the cause is being eliminated, but seek first to naturally balance out your life, your body, and your thinking, so you can achieve lasting relief. Realize that overeating and gaining more fat make it harder to resolve depression.

Depression can easily be caused by a poor diet, especially one lacking in the B-complex vitamins. Processed foods are severely deficient in these vitamins so vital to the health of your brain and nervous system, and low-calorie diets often fail to supply adequate B vitamins. Alcohol is a depressant and it, sugar, processed grain products, birth control pills and other medications deplete your body of these important nutrients. Remember that a minor deficiency of the B vitamin niacin can cause a loss of the sense of humor. This could certainly be a part of many people's depression.

Research indicates that obese people cannot use carbohydrates as well when they are depressed. This makes it easier to gain fat. Hypoglycemia, hypothyroidism and hormonal imbalances can create or intensify feelings of depression. Many people binge on *processed* carbohydrates (no one binges on broccoli) when they are depressed. People keep eating these empty foods to get the temporary rise in blood sugar that they produce. Unfortunately, these foods do not supply the nutrients people need to feel better, and make the depression worse by depleting the nutrients needed to feel good. This starts a negative cycle. Physical health problems usually cause some degree of depression and being fat causes many health problems. This starts yet another negative cycle.

Having excess fat and being unable to lose it can make you depressed. You already know that physical imbalances affect you emotionally and vice versa. Therefore, if a physical imbalance is causing your body to be fat, then failed attempts at losing excess fat may be the cause of your depression. Ask yourself if you are fat because you are depressed or depressed because you are fat. Supplying your brain with good nutrition increases the chance that your depression will end before or while you are losing your excess fat.

Physical exercise improves how you feel physically and emotionally. As you have learned, the physical, spiritual, mental and emotional aspects of your being are interrelated and affect each other to varying degrees. Find some emotional and physical activities that make you feel good. Doing something nice for someone else is one of the best ways to help yourself feel better about life and who you are. The right form of exercise can often lift your spirits and make you feel more alive and positive about yourself and your life. Many books with uplifting and insightful messages are available to help you realize that you are far more than you think you are. Having positive thoughts or partaking of some soul food can often lift depression.

Lack of joy is usually the root of all depression. Find out and eliminate what is causing your lack. It can be physical or emotional. Is it the breakup of a loving relationship? Is it the loss of a job or failure in business? Is it a physical imbalance, injury or illness? Don't just sit around feeling lonely and sorry for yourself—do something uplifting for yourself or someone else. Take action to resolve your depression and get back into life.

Not enough balanced light (sunlight or supplemental full-spectrum light) may be causing some (perhaps all) of your depression. Follow the guidelines you have learned and let Nature light up your life and lift your depression.

Laughter can be tremendously useful for lifting your spirits and getting rid of depression. Read some joke books or comics or watch some videos of old television programs or movies you find especially funny. Laughter really is good medicine and few of us laugh enough.

Learning to love yourself is the best way to break out of depression coming from an emotional cause. Of course, physical imbalances can also cause depression. Natural remedies can often restore physical balance, but sometimes medication is necessary. This should be your last resort, because medications have side effects that create new problems. Your depression may even be caused by a medication, as this is a common side effect of many drugs. Who wants to take a drug that solves one problem but creates a new one? It could be a never-ending cycle. Take a second pill for the side effects of the first one, a third pill for the side effects of the second one, and so forth. It can become complicated and is often seen in the lives of older people. They start with one problem but take ten different pills every day. This is unhealthy and can even be life threatening. Too many people see a television commercial or magazine ad promising relief if they use a particular drug. Unfortunately, most doctors simply give people what they ask for, because the doctor will not take the time, or does not know how, to figure out and eliminate the cause of their patient's problems. If you do use medication, never stop looking for a way to resolve the problem or at least a natural way to treat the symptoms.

Depression often develops from past emotional or mental programming. Various techniques can help you discover and eliminate programmed behaviors. Being self-aware is an excellent way, because each time a programmed behavior starts, you are conscious of it. You can then often see the past events that created it, the reality of current circumstances, and act accordingly instead of simply reacting. This can gradually release the control your programming has over you. Accepting yourself unconditionally makes it easy to eliminate false programming and to express the real you in each new moment. Hypnosis, if done properly, can usually help identify and eliminate past programming. In essence you have hypnotized yourself into believing certain things and behaving in certain ways. Effective techniques de-hypnotize you and free you from your programming so your inner spirit can express itself without distortion. I have developed a technique, which I plan to explain in a future book, that has helped people eliminate past programming that was causing them to react the same way to certain conditions instead of acting new, fresh and true in each situation.

You have learned that perfectionism is stressful and negatively affects your self-worth, because you or anything you do will never be good enough. This may be all or part of the source of someone's depression.

Positive ions are generated by electronic equipment like televisions and computer monitors. An excess of these ions can cause fatigue and depression. An air purifier (not filter) or negative ion generator can help restore balance.

If you eat when you are depressed and eat when you feel good, then depression is not your primary cause of overeating. People who overeat at both times have another cause and use any excuse to justify eating to excess or making poor food choices. If this sounds like you, chances are you will find the emotional cause of your poor eating habits elsewhere in this chapter.

Not Accepting Responsibility

Some people never accept responsibility for their own lives. They waste much of their time complaining and blaming others for their past and present problems. They do not understand that they created their lives and circumstances and that they, not others, are the only ones who can change them. Once you realize that no one can make any real changes in your life except you, life gets a great deal better. You will be able to see that if you complain and blame, your mind will continually create new problems for you to complain about. It creates what it thinks you want. On the other hand, if you give thanks for what you have, your mind will create more for you to be thankful for and enjoy. Start seeing and appreciating what's good in your life. You attract what you focus your attention on, so think about what you do want, not what you don't want. Think about what you don't want only long enough to help you see what you do want.

Not assuming responsibility for their own lives and actions can affect people in many ways, including being fat. If they are fat, they can blame their parents for their genetics or their poor eating habits. They may just say, "That's the way life is," or blame work schedules or other circumstances. These excuses and complaints perpetuate and worsen the problem. These people simply eat whatever is handy and let whatever happens, happen. If they get fat, they just think it is a natural part of life that they can do nothing about. If this is what they believe then there is nothing they can do about it—at least not until they realize that getting and staying lean is their responsibility and their responsibility alone.

If you believe that obesity is a disease, instead of feeling helpless and doing nothing, realize that you now know how to cure it. You just have to assume the responsibility to administer the cure.

Some people never take responsibility for their excess fat because they believe that they have a "fat" gene and therefore no control over it. Studies with identical twins have shown that some are fat and some are lean, even though they have the same genes. I once saw a story on a popular news program about identical twin brothers. One of them weighed 40 pounds more than the other one. They had the same genes but one had much larger jeans. The lean brother does a bit more exercise than the fat one, but the main difference was in their food choices and the quantity eaten. This was easily seen when they were taken to an all-you-can-eat restaurant. The lean brother chose the more healthful foods and ate less than his brother. It was apparent by what he said that the lean brother made different food choices because he wanted different results than his fat brother did. It was also clear that the fat brother felt like he would be missing something or giving up something "good" if he did not eat a larger amount of the unhealthful, higher-calorie foods. The difference in their body fat percentages came from their attitudes about food and the choices they made, not genetics.

Another theory you have probably heard on television or read about in magazines is that the obesity problem in America started in prehistoric times. You will hear that we love sugar, salt and animal fat because of our genes that have developed over millions of years. Some people use this kind of information as an excuse to be fat, but you now know better. Billions of people with similar genes are leaner and healthier than most Americans and many of them rarely eat much animal fat and quite a few *never* eat sugar or salt. Americans who are lean and healthy are that way because of the choices they make. Making unhealthful choices is the real reason for the obesity epidemic and one that has been evolving for only the last forty or fifty years. It is also a reason that you can change any time you choose. Nature has not programmed you to eat processed sugar, high-fructose corn syrup, processed grains and artificial foods that are nutrient vampires. You have programmed yourself (with a lot of help from others) to eat these unhealthful "foods."

You may have heard about the hormone leptin and other substances in our bodies that lead to obesity. These chemicals are not the problem. It is the distortion of appearance and function that people create in their bodies that causes the chemicals to not produce their normal effects. They work fine in the people who eat relatively well and do physical labor or exercise. Of course, drug companies are trying to develop drugs to manipulate these chemicals to cheat the laws of Nature and help people lose excess fat. If they succeed they will make millions of dollars from the sale of these drugs that will most likely have serious side effects or only temporary effectiveness.

Contrary to what you will read elsewhere, the human body has not evolved to be fat. Look at African people who live in the jungle and eat their natural diets. They are lean and not plagued by cancer and other man-made diseases. Now look at African Americans who eat hamburgers, fries and pizza and drink milk, beer and sodas. The design of our bodies is not the problem; the problem is the design of the man-made foods and drinks that people consume.

Being obese is unhealthy but according to the evolutionary theory, the strongest survive not the fat and sickly. Therefore, evolution did not design our bodies to be fat nor would a Higher Power design them to be unhealthy.

When I was growing up, I rarely saw an obese person. Now, I rarely see someone who has an attractive body. My family and the people that I knew all had plenty to eat but very few were even moderately overweight. We weren't driven to eat everything in sight by millions of years of evolution. If the gene theory had any validity, we all would have been obese and we still would be. What was the difference between then and now? Were most of these people a lot more physically active than people are today? No. Were we all very good at fighting millions of years of evolution? No. Did most of us exercise frequently? Definitely not. The primary difference was the ratio of real foods to processed junk foods and fast foods. Back then we ate approximately 75 to 85 percent real foods and only 15 to 25 percent junk foods and fast foods. There wasn't a fast-food outlet on every corner, people ate at home more often and we were not constantly bombarded with advertising for fast foods and junk foods. There also weren't as many different fast-food outlets and junk foods to choose from. People went out for fried chicken or a hamburger and fries once a week, not to a different fast-food chain every night. Here's the bottom line on obesity. The primary cause of the obesity epidemic in America that is fast spreading to other parts of the world is that the ratio of what people eat is now approximately 75 to 85 percent fast foods and junk foods and only 15 to 25 percent real foods. As that ratio has reversed so has the ratio of fat to lean people. Reverse that ratio and your problem with excess fat could soon be history.

Here are a couple of more questions to ponder if you still think that genes cause obesity. If genes are the cause of obesity, why can people be lean at age thirty and obese at age forty-five? They still have the same genes. Why also can an obese thirty-year-old man be lean and healthy at age thirty-two if he changes to a healthy lifestyle? His genes didn't change.

When your body tells you to eat something sweet, *choose* to eat a peach or a bowl of blueberries instead of a donut or candy bar. When your body craves fat, *choose* to eat some nuts, seeds or eggs instead of chocolate, potato chips or other fat-fried snacks. *Choose* to do two or three one-hour strength-training sessions a week instead of sitting in front of the television eating junk food. If you make healthy choices, you will be lean and healthy. If you make unhealthy choices, you will be fat and unhealthy. It really is that simple and it is *all* up to you.

There are researchers currently working to prove that a virus causes obesity. Some of them may have good intentions but a company that wants to assume responsibility (for a price) for your excess fat is most likely funding the research. According to a July 2004 article in *Reader's Digest* magazine, Nikhil V. Dhurandhar, a nutritional biochemist at Wayne State University in Detroit, believes that human adeno-virus-36 can cause obesity in people. He says that fat cells begin to multiply in animals injected with the virus. I do not believe that it does the same in humans for a few reasons. Where was this virus fifty years ago when most Americans were not obese? Why does it seem to be most prevalent in countries where people eat mostly processed junk food and do little strenuous work? And, why do people who exercise regularly and eat well seem to be immune to this "fat" virus? Even if a virus does make fat cells multiply, it still does not mean you have to eat excessively to fill up those cells with fat. Some people with three times more fat cells than average are lean and healthy because they make healthy food choices. Please do not use a virus as your excuse for not accepting responsibility for your excess fat.

A greater percentage of low-income people are overweight or obese compared to people with higher incomes. Some people believe that part of the reason is that good foods cost more. I disagree. You have learned that the fast and processed foods are the expensive foods. For about one dollar you can buy what makes six to seven pounds of nutritious and filling brown rice. The same amount of unhealthful processed cereal would cost $15 to $38. Who do you think pays for the millions of dollars worth of advertising that is done for fast foods and junk foods every day? For five years during the late nineteen eighties and early nineties my rent was $350 a month and my total monthly income was less than $750 but I still managed to eat well and stay lean. Even now, my food bill is less than $400 a month and I eat organic fruits and vegetables, legumes, fertile eggs, whole grains and good meats. Many obese people spend more than that on junk food that supplies little of the nutrition that their bodies need. A lack of knowledge of how to eat well is the reason why low-income people have more excess body fat, not a lack of money.

Another reason given for why low-income people have more excess fat is that the parents make their children stay indoors to keep them from playing in unsafe streets. The children spend most of their time in front of the television being influenced by fast-food and junk-food commercials. I believe that this reason also comes from a lack of education. Educated people are less influenced by television commercials, know more about eating well, and encourage their children to use their time indoors more wisely. Some of them teach their children how to prepare nutritious meals. When children are indoors they can do their homework, read good books, practice musical instruments and do many other positive activities that feed their minds and souls. They do not have to sit in front of the television all night eating junk food.

Another reason given for low-income people being fat is that they work long hours and are too tired or do not have time to make healthful meals. Once again, I disagree. I often work 10 to 11 hours a day and still manage to eat nutritious meals and snacks all day. You have learned that it does not take much time to put together nutritious meals and snacks. Many of my meals take less than 5 minutes to prepare—less time than most people wait for food at a fast-food restaurant.

You learned in chapter eleven about numerous physical reasons why one person may gain fat more easily and lose fat slower than someone else does. I believe that almost all of these reasons can be eliminated or compensated for in natural and healthful ways. Accept responsibility for the care of your body, discover and eliminate your causes and then get on with the process of enjoying your life.

Before you can assume responsibility for your own life and actions, you must let go of the past and forgive everyone you are blaming. Your parents may have fattened you up when you were young, but it does no good to blame them for your excess fat or for other problems you may feel they created. They always did their best, just as you did. You created the emotional programming that is causing your problems, not them. Luckily, you have the power to change and eliminate this programming whenever you choose. Life is change and now that your best has gotten better, you can correct and eliminate what you created in the past. As you should know by now, the most important person to forgive is yourself. When you stop blaming, your mind is freed to create constructive changes. If you spend (waste) all your time complaining and blaming others, no time is left to make the changes necessary to improve your life. Spend (invest) your time wisely creating the happy and healthy life you deserve.

There are groups of people trying to force automobile manufacturers, airlines, and other transportation companies to accept responsibility for the excess fat of their customers and passengers. They want cars, buses and airplanes to have larger and stronger seats for fat people. This was not necessary in the past. Why is it necessary now? If airlines complied, what might happen? After seats for 300-pound people were installed, people who weighed more than that would complain. Soon the doors would have to be made larger and special forklifts might even be requested to load people into the planes. Do you see the absurdity of this way of thinking? Installing larger seats on planes would decrease the total number of seats available and this would inconvenience and increase costs for everyone. It would also take away any incentive some fat people may have to be responsible for themselves. And what about restaurant chairs, seats in movie theaters and the seats at other entertainment venues. Would they all have to be larger? If these people put half as much effort into eating and exercising healthfully and productively as they do into trying to make the world change to fit their fat bodies, they would solve their own problems.

The previous paragraph was not meant as a putdown or to hurt anyone. It was written solely to express the absurdity of certain ways of thinking. If people believe that being obese is out of their control, they will never assume responsibility for their excess fat and then learn and do what it takes to get rid of it. The truth is, if my lifestyle and eating habits were the same as most obese people, I would be obese. I feel sympathy for the people with excess fat who have tried desperately to lose it and regain some dignity and a healthy self-image. It is mostly for these people that I have written this book. Sadly, many of them have given up because their efforts have failed. They failed because their attempts at permanent fat loss were based on fad diets, ineffective drugs and supplements, an abundance of misinformation and others saying that for a price, they will take responsibility for getting rid of these people's excess fat.

I hope that many of the people in these groups will use the truths found in this book to help themselves and each other to win their battles with fat. Then they can spend their time expressing their love and creativity in positive and rewarding ways instead of trying to convert many things in the country to extra large.

Some people have sued fast-food restaurants because they or their children have eaten the fast food and gotten fat. If alcoholics keep ordering drinks, they will continue to be served and if fat people keep ordering fast foods, they will continue to get it. I do not think that there will ever be "fat" police to prevent you from buying unhealthful and fattening foods. *You* are responsible for what you and your children eat and drink, not the fast-food restaurants you frequent or supermarkets that sell you candy and ice cream.

Why do some people grow up in poverty and negative environments but become successful and happy, while others grow up in luxurious and positive environments but end up living unhappy and unsuccessful lives? The ones who are happy and successful chose to assume responsibility for their lives. They focused on what they wanted and did what was necessary to get it. Those who failed chose the role of victim and blamed others for what happened to them.

Another way to avoid responsibility is to simply not choose. Being lean and healthy does not happen by default. If you do not choose for yourself and then act on your choice, life will choose for you and I doubt if you will like what you get. It is like sailing a ship on the ocean without steering to your desired destination. You will end up shipwrecked on a deserted island instead of in Hawaii where you wanted to be. Once you choose to be lean and healthy, your lifestyle choices are easy. You just do the activities and eat the foods you know are going to create the results you want. By choosing the foods that make you lean and healthy, you will soon be feeling so good that unhealthful foods will not even be a part of your life. Someday you may not waste a moment of your precious time even thinking about them.

Alcoholics, smokers, drug users, overeaters and other addicts quit abusing their bodies and their lives when they accept responsibility for their actions and the consequences created by those actions. They must actively choose different results before anything can change. Once they do this, they can then learn what actions will create the results they want.

No one can make you sad, happy, fat or lean. It all comes from within you. Your own thinking generates feelings that attract what you want. No one else can exercise or eat for you and no one else can do anything for you to make a permanent change in your life. You have been given the gift of life and a body and mind to experience its many joys and wonders. You have also been given the freedom of choice. You can choose to assume the responsibility to take care of your body and mind and create the life you want, or not. You have choices that can greatly influence the quality and length of your life.

Do not leave the responsibility for your health and well-being up to your doctor. Very few of them know how to restore balance and lost health or how to help you maintain good health—even the ones who claim they do. They usually just treat your symptoms with drugs that have damaging side effects. Also, do not wait until you have a health problem before you do anything. It may be too late. Make the decision now to do what is necessary to enjoy a lean, healthy body.

Some people do not take responsibility for their own bodies because they lack the knowledge of how to do it or do not realize they have the power to greatly influence how they look and feel. You now have a good idea of what can be done and the knowledge of how to do it. If you created a fat body, you can create a lean one. It is simply a matter of accepting the responsibility.

Attitudes about Food and Eating

We all pick up attitudes about foods and eating from our parents, family, friends, health "experts" and role models. This is why advertisers use parental figures, peers, celebrities, doctors, athletes and other role models to sell processed breakfast cereals, milk and other unhealthful foods.

Some people develop the attitude that if you have an abundance of money you should eat rich foods. I believe many people attempt to make themselves feel rich by eating the gourmet, high-calorie and high-fat foods they believe rich people eat. In past eras, kings and other royalty were often fat, because they overindulged in meats, pastries and other rich foods. Perhaps they got the name "rich" foods because only the rich could afford them. On the contrary, the peasants could not afford to overeat and ate whole, natural foods such as fruits, vegetables, legumes and whole grains. The peasants did physical labor so they got more exercise than the royalty usually did. It is not hard to see why most of the peasants were leaner, stronger and healthier than the kings and wealthy people.

Another learned attitude is seeing food as a reward. Your parents helped you develop this attitude if they gave you candy or a cookie as a reward for being quiet or behaving as they wanted you to behave. Like using food to train a dog, they controlled your behavior by bribing you with unhealthful and fattening foods. As many of us get older, we eat these types of foods whenever we feel we have behaved well and therefore deserve a treat. You deserve a cocktail after work or ice cream after dinner because you have been a good boy or girl that day. There will always be a reason to eat unhealthful foods if you have this attitude.

You need to realize that you are grown up now and have the power to change your thinking and behavior. You must eliminate your false and unhealthy thinking and behavioral patterns by developing new, healthy ones based on reality, facts, your goals, and nutritional knowledge. An old dog *can* learn new tricks. Develop the attitude of being lean so you can enjoy all the rewards being lean has to offer. Your treats can then be improved health, longer life, a more pleasing appearance, greater energy, improved self-image, better fitting clothes and an improved way people react to you. If you choose, these and the many other rewards we have discussed can be yours all day, every day.

Reward your children with positive attention and your time. If they behave, praise them for it and reward them with a promise to read them a story later, play catch in the back yard or take them to a park or somewhere else you can spend quality time together. Be aware that whatever you promise, you must do or you will lose their trust and future promises will mean nothing. Show honest interest in what they do, what they like, what they think and how they feel. They will know if you are faking it. Sit down and talk to your children (listen mostly) and touch them often with a loving hand and with all the things you do for them. Love and positive attention is what they all truly crave. If you give them this, they will not have to create negative behaviors to get your attention and you will not have to give them junk food to get them to behave. Even a dog can be trained just as well (I believe better) with praise and love instead of food treats.

Some parents tell their children that having a cookie before eating will ruin dinner but think nothing of giving them one right after. This adds more calories to a meal that may have already contained too many. It would be healthier if they ate the cookie an hour or two before dinner, but clearly the best choice is not to eat it at all.

Many people are conditioned to believe that after eating dinner they have to eat a dessert of some kind or the meal is incomplete. Why would you want to create such a poor food combination and add all those extra calories to what may have been a nutritious meal? This is like filling up your car's gas tank with premium fuel and then adding sugar or something else that is harmful to the engine. If you do ever choose occasionally to eat a dessert of some kind, it is best to do it in the afternoon two or three hours after eating lunch.

Another common learned attitude is that a celebration means a time for overeating and indulging in high-fat foods, cakes, pastries and other desserts. Thanksgiving, Christmas, New Year's Eve, birthdays, weddings, anniversaries, other holidays and special events are celebrated by eating and drinking, usually to excess. These times are often used as an excuse for eating unhealthful and fattening foods. Drinking alcoholic beverages is a part of celebrating for many people. Alcohol has a large number of empty, fat-producing calories and, as you have learned, many negative effects on your physical and emotional well-being. It has ruined parties, evenings out, marriages, families, and often puts people at risk of injury or death—not exactly things to celebrate.

The aforementioned events usually include getting together with family and friends to celebrate. Think about it. What is the essence of celebrating? Is it the company of friends and family, or is it overindulging in foods and drinks that cause fat gain and poor health? The true meaning of many celebrations is lost because more attention is paid to the food and drink than to the event itself. The person having the birthday, the couple having the anniversary or the true meaning of the holiday frequently take a back seat to the food and drink.

I believe it is possible to enjoy these times far more by remembering why you are there and sharing the ideas, merriment, dancing, conversation and other activities with the people who are also celebrating. Keep your focus on what is really important and eat a moderate, simple meal. Then you will not need a drug to treat the unpleasant symptoms of poor food choices or overeating. Especially avoid the alcohol. It does nothing but create problems and increase the risk of you or someone you care about being hurt or killed. Partake of more mind and soul food and less body food. This is where most of us are deficient.

Eating well is actually not difficult even when everyone else is overindulging in food and alcohol. Remember that most people will not even pay attention to what you are doing, some will respect you, but others will try to tempt you. Some may do it just for something to say. For example, if a man at a party offers you a piece of cake or tries to get you to eat excessively, politely decline and then simply change the subject. Compliment him on his clothes, an accomplishment, his new baby, or whatever else you can compliment him on or ask a question about his work, hobby, or about another interest he has. He will like you better and think you are a great conversationalist. You may even learn something useful or interesting. This way, you can enjoy the party without getting fat.

If you are on a cruise ship or at an all-you-can-eat restaurant, the best thing to do is to eat moderate amounts of the healthful foods available. You may want to taste some of the many different foods. This is not that bad if you try a few at each meal. You will enjoy the experience more if you do not eat excessively and make yourself uncomfortable and fat.

"Eat, drink and be merry, for tomorrow we die" is an adage some people use as the basis of their actions. If you think about it, being fat does not make most people merry—not if they are honest about how they really feel. You also know many of the negative effects of drinking. If this way of life is followed, the tomorrow when they die will come much sooner. Reject this irresponsible and negative thinking. It will bring only pain and suffering into your life. Live with a childlike enthusiasm for each new day as you partake of healthful foods and drinks, feed your mind positive thoughts and enjoy much love and soul food.

See eating as a means to an end, not an end itself. Eating has a purpose— to nourish your mind and keep your body lean and healthy. It is not intended to calm you, comfort you, give you something to do with your hands and mouth, or fill in the gaps in your life created by a lack of mental stimulation, emotional imbalance or deficiency of soul food. Whenever you eat, think about what your body needs for good clean-burning fuel and for rebuilding and maintenance. Give it good care and it will give you good service. Remember that eating healthfully provides true physical *and* emotional satisfaction.

Programmed Thinking

You have created thinking and behavioral patterns based on ideas implanted in your mind by books, magazines, radio and television programs, advertisements, family members, friends, acquaintances and your own thinking. Some of this programmed thinking is part of other emotional causes. In this section I want to concentrate on your attitude about yourself.

As you go through your day, notice if you think or say things like "I look at food and gain weight," "I've always been fat," "I can't lose weight, no matter how hard I try," or "It takes will power to lose weight and I don't have any." This is the kind of negative self-talk you must become aware of and eliminate. These things are true only because you have brainwashed yourself into believing they are, and these thoughts constantly reinforce the programming. Change your thinking and you can change your body composition and your life.

It does not take years of psychoanalysis or work to change your thinking. You created your conditioned thoughts and behaviors and you have the power to start fresh at any moment you choose. Ebenezer Scrooge changed his thinking, behaviors and life overnight once he realized what his life would be like if he didn't. Scrooge was a fictional character, but you probably know or have heard stories of people who made similar changes in their behaviors. You are not your past behaviors, but chances are you are being controlled a great deal by past programming. Realize that you have the power to change your thinking starting right now and create a new present, which will gradually become your new past that originates from this point in time.

When you were a child, did your parents frequently tell you to be a "big" boy or girl? This is common and may have conditioned you into believing that you should be big (fat). If you have children of your own, please do not use expressions like, "Be a big girl" or "Big boys don't cry." You could be helping condition them to be fat. If they fall down and are crying say, "Be a brave girl" or "Be a strong boy" instead. Replace the word "big" with something positive or better yet tell them everything is all right and how much you love and care about them. Giving them physical affection at the same time would be helpful and nurturing for both of you.

If you were given ice cream, candy, a cookie or other sweets when you were emotionally upset or physically hurt as a child, you may still be doing it. This is more programming that must be eliminated. Get rid of it and then do not program your children to see food as a source of comfort when they are hurting. Help them to deal with their problems with soul food, physical exercise, mental exercise and in other healthy ways.

Do not create your own excuses and problems. Stop thinking or saying things like "I have a slow metabolism" or "I have a gland problem that makes me fat." This instructs your subconscious to create a self-fulfilling prophecy. Start thinking and talking about the truth, like excess body fat being unhealthy, abnormal and unwanted. Besides, excess fat and internal waste cause most gland problems, and you can do numerous things to normalize your metabolism. Your body wants to be lean and will help you achieve that goal, but you must first stop creating the fat with your "fat" talk, thoughts and feelings. Remember that you did not need will power to make your body fat and you do not need it to make your body lean. Because your thoughts and feelings can create whatever you want, all you need to do is change what you want. This will change what you think and how you feel. Keep your focus on what you want and talk about, think about, and feel what it will be like when you have it. Your subconscious (true self) will then guide you to complete the necessary actions. You will be a spirit living in a lean body, instead of a spirit living in a fat body. This may seem simplistic, but the truth, whenever you find it, is always simple. You will learn that being in a lean body is no more difficult than being in a fat body.

Never focus on your goal not having materialized yet, because this creates negative energy and blocks what you want from coming. Once you stop *being* fat, you will stop doing what people with fat bodies do and when you start *being* lean, you will start doing what people in lean bodies do. It is *entirely* up to you. You created the fat image, the fat thoughts, the fat feelings and the fat body. You can just as easily create a lean image, lean thoughts, lean feelings and a lean body.

The word "try" is negative and has a weakening effect on the body that can easily be demonstrated with applied kinesiology. Avoid using it as much as possible. Do not say "I'll try to eat healthier" or "I'll try to resist the dessert." The word try implies failure, so be aware of what you are thinking and saying. Replace "try" with "do my best" and say things like "I'll do my best to eat healthier." Better yet just make a statement of what you are doing or plan to do. Say things like "I'm eating healthier" or "I do not eat dessert" or "I am not having dessert tonight." Avoid talking about how well you are *going to* eat or what a great exercise session you are *going to* have tomorrow. Tomorrow never comes; there is only now and it is a precious gift. Do not let the past *or* the future control you.

One way to eliminate your fat programming is to pretend you have been playing a role in a movie that required wearing something to make you look 50 pounds heavier. All you have to do is stop playing the role and the fat can now be taken off. Sadly, many fat people have chosen to accept their roles permanently. They do not feel worthy of playing the part of the dashing leading man or beautiful leading lady.

In reality you are the writer, casting director, producer, director and star of the movie called *My Life*. You can play any part you like, rewrite the script at any time and choose the other main characters. You have the power to change what you don't want into what you do want. If you have cast yourself in the role of a fat character, write the sequel and cast yourself in the role of a lean and healthy character. For once, the sequel will be better than the original.

You must always remember that you have done nothing wrong. If you have a fat body, it is not wrong. Being lean is not right; it is simply the natural way of things. Do not judge and label either one as right or wrong. You are not your body, but how you see yourself, feel about yourself, and treat yourself is reflected in your body. The physical reflects the spiritual and emotional like a mirror. You must lose weight from within by changing your thoughts and eliminating the false emotional programming that created your excess fat. Then, the physical actions of exercising regularly and eating whole, natural foods will be easy. You must trust that the spiritual being inside your body— the real you—will create the best possible vehicle. You do not have to search for the truth; it is already within you. You need only to eliminate the false programming so your truth can be physically expressed.

Labels, judgments, negative emotions and false thinking must be eliminated—not just to create the lean body you deserve, but to give you the satisfied feeling inside that you are being true to your inner nature. This is the feeling many people seek to experience by eating. As more guilt, fear and self-condemnation are eliminated, it will become easier to create and maintain your lean, healthy body.

Emotional Addiction

You have learned how to cleanse your body of the residues of the fattening and unhealthful foods you have eaten in the past. Once this has been done, your physical addictions and cravings will be gone. Now, the only thing that can cause you to overeat, or eat foods you know will make you fat and unhealthy, is an emotional addiction. Therefore, you must also cleanse your mind of any emotional addictions and cravings.

Some of the causes of emotional addictions are environment, learned bad habits, hormone imbalances, stress, learned attitudes about foods, programmed thinking and others we have already covered. The thought that you are missing out on something perhaps leads to emotional addiction more than all others. Do you remember when you were a child and did not want to go to sleep because of what you thought you would miss out on, and how if a sibling or friend got something then you wanted it also? This thinking pattern can be observed at a smorgasbord by looking at the plates of people who have to eat some of every food. They do not want to miss out on eating even one food. Some fill their plates to overflowing even though they can go back for more as many times as they want. People often eat dessert because they feel as if they would be missing something if they do not. It is time to rethink this childish belief and see that you need only what is right for you. Realize that you always have what you need to progress to the next step in achieving your goals. Live a healthy, balanced and loving lifestyle and you will not miss out on a lean and healthy body, positive mind stimulation and an abundance of soul food. These are the things that make up a happy and satisfying life.

To a small child, everything is "mine, mine, mine." While growing up, you should learn that you do not need everything and that plenty is available for everyone. For example, you may have a goal to retire early. You would save and invest as much as possible and may have a part-time business along with your job or regular business. If people you know spend their money as fast as they can, you cannot do the same and accomplish your goal. You cannot save money if you spend it all. Let their goals be theirs and your goals be yours. It is impossible to work as a full-time doctor and a full-time lawyer. Unfortunately, being stuck in the thinking pattern of wanting it all can easily lead to making poor food choices and overeating.

If your goal is to be lean and healthy, you cannot have the goal to be fat and unhealthy. If people have the goal of staying fat, they will eat cake, pie and other fattening foods. If your goal is different, your eating habits and actions must be different. If you go to dinner with someone who makes poor food choices, overeats, drinks wine and eats dessert, do not think you are missing out on anything worth having. Face reality and think about what you will really be missing. Things like indigestion, excess body fat, putrid body odor, bad breath, constipation, poor complexion, lack of energy, poorly functioning body and mind, feeling unattractive and weak-willed, frustration that your clothes do not fit, body aches and pains, colds and other diseases, depression, bad teeth, premature death and many others. Do you really want any of those things? Many people waste a great deal of time and money attempting to get rid of the problems they caused with the childish belief that they are missing something if they do not eat some cake or ice cream.

Some people can eat a piece of cake occasionally and not have a problem, but many people seem to have addictive personalities. For some people, eating one piece of cake is like a true alcoholic taking one drink. A cycle of negative and destructive behaviors is quickly created. It is like dropping a match into a pool of gasoline in the middle of your living room. People soon find themselves out of control and on the way to creating more physical imbalances and addictions. The poor nutrition to their minds and bodies then makes everything spiral downward faster and faster. If you have an addictive personality, you must realize that you cannot have even one dessert or you will be in for trouble. Always think about the effect that the food you eat is going to have on your physical and emotional health. It is especially important when you are feeling a little down or stressed out to remember that healthful foods will make you feel better and unhealthy choices will make you feel worse.

Keep in mind that the satisfaction people believe they get from eating sweets is short lived. This is why they have to keep doing it. It is like using a drug. This false satisfaction does harm by making them feel weak-willed and unloved. In contrast, the feeling of power and control over how your body looks and feels is a truly satisfying soul food that can help eliminate emotional addiction to unhealthful foods.

Boredom

It always amazes me when I hear people say that they are bored and have nothing to do. With the thousands of hobbies and activities we can do, the millions of things available to study and learn, and a multitude of creative pursuits, how is it possible to be bored? It seems impossible, but boredom is a common reason why people overeat. It is sad that so many people lack the mental stimulation necessary to distract them from constant eating. Now, tell me that eating all day isn't boring.

The problem is, these people's minds are starving for a challenge or worthwhile activity. The common saying "Use it or lose it" refers to your mind as well as your body. Exercising your mind is as important to feeling young and energetic as exercising your heart and skeletal muscles. Remember that your mind is a part of your body and that you are a part of the world. If you improve your mind, you improve the world. Use your mind to help you understand the meaning of, and appreciate the value of life, and to express your true spirit to the world around you. Refer back to the emotional health section in chapter nine for more ideas about feeding your mind.

Laziness can cause boredom, lack of meal planning, low self-worth, limited creative expression and a lack of soul food. All of these can lead to overeating, making poor food choices, or alcohol and drug abuse.

Boredom can create a feeling of emptiness and low sense of self-worth because you feel like you are not accomplishing anything worthwhile with your life. This may cause you to be unhappy in your work or personal relationships. After all, what does it matter if you end up broke, divorced or lonely? That is what you feel you deserve and you have the power to create what you deserve. Boredom is also a major cause of depression and you already know what it leads to.

Lack of Soul Food

You will experience a feeling of emptiness if you do not nourish your true self with enough soul food. Eating in an attempt to fill up this empty space leads only to frustration, despair and more feelings of emptiness. Many people turn to alcohol or other drugs when their souls are starving. People also often use foods, drugs or both to escape from feelings they do not want to feel. This creates a negative cycle, because when the deadening effect wears off, they have more feelings they do not want to feel. Attempting to escape is part of most other emotional causes: low self-worth, stress release, fear, depression, not accepting responsibility, boredom and loneliness. Reverse this negative cycle by creating a positive cycle of thoughts and feelings that make you feel good. Instead of deadening your feelings—life is extremely unfulfilling if you do—stimulate and enjoy the positive feelings generated by soul food. This will help you more than anything else and is important to keep you eating healthfully and exercising regularly.

Some people use drugs and stimulating foods in an attempt to feel good, or to feel anything at all. This may appear to work sometimes but is temporary and starts another negative cycle. Once again, the key to reversing this cycle and experiencing true satisfaction and sense of well being is to get an adequate amount of soul food.

If you are unhappy in your job, relationships or life situation, find positive ways to get the fulfillment you need to be healthy. The negative effects of eating unhealthful foods, excess food, drinking or taking drugs will only make *everything* worse.

You lack soul food if you are not experiencing happiness and a sense of fulfillment. Ask yourself some questions and you should be able to figure out what you are missing and then formulate a plan to get it. Do you leave work with a sense of pride in a job well done? Are you fulfilled emotionally and sexually if you are in a romantic relationship? Are your other emotional needs being met? What are they? Do you feel loved, liked and appreciated by yourself and others? Do you feel worthy to be loved? If not, why not? Are you expressing your creativity in your job or in a hobby? These are just a few examples to get you started. You know what makes you feel happy and fulfilled. Write them down and then make a list of the soul food you are getting and what you are missing. Then figure out how to get more and a variety of different kinds. Refer back to the soul food section in chapter nine for more ideas.

The greatest soul food you can experience is feeling loved. This is why you must love yourself and realize that you do not need anyone else's acceptance and approval. Accepting yourself as you are starts numerous positive cycles and improves your life in countless ways.

An Unbalanced Life

Your life is unbalanced if the physical, mental, emotional and spiritual aspects of your being are unequal. If you view each one as a leg of a table, to keep your table level (to keep yourself balanced and healthy) each leg must be kept approximately the same length. Each aspect requires a different amount of time, but it is the balance among them for which you should strive. If the legs are equal in length, the table will be stable and can support a great deal. If your table has legs of different lengths, it will be tilted and unstable. Similarly, it will be difficult to handle life's changes and problems if your four aspects are unequal, but if they are the same, you will have balance in your life and be able to deal more easily with the trials and challenges you create for yourself. Overcoming obstacles is how we learn and get stronger. If you are balanced, you can turn your stumbling blocks into stepping stones as you grow and progress.

If your life is balanced, it is easier to handle the success and happiness you create for yourself. Some people are unable to cope with success. They sometimes turn to drugs and alcohol, which create greater imbalances and a decreased ability to think clearly and act rationally. Some people turn to food and get fat. For example, if a man works hard for his family and makes a large amount of money, he will sabotage his life if he does not feel that he deserves it. If he feels like his family deserves it but not him, he may neglect his health and work himself into an early grave. But, he will leave the money behind for a family he may have also neglected. What do you think his family would prefer, him or the money? It may be difficult to handle the success of losing your excess body fat if your life is unbalanced.

Financial success can lead to obesity. First, it supplies the money to buy excess food and to eat out more often. Second, transportation can be purchased that requires no muscle power. This is more of a factor in certain countries. Third, working excessively steals time so none is left for regular exercise, learning who you really are, or for getting enough soul food. Fourth, too much work causes physical and emotional fatigue and stress. This may stimulate you to eat or use drugs to regain your energy or use alcohol or other drugs to reduce your stress, when most often all you really need is a brief change of scenery and activity. Remember that Nature wants you to experience success in all areas of life, not just the financial.

Being unbalanced is essentially malnutrition of one or more of the aspects of your being and any part that is out of balance has detrimental effects on the others. If you want to be a whole, balanced and healthy person, they must all be in balance. Your physical body will malfunction and be unable to reflect your spirit accurately if it does not get the nutrients and exercise it needs. If you are tired or hurting, you will not have the patience to act with love from your true spirit. If you fail to keep your physical body healthy and strong, it will be difficult to handle the mental, emotional and spiritual stresses you experience. Physical health helps keep your spirit in tune with your environment and the people and other creatures around you. Besides affecting your spirit, a physical imbalance has a negative impact on your mental and emotional well-being. An athlete who overdoes the physical at the expense of the others may end up a financial failure due to a lack of education, or may create destruction in his life because of emotional immaturity or a lack of meaning in his life.

If your mental growth and stimulation are lacking, it will have a negative impact on your physical, emotional and spiritual well-being. If you do not learn how to take care of your body, your diet will be poor and you will not give your body the exercise it needs to function normally. As you have learned, this will be detrimental to all parts of your being, including the mental. You will be bored if you are not challenging yourself mentally. This often leads to overeating and negatively affects all four aspects of your being. Some people spend excessive time on mental development at the expense of the others. They may be brilliant, but lonely and sad because of bad health, poor social skills or a lack of purpose in life. Are you starting to get the picture of how important it is to have balance among your four aspects? Some of this may seem redundant but this principle is so important that I want to make sure you truly understand it.

Unless you strive to understand and properly express your emotions, you can cause terrible havoc in your own life and the lives of those around you. All aspects of your being will suffer. You already know what a tremendous impact a minor nutritional deficiency can have on us emotionally and how physical exercise makes us feel better emotionally. Now, consider this: our emotions also need exercise. Unfortunately, many of us either rarely exercise our emotions or do it improperly. It is important to learn to enjoy our positive emotions and to understand and express our negative emotions in healthy ways. The positive emotions of joy, curiosity, fulfillment, accomplishment, laughter, appreciation, satisfaction, happiness, love and others need to be used or they will become weak and ineffective. Without these feelings, it is impossible to live a satisfying life. Like physical exercise, emotional exercise has numerous benefits. The feelings we have while experiencing positive emotions uplift us mentally. This makes us want to do something creative with our mind, improves our physical health and brings joy to our spirit. Your spirit rejoices when true positive emotions are felt, because it is being accurately expressed at that time. The feelings we have when exercising our positive emotions are vital nutrients for our entire being. Sadly, many of us are extremely deficient in these nutrients.

What about the influence our negative emotions have on us? In essence they are all forms of fear created by self-judgment. We have already discussed the need to stop being judgmental, but we must also understand the emotion of fear. When we experience negative emotions, we need to express them in positive ways by learning to see the truth of the situation. For example, if a man is afraid to lose the love of his wife, he may verbally or physically abuse her whenever anything happens that triggers his insecure feelings. When his wife finally gets tired of the abuse and decides to leave him, he will be either afraid to face that fact, afraid to be alone, or afraid to face the reality that he has driven her away with his fear-based behaviors. One fear often creates something else to be afraid of and starts another negative cycle.

When you face and eliminate your fears with love, you can rid yourself of the consequences of these negative cycles. If this man truly cares about his wife's happiness, he will talk to her rationally and find out what she is feeling. He may find out, if he shares his feelings honestly *and* really listens to her, that his abuse is driving her away. He now has the choice of eliminating his destructive behaviors and perhaps resolving the problem. If he is afraid of being alone, it is because he has imbalance among the four parts of his being. If he does not feel worthy of the love and companionship she gives him, he will sabotage the relationship to punish himself. He may find that their goals have changed and they do not want the same things anymore. This may have been one of his fears. If this is the case, the best thing to do is split up so each can have a chance at finding happiness. It may be emotionally painful for a while, but in the long run will be the best for both of them.

The underlying cause of these problems is the lack of the man's emotional development. If he has not exercised his negative emotions properly throughout life and learned to understand and express them in a constructive way, he will react similarly to the way he did when he was five years old. Now, however, the temper tantrum designed to get his way (to eliminate his fear) takes the form of physical or verbal abuse of his wife instead of crying or lying on the floor kicking his feet and holding his breath. If this man had exercised his negative emotions and learned to experience and express them truthfully, he would be more emotionally mature and probably not having problems in his relationship. It would have improved the physical, mental and spiritual aspects of his being as well.

We all have masculine and feminine sides. When a woman is stuck in her problem-solving male side, her most common reaction is to eat if she fails to get the nurturing and support she needs to move back into her female side. Unfortunately, this just temporarily suppresses her painful feelings of insecurity. Eating becomes an easy replacement for love, but just treats her symptoms and can easily become addictive. Loving herself, learning to express her own emotions properly and getting adequate soul food will help her tremendously. To learn more about how to resolve this problem and to understand the new challenges that face us in male/female relationships I highly recommend the book or audiocassettes, *What Your Mother Couldn't Tell You & Your Father Didn't Know*, by John Gray, Ph.D.

Many more examples could be given of how negative emotions are expressed in harmful ways, but why don't you exercise your mind and think of some yourself. Write down the ones that are causing problems for you. Here are a few negative emotions to get you started—apprehension, fright, concern, discouragement, panic, frustration, rejection, despair, dread, anxiety, misgiving, jealousy, disappointment, foreboding, hate, fear, envy, dismay, guilt, worry, regret and even conditional love. An especially destructive one is blame. Regret is blame toward yourself. Asking yourself what you are afraid of often makes the true problem clear. Once you see the reality of any situation, you can then formulate a plan to resolve it. Remember our invisible monster with no teeth? You have been given numerous examples of how fear can be the cause of overeating and some ideas about how to eliminate your fears.

Do not keep your emotions, good or bad, bottled up inside. This is harmful to your health and negatively affects your self-image, leading to overeating or other destructive behaviors. Learn to define, acknowledge and accept your emotions and feelings. They are a natural part of you. Relax and let them flow through you, but do not just react like a programmed machine. Act instead of react and think before you act. Postpone doing anything until you have determined a positive way to express what you are feeling. Learn to express your emotions truthfully with acceptance of yourself and others. If you are frustrated with your boss or with rush-hour traffic, do not go home and yell at your spouse and children or kick your dog. Discuss your frustration with your spouse or a friend and determine together how to resolve the situation. Learn to communicate your feelings tactfully and lovingly to others and yourself. Remember that self-judgment is the source of your negative emotions, so do not put yourself down for all your perceived faults and failures.

Keep in mind that we always do our best and that our best is constantly fluctuating based on what we have eaten, how rested we are, circumstances of the moment and numerous other variables. Understanding this can help you to stop judging and putting yourself down. What we should all strive for is to make our best progressively better.

Whenever you experience a negative emotion, be thankful for the opportunity to understand yourself better and to grow more emotionally balanced and mature. Learning how to deal constructively with negative emotions helps you to eliminate or control them instead of letting them control you. There will be many benefits from doing this. Because faith created by love is the opposite of fear, love is the way to overcome all fear-based emotional causes for being fat. Keep this in mind as you strive to find and eliminate yours. Replace negative emotions and feelings with positive ones like wonder, curiosity, enthusiasm and the most powerful—appreciation. Learn to appreciate everything and everyone in your life no matter how insignificant it or any person may seem. Eliminating negative emotions reduces your stress tremendously, and experiencing more positive emotions adds to your enjoyment of the precious gift that we call life.

People may have put a great deal of effort into learning to lovingly express their negative emotions. They may be relatively balanced in the emotional part of their lives if they have also learned to experience joy from their positive emotions. Unfortunately, some people have concentrated so much on their emotions that the other parts of their being have been neglected leading to unbalanced lives.

You already know how important it is to get enough soul food. Now you should be able to see how important it is to your physical, mental and emotional health and well-being. Feeding your spirit with positive feelings helps you to understand Nature and the wonderful balance it has created. It helps you to see your place and to be a well-rounded and balanced part of your world. When you are in harmony with Nature, life has meaning and great value. It is easy to understand why things happen the way they do and to know that you have the power to create the life you want. The key is to let your true spirit create your life, because it alone knows what is best for you. Your false worldly programming can never create all you need to be happy. You can create many of the things your programming tells you that you want, but it will never be what you really need. You will still have the feeling that the true key to happiness is missing. Even if you have fame, fortune and companionship, there will be no meaning to, or satisfaction in your life if your soul is starving. If you are expressing your true self, you should primarily experience only one emotion—joy.

A good way to stay balanced is to avoid extremes, because an excess of anything causes an imbalance of some kind. Too much of a certain mineral causes an imbalance among it and other minerals. Excess food creates imbalance between the muscle and fat composition of the body. Overworking produces imbalance in the lives of those who do it and in the lives of their friends and family members. Excessive speed in a car leads to an imbalance between the skill of the driver and the driving conditions. Too much or too frequent exercise can cause injuries and joint imbalances that lead to chronic pain and suffering. Even an excess of money can create an imbalance between what people have and what they feel they deserve. You may have heard of at least one person who has millions of dollars but lives in extreme filth and poverty. I recently saw an example of this on the news and the woman had a number of advanced college degrees. The bottom line is that any imbalance is detrimental to your health and happiness.

You will be unbalanced if one or more aspects of your being fail to keep up with the others. It can also happen if one or more are overdone. If a man is obsessed with health, he may exercise excessively and be fanatical with his diet. He may have a great body but be sadly lacking in the other aspects of his being. Think about the stereotypical absent-minded professor who is so engrossed in the mental that he is extremely lacking in the physical, emotional and spiritual components of his life. You already know how various emotional excesses can prevent us from developing in other areas.

Even the spiritual can be overdone to the detriment of the others. What happens if a man does mostly spiritual study or meditation? He may be limited in how to deal with his emotions, deficient in mental growth and stimulation and have an out of shape, fat body. If he is fanatical, he will be unbalanced and will create problems for himself and others. What good is spiritual knowledge if he is unhealthy, illiterate or unable to communicate his insight to others? How close to Nature is a man who defiles the temple (body) he has been given by eating junk food or eating to excess? If he is in tune with Nature, he will have all the legs of his table even and be living a happy, productive and balanced life.

Physical, Verbal or Sexual Abuse

Being physically, verbally or sexually abused either as a child or as an adult can cause people to get and stay fat for one or more of the previous reasons. They may feel the need to punish themselves for what they label as "bad" behavior or for being unable to prevent it from having happened or from still happening. Being less attractive reduces the amount of attention a woman gets from men and reduces feelings of guilt, fear, blame and anxiety. These people may lose fat when the desire for an intimate relationship gets strong, but when they start looking good, their negative feelings increase and they gain it back. The yo-yo effect this causes is harmful to the self-image and the body.

For many people, abuse causes depression and lowers their self-worth. It can make them feel unworthy of being loved or of enjoying the benefits of a lean and healthy body. Gaining fat could be a form of protection or an attempt to make themselves less attractive, thereby reducing the chance of being sexually assaulted. It may give some a feeling of power to resist future attacks. Others may feel emotionally weak and unable to take responsibility for the health of their bodies. Some abused people may deprive themselves of soul food and live unbalanced and unhappy lives.

Some people may be able to use self-help books and audiotapes to rid themselves of the negative feelings created from abuse. Many people, however, will need professional assistance to eliminate the destructive feelings they are directing at themselves.

Loneliness

Being alone is a physical state that has nothing to do with feeling lonely. Some people can be alone and feel happy and fulfilled, yet others can be surrounded by a crowd of family and friends and feel terribly unhappy, isolated and lonely. We are social beings and need interaction with others to varying degrees. Some of us, however, have learned to be happy just being with ourselves, but others have not. Take a look at your soul-food list. Some of the activities can be shared with others but many cannot and almost all can be done alone. If you think about it, you will realize that we are always alone in our own private world created by our past thoughts and current perceptions. You may share a physical event with someone but you will each experience it very differently.

Feeling lonely can cause stress and feelings of inadequacy, not belonging, being unworthy, not being loved, being misunderstood and numerous others. Any of these negative feelings can lead to alcohol and drug abuse, overeating, or not caring enough to make wise food choices. Some people may see food as their only friend. Many people use "comfort" foods—usually stimulants—in an attempt to feel the healthful stimulation that comes from leading a positive and productive life, from enjoyable activities (alone or with others) and from feeling loved. I believe that many people are uncomfortable being alone because they need constant feedback from others to feel that they are all right. You need to learn to understand yourself and know who you really are. Once you love who you really are, you will not need frequent feedback and support from others because you will not be constantly doubting or putting yourself down and because you will be getting positive feedback and loving support from yourself.

Your conditioned self may feel lonely but your true self is not because it is in touch with and a part of Nature. This is another reason why it is important to discover and live as your true self. When you no longer feel lonely, you will find yourself enjoying everything in your life more fully. It will not matter if you are alone, with one person or in a crowd. You will feel more in tune with everything and everyone. You will eventually realize that you are a vital part of Nature who came into this world alone, lived in your own private world alone and will someday leave this physical world behind—leaving alone, but going once again to be with others.

Be cautious with whom you associate, and never give your company or your
confidence to those of whose good principles you are not sure.
William Hart Coleridge

The happiness of your life depends upon the quality of your thoughts,
therefore guard accordingly; and take care that you
entertain no notions unsuitable to virtue and reasonable nature.
Marcus Antoninus

The most wasted of all days is the day when we have not laughed.
French Proverb

If there is to be any peace it will come through being, not having.
Henry Miller

Better face a danger once than always be in fear.
English Proverb

Two things a man should never be angry at:
what he can help and what he cannot.
English Proverb

thirteen

Being Lean

You have learned how to eat healthfully and about many reasons why people gain and maintain excess body fat. Now it is time to develop a specific plan to lose your excess fat and to then easily maintain your new lean shape. You have seen repetition of certain ideas throughout this book. I did this on purpose, because most people need exposure to these key concepts a few times before they finally sink in and become a part of their "inner knowing." You may understand a concept when it is explained a certain way, but someone else may not grasp it until it is expressed in a different way. You may have to read the chapters dealing with causes several times before you finally determine your reason for having excess fat. It may take that long to recognize it, develop the honesty to accept it, or find your reason to take action. If it takes a while, do not feel slow or stupid and put yourself down. It has nothing to do with your I.Q. or learning ability. Accept yourself completely and without judgment. Remember that all success is based on repetition and that I want you to be successful. If you are not, reread your highlighted areas or the entire book. Keep reading until you finally *learn* what you need to know to succeed.

Most people fail to lose fat permanently because they have not learned how to use the tremendous powers at their disposal to work for them instead of against them. They follow the latest fad diet or waste money on "miracle" potions they are told will magically melt away their fat. They do not eliminate the root cause, because this requires something most people fear—changing themselves. Some of these diets and potions help people lose weight, but the results are short-lived because they usually go back to the old habits that made them fat in the first place. It is easy to see why most people fail. It is like giving all the rich people's money to the poor people. It would not be long before the rich people had the money back, because they know how to make and keep money but the poor people do not. Likewise, if you transferred all the fat people's excess body fat to the lean people, it would not be long before the lean ones were lean and the fat ones fat again. That's because lean people know how to be lean and fat people do not. The key is attaining the knowledge that gives you the power. If you were poor and learned what rich people know about money, you may be able to use that knowledge to get rich. You now have the knowledge of how to lose your excess fat and stay lean. You have the power—*all you have to do is choose to use it.*

You now know that accomplishing your goal is simply a matter of finding a reason, eliminating the cause, learning how to eat properly, using your six powers to work for you, exercising regularly and correctly, and feeling you deserve to be lean and healthy. To help you find a reason, you have been given a tremendous number of benefits you will enjoy if you lose your excess fat. You know how to develop the right eating program for your body, have learned how to discover and eliminate your cause and have been given many ways to develop the feelings that you deserve a lean and healthy body. You know that following a natural and balanced way of eating has kept people lean and healthy for thousands of years.

We are going to go over the six steps to accomplishing your goal of achieving and maintaining a lean and healthy body. Then I will teach you more about being lean and healthy for the rest of your life.

Here are the six steps to permanent fat loss and super health:

1. Find Your Reason to Be Lean
2. Discover and Eliminate Your Causes for Excess Body Fat
3. Learn What, Why, How and When to Eat and Drink
4. Harness the Six Powers that Make People Fat to Make You Lean
5. Shape and Strengthen Your Body
6. Be a Lean Person

Step 1—Find Your Reason to Be Lean
[Desire]

The first step to achieving permanent fat loss is to find your reason to be lean, because until you have a good reason, you will not even start looking for the cause. As you read on, keep in mind that it should be easier to have a reason to be lean than to have a reason to be fat.

Many of us find motivation by thinking about attaining and enjoying what we want. We are goal-oriented and work toward acquiring what we feel has value. If this is how you are motivated, write down all the benefits you will enjoy from being lean and healthy. Under each benefit list the reasons why you want the benefit. One major advantage is living longer and being in better shape as you get older. Life can be as enjoyable when you are old as when you are young if you are healthy and fit. Think about it. What is worth more than health and life? How much would a billionaire pay for another year or two of *vital* life?

Think about why you want to live longer. Perhaps so you can accomplish more with your life, or so you can travel more and do all the other things you have been postponing until you have the time and money to do them. Your reason may be to spend more time with your spouse or not to become a burden to anyone. Maybe you want to be there for your children and grandchildren. List everything of value to you in order of its importance. List what truly motivates you and makes losing your excess fat a high priority in your life. Doing it *for yourself*, because you know you deserve all the benefits, must be included. If it is not, you do not feel worthy and will surely fail.

Another good reason for being leaner is to be healthier throughout your *entire* life. You can be more physically active if you are leaner and stronger. In fact, more physical activity is what helps keep you lean and strong. Carrying less fat around will decrease, or prevent, pain and excessive wear and tear in your knees, hips, feet and other joints. Because excess fat increases the risk of almost all health problems, being lean lowers your chances of developing minor diseases as well as life-threatening conditions such as heart disease, stroke, diabetes and cancer. Your sex drive and performance will be better and you will be able to keep participating in sports and other physical activities you enjoy. Add these and other benefits that are important to you to your list.

Another reason for being leaner is to be more attractive. Your beautiful spirit will be expressed more closely through your physical body and you will be able to wear more flattering and fashionable clothes. Remember Dr. Maltz's examples where altering someone's nose slightly or making other physical changes led to dramatic self-image improvements. The physical changes were usually minor but often had tremendous impact on how his patients felt about themselves. Their lives changed dramatically for the better. Losing 10 pounds may make you feel so much better about yourself that the next 30 should be even easier to lose. You may have seen before and after photos of people who have lost 50 or more pounds. Their appearances often change so dramatically it is almost unbelievable. Imagine the positive effect this change has on how they feel about themselves. Think about how much better you will feel physically *and* emotionally. Your improved self-image will enhance all areas of your life and make it easy to live a natural, healthy lifestyle.

You may be a person who considers your body as a temple that houses your spirit. If so, keeping your temple clean inside and attractive outside is important for the health of your spirit and improves your harmony with Nature. If you think of your body as a vehicle that carries your spirit, you can take care of it and get good service for a long time or you can abuse it and it will soon be falling apart and ready for the junkyard (graveyard).

We are moved to action by wanting to belong, feel secure, be admired, and feel warmth and love. Understanding this may help you to find your reason or reasons to be lean. Refer to chapter one for more benefits of losing excess body fat and add to your list the ones that are important to you. After you find your reason(s), keep your list so you can use it during the visualization sessions explained in chapter fourteen.

As you search for your reason to be lean, keep in mind that most of us have been conditioned to believe that wanting is bad or selfish. Because most of us do not want to feel like we are bad or selfish, we often avoid these uncomfortable feelings by not wanting. Sadly, this often leads many people to not want to be lean and healthy.

Not everyone is motivated by striving to achieve goals. Some people's motivations come primarily from avoiding what they do not want. They want to avoid the stares and laughter of others or eliminate suffering with painful feet and knees. They may not want the excess sweating, bad breath and bad body odor that come from a poor diet and excess fat. A good way to find things you want to avoid is to reverse the benefits. For example, if you are goal-motivated, you may want smooth, healthy skin, but if you are avoidance-motivated, you may want to avoid ugly, oily and loose skin, premature wrinkles and age spots. If you are avoidance-motivated, you may already know many things you do not want. Think about all the negative things that losing your excess body fat and internal waste will eliminate. Make a list of what you want to avoid so you can use it during your visualization sessions. Also include why you want to avoid the things on your list. You may end up with a list of things you do want and another list of things you do not want.

Do not use fear as a motivator. Fear develops in the absence of love and you want the motivation for everything you do to come from love. Fear is extremely negative, harms our health, and does not work that well as a motivator. Think about the person with emphysema who continues to smoke. Even when fear motivation seems to work, the results are usually only temporary. Both motivation methods I have explained are positive and developed from what we want; they just go about getting it differently. Each one works, because it stimulates you to action. Use the better one for you or perhaps a combination of the two. Your spirit and mind work only in positive ways to create what you want, so your new thoughts and behaviors should come from focusing on the positive side of everything.

Many people give up on losing excess fat after failing one or more times, because the methods they use are not natural, balanced, healthy or positive. Almost all "weight-loss" programs create struggle and conflict, which are two things the majority of us want to avoid if we can. Most people have enough things in life they are struggling against, so losing body fat is not another one they want to face. It is often a low priority, because they feel they will never win the war even if they do occasionally win a battle. Many of our struggles help us to grow and get stronger, but temporary weight loss makes us feel weaker. You now know that it should not be a struggle or require will power. Just find your reason to be lean and then make it a priority in your life.

The other steps should then follow naturally and put you on your way to enjoying the benefits of being cleaner and leaner.

Some people are unable to find or eliminate their causes for being fat. They may be unable to do it on their own or may never get the right help from someone knowledgeable. If you cannot eliminate your cause, do not give up hope, because an alternative exists. It is not as natural as eliminating the cause, but it can help you. It is a simple concept. You will lose your excess fat if your reason to be lean is stronger than your reason to be fat. There may be a bit of struggle occasionally but the combination of working toward an important goal and having a powerful reason can often overpower the cause. After you lose the fat, the cause may simply drop away or be easily eliminated. For example, if your cause is a low self-image, after you lose the fat your self-image will improve and the cause will be gone. Numerous physical causes may be resolved as your body cleanses out fat and internal waste. Finding your reason to be lean must be your first priority, because it is the key to achieving your goal.

Step 2—Discover and Eliminate Your Causes for Excess Body Fat
[Non-resistance]

Eliminating your causes for having excess fat is the second step and a vital one. As you just learned, this step may be skipped initially, but it is much better if it is completed as soon as possible. I am sure you noticed the word "causes" was used instead of "cause." This is because a physical cause such as hypothyroidism leads to fatigue, a slower metabolism and easy weight gain, which in turn causes depression and lower self-worth. On the other hand, depression and low self-worth can lead to overeating and excess fat that cause fatigue, inefficient thyroid function and a slower metabolism. Therefore, everyone has at least one physical and one emotional cause for having excess fat.

One primary cause generally starts the negative cycle, but after they are created, all causes must be eliminated or the whole cycle could start again. If you do not determine and eliminate your causes, you may make temporary progress and even maintain it for a long time by following the eating guidelines in this book. But it will be a constant struggle to eat well. Remember that being lean is the natural way of your body and should be as simple and effortless as breathing. If you are struggling, you are fighting against a cause of some kind. Eliminate it and keep in mind that you now know how to reverse the effects of different negative cycles by replacing them with positive cycles.

If you have not determined your causes yet, reread chapters eleven and twelve. Going through them with a trusted friend is often helpful. A lean friend may be best, but it doesn't matter as long as your friend is completely honest with you. If your friend is fat, it would be helpful if you are both reading this book. This way, you can help each other in looking for your individual causes. You can support one another with this step and perhaps some of the others.

Write down your feelings about being fat. Describe how it makes you feel about yourself, your life and the people around you. Write how you believe others see you and about other aspects of your life affected by your body being fat. Then start a paragraph with "I am fat, because…" "I deserve to be fat, because…" or "I do not deserve to be lean and healthy, because…" What you write may furnish the clues to discover why you are fat.

Another way to develop insight into your emotional reason(s) is to look yourself in the eye in a mirror and say out loud, "I accept myself 100 percent unconditionally as I am now." Then just be quiet and listen to the voice in your head (your false programming) telling you why you cannot do it. Your false programming will give you reasons why you are not good enough to be accepted as you are. I hope by now you are starting to truly believe and feel that you are good enough and that you always have been.

You may want to express your feelings to your personal Higher Power or to yourself while looking in a mirror. Share your secret fears, angers and wants. Talk out loud and you may determine your emotional cause for being fat.

You may have said or heard, "She's fat but has a pretty face." Many fat people do have attractive faces and would have attractive bodies if they let go of their excess fat. Yes, you read correctly. They must *let go* of their excess fat before it can be eliminated. You may lose some weight with every diet you go on, but will always gain it back if you have an emotional need to be fat. The diets are done only to create the illusion that you want to lose your excess fat. Therefore, you must make sure that you eliminate your cause once you find it.

You may want to seek help from a qualified hypnotherapist if you cannot find your emotional cause. Some people use hypnosis to "lose weight." It is often done primarily as an attempt to fight against an unknown cause or to program you to eat in a particular way that may or may not be healthful. I believe this is an ineffective way to use such a powerful tool. The weight-loss protocol normally followed is a form of programming. Remember that your self-hypnotic programming is what created your emotional cause. Programming the subconscious mind to fight against a hidden cause may create an inner conflict that leads to frustration and overeating. It is best to get rid of the conditioned behaviors you already have, not create more.

Hypnosis is one of the best tools (if you choose to use it) to help determine and eliminate your emotional cause(s). You can use it to rid yourself of the programming that is keeping you fat. Doing this in conjunction with applying the eating and exercise advice found in this book could be an unbeatable combination. If you know of another method of communicating with your subconscious mind, use it to help find and get rid of your emotional cause(s). I sometimes use applied kinesiology for this purpose.

If the primary cause for your excess fat is physical, you need to find a competent doctor to help you. Look for someone who has the knowledge and methods to permanently restore the lost balance in your body and return it to proper function. The doctor should do this in a natural way by reestablishing normal nerve and blood flow to your internal glands and organs and by having you use whole foods, herbs and other natural products.

Normal function can usually be restored using one or more of the healing therapies I practice. Unfortunately, not many doctors practice Neurovascular Dynamics and as of this writing, I have trained only one other doctor to do PMBT, the only therapy I know of that can restore normal nerve flow permanently. A few effective emotional clearing and balancing techniques are available, and doctors who use applied kinesiology properly or who are skilled in electroacupuncture testing can determine the right foods and supplements for you. Drugs should be used only as a last resort, because they almost always create imbalance and new problems.

Step 3—Learn What, Why, How and When to Eat and Drink
[Knowledge]

If you have read the previous chapters of this book, you have learned what, why, how and when to eat and drink. You now understand the simplicity of eating healthfully and know that following my program will gradually reduce your internal waste and excess body fat as you move toward your normal, natural body composition. You know how to reverse the negative cycle of inefficient digestion and utilization. In chapter six you learned why it is important to develop an eating program to supply the unique needs of your body. You also learned ways to determine what is best for you. Most of the meals you share with others can be similar except for occasional minor differences determined by each person's specific needs and digestive capabilities. Ideally your whole family should follow this program, because it is difficult if one person is eating foods loaded with unhealthful fat and refined sugar and the others are eating nutritious foods. It is even harder if only one is eating healthfully. Everyone eating well not only helps the fat ones to lose excess fat but keeps the others from gaining.

You have learned that if you follow the nutritional laws of Nature that you will reap the benefits of a lean and attractive body, better health and most likely a longer and more vital life. You also know that if you break these laws that you will suffer the consequences of living in a fat body, having poor health and dying many years premature. You have also learned that the choice is yours. Which results are you going to choose?

Step 4—Harness the Six Powers that Make People Fat to Make You Lean
[Creation or Control]

Throughout this book you have been learning various ways to harness the awesome powers of Nature, habit, inertia, momentum, your subconscious mind and love to work for you instead of against you. In upcoming chapters I will explain even more about using these powers to create positive cycles to reverse the effects of the negative cycles currently working against you.

Step 5—Shape and Strengthen Your Body
[Work, Use or Action]

You have learned that your body was designed to be used and will weaken and age faster if it is not. Exercising to build and maintain strength and muscle mass helps keep your metabolism normal and your body looking and feeling younger and more attractive. It also makes you more capable of physical work and play and more resistant to injury, stress and other physical problems.

You must exercise regularly if you want to be lean, healthy and stay vital as time passes. Exercise can help you reach your goal whether you enjoy it or not. If you hate to exercise, you may eat better so less exercise, especially fat-burning exercise, will be needed to accomplish your goal. Some people say they love to exercise because it feels so good when they stop. If this is your motivation, it's fine. Over time, you may start to enjoy exercising, because of how it makes you feel—strong, vital and alive. If you vary your exercise routine and do many activities you enjoy, it will not get boring and your body will respond better. A productive workout reduces stress and gives you a healthy sense of accomplishment.

I cannot stress enough how important regular strength-building exercise is and, contrary to what you may have heard or been taught, it does not take a great deal of time if done efficiently. Initially you should do a strength-training program to rebuild or increase your lean body mass and normalize your metabolism. Building some muscle makes your body look shapelier when the fat is gone and helps you lose body fat faster. You will be stronger and more capable of doing physical work or play and your body will be more resistant to disease and traumatic or overstress injuries. Until you have lost your excess fat, you may also want to do some fat-burning exercise. After you reach your goal, it is a good idea to do some cardiovascular training in addition to your strength training. You will no longer need to do fat-burning exercise.

Exercise is a vital part of the physical aspect of your being and helps keep it in balance with the mental, emotional and spiritual aspects. Strength-building exercise also reduces emotional and mental stress.

Step 6—Be a Lean Person
[Being]

Most of us have been programmed to believe that we must first *have* something, such as a lean body or a million dollars, before we can *do* what lean people or millionaires do and only then can we *be* lean or *be* a millionaire. This is like swimming upstream. It is difficult to achieve anything this way, because it is opposite of the truth. The way of Nature is BE—DO—HAVE. This means you must first *be* something, then *do* what they do before you *have* what they have. Be a lean person, then do what lean people do and you will have what they each have—a lean body.

Developing thinking patterns based on the truth will change your behaviors, your body and your life. This section gives you ideas about how to eliminate your unhealthy thinking patterns and behaviors and develop a lean consciousness and new health habits. You will learn how to be a lean person instead of a fat one.

You experience positive or negative consequences from everything you eat and drink and from how and when you consume it. Therefore, a simple health habit is to look at everything you plan to ingest and ask yourself one simple question: "Will ingesting this food or drink at this time help me get leaner, healthier and live a longer more satisfying life?" You should have enough knowledge by now to know whether something is going to help you or hinder you. Keep in mind that junk food takes up space where nutritious food should be and has negative effects on your health and well-being. Eating it makes you feel weak-willed and discouraged, so you may also want to ask yourself how every food and drink is going to make you feel emotionally.

Another helpful activity is to share your knowledge and experience to help someone else lose their excess body fat. When you help others, you get as much benefit or more. Helping friends or family members discover their causes for being fat and their reasons to be lean may help you determine your own. Helping others makes you feel better about yourself and improves your self-image. This may be what you need to break your own inertia and get you moving toward your goal. And, whenever you teach someone else, you develop a better understanding at the same time. If someone you are helping looks up to you as a role model, your success is going to motivate that person, especially in the beginning when it is needed the most. If a celebrity loses some fat, millions of people have an interest in how it was accomplished. Even though you may not be famous, you never know how many people you may inspire by your success. You may even end up on television telling your success story to millions.

Create a Lean Mental Attitude and Lifestyle

Because thinking always precedes action, you must change your thinking and mental attitude before any physical transformation can take place. As your attitude and thinking (mostly about yourself) improve, so will your lifestyle.

You will not eat a quart of ice cream every night in front of the television or have a cookie jar in the kitchen that always seems to need replenishing. Instead, you will start exercising regularly and developing other healthy habits.

Any permanent alteration in you or your life causes a change in your lifestyle. If you get married or divorced, your lifestyle changes. If you move from an apartment to a house, get a new job or move to a new city, your lifestyle must be modified. Every life change requires an alteration of lifestyle. Never fear change. Life is nothing more than one evolution, or change, after another. This is what keeps it fresh and exciting. Children usually find life more exciting than adults do, because they experience more changes in their lives and in themselves. People who resist change get bored with their lives and live in depressing ruts that are nothing more than long graves. Many of these people become bitter, antisocial and unhappy. A large percentage of them get fat and create other health problems with their negative and destructive emotions.

You will stay fat if you fear change. It may be fear that is keeping the fat locked in the body you now inhabit. Remember that you are not your body but you do have a great deal of control over what it looks like and how well it functions. It is up to you to decide to change what you dislike. The decision itself empowers you and eliminates your fear. Now, not only will your body transform by getting leaner and healthier, but your entire life will also blossom. You will climb out of your rut and start enjoying more of the wonderful experiences life has to offer. Life becomes a joy and starts giving you everything you need to create and maintain the lean, healthy body you want.

Most fat people tend to have similar habits that are usually opposite of the habits of most lean people. Below is a list of the most common ones. Many people have all the habits that cause excess fat gain but few people have all the habits that make and keep us lean. Comparing them will give you numerous ideas about habits that need changing and how they need to be changed. You will probably do fine if you change most of your habits to those in the right column. For example, I often work late and do not sit down to dinner until eight or nine p.m. This is a bad habit but I easily stay lean because I follow the other habits of lean people and eat earlier on my days off.

Common habits of fat people	versus	Common habits of lean people
Skip breakfast or have a donut and coffee		Eat a relatively nutritious breakfast
Eat concentrated, high-calorie (acidic) foods		Eat mostly natural, low-calorie (alkaline) foods
Rarely, if ever, exercise		Exercise regularly
Do some non-productive exercise		Do strength-building exercise
Usually eat dessert		Often skip dessert

Eat a few large meals every day	Eat five or six smaller meals daily
Eat most foods in the afternoon or evening	Eat foods throughout the day
Eat dinner late	Eat dinner early
Eat everything and often have seconds	Often leave some food
Eat foods fast	Eat foods slowly
Eat unhealthful snacks in the evening	Eat healthful snacks during the day
Do not chew foods thoroughly	Chew foods thoroughly
Eat a limited variety of foods	Eat a wide variety of foods
Talk and think about food frequently	Talk about, think about and accomplish creative and productive pursuits
Play the role of the victim with no responsibility or control over personal health	Accept responsibility for and take control of personal health
Eat more fatty red meats	Eat fewer, and leaner, cuts of red meat
Give children excess food and eat the leftovers	Do not give their children excess food
Eat more dairy and processed foods	Eat less dairy and processed foods
Often eat at or order out from fast-food chains	Usually eat at home or eat at good restaurants
Often drink junk liquids	Seldom drink junk liquids
Often have a late night snack	Rarely eat late at night
Wear baggy, unflattering clothes	Wear more form-fitting, attractive clothes
Live to eat	Eat to live

It should be fairly easy to see why fat people are fat and many of the lean ones lean. I want you to take the time right now to go over each habit on these lists and explain to yourself why it creates either fat gain or fat loss. If you cannot explain them, finish reading this book and do the lists again. If you still cannot explain them, start at the beginning and read your highlighted areas and then do it again. Unless you are a super genius, chances are you missed a great deal the first time through. Remember that this book is like a textbook designed to impart knowledge that will benefit you for the rest of your life. The material must be studied until it is *learned*, not just read once.

Make a list of all the habits you have and the new ones you want to develop. Do not forget to list any unique habits you may have. Then determine the most important ones and what you want to change first. The body thrives on the regularity and balance that good health habits help maintain.

If you do not change your mental attitude, thinking patterns and lifestyle, you may lose some fat but will just be a fat person in a thinner body. It will be a constant struggle to maintain your fat loss and you will feel like an impostor. This lowers your self-image, decreases normal body functions and inhibits your enjoyment of life. You may associate with people less because of your fear of being exposed. You may get depressed because you feel like a phony. You could easily become pessimistic and prevent yourself from accomplishing many goals you have the talent to achieve. These feelings can cause you to quickly gain back fat to avoid what you fear.

Do not think of yourself as a thin person living in a fat body. You must drop any labels, because they are all false and limiting. You are a spiritual being, neither fat nor thin. Your body would be lean if you were physically expressing your true nature, because it is the healthiest and most efficient way. It is how your body was designed to be. Being leaner should help you get more in touch with your spirit and help you drop the false worldly programming that is controlling you and creating a life incapable of producing happiness. True happiness and inner peace are never experienced unless they are created from the truth within you. If you let yourself just *be*, your spirit will create for you the things in life that will lead to inner peace, harmony and happiness. You will enjoy lasting fat loss. Worldly programming can attract great wealth and power, yet there will always be a feeling of emptiness inside begging to be filled. Some countries' leaders constantly seek attention and more power in an attempt to give their lives meaning. Sadly, they often fail to improve the lives of their people, which is what would give them what they are missing.

Get excited. You are about to embark on a wonderful adventure—a metamorphosis like the slow-moving, always-eating, fat caterpillar becoming a lean, beautiful butterfly soaring high and expressing its true nature.

Avoid Fad Diets and Unhealthful Weight-Loss Products

You may be tempted to follow a "crash" diet that promises you will lose excess body fat quickly. Most of us are exposed to at least one a day in some way or another. I strongly recommend against following fad diets or going on weight-loss programs that require you to buy special foods. Following the latest diet craze or buying expensive foods do not help you learn how to eat healthfully. Most of these diets and programs are unhealthful, costly and incapable of providing permanent fat loss. You should be learning to think, feel, act and eat healthfully, and how to maintain or increase your lean body mass.

As far back as the mid-1970s there were more than 17,000 weight-loss programs on public record. Imagine how many there are today, yet more people are fat now than ever. Clearly, what is out there is not working. Even the programs based on sound dietary principles rarely produce lasting results, because they seldom help people to determine and eliminate their physical and emotional causes. Most of them supply only a few of the pieces necessary to solve the permanent fat-loss puzzle.

Some diet programs claim you can eat cakes, pies and other unhealthful and fattening foods and lose weight. Please never fall for this one. It should be obvious they are just trying to sell you something. Sales pitches are used that prey on your vanity or desire to feel better. Magazine and newspaper sales are increased if the headlines are about sex, celebrity gossip, tragedy or "miracle" weight loss. Do not let the media mess with your mind and take away your hopes and desires with empty promises. If it sounds too good to be true, chances are it is. Americans spend more than $33 billion a year in the search for lasting weight loss, yet the number of fat people is growing rapidly. An estimated $117 billion more is spent each year treating health problems caused by excess fat. Stop letting your money be a part of these rapidly growing statistics.

Most fad diets cause a loss of lean body mass that leads to a slower metabolism. This is why most people end up gaining back more fat than they had before. Regaining body fat is especially defeating mentally, because it reinforces negative thinking patterns—the ones that make you believe you are a failure at fat loss, doomed to live in a fat body the rest of your life or that you will always gain the weight back so why even attempt to lose it. Your positively oriented mind resists dieting, because dieting is negative and is trying to make you a "loser."

Some people go out to lunch and order just a salad because they think it is a good way to lose weight. What they usually end up eating is a 500-calorie meal of fat that comes from the salad dressing. The salad provides some vitamins and minerals to help digest and utilize the fat, but *a salad is not a meal*. This is an unhealthful attempt to lose excess body fat, because the fat being ingested is acidic and because many vital nutrients are missing. The body will then often stimulate more eating in an attempt to get those nutrients. A salad is a delicious and nutritious addition to a protein or complex-carbohydrate meal.

Fad diets do not supply the balance of nutrients your body and mind need to function normally. If you crave certain nutrients or cannot think straight, you may overeat because of not caring or as an attempt to get the nutrition your body needs. Some of these diet programs claim you are getting all the vitamins and minerals that scientists have determined you need. This may be true, but mankind's knowledge is sadly lacking, the nutrients are usually artificially added and you will not get all of the enzymes, phytonutrients and other synergistic health-building nutrients that whole, natural foods contain.

Most dietary programs are expensive because you pay for processing, packaging and costly advertising to market their pills or so-called healthful, low-calorie foods. These products are low in calories, but most of them are like processed TV dinners. They have no life force, they have no balance, and they have no place in a healthful nutritional program.

Prolonged dieting creates imbalance in your body's sensitive weight-balancing mechanism. This makes it more difficult to generate or maintain fat loss. Frequent dieting also leads to worry, stress and nutrient deficiencies that often stimulate bingeing or overeating. This in turn leads to guilt, lower self-esteem and even more overeating.

Chances are you have followed more than one diet in your life and already know that they do not work. If any had worked more than temporarily, I doubt you would be reading this book. Let's go over some of the specific reasons why diets fail so you can see why it was not your fault and so you will not be tempted to follow others in the future.

Counting Calories is Negative

I strongly recommend against counting calories. First of all, it is extremely negative and your mind is positive. It forces you to focus on what you are not getting and how limited your nutritional choices are instead of what you are getting and the vast and varied choices you do have. Second, counting calories is time-consuming so few people will keep doing it. Third, it does not usually work—at least not for long—because your body simply adapts to the lower calories. Then, if you eat more calories, you can easily add fat, even though you are eating a relatively low number of calories. Nowadays, most people who recommend counting calories tell you to vary the number of calories you eat each day. This helps some but still causes the body to conserve and slow the metabolism.

Another thing I dislike about low-calorie diets is that someone can have a low-calorie intake of junk food containing hardly any nutritional value. This makes matters worse, because if the body is starved for nutrition, it cannibalizes its muscles to survive and this slows the metabolism even more. The efficiency and general health of the body is also severely compromised. People will feel terrible and stop caring, because their bodies and minds are not getting adequate nutrition. Their bodies will most likely also be storing fat as a protective mechanism. When a diet like this is ended, their bodies usually stimulate them to eat everything in sight in an attempt to get the nutrition needed. This leads to rapid fat gain. Therefore, the end result of their efforts is less lean tissue and more fat—the opposite of their goal.

The Low-Fat Craze

A program that comes and goes in popularity is the low-fat diet. Reducing fat in the diet has helped many people, but often keeps them from getting the healthful fats needed for good health. You have learned why an adequate amount of essential fatty acids is an absolute necessity for normal bodily function and that a low-fat diet may contribute to the development of osteoporosis.

Healthful fats are an excellent energy source for most of us. A low-fat diet can lead to a lack of these fats we need for energy and their other important functions. Other deficiencies are created if the body does not get the essential fatty acids it needs, and unhealthy cravings for saturated fats and greasy fried foods often develop. Some people give in to these cravings and end up eating unhealthful fats instead of healthful ones. Science has not determined a correlation between total fat intake and the risk of disease. Health problems come primarily from the type of fat, not the amount.

Because many people on low-fat diets do not get enough energy from good fats, they often eat an excess of sugar, artificial sweeteners and processed grain products. You know that the acidic condition this creates makes the body want to store body fat, not burn it. It also increases inflammation in injured areas and increases the degeneration of various parts of the body. Processed grains can increase the amount of triglycerides and cholesterol in our blood and often increase blood sugar levels rapidly, leading to a release of insulin that causes the excess sugar to be stored as fat.

Low-fat diets are bland, because fats supply most of the taste we find appealing in many foods. People often compensate for the lack of taste by adding salt and sugar to most of their meals. Of course, this is not healthful or helpful for the fat-loss process. People tend to tire quickly of a low-fat, low-taste diet. The whole foods recommended in this book have naturally good tastes. The fruits are sweet and the eggs, nuts, seeds, whole grains and certain other foods contain healthful fats for a pleasing taste. Many of the other foods have unique combinations of appearance, taste, smell and texture that make them appealing and pleasant to eat.

The Calorie-Restriction Diet

A calorie-restriction diet is a combination of low calorie and low fat. The primary reason people follow this program is to extend their life spans. Calorie restriction (CR) is the only thing proven to dramatically lengthen the life of animals. Remember the hundred-year-old mouse? Because free radicals are formed when our bodies digest food, the theory is that the less you eat, the fewer free radicals there will be to damage and age your cells.

Mice and monkeys on the CR program look healthy but the ones being fed "normally" look fat. Some humans on the program look like walking skeletons ready to die at any moment. They look extremely unhealthy and I definitely do not think Nature intended us to look like that. I believe that these people are following the program to an excessive (and unhealthy) degree. They probably think that the more they restrict their calories the longer they will live, but you have learned that more is not always better. They are able to live on few calories, because they have hardly any muscle left to maintain. Their bodies have cannibalized most of their muscle tissue to keep their internal organs healthy. A man on the CR diet made the comment on a television program that he often feels hungry. His body is telling him that it needs more

nutrition but obviously he is not listening. The repair and health of internal
organs can be compromised if there is not enough muscle left to scavenge the
necessary raw materials. People may become deficient in the healthful fats
and other nutrients needed for proper function. I doubt if most people on the
CR program are eating any seeds, nuts or eggs, which you know are my
preferred sources of healthful protein and fats. These people may have good
energy levels, because their bodies will not be using much energy for digestion
and due to minimal friction from internal waste. This is a benefit, but can be
enjoyed without starving the body for the nutrients it needs.

When following my program, you will eat a variety of highly nutritious
foods when your body tells you it is hungry. You will get maximum nutritional
value from a minimum amount of food. Free radical creation will be low,
because you will eat less and consume mostly foods that are easily digested.
And, many of the foods contain nutrients that neutralize free radicals and
prevent them from doing damage. This is how the long-lived peoples of the
world eat and most of them do not look anorexic. These people usually live in
environments that have fewer free radicals from air pollution, chemicals and
other sources. If you take a good multivitamin and mineral and a potent
antioxidant, you should have hardly any damage from the free radicals found
in your modern environment and those created by eating.

If you follow my program, you will not overeat *or* undereat but get the
type and amount of food that Nature intended so you can enjoy optimal
health and longevity. You will have the amount of muscle mass needed for
your activities, just the right level of body fat and an abundance of energy
because of minimal internal waste and because you will be eating good clean-
burning energy foods. The program will maintain a balanced pH of your
blood so your body will not want to store or lose fat and you will not lose
calcium from your bones. You should be extremely resistant to disease and
your health statistics (cholesterol level, blood pressure and so on) will be so
uncommonly good that your doctor will be amazed. Mine is.

High-Protein Diet

Some best-selling books and various dietary programs recommend a high-
protein, low-carbohydrate diet. The popularity of this diet comes and goes
depending on who is currently promoting his or her book on the talk shows.
A well-known doctor wrote one of these books back in 1972. If it had been
effective, don't you think that many people would have used it and we would
see a nation of lean people instead of an increasing number of fat ones? The
same doctor wrote a similar book in the 1990s and another book in 2003 that
says you can now eat more carbohydrates with the protein. Junk-food
companies, beer producers and fast-food chains are currently exploiting the
low-carb craze to increase their profits and many low-carb products are now
available. I do not recommend any of them because they are expensive,
processed, often high in bad fat and many contain unhealthful ingredients

such as chocolate. This fad ended back in the 1970s and it will end again when the current generation realizes that it does not work any better than other diets they have followed.

High-protein diets are lacking in many vital nutrients and are extremely stressful on the body. They do not make sense when you know that most of the foods humans are able to digest and use are carbohydrates and that the only foods that stimulate *healthful* fat burning are carbohydrates. Most of the foods that I eat are carbohydrates and my body fat percentage is less than 10 percent. The vast majority of lean people in the world eat *low*-protein diets.

Because fats supply long-lasting energy, satisfy the appetite and taste good, I agree with the high-protein advocates that we should have more fat in our diets. I do not agree, however, that so much of it should come from saturated animal fats and from processed meats that contain carcinogenic chemicals. You already know that I recommend healthful fats primarily from nuts, seeds, eggs, whole grains, avocados and healthful oils—foods that supply fat without an excess of protein.

Promoters of a high-protein diet often mention that ancient, primitive humans ate large amounts of meat. This was true for those living in cold, harsh environments, but those living in hot climates would have never survived without eating the fruits, root vegetables and grains that grew where they lived. Eskimos do well on a high-protein, high-fat diet like their ancient ancestors ate, because it is what they need to survive in a cold, harsh environment. I doubt, however, that you live in northern Alaska. If you do, and you spend time doing physical work outdoors, eating more protein will be best for you. If you live in Texas, Florida or California, I do not recommend it. Even today, primitive peoples living in hot climates subsist largely on root vegetables and fruits. They eat meat occasionally when they are able to kill an animal. I have already explained eating for your environment and for the different seasons so you should understand the concept by now.

High-protein diets often consist of large amounts of meat and this increases cancer risk. This is because many processed meat products (like bacon) contain carcinogenic chemicals and it may also be because fewer of the carbohydrate foods that protect us from cancer are being eaten. The protein you eat should come from natural, chemical-free meats and from the other healthful sources I have previously mentioned.

Eating excessive protein, especially in the absence of adequate B vitamins, can elevate homocysteine levels in the blood. You have learned that excess homocysteine causes inflammation and damage to your arteries, which increases the risk of a heart attack and other vascular problems.

A high-protein diet forces the body to use stored glycogen and muscle protein for energy. Fat is also used for energy, especially after the first ten days. This causes an accumulation of ketone bodies in the blood, because the fat cannot be burned completely. Ketone bodies make the blood more acidic, stressing the body and making it want to store fat, not burn it. The acidic condition also causes a loss of calcium from the bones. High levels of nitrogenous waste in the form of ammonia, an extremely toxic chemical, are formed from the muscle protein used for energy. The liver converts the ammonia to urea, which is less toxic but still must be eliminated by the kidneys. Parts of the body are exposed to ammonia and urea, and more stress is placed on the liver and kidneys. On the contrary, metabolizing fats and carbohydrates uses less energy, is not stressful and produces only water and carbon dioxide as by-products.

A high-protein diet initially causes a large loss of water and sodium. This creates rapid weight loss, but is dehydrating and unhealthy. After two or three weeks, the body starts to retain water, causing a weight gain. A high-protein diet can lead to high uric acid levels and hypokalemia (low potassium levels). The combination of ketosis and these two conditions can lead to sudden death. Sadly, some people attempting to lose weight using only liquid protein found this out the hard way. High uric acid levels can also cause gout.

A high-protein diet works for some people because it takes many calories to digest the protein and convert it into glucose. This increases the metabolism more than a meal of carbohydrates or fats would because of what is called the specific dynamic action of protein. But, as you have learned, it is extremely stressful on the digestive system and other internal organs. This can lead to a physical breakdown and development of hypoglycemia (it is what caused mine) and other physical and emotional problems. Some people get irritable, destructive and violent when eating large amounts of protein. People often eat less on a high-protein diet, because the fat content satisfies their hunger longer and because it is boring. Because the diet is so stressful, the body slows the metabolism down as soon as it can to be able to subsist on fewer calories. Guess what happens when the diet ends and old eating habits are resumed?

Some people who go on high-protein diets feel like they have more energy. This occurs because the protein is keeping their blood sugar levels more constant and treating the symptoms of hypoglycemia. You have learned, however, that the excess protein is also stressing certain glands and organs, and making the condition worse without people realizing it. Many people believe that eating carbohydrates makes you hungrier and stimulates overeating. This is only true if the carbohydrates are made from processed grains, which contain little nutritional value. Eating *whole* complex carbohydrates will keep your blood sugar level normal, satisfy your appetite, provide easily digested, clean-burning energy and supply many of the nutritional needs of your body.

Many doctors and nutritionists advise people with excess fat, hypoglycemia, cancer, osteoporosis and other serious conditions to eat more protein. They often recommend using processed protein supplements. This is unhealthy advice, because the protein uses up vital energy to be digested and causes an acidic condition that makes the problem worse. The processed products create other imbalances and problems. Converting protein to energy most likely creates far more free radicals than getting energy from carbohydrates and fats, and this adds to the negative effects of eating the protein. What almost all of these people need is to eat less complete protein and to get what they do need from natural foods.

I have already mentioned that high-protein diets are expensive. To see how expensive, cook up one dollar's worth of dried beans, whole grains or potatoes and compare it to the amount of fish or beef you can get for a dollar. One reason for this is that far more land is needed to produce most protein foods as compared to carbohydrate foods. For example, a large amount of fruits, vegetables or grains can be grown on an acre of land but it will not support many sheep or cattle.

Carbohydrate foods such as whole fruits, whole grains, legumes and vegetables are the healthiest foods you can eat. They are loaded with essential vitamins, minerals, enzymes and phytonutrients. Eliminating them from the diet is unhealthy and ridiculous. Some people lose weight on a high-protein diet because they stop eating the unhealthful and fattening carbohydrate foods made from processed grains. You now know that this is the source of carbohydrates you should avoid.

Other Weight-Loss Ideas

I do not intend the upcoming comments as a putdown to the authors of "diet" books. Most of them, like you and I, are searching for answers and want to share their beliefs and discoveries. They want to help others and this is admirable. Unfortunately, numerous problems and confusions arise for their readers because of the incompleteness or errors of most theories. They often contradict each other and this compounds the problem. My comments are made only to inform you and help end your confusion.

I believe that these authors usually have only five or ten pieces of a 100-piece puzzle. None have enough to complete the puzzle and see or understand the big picture. It reminds me of the story of the five blind men asked to describe an elephant. The man feeling its tail says an elephant is like a rope but the one touching its side believes it is like a wall. The man feeling the elephant's trunk envisions it like a snake and the one touching its leg says it is like a tree trunk. The fifth man feels the elephant's ear and thinks it is like a large leaf or fan. Each man has part of the picture but not enough of it to be even close to the reality of an elephant. All of these men are being truthful in describing what they are experiencing, but they all have incomplete information. Each one disagrees with all the others. Even if one of them touched all five parts, he would still not know how to put them all together and correctly describe the elephant. With the knowledge you now have, you should be able to see how limited most of the authors of weight-loss books are in their understanding of healthful eating.

One author recommends what people should eat based on their blood type. This may give some people a few ideas about what foods their bodies will do best with, but does not address removing the causes or reversing all the negative cycles people create. It also does not address the many other variables involved in determining the right foods for each person. Do you think Nature intended humans to be fat and unhealthy for thousands of years until the blood-type diet was developed? Do you think an Eskimo and an African tribesman should eat the same foods if they have the same blood type? How long do you think a vegetarian Eskimo would survive in northern Alaska? Another question we can ask is "How have millions of people stayed lean and lived long lives without even knowing their blood type?" The answer is simple—they ate the whole, natural foods available in their environments and did strenuous physical work.

Even if your blood type does have something to do with fat loss, it is only one of many variables. The blood-type diet book indicates that a cup or two of coffee may be good for blood types A and AB, because it increases the production of stomach acid. You already know coffee is not good for anyone and you have learned how to increase your stomach acid healthfully, if necessary. The author of this book even tells people they should exercise differently according to their blood type. This makes no sense, because, as you have learned, every "body" primarily needs strength-training exercise and some cardiovascular training regardless of blood type, body type, or anything else.

I looked at the diet recommended for someone with my blood type (type A). Some of the foods were cornflakes, rice cakes, coffee, red wine, tofu and yogurt. I would never ingest any of the preceding except tofu, and that only in moderation, because my body does not do well with soy products even though the book indicates that it should. None of my ancestors, including my parents, ever ate any soy product. Red meat is supposed to be completely avoided but I have joint pains all over my body unless I eat some about once a week. People with blood type A are supposed to thrive as vegetarians, but while I was eating a vegetarian diet for almost two years, I lost more than 35 pounds of muscle and could barely function. Small cuts took weeks to heal and my muscles stayed extremely sore for many days after exercising them. Some of the foods supposed to be highly beneficial for me have caused problems in the past (so I no longer eat them) and some of the foods I am supposed to avoid have never given me any problems. Almost all the sample meals included water, herbal tea, coffee or red wine. As you know, drinking anything with meals reduces your body's digestive efficiency. The sample meals were also poor food combinations.

The blood-type diet book indicates that because my blood is type A, heavy exercise will exhaust my nervous system, make me tense and leave my immune system open to illness or disease. I disagree. I have been doing heavy weight training three to four times a week for more than thirty-seven years and I physically work long and hard. I am calm almost all the time and have not even had a cold for almost thirty years. The suggestions in this book may be more accurate for other people with type A blood, but I would never ingest (or recommend) many of the foods listed or do most of the exercises claimed to be the best for me. I have had patients tell me that this program did not work for them either. I could write the hair color diet or astrological sign diet and be as accurate as this program seems to be.

The author of another popular book tells us that each meal or snack should contain 40 percent carbohydrates, 30 percent protein and 30 percent fat. You are supposed to drink at least eight ounces of water or sugar-free decaffeinated beverage with every meal and snack. I guess you could drink quite a few soft drinks sweetened with aspartame or saccharin. I do not recommend it and you already know what drinking with meals causes. The sample meals sometimes include eating fruit with meat. You already know that's a terrible combination. Three meals and two snacks are suggested for the average person. The recommended combinations would satisfy your appetite for a long time, because they will take a long time to digest. This would overwork your digestive organs and make it difficult to eat five times a day unless you were constantly eating when you were not hungry and putting a new meal into your stomach along with a partially digested one. You have learned that neither of those habits is healthy.

Another problem with this plan is that someone can eat mostly junk food but still maintain the recommended ratio of fat, carbohydrate and protein. The author even gives fast-food recommendations that he considers good combinations. What about supplying the body with some nutritional value? He states that it is easy to determine the ratios his plan calls for, but that is not what I have heard from people who have tried it. I have not seen anyone follow this program for more than a month or two. What complicates matters is that most foods are a combination of protein, fat and carbohydrate. For example, an avocado has 5 grams (g) of protein, 37g of fat and 13g of carbohydrate. A cup of oatmeal has 2g of protein, 2g of fat, and 23g of carbohydrate. A cup of red kidney beans has 15g of protein, 1g of fat, and 42g of carbohydrate. Three ounces of beef liver contains 22g of protein, 9g of fat, and 5g of carbohydrate. You already know that more healthful fat is needed during cold weather, but the author does not adjust his ratios for different seasons. We can also ask most of the same questions we asked about the blood-type program about this one.

The author of this program also says that we should not eat grains because they have not been around long enough for our bodies to have adapted to using them well. I do not advocate eating an excess of whole grains and I recommend against eating any processed grain products, but I disagree that grains are unhealthful. The body of a frozen 5,000-year-old man was once discovered whose stomach contained some wild grain. Just because people have not been planting and cultivating grains for that many years relative to how long humans have existed does not mean that they were not eating wild grains. After all, Nature created the grains, not mankind. Eating whole grains is associated with a decreased risk for many cancers, and grains are a staple food for many groups of people who live long and healthy lives.

This author's primary goal is to keep blood glucose levels normal because, as you have learned, high levels increase insulin secretion causing the glucose to be stored as fat. This is a good goal but a poor way to achieve it. Low insulin levels can lead to development of a fatty liver. I do not know if his eating plan will cause this, but it may be a possibility. Being lean and healthy should not require a complicated eating plan to manipulate your insulin levels. This is unnatural and unhealthy. By following my dietary and exercise recommendations, your glucose levels should stay normal most of the time. Remember that exercise decreases insulin levels and at the same time increases your sensitivity to it, so you do not need as much. And, exercise stimulates glucose to be stored as glycogen instead of fat.

Some authors tell us to eat only foods with a low glycemic index. The question is, who did Nature intend to eat all the high-glycemic foods? A doctor I know read a book about glycemic index and told a friend of mine he would be better off eating potato chips (GI of 54 due to high unhealthful fat content) than a rutabaga (GI of 72). He also said that a Snickers® candy bar (GI of 41) would be better than some cantaloupe (GI of 65), because the junk food has a lower glycemic index. What do you think? Slightly reducing the intake of high-glycemic foods may have some validity for a diabetic, but unhealthful food with a low glycemic index is still unhealthful.

Some authors write that eating low-glycemic foods helps prevent diabetes. This has hardly anything to do with it. People get diabetes because they eat fattening foods that contain hardly any nutritional value—processed foods. Many people have gotten fat eating low-glycemic foods like potato chips and candy bars. Potatoes have a high glycemic index but have been a staple food in some countries for hundreds of years and these countries are not filled with fat diabetics. What saddens me is that these authors tell diabetics they can eat unhealthful foods as long as the foods have a low glycemic index. They sell their books or courses by telling people they can eat foods loaded with sugar, because its glycemic index is low. This is true, but people eat such high concentrations of sugar that it all hits the bloodstream at the same time and that's when the trouble starts. You know that processed sugar is detrimental to the health of anyone. Apparently, these authors do not know that the body needs good nutrition to be healthy, not just some junk food releasing energy at a slow rate.

Glycemic index gurus usually say that if you eat high-glycemic foods, your blood sugar level will crash and you will feel hungry shortly after eating. This may be true if you eat unbalanced, processed foods, but is not true if you eat whole, natural foods. I often eat steamed vegetables (with potatoes sometimes) for lunch with a salad and some olive oil. This maintains my energy to do mentally and physically demanding work for many hours. I often do not get a chance to eat again for five or six hours but have abundant energy and rarely feel hungry. And, as you know, I had severe hypoglycemia when I was younger.

Numerous books and dietary programs are based on the glycemic index of foods so let's take a look at the reality of this concept. To determine the glycemic index of a carbohydrate food, volunteers eat 50-gram portions. This is usually a large amount. For example, it is about a pound and a half of carrots and more potatoes than most of us would eat in two or three meals. Labeling a food healthful or unhealthful based on its glycemic index is ridiculous, because most of us eat a combination of foods at one meal. One may be converted to glucose fast, one medium speed and another slowly. The result is a balanced (timed) energy release. A mixed meal of whole, natural foods will usually have a moderate to low glycemic index. How often have you eaten a plate full of potatoes and nothing else or sat down to a pound and a half of carrots? Even someone eating a mono-diet (one food at a time) would not eat such large quantities and would rarely follow the program for long. Eating fruit separately is fine, because fructose has a low glycemic index, the concentration is low and the nutrients necessary to use it for energy are also in the fruit. Do you think Nature planned it this way? Of course, because the way of Nature, the universe and truth is simplicity.

One well-known author gives reasons why other popular diets are unhealthful and has some good information about foods in his books. The meals he recommends, however, contain unhealthful foods and are often poor combinations. He states that drinking with meals will not affect your digestion. He also believes that processed sugar is not a problem. Perhaps he should read the section about sugar in chapter four of this book. He says dark chocolate can be eaten because the fat in it is a healthful form. The caffeine, theobromine and oxalic acid in the chocolate do not seem to bother him. They will, however, bother you and your children despite what this well-known medical doctor says. He states that he takes a baby aspirin every day. This is an unhealthy habit, because aspirin can cause gastrointestinal bleeding and may contain aluminum. This author does not seem to have faith in his dietary program's ability to prevent heart disease and stroke.

The authors of most "weight-loss" books generally focus on a single idea like glycemic index, food combining, insulin levels, high protein, low protein, no sugar, low fat, blood type or body type. This is like saying your house is clean if just the garbage cans are emptied or just the mirrors cleaned or just the kitchen floor mopped. I hope you're getting the picture. Healthful eating consists of a number of things just like cleaning your house. But this does not mean it is complicated.

Like the blind men describing the elephant, these authors do not seem to agree on many things. Most of them seemed to have stumbled upon something that worked for them (at least temporarily) and then wrote a book about it. All the ones I have seen recommend foods that will *absolutely not* create the "optimum" health they usually promise. Most of them tell you to eat the enemies we covered in chapter four. They seem unconcerned with the nutritional value someone gets or the negative effects the foods create. Some of them sell processed "foods" based on the dietary concepts found in their books. Ice cream, food bars and other products I would not recommend. Some of these authors write follow-up books to clarify or simplify their first books. The follow-up books are often filled with a bunch of recipes most people will never make. These authors fail to address the physical and emotional causes for overeating, negative cycles and how to reverse them, eating for the season and the principle of timing. They usually also fail to address individual needs based on environment, age, activity level, gender, body efficiency and most of the other important keys to permanent fat loss and good health explained in this book. Some of them have discovered a few truths but still lack too many of the pieces to be able to see—or teach *you* how to see—the big picture. I believe that they are intelligent, well-meaning people. They just lack the completeness of knowledge necessary to help most people. This is one reason why there are more fat people than ever. As you have learned, just because people have Ph.D. or M.D. after their names does not mean they know much about healthful eating.

There is even a book that claims to help you decide the best "diet" for you. I do not recommend it, because I believe all the diet books are incomplete and confusing.

About June of 2003 I saw a "health" newsletter written by a medical doctor. He started this newsletter by saying how unhealthful eating a high-protein diet was and that it was not that effective for losing weight. He then briefly described the Pritikin diet and said that it was extremely healthful and effective at fat loss, but a little difficult to follow. Then he disclosed that he was 50 pounds overweight and was planning to go on a diet. The diet plan he then said he was going to follow was a high-protein plan. This made no sense after his previous statements. This doctor has also written a weight-loss book in the past. I wondered why he was obese and why he did not follow the advice of his own book. What do you think?

In her book, *Linda Goodman's Star Signs*, the author describes programs designed to balance your aura (subtle energy field around your body). She believes that if the aura is balanced, your body will follow suit and lose or gain weight depending on which procedure you follow. I have studied the aura and learned aura-balancing techniques. My belief and experience is that the aura reflects our inner states, it does not create them. Your aura is green if you are envious and red if you are angry. You are not envious because your aura is green or angry because it is red. The idea of the aura controlling the body and mind does not make sense and if it was true, balancing the aura could easily solve all our problems. My question is this: if our inner state does not create the colors of the aura, then what does? Another reason Ms. Goodman's idea does not make sense is because it is far from simple. Being your normal body weight should not require completing the complicated procedures she recommends. It is not the way of Nature. I enjoyed her book, but disagree with her weight-control plan. Balance your body, mind and spirit and your aura will be balanced as a natural result.

The authors of these weight-loss books usually claim you will experience optimum health, achieve maximum physical performance, lose weight permanently and enjoy many other benefits. One of them claims you can achieve optimum health in just two months. Do not believe it. It will take longer than that even if you follow the much healthier guidelines found in this book. It should be easy to see that you will never obtain what they promise by eating as they recommend. I know people who have followed the high-protein diet, others who followed the blood-type diet, and others who had followed one of the other popular diet programs. They all lost some weight, but it was not long before they had gained it back and usually added more.

A vegetarian diet works well for some people, but creates an unbalanced condition in those whose bodies cannot get enough protein from the vegetarian foods. I have followed high-protein and vegetarian programs and created severe health problems with each. Diets relying on eating large quantities of one particular food (pineapple for example) also create imbalances and poor health.

A negative aspect of all "diets" is that the dieters have to eat differently than the rest of their family. This can make it difficult. By following the program in this book, most family members should be able to eat about the same while losing fat or maintaining healthy body fat levels. The main difference will be the quantity eaten.

I saw a story on a well-known television news program about the city of Durham, North Carolina. This city is called the "Diet Capital of the World." Thousands of people from all over the world go there every year hoping to lose their excess fat. Some sell their cars or homes to get the money—three to eight thousand dollars a month—to stay long enough to accomplish their goals. About $80 million a year is spent at the weight-loss centers of Durham. I do not know everything about all of these places but based on what I saw, people are not getting much for their money.

There are three main diet centers. At one of them, people are fed a bland diet of rice and fruit. People lose some weight, because they get bored and eat less and because other foods are unavailable. Let's think about this diet for a minute. First of all, the rice (probably processed white rice) is acidic so does not stimulate healthful fat burning. The fruit is alkaline but much less concentrated so the overall meal will leave an unhealthful acid ash. The forced fat burning creates more acid, which causes calcium loss from the bones. Second, their bodies are stressed tremendously, because they are being forced to burn fat and not supplied the nutrients needed for fat burning or most other vital functions. Third, the people eating these meals will lose muscle mass, because they are not getting any complete protein. Their muscles will be cannibalized to supply the protein needs of other parts of their bodies. This will slow their metabolisms and make it easier to gain fat when the diet ends.

Fourth, they are not getting any satisfaction from eating, because the meals supply few vital nutrients and hardly any stimulation to their five senses. Fifth, they are not learning how to prepare and enjoy healthful, balanced meals (the kind that would help them maintain or lose even more) so will return home and eat close to the same way they did before (i.e., the way that made them fat). I cannot imagine any of them continuing to eat fruit and rice most of the time, nor would I recommend it.

Another diet center puts people on a low-calorie diet. You have learned how detrimental that is to your physical and emotional health.

The news program only showed people being weighed. There was no mention of body fat testing. They did not show anyone doing any fat-burning exercise except walking. Some people were walking for about two hours a day, which is something I am sure few of them will have time to do after they return home. There was no mention of strength training—which takes only a few hours a week and could be continued at home—to build or maintain muscle mass and normalize the metabolism.

A class was shown where people were being taught to read labels and purchase low-calorie *processed* foods. You know that these foods are lower in nutritional value, so their bodies will make them eat more in an attempt to get the needed nutrition. Most of these processed foods also have harmful additives. I heard nothing about eating whole, natural foods—foods that do not have labels or harmful additives. Another class was teaching people how to eat only one piece of pizza. This is not difficult if there is one pizza cut into ten pieces and there are ten people in the class and they cannot get any more. But what will happen when they order a pizza at home? Are these people going to eat just one piece and let their other family members eat the rest? I doubt it, because the unhealthful ingredients in the pizza will stimulate them to eat more. What if they live alone? Are they going to eat one piece and throw the rest away or eat one piece every day for ten days? What is going to happen when they buy one pizza and get a second one free? These people should be learning how to eat great-tasting, nutritious foods, not one piece of fattening and unhealthful pizza.

Most of the people interviewed said they needed to get away from their normal environments before they could lose weight. You do not have to be a rocket scientist to figure out what is going to happen when they return to those environments. And, most of them will be under increased stress because of the debt incurred from going to Durham. What these people need to learn is how to eat healthfully and develop thinking and behavioral habits that will improve their normal environments—primarily their internal programming. This will not only change how they feel about themselves but will help them to associate with more positive and healthy people.

One interview was with a woman who had gone to Durham thirteen years earlier and lost 100 pounds. She has lived there ever since and has researched dieting for many years. She has even written a book about it. She said that if you cannot lose weight in Durham, that you just cannot lose weight. She seemed like a nice person, but is still fat after thirteen years. Why? The answer to that question should be obvious.

At the end of the news program they mentioned a few people they had profiled in the show. One had gained back 20 pounds and another had gained 15 pounds. If they had learned anything useful, they should have continued to lose more fat, not started gaining it back.

Even at the famous weight-loss centers of the "Diet Capital of the World," the meals were unhealthful and not something people would continue to eat, people were only weighed, not tested for body fat percentage, and there was no strength training. People were not taught how to make nutritious meals from whole, natural foods and their causes for being fat were not determined and eliminated. This "ultimate" weight-loss city perfectly illustrates my point that most of the information being dispensed about "weight" loss is inaccurate or extremely incomplete.

I saw another television news program about three high-school students who attended a fat-loss camp for the summer. It was their third summer because they had all gained back the weight they had lost during the two previous summers. I do not know why they thought it would work the third time.

These students followed a low-calorie diet and did up to six hours of exercise every day. They lost some weight but eventually stopped losing. No one seemed to know why, but you should. It was explained in chapter two. The following summer they returned for a reunion. One had gained all of the weight back, if not more, and the others had gained back some. One of them gained some weight even though he was doing all he knew how in an attempt to lose more. They all failed because they had not learned what to do to succeed. They were shown eating sandwiches and drinking soft drinks at the reunion. Is that healthful?

They all returned to bingeing and poor eating habits because they had not learned good eating habits, how different foods affect the body, or how to eliminate their emotional reasons for bingeing or how to replace it with healthy activities. They had lost water and muscle along with some fat when they were dieting. The muscle loss slowed their metabolisms making it easier to gain the weight back. The hours of exercise they did at the camp were almost worthless and could not be continued after they left because of the time demands. The weight training they were shown doing was poor form and of low intensity. These students had not learned how to build and maintain their muscle mass with a few short strength-training workouts a week. None of them had physical education classes at school and only one of them continued to exercise occasionally. The young girl said she had no time for breakfast, but had time to stop at a restaurant for a bagel. Is that what she learned to eat for breakfast? If she had to leave early because her mother was giving her a ride, why didn't she just get up earlier? It does not take much time to fix and eat a healthful breakfast or to fix it and take it with you. This is another example of the misinformation or lack of information that is making the people of this country fat and unhealthy.

Many authors of articles about weight loss tell you that you must walk if you want to succeed at losing weight. They often have stories of people who lost weight and are keeping it off by walking an hour a day. This is extremely discouraging to many people because they do not have an extra hour of time every day to walk. Certainly, walking is good exercise and often provides a healthy dose of soul food, but it is absolutely *not* necessary to lose excess fat and to easily keep it off. My body is extremely lean and I do not walk much. I also know many lean people who do not do much walking. Some of them eat well and do strength training and others just eat well. I also know many people who walk frequently for 30 to 60 minutes at a time and they have fat and flabby bodies.

Walking is not the miracle "cure" for excess fat that many people claim. Let's take a closer look at it and I think you will agree. Walking at a moderate pace (3.5 mph) burns 5.6 calories per minute or 336 calories per hour. Weeding your garden burns the same number and driving your car burns half as many. A small slice of cherry or apple pie contains 350 calories, a cookie has 120 and a cola soft drink has 145. Because of the lag time before your body starts to burn fat, you would have to walk for an hour and twenty minutes to burn off 350 calories of stored fat. That is a lot of work to eliminate the fat from one small piece of pie. It is far easier to not eat unhealthful and fattening foods than it is to attempt to walk off the fat they create.

Many people indulge in junk food and then attempt to work off the calories with exercise. Most of them do not succeed. A few people can maintain their weight by doing this but chances are that most of them do not consider the damage those unhealthful foods are doing to their bodies. Even if you burn off the calories later, the damage done to your body is often permanent. Keep this in mind when you are having a pig-out meal. Overeat on relatively healthful foods instead of eating unhealthful foods.

Now let's look at what gaining some muscle (regaining for most people) will do for you. If you gain five to seven pounds of muscle, your body will burn the same number of calories every day as walking for one hour would. Increase and maintain your lean body mass with two to three hours of strength training every week and you will get the calorie-burning effect of seven hours of walking in addition to all of the many other health benefits that come from strength training. The increased muscle will help you to lose excess fat faster, make your body more efficient and shapely, and allow you to eat more every day while easily maintaining your weight.

Some people say that we primarily need more physical activity to stay lean. I agree that physical activity is good for us in many ways, but you have learned that most people do inefficient exercise and activities if they do any at all. One of the reasons physical activity is helpful is that you cannot eat junk food while you are playing basketball or swimming. Other people believe that our cities need to be changed so that many of us can walk to restaurants and stores instead of driving. This would be wonderful but do not wait until that happens before you get some exercise. Many fat people will still drive because their feet and knees hurt when they walk. Also, it will not make much difference if people walk to fast-food restaurants to eat and continue following other fat-producing habits. People in many foreign countries are generally more physically active than most Americans but stay leaner primarily because they eat fewer processed foods and do not overeat.

There are people who believe that watching television and sitting in front of computers is a major reason why so many Americans are fat. Certainly, many people do watch an excessive amount of television but the real problem is that they eat fattening junk foods while they are watching. Some people watch an educational television program while walking on a treadmill or pedaling an exercise bike. Watching television has negative consequences if it prevents you from getting adequate mind and soul food, if you eat junk foods while watching and if you watch programs that are disturbing to your mind and inner spirit. Watching murder after murder in gruesome detail is extremely damaging. Once again, it comes down to the choices we make.

I often see the advice to eat less and exercise more. For the people who need it the most this advice is completely worthless. Eating less is not what people with excess fat need to do. They need to eat the right foods, in the right combinations and at the right times. They could eat far more and lose fat and improve their health. Eating less junk food is not going to help much and will not last long because the body will stimulate eating because it is starving for nutrition. Exercising more is not going to help many people either because very few know the best kind of exercise to do or how to do it to produce the desired results.

Many of the authors who write articles about weight-loss are most likely struggling to lose their own excess fat. They often write that losing weight is hard and that keeping it off is harder. It is clear that they do not know how to lose fat naturally and healthfully or they would not write such things that just provide excuses for many people not to do anything.

Weight-Loss Products

Numerous products claim to help you shed excess fat without changing any dietary or lifestyle habits. Others say a few minor modifications are necessary until after you have lost the weight. Let's take a quick look at some of the most popular weight-loss products. Keep in mind that more people are fat now than ever.

Millions have used various diet shakes in an attempt to lose excess fat. You are told to replace one of your meals with a delicious shake and then eat a "sensible" dinner. I wonder what they mean by that. First of all, if people were able to eat sensibly, they would not be fat. Second, these shakes are usually made from sugar, cocoa, milk and other unhealthful ingredients. Third, if your causes are still there, you will just get fat again after you stop using the product. Some are labeled "balanced and complete." Balanced and complete what? It is certainly not balanced and complete nutrition. If it were, they would not have to add a caution telling you not to use it as your sole source of nutrition.

Some weight-loss products are designed to suppress your appetite. They usually contain a chemical called phenylpropanolamine (PPA). It is a stimulant like caffeine and does reduce the appetite temporarily. Now people will eat less junk food than before and be even more starved for healthful nutrients. Does this sound like a good idea? Once people stop using the product and start eating more again, chances are their weight will soon be more than it was before they started. The FDA recommends that consumers avoid using products that contain PPA because of the health risks associated with it. This chemical will probably eventually be banned.

Other weight-loss products are candies designed to curb your appetite by raising your blood sugar level. These are expensive, stimulate insulin release and confuse your mind. Eat candy to lose weight. Does this make any sense? Other products contain benzocaine, a local anesthetic. These are supposed to deaden your taste buds. Does not tasting your meal sound enjoyable? This may make people eat foods high in sugar or salt in an attempt to taste something. The previous two products have not been proven to be effective. Some products contain methylcellulose that is supposed to swell up in your stomach and make you feel full. Unfortunately, it doesn't swell until it is in your intestines, so it does not work. Certain other products have a diuretic effect, causing the user to lose water. These can lead to dehydration and a loss of potassium, both of which are unhealthy conditions. It is not hard to imagine how short-lived this "weight" loss will be.

Another product becoming popular is indigestible fat. The idea is to get the taste of fat without the weight gain. This may sound great, but this product takes up the space where nutritious foods should be and can lead to nutritional deficiencies and poor health. It can leach out fat-soluble vitamins, causing an even larger deficiency of vital nutrients. Eating indigestible fat causes diarrhea, because the body is attempting to get rid of this unnatural substance. Indigestible fat can also cause abdominal cramping and may even contribute to the development of heart disease, cancer and blindness. This product was approved by the FDA, even though many leading food scientists told them it was unsafe. Foods containing it must have a warning on the label. That should be your first clue it is not good for you. I recommend avoiding foods containing this product.

Some doctors claim that the majority of Americans are fat because there is not as much conjugated linoleic acid (CLA) in our foods as there was in the past. The primary sources of CLA are beef and dairy products. CLA supplements are also available, but I do not recommend them. You already know how unhealthful dairy products are, and that most of the lean people in the world do not consume dairy products or beef. You have also learned the truth of why so many Americans are overweight or obese. As usual, however, there are companies trying to figure out ways to increase the CLA levels in milk, butter and cheese so sale of these foods can be increased under the guise that they will help you lose fat.

One weight-loss product's advertisement claims that stress causes overproduction of the "fat-storing" hormone cortisol (hydrocortisone). It is true that cortisol is produced from stress, but I do not believe that all the lean people in the world lead stress-free lives. Do you? This product's advertisement also claims that it will help you to lose stubborn fat cells from your abdomen. I disagree with this claim because cortisol causes fat to be stored on the chest and face, not the abdomen. Take a look at someone who is taking hydrocortisone drugs and you will see.

I recently received a sales booklet in the mail announcing another weight-loss product. This one's main ingredient is theobromine from chocolate. It has a few herbal ingredients, one of which helps calm you. I find that interesting, because theobromine is a stimulant similar to caffeine. This product contains a stimulant and a calming agent. Keep in mind that the dictionary defines theobromine as a *poisonous* powder.

Many weight-loss products contain harmful stimulants. Some of them used to contain ephedra, which is the natural source of the stimulant ephedrine. The FDA has banned the sale of ephedra because serious side effects can be experienced. Some people recommend drinking numerous cups of coffee every day to stimulate weight loss. Using these products may help stimulate some temporary fat loss but none of them are good for you.

Be wary of products claiming to produce weight loss with no effort or change of diet. Eat all you want, and anything you want. This may be what made you fat in the first place. How is it now going to make you lose excess fat? The answer is: It's not. It goes against the laws of Nature and is clearly too good to be true. These products or diet plans are just out to get your money and will tell you what they know you want to hear in order to do it.

Let's pretend for a moment there really was a product that helped people lose weight while eating anything they wanted. Instead of millions of unhealthy fat people there would be millions of unhealthy lean people, because their bodies would still not be getting the nutrients necessary for good health. Remember that the foods that make and keep you lean also keep you healthy. Eat to be healthy and you will naturally be lean.

Many "weight-loss" products are currently being sold over the Internet. Unfortunately, many of them are not regulated for safety in any way. One example is 1,4 butanediol. This product was taken out of health-food stores about 1998 but is still sold online as a dietary supplement to lose weight. It is used as an industrial solvent and that should be a red flag that it is not something you should ingest. It is highly addictive and had killed 158 people up to early

2001. You can have a "body to die for" without dying. Why not learn and follow Nature's laws and have a "body to live for"?

I am constantly solicited to sell the latest and greatest "miracle" weight-loss products. Most of them are expensive products sold through multilevel marketing. Do not worry about missing out on one of these miraculous new discoveries. If one of these products ever works as well as claimed, everyone will hear about it and all the distributors will be rich. Do you think Nature intended us all to be fat unless we use some product processed with a complicated technique, found only on a tropical island or in one small lake in the entire world? Recently, someone gave me a so-called weight-loss food bar along with literature about it and other "health" products. I read the ingredient list and did not see even one I consider healthful except for the added vitamins and minerals. If the main ingredients were nutritious, they would not need to add artificial vitamins and minerals. The man kept telling me how healthful this bar was, but I disagree. The negative effects of the main ingredients far outweigh any benefits of the added vitamins and minerals.

Many weight-loss products and fad diets show before and after pictures of people who have used the product or followed the diet. A few of them may have gotten rid of their emotional causes, but I believe that this is rare. Most of the small percentage of people who keep the weight off had gained it originally because of creeping obesity. The others will gain back all they lost or perhaps even more. This is why you rarely see pictures of people six months after they stop using the product or following the diet.

Remember that the primary purpose of most weight-loss products is to take advantage of people's lack of knowledge about healthful eating and to make money for the manufacturer of the product. Also keep in mind that there will always be another weight-loss product coming on the market because a great deal of money can be made from its sale, and that the next "miracle" product will not work any better than the last one that just wasted your money. Many years ago, tapeworms were sold to desperate people who wanted to lose excess fat. Most of these new "scientific" products are not any better.

Many people who lose weight using various weight-loss products do so because they just pay more attention to what they are eating. It has a placebo effect something like the "magic" feather Dumbo the elephant held that he believed gave him the ability to fly. He could fly because of his big ears, not because of the feather, and most people would lose the same amount of weight just by paying attention to what they are eating and drinking.

A statement often found in the fine print of the literature of most weight-loss products goes something like this: "Works when used in conjunction with a diet containing more fruits and vegetables and when following a regular exercise program." If you are going to eat well and exercise regularly, why do you need the "magic" product? You should know by now that the real magic is found within you and in the way and balance of Nature.

Weight-Loss Drugs

What about the prescription drugs used for weight reduction? The long-term success of these drugs has not been good. When fen-phen® (the fenfluramine-phentermine combination) was developed, it seemed to many that the magic weight-loss pill had finally been found. More than eighteen million prescriptions were filled in 1996. But, like most drugs, there were side effects (some severe) and it is no longer available. A large number of lawsuits were filed against the manufacturer and some people believe their loved ones died because of this drug. Fen-phen usually had to be used continually for the results to last. During test studies using fen-phen along with diet and exercise, the results were better than diet and exercise alone but tended to plateau after five to six months. The only people able to maintain their weight losses were the ones who made significant changes in their eating habits and lifestyles. That should not surprise you. I know someone who used fen-phen and lost weight. She looked good for a short time, but is now fatter than ever. Do people truly believe that they can eat high-calorie, nutrient-deficient foods and never exercise but have a lean, energetic and healthy body? I do not believe mankind's attempt to cheat the laws of Nature is ever going to work, because a pill will never be developed that can reverse all the laws of how your body functions. It would be easier to invent a pill that could make you fly.

Another diet drug no longer on the market is Redux® (dexfenfluramine). It is related to fenfluramine and has been linked to pulmonary hypertension, a potentially fatal lung condition. Numerous other drugs have been used to stimulate weight loss, and they all have uncomfortable and dangerous side effects, because of the imbalances they create.

The drug Orlistat® is designed to block fat absorption. It can cause diarrhea and perhaps some of the same problems associated with non-digestible fat. Using it may lead to a deficiency of antioxidants, fatty acids and fat-soluble vitamins.

Meridia® is another currently popular diet drug. It suppresses the appetite by working as an antidepressant. It helps some people because, as you know, depression can cause overeating and poor food choices. This drug may not help you at all if your cause is different. You probably won't need it, because you have learned numerous ways to stop creating depression or to rid yourself of it without drugs. Meridia will no doubt soon be replaced by another drug I am sure some scientists are working to develop. Because these drugs have side effects and health risks and you have to change your lifestyle and eating habits anyway, why not just follow the guidelines in this book and achieve *permanent* victory over fat.

More Unhealthy Weight-Loss Ideas

Some people get so desperate to lose weight that they resort to fasting or starvation. Others think it will help them to lose faster. Cleansing and fasting can be helpful if done correctly and for the right reasons, but for most people it is ineffective for creating fat loss. For many of them, their excess fat is a result of their bodies being starved for healthful nutrients. They should be feeding their bodies, not starving them. As you have learned, it is possible to lose fat faster by eating large quantities of the right foods than by starving. Alkaline foods stimulate fat burning and supply the nutrients needed to produce and assist the enzymes, hormones and other internal chemicals necessary for burning fat. By eating correctly, you burn excess fat, supply healthful nutrition to your brain, muscles, internal organs and glands, and maintain a normal metabolism. Not eating causes your body to conserve energy and burn up lean body tissue, both of which slow your metabolism.

Anorexia nervosa is a condition that has killed many people. I believe that most of the people who have this condition feel that they are not good enough. Even though they see skin and bones in the mirror, they keep starving themselves, because they still do not think they are thin enough. They do not feel loved, accepted or worthwhile and fail to realize that they are not the body they see in the mirror. Clearly, self-image or other emotional problems need to be discovered and corrected. For maximum physical attractiveness, a good ratio of muscle and fat is necessary. That is what Nature intends, because it is best for the optimal health and function of our bodies. We are not supposed to abuse our bodies in an attempt to look like Popeye's girlfriend or a stick figure. Women should strive to look *their* best instead of like some models or actresses who are built like coat hangers and most likely starving their bodies to look that way. Sadly, these people often cannot be helped, because their brains are being starved for the nutrients needed to function normally. Therefore, correct nutrition is vital but is often overlooked or unknown. All the counseling in the world will fail if nutritional deficiencies are preventing someone from thinking clearly and rationally. For some of these people, the true cause is never determined or eliminated, so it causes a lifetime struggle. I believe that other eating disorders have similar causes and cures.

Some people have used powdered or liquid protein supplements while abstaining from all food. This may decrease the loss of lean tissue but, as you have learned, protein leaves an acid residue that makes burning fat even more stressful. A number of people have died following these extremely unbalanced and stressful programs.

Short fasts with fruit or juice are excellent for cleansing the body and giving overworked internal organs a chance to rejuvenate. Most people will probably never want to do more than a three-day apple juice cleanse and that is fine. If it is done enough times, this cleanse will eventually detoxify someone with extremely high levels of internal waste. I believe that the body rejuvenation that cleansing provides may help balance people's hormone levels and restore their appetite control centers to normal function. I highly recommend against cleansing for more than ten days or fasting with just water, because I believe that doing either of these has the potential to stress the body so severely it can become unbalanced and perhaps be permanently damaged. Most imbalances created could be normalized with a few Neurovascular Dynamics treatments, but any permanent damage would remain.

Some people smoke cigarettes to curb their appetites and prevent weight gain. As long as they keep smoking, they stay lean. This is an extremely unhealthy practice that creates even greater health risks than being fat. People who do this are not eating a nutritious diet, because if they were, they would not need to smoke to curb their appetites. Poor eating habits are why most people gain weight after they stop smoking, although some of the gain is muscle tissue. Following the guidelines in this book can eliminate the physical addiction to smoking by cleansing the body of nicotine residue and also eliminate the emotional need to smoke by getting rid of the fear of gaining weight after smoking is stopped. For some people, smoking satisfies the oral urge they have not outgrown. Instead of satisfying it with food all the time, they do it by sucking on a cigarette. Some people chew gum all day for the same reason. If they eat the right foods, these people can stay lean while eating enough to satisfy an excessive oral need or to help them reduce the need to normal.

Some obese people have had their jaws wired shut so they could not eat. They could only drink broth, juices and other liquids through a straw. They lost weight but I am sure you know what happened when the wires were removed and they started eating again.

Extremely obese people sometimes get so desperate to lose fat that they resort to surgery. I knew a woman who had her stomach stapled to make it smaller. She lost some weight but then got fat again. She ate high-calorie junk food more frequently and stretched the small section of her stomach until it became larger. I saw a television program about people who had gotten their stomachs surgically reduced in size. They all lost weight, because their stomachs were so small that they could eat only a few bites at a time. This does not sound like a healthy way to lose fat and because they cannot eat as much, these people may not get enough of the nutrients necessary for good health. Their health may suffer even more because, as you have learned, the foods that keep you lean also keep you healthy and rarely do any of these people learn how to eat to stay lean. I would be willing to bet that they will all have side effects from this surgery and that many will get fat again from eating high-calorie junk food every 20 to 30 minutes. I believe this because even after people's entire stomachs have been taken out they still experience psychic sensations of hunger. Another thing I noticed was that they were eating things like french fries and other junk foods during the interview. It seemed fairly obvious why they had gotten so fat in the first place. None of them had eliminated their causes for being fat or had learned to eat healthfully and exercise correctly. Drastic stomach reduction surgery has about a one percent mortality rate.

More and more obese teenagers are using adult diet drugs and resorting to risky surgeries to lose weight. One television program told the stories of a few of them who were having their stomachs reduced in size by about half. One was shown eating her "last" fast-food meal prior to her surgery and it was said that they all had to adhere to strict diets after the surgery. My question is: Why will they be able to resist fast foods and follow a strict diet after the surgery when they couldn't before? If they ate like that, they would get the same results without the surgery. And, having a stomach half as big will not make much difference if they continue to eat high-calorie junk food. These teens will lose weight but few, if any of them, will be taught how to eat for good health or how to exercise correctly to build or maintain muscle mass.

Another surgery frequently being done is liposuction, where subcutaneous fat cells are sucked out from under the skin. I do not recommend this surgery for many reasons. First of all, it should be unnecessary if the guidelines in this book are followed. Second, it is an attempt to cheat Nature's laws and this would have a negative impact on your self-image. Third, no nutritional or lifestyle changes are necessary, so the results may be temporary. Fourth, the causes of why you were fat are still there so you would start gaining again. This is discouraging and negatively impacts your self-image even more. It would make you feel powerless to control your weight. These physical and emotional effects can cause you to overeat and make poor food choices. Last, but certainly not least, numerous people have died after having liposuction, especially when an excessive amount of fat was taken out at one time. Liposuction may be an option for people who developed excess fat cells when they were children but these people should first eliminate their causes, change their eating patterns and lose most of their fat. After they have done all they can do naturally, they may look fine and be happy. If not, removing the excess fat cells may be desired by some. I would not recommend this option until the eating and exercise habits taught in this book have become a part of someone's lifestyle.

A woman I used to know ate well and exercised regularly. She had a great body, but did not like the small amount of fat on her lower abdomen that would just not go away. She had liposuction on that area and promptly gained a "love handle" on each side of her abdomen. Her body wanted extra fat there (which is normal for women) and was going to store it one place or the other. She was more unhappy after the liposuction than she was before.

I once saw a television program about a woman who weighed more than 1,000 pounds. She was so huge she could not even get out of bed. It was easy to see the reason why when they showed what she was eating every day—entire chocolate cakes, a pie or two, pizzas, hamburgers and loads of other high-calorie junk foods. She ate more desserts and junk food in one day than the average fat person eats in a month. Can you imagine the cost of feeding her? She ate few foods with any nutritional value or that would be helpful for losing excess fat. It seemed strange that she kept eating the way she did when she said that she wanted to lose fat and regain a normal life. I do not understand why her loved ones continued to give her all that fattening and worthless food. Why not give her some fruits, vegetables and legumes? I doubt if she was taking any nutritional supplements that would supply at least some of the nutrients her body needs. Even that woman should be able to return to a normal body weight by following the advice in this book. The only surgery needed would be to eliminate her excess skin.

There is a device currently being tested called a gastric stimulator. It is implanted in the wall of the abdomen and has electrodes that go to the stomach. It works something like a heart pacemaker and is designed to make your stomach feel full faster. This device may make someone eat less but does not effect what they eat or when. They could still just eat less junk food and not supply their bodies with the nutrients needed to be healthy. They could also eat more frequently. This device could have serious side effects if people do not eat healthful foods. This could happen to many of its users because if they knew how to eat healthfully they would not need the device.

The bottom line is to trust in Nature and its perfect balance instead of risky surgeries, gastric stimulators, diet shakes, low-calorie processed meals, diet drugs or some "scientific" weight-loss formula that costs you hundreds of dollars a month. The truth is, there is only one healthy way to lose excess fat and keep it off—Nature's way. Get yourself more in tune with Nature and then trust yourself and a balanced (you now know what this means) eating program of whole, natural foods—the foods Nature created to keep your body lean and healthy. Your body needs to be used regularly and strenuously, so make exercising intensely a regular part of your life and stay active with physical work and play. It makes you feel strong and alive. If you sit on the couch like a potato, your body will soon end up looking like one and you will end up feeling like one.

If for some reason you still feel the need to follow some "special" diet program, please do it under the guidance and supervision of a lean (not skinny) and experienced health professional. You will get advice soon on how to find a good one.

Avoid "Loser's Clubs"

Because excess fat is such a common problem, thousands of weight-loss products, diet centers, support groups and aerobics classes have been designed to aid people in their weight-loss quests. I say "weight loss," because most of these groups are not concerned about what people lose and few focus on the correct type of exercise to accomplish the goal. This section is not meant as criticism of anyone, but is written only to educate *you* and to save you time, money and frustration. Most of these diet centers and groups have limited success helping people achieve their goals. For a price, you can get consulting, support, and "diet" foods. You already know, however, that about 95 percent of the people who lose on these programs gain back at least as much fat as they lost. They fail because they do not work in harmony with Nature, do not teach you how to eat nutritious meals of whole, natural foods, do not help you design the best meals for your unique body, do not teach the best exercises for building muscle and losing fat, and do not teach you how to eliminate the physical and emotional causes of why you are fat.

Some of these groups can make you psychologically dependent on their meetings, products or exercise classes. If you enjoy socializing with many of the people there, why would you want to get and stay lean? If you did, you would not get any attention at this social event and you would see your friends less often or not at all. Some groups can be tremendously influential at keeping you fat, or your weight may fluctuate up and down as you attempt to fool yourself into believing they are helping. As you have learned, continually losing and gaining is extremely unhealthy, physically and psychologically.

You are told at some dietary centers that you have no control over your excess fat because it is genetic or because you are an addict. For a price, however, *they* will assume responsibility for your excess fat. They cannot change your genetics and I doubt if they know how to help you stop being an addict. But they will keep trying as long as you keep paying. Do not keep spending money to buy an excuse for your excess fat. You already know that you will not enjoy permanent results until *you* accept responsibility for having your excess fat. What incentive do those selling weight-loss products or working at dietary centers have to tell you that?

Do not misunderstand me when I comment about dietary centers or groups. Many of the people operating them have good intentions. Their methods are simply ineffective because they do not know how to help you achieve permanent results. Remember that your dietary and psychological needs are unique. What works for someone else may do nothing for you or could even make your problem worse.

A few years ago I met a man who had recently sold a large chain of well-known weight-loss centers. It seemed strange that he was following the unhealthy suggestions of the current fad diet in an attempt to lose his own excess fat. Why would the former owner of these diet centers be fat? Clearly, his own centers had failed to develop an effective program for him.

You may have gone to a weight-loss center or support group in the past, and now, armed with your new knowledge, you may want to go back if you feel it will help you accomplish your goals. You should not need it after you have reached your goals. Learn from the positive aspects found there but be forewarned of some of the negative aspects you will often find. Here are some of them.

Some weight-loss centers are expensive. They may charge a fee just to weigh you. If all they do is check your weight, they are unaware of how to help you accomplish your goals because, as you now know, weight is the most inaccurate way of determining if you are making positive changes or not. Some of these centers are inexpensive to join but sell expensive foods or dietary products you have to buy if you follow their programs. Most of these foods and products are not good for you even if they are low in calories and low in fat. If it is processed, chances are it has lost much of its original nutritional value. It may help some people lose weight, but did they lose fat or muscle? Remember our 110-pound woman who believed she was healthy, yet had 40 percent body fat? Her low weight created an illusion of health. She was deceiving herself and setting herself up to develop diabetes, heart disease, stroke and other serious diseases linked to excess body fat. And, as you have learned, processed foods are not helpful at building health and preventing disease. Not everything we need can be artificially added, and if your body does not get adequate nutrition, it will continue to ask for more food. This can lead to overeating. Using these "weight-loss" meals does not help you learn how to make nutritious meals from whole, natural foods. And, will you have to buy these products for the rest of your life to stay lean? You now know that you do not need "special" foods to be healthy and lose body fat quickly and easily.

There are dietary centers where particular point values are given to different foods. This plan lets you eat a certain number of points each day. This is like counting calories—the numbers are just smaller and easier to add up. A piece of pie may have the same number of points as two scoops of ice cream. Neither is healthful so it doesn't matter which one you choose. You could still end up eating foods lacking in nutritional value all day long. It should be easy to see that substituting processed pasta for processed bread is not going to help you achieve your permanent fat loss goal. Remember that the goal of eating is to satisfy some of your physical and emotional needs, not just fill up your stomach. If you fill your car's gas tank with water, there is no room for gasoline to fuel the engine. Likewise, if you fill your stomach with worthless food, there is no room for nutritious food to supply energy and build health. Fill your car's tank with high-octane gasoline and your body's "tank" with highly nutritious food.

Some weight-loss centers and groups have exercise recommendations or classes as part of their programs. You are often told that because a pound of fat contains 3,500 calories, if you attend seven exercise sessions and burn five hundred calories each session, you will burn up one pound of body fat. This is true if you are doing fat-burning exercise and not eating more than you were, but most classes are aerobic programs that raise your heart rate so high that you do not burn any fat. You may be expending five hundred calories but the calories are not coming from fat being burned. They are coming from glucose and stored glycogen that will be replenished the next time you eat. The truth is, you can burn five hundred calories every session for seven sessions, seventy sessions, or seven hundred sessions and burn absolutely zero body fat. Do not be fooled by this illusion. If your exercising heart rate is more than 120 beats per minute, chances are you will not burn much body fat. This is why so many people never lost any fat doing aerobics for years and why millions have given up on exercising.

Some exercise classes are called muscle toning. They use large rubber bands or extremely light weights for resistance. These classes are so ineffective at toning and firming your muscles that they are essentially a waste of time. You can accomplish more in a few weeks of correct strength-training exercise than you could in fifty years of these classes, because the intensity is so low there is no gain of lean body mass. Therefore, your metabolism is not increased and you have accomplished nothing to help you reach your goals. Instead, you have wasted time and made yourself more discouraged. Most of these classes will not even prevent you from losing muscle mass. These light, pumping exercises may stimulate your appetite and actually increase your fat level if you do not eat correctly.

Unless you have been doing heavy strength training, your body has the potential to be much stronger than it is now, and if you want it to be lean and healthy, you must use it. You have to make your muscles work against gradually increasing resistance. Otherwise, you are just deceiving yourself and getting almost no benefits for your time and money. Developing your physical strength has another significant benefit beyond keeping your bones and muscles strong and your body leaner, firmer, healthier, more physically capable and more resistant to injury. As you get physically stronger, you start seeing yourself as a stronger person. Your mental strength increases and this can help you in countless ways. It is easier to replace destructive habits and behaviors with healthy ones, and as you progress your self-confidence will grow and your self-image will improve. A positive cycle will start that will make you feel more capable of handling whatever difficulties or opportunities you create for yourself.

Perhaps the most destructive part of some "Loser's Clubs" is what you hear from others. People stand up and tell their stories or offer support. This can sometimes be motivating but is usually short-lived. The problem is that the people who go to these groups are struggling. They do not know how to eat or exercise properly, have not found and eliminated their causes for being fat or are unwilling to face and eliminate them. They are deceiving themselves and they go to these groups and talk to others who are also deceiving themselves and doing all the wrong things to accomplish their goals. Some may feel a bit better after they leave each meeting because they see other fat people in the same rut with the same problem they have. Birds of a feather flock together. Sadly, they also stay fat together. You may feel like you belong to a group like this, but you do not. These are the thinking and behavioral habits you need to eliminate. Listening to fearful people who do not know how to accomplish their own goals is not going to help you accomplish yours. The information disseminated is often misleading or incorrect and much of the talk is empty. They analyze and discuss but perform no action other than meeting periodically and having the same old discussions. This is why the vast majority of people who go to these groups never achieve lasting results.

You may occasionally hear someone speak who inspires you to action. The problem is, without the knowledge of what to do, your actions will produce only more discouragement. Keep in mind that what worked for that person may not necessarily work for you—not unless you both have the same physical and emotional causes, the same body types, the same digestive capabilities, the same nutritional needs, the same metabolism, the same activity level and so forth. Do you get the picture? Your unique program must be developed from a number of variables. Unless you hear about finding and eliminating causes and learning how to eat healthfully, naturally, and balanced, the greatest favor you can do for yourself is never to go back. If you were to return in six months with your new lean body, you would see most of the same sad faces listening to the same stories, supporting each other and keeping each other fat. They cannot help each other get lean, because none of them knows how.

Some groups talk about accepting yourself and being content and happy with your fat body. They help each other to believe that being fat is what they want or that it is okay to be fat. It is okay to be "you," but "you" are not fat, your body is, and you now have the knowledge and power to change it anytime you choose. As you have learned, accepting yourself unconditionally as you are (loving yourself) is the most important goal you can achieve. Loving yourself is the key to everything good in life, but you must remember that loving yourself is not the same as liking your behavior, your body or anything else. You are the spirit *in* the body, not just the body. Your mind may think fat-creating thoughts and your body may be fat, but your spirit is not. Your false thinking and behavioral patterns have created excess fat in a body designed to be lean. Armed with the truth, you can now eliminate your false thinking, change your behaviors and watch your body change to reflect the real you inside.

Some people go to weight-loss groups to get attention. First they lose some weight and then they gain it back so they can lose it again and get more attention. It is an unhealthy way of attempting to achieve the love they are craving—the love that first must come from within.

Time is our most valuable commodity and the primary reason why I have seen people give up on going to weight-loss centers. They no longer wanted to waste time in meetings and nonproductive exercise classes. I have known many people over the years who have tried these programs. Most of them lost some weight in the beginning but then got discouraged due to their lack of continuing progress. They all then regained at least as much as they had lost.

If you have friends who go to these groups, buy them a copy of this book and start your own club—a "Winner's Club." They, like you, are good but frustrated people searching for the truth. They are beautiful spirits; they just do not know it yet. Two or three of you reading this book and working together may be the best support group ever. Rapid results should be achieved, because you will be motivating each other based on the truth. You can help each other determine and eliminate your causes for having excess fat and learn together how to eat in a healthier way. You can share meal ideas and other discoveries.

You may be able to exercise together and help each other train at a higher intensity. You will be supporting each other as all of you accomplish your goals. It could be extremely motivating and exciting. And, once you learn the truth, you can be free from your excess fat forever.

Be careful not to let yourself become dependent on someone else. Always remember that your success or failure depends on you alone. You do not need anyone else to accomplish your goals just like you do not need anyone else's love but your own. The knowledge is within you now and the only one who can stop you is *you*. Support from others can be a great boost when learning and starting out, but you must claim your independence as soon as you can. If your friends feel unworthy or lack a good reason to be lean and healthy, they will quickly fall by the wayside. You must be able to do it on your own so they do not drag you down with them. If they want your help and are making an effort, continue helping them, but mainly just never stop being a good example for them and others. You owe this to yourself and those who look up to you. If you are on your own, your gym or health club can be seen as a "Winner's Club."

There may be groups that do challenge people to take an honest look at the reasons why they are fat and help them change their thinking and appearances permanently. I am not aware of any, but if you find one like this, it may be helpful. I still recommend developing your inner strength and convictions so you do not become dependent on others. Some people may need a support group for the rest of their lives. If you do, please do not condemn or judge yourself in any way. It is just a need you have much like a diabetic who needs regular injections of insulin.

If You Seek Professional Help

Complete this book and review it once. Then, if you feel you need professional assistance to help you develop your nutritional program, read the following suggestions on how to find someone who can truly help you.

The first thing to do when interviewing doctors or nutritional counselors is to look at them. If they do not have a lean and healthy appearance, do not even waste your time. No matter what they seem to know, if they cannot help themselves, they cannot help you. Ask them to explain their nutrition and exercise philosophies. Do not be influenced if they start spouting off impressive-sounding gobbledygook. The more technical jargon they use, the less real truth they usually know. People who know the truth should be able to explain things in simple, easy to understand terms. If they recommend eating a variety of natural foods, getting rid of the causes, and exercising with relatively heavy resistance, they may be able to help you. They should sound like they have read this book. If they talk about eating something from each of the four food groups at every meal, drinking protein shakes, learning to read the labels on *processed* foods, or exercising with light resistance, run the other way.

Keep in mind that many professional dietitians have only a few pieces of the permanent fat-loss puzzle. A large number of them are struggling to lose their own excess body fat. They went to college, but most of them never learned what, how and when to eat in a healthy, balanced way. Many of the instructors teaching the nutritional courses are fat, unhealthy people simply repeating the same information they memorized twenty or thirty years ago when they were in school. Some of these "dietary specialists" design hospital meals that are so unbalanced and unhealthful it is absolutely absurd. Even people who know almost nothing about healthful eating usually recognize that these meals are extremely unhealthful. Most hospital meals are poor combinations of primarily acidic foods that increase inflammation and slow healing. They consist of white bread, pastries, soft drinks, milk and a conglomeration of overcooked "dead" foods with rarely, if ever, anything raw to supply any healing life force. Hardly anything can be found that would help someone regain lost health. A regular diet of hospital food would make healthy people sick and fat. Take a look at the people working in hospitals. Most of the ones I have seen are fat and out of shape.

Many people believe that medical doctors know about nutrition, but the majority of them have never attended even one nutritional class. They are perhaps the worst source of information about fat loss and healthful eating. Doctors of chiropractic and osteopathy have some nutritional classes but rarely learn how to help someone design a healthful nutritional program. There are doctors who have studied nutrition extensively and perhaps even use it in their practices, but this is definitely a rare exception and not the rule.

Be wary of counselors who are extremely thin. If you do not hear about finding and eliminating the physical and emotional causes of why you are fat, learning to eat in a healthy, balanced and unique way for you and exercising against a challenging resistance, again, save yourself and your money by running the other way. The counselor is most likely lean because of a fast metabolism.

If someone told you to wear a shoe with a four-inch heel on your right foot and a shoe with a one-inch heel on your left foot, would you do it? Probably not, because it is easy to see what an extreme imbalance this would cause. Remember this if someone tells you to drink fruit juices or to eat egg whites, processed flour products or other incomplete and unbalanced foods.

Be skeptical if the person you interview has some "miracle" product to sell. If this product takes the place of eating a wide variety of natural foods, look elsewhere. Nature's foods supply the substances you need that scientists have not even discovered yet, along with the ones they have. Some herbal formulas are helpful for cleansing and fat loss, but you should not need to continue taking them to maintain. If you do, it most likely contains some kind of stimulant. Avoid using stimulants. If the cost of a product is excessively high, be wary of it. Avoid using protein powders, protein bars, meal replacements and engineered foods, especially the ones claiming to be better than real food. If doctors or nutritionists recommend these products, they do not understand good nutrition regardless of their reputations. The only way to lose and then maintain your fat loss *healthfully* is to learn to eat *real* foods in good combinations and at the right time.

You should now know how to develop your own healthful eating program. You may need professional help only to determine and eliminate your emotional or physical reasons for having excess fat.

Set Realistic Goals

To complete the journey from living in a fat body to living in a lean, clean, healthy machine (body), you must set goals. The first thing to determine is where you are now. Record your weight, measurements, clothing sizes, and most importantly, your body fat percentage.

Use a cloth or plastic tailor's tape to take your measurements. Put it on your skin around the largest part of the area you are measuring and flex the muscle. Even though it may not feel like it, you do have muscles under there. Measure your neck, chest, waist, upper arm, forearm, hips, thigh and calf. Record them along with the date. You most likely lack the experience to set measurement goals and they are really unnecessary, but checking your measurements is a good way to see and chart your progress.

Your body fat percentage can be checked easily using body-fat calipers. These can be purchased for less than $30 and include instructions. Many gyms and health clubs offer this service free or for a small fee. Scales are available that measure your body fat percentage when you weigh yourself. They use the bioelectrical impedance method and are inexpensive. Some are not extremely accurate but you can see if the percentage is going up or down and that is all you need. Hand-held body fat testers are also inexpensive and easy to use. Keep a record of your body fat percentage along with your weight, clothing sizes and measurements.

The most important and accurate feedback of your progress will come from rechecking your body fat percentage. I suggest doing it approximately once a month. Many health and fitness authorities believe that a healthy body fat percentage for men is 15 percent and for women, 22 percent. I recommend about 10 to 12 percent for men and 18 to 20 percent for women. These percentages are not only healthier but can easily be achieved by the average person who eats relatively well and does strength-training exercise two to three times a week.

Sit down and think about some realistic goals for yourself. Weighing 110 pounds is not a practical or healthy goal if you are a 5'10" tall woman with a large bone structure. Be realistic and use some good sense. Keep in mind that the amount you weigh should not be the primary focus unless you are extremely obese. A woman weighing 130 pounds with a high body fat percentage will look large and unshapely while the same woman at a low body fat percentage but still weighing 130 pounds will look shapely and much smaller. She will have lost many inches, because muscle is much denser than fat, and well-developed muscles are what give the body its most natural and pleasing shape.

There may have been a time in high school, college or the military when you were in good shape and at your best weight. This can give you a realistic weight goal. Height and weight charts may help you but they are inaccurate for someone who has more muscle than average. When you reach a healthy body fat percentage, you will be at the best weight for your body. Therefore, a body fat percentage goal is all you need, but you may want to set other goals as well.

As you set your goals, keep in mind that you are a unique person in a one-of-a-kind body. Your best will be better than the best of some people but not as good as others. Comparing yourself to someone with the genetic potential to have a much better body than you or with someone who is using dangerous and unhealthy drugs may make you feel terribly discouraged. Never compare yourself to anyone else, only to your own previous best.

Many young women create a tremendous amount of grief and unhappiness in their lives by comparing their bodies to those of models, actresses or even a Barbie® doll. They deprive themselves of the nutrients they need to think straight and feel good physically and emotionally. You must understand that models need to be thin so clothes will hang on them like a clothes hanger; and because the camera adds 10 to 15 pounds to someone's appearance, an actress has to be excessively thin to look normal on screen. The need to be overly thin not only wreaks havoc on the lives of many who look up to them as role models, but on the lives of those in, or striving to be in, these professions.

Avoid comparing what you eat with what others eat. Your friend who seems to subsist on candy and other junk food may have a fast metabolism and be thin, but will not be healthy. Your goal should be to have a lean *and* healthy body. You may feel like you eat less than people with lower body weights do. There is a simple answer. If they have more lean body mass—even if you outweigh them by 50 or more pounds—their bodies need more calories than yours does. Muscle is lean working tissue requiring energy, but fat uses hardly any calories so is just excess baggage. Another possibility is that you are eating a small amount of food that contains a large number of calories and the person you are comparing yourself to is eating a larger amount of food that contains fewer calories.

We each have a body fat percentage that is right for our unique body. A small-boned ectomorphic (slender, fragile body type) man may have the potential to have as little as 5 percent body fat, but a large-boned endomorphic (soft, round body type) man may never be able to get below 20 percent. No matter how much we restrict our diets or increase our exercise, we will not lose any more fat once we reach our genetic limit. This is because our bodies have a hormone-regulated feedback mechanism that prevents us from depleting the fat level below what is necessary for survival and optimal health. Once you reach your best body-fat level, your body will stop burning stored fat and start burning muscle tissue. Bodybuilders, athletes or others who use anabolic steroids can keep burning body fat until it gets to unnaturally low and unhealthy levels, because the drugs block the body's normal feedback mechanism. These extremely low body fat levels are physiologically impossible without using certain drugs. Be especially careful never to compare yourself with people who use these drugs.

Accept yourself and be happy with your current best while continuing to make it better. Do not make yourself crazy by setting unrealistic goals. A five-foot tall man could ruin his life if his goal is to be a professional basketball star. Set goals to improve and move closer to your personal potential. If you are a large-boned woman with 27 percent body fat (the lowest your body can go), rejoice and be glad. Maintain it and have a happy and productive life. Do not constantly put yourself down because your body fat level is not 26 percent. The stress and negativity you create will sabotage your ability to easily maintain your current (and healthy for you) fat percentage.

Your weight is a rough guide to your progress and something I recommend checking every day, because it helps you adjust your food intake. Weigh yourself every morning and then *choose* to eat well enough that day so you will weigh a bit less the next morning. It is vital that you understand, however, that your weight will fluctuate up and down as you lose fat. You may weigh 170 pounds on Monday, 168 on Tuesday, 170 on Wednesday, 167 on Thursday, 168 again on Friday, 165 on Saturday and 166 on Sunday. The next week may be similar but will end at 162 pounds on Sunday. These fluctuations occur because water is formed when fat is burned. On the days your weight goes up, your body is just retaining excess water. Your weight goes down when the water balance of your body is reestablished. This up and down pattern is normal, so do not be discouraged. The average of the fluctuations should gradually become less. Use your daily weigh-in to motivate you, not discourage you. Remember that everything about your lifestyle must be positive. If these normal fluctuations discourage you, your thinking needs to change so a daily weigh-in helps you instead of hinders you.

It may be helpful for you to know that fat cells store mostly triglycerides in liquid form and that a constant turnover occurs. This means that fat is burned every day and the way people eat causes the amount to increase, decrease or stay the same. Because fat is always being eliminated, all you have to do is eat in such a way that less fat is stored to replace what is being used. See how simple it is to lose fat?

If you have never exercised or have not trained correctly to build strength and muscle, you will most likely be gaining muscle mass and losing body fat at the same time. Your weight may stay the same or even increase if this is happening. You will, however, be measuring a lower body fat percentage, losing inches and wearing smaller clothing, so you should know that positive changes are happening and not be discouraged. Your muscle gains will slow down after a while but your body fat loss will continue and the scales will then show more of a change. If you are obese, you will see a decrease in your weight right away. Some people will end up weighing the same but have an extremely improved appearance and much less body fat. Think about how great our 110-pound obese woman would look at 110 pounds if she had 20 percent fat instead of 40 percent.

Take your measurements about once a month and keep a record of the changes. Be aware that changes in your measurements can be misleading, because some areas may initially get larger due to muscle gain and an area will stay the same if it is gaining muscle and losing fat equally. Some areas will get smaller, tighter and firmer right away. Like your weight, your measurements will eventually start to change. Once again, the power of knowledge should prevent discouragement.

Some people start relatively productive exercise and nutritional programs but believe nothing is happening if they do not see changes in their weight or measurements in the first month or two. A number of positive changes may have taken place, but because of their lack of knowledge they assume the program is not working and abandon it. This is unfortunate, but shows you how important it is for you to know what changes are taking place.

Never be afraid that you might become overly muscled. Developing large muscles takes men a number of months—generally years—of intense training. If you are a woman, it is even more difficult, because you have far less testosterone production and muscular potential. You are not going to complete a few heavy workouts and look like Arnold Schwarzenegger did in his prime or like some female bodybuilder who has trained hard and taken anabolic steroids for years. Many women who take steroids have smaller measurements of most body areas than most fat women do, because they have less body fat. Never be afraid to train as hard as you can. Because building muscle is a slow process, you will *never* get bigger muscles than you want. And, if you ever want them to be smaller, it is easy to accomplish.

If you are a woman, you need not fear getting too lean from working out hard. A woman's body has a natural layer of fat all over that a man's body does not. This is regulated by hormones and is important for childbearing purposes. The point is, do not be afraid of looking like a man. Larger muscles just give you a more attractive feminine shape. Few women can get extremely lean and have much muscle size without using anabolic steroids or similar illegal drugs. Do not believe female bodybuilders who look like men when they say they do not use drugs. It is physiologically impossible for a woman to have large muscles and be extremely lean.

Do not believe the old wives' tale that lifting light weights for higher repetitions creates definition and lifting heavy weights for lower repetitions builds "bulk." The truth is, you must train as hard as you can if you want to get stronger and build lean body mass. What most people will gain initially is the muscle tissue they have lost through inactivity. Most women will gain only a few pounds of new muscle in their first year or two of strength training. Continuing to exercise may build a little more but will primarily just maintain their strength, muscle size and shape. Those not doing strength-training exercise will continue to lose muscle tissue each year and most will gain fat in its place. High repetitions with a light weight cause a loss of strength and muscle, and will not spot reduce a part of your body. Muscle definition is achieved by losing subcutaneous fat, and that is done with correct eating and fat-burning exercise.

Excess fat stretches the skin, causing it to be loose after the underlying fat is lost. This loose, flabby skin can make people feel like they are getting fatter or looking worse. They may get discouraged and abandon a successful fat-loss program. Do not let this happen to you. With correct exercise, good nutrition and time, your skin should gradually tighten, at least to some degree. A tablespoon of liquid pre-digested collagen protein taken just before bedtime seems to help the skin tighten faster. Someone who was extremely obese may need surgery to eliminate the excess skin.

To avoid discouragement you must understand that the first place your body stored fat will be the last place from which you lose it. For men, this is generally the abdominal area. Some women store it there but most women store fat first on their hips and upper thighs. Do not worry; it will eventually go away in these areas as you follow your healthy lifestyle.

If you do some cleansing or follow most of the recommendations in this book, you could lose a great deal of unwanted weight in a short time. Many of my clients have lost 10 to 20 pounds in just a few weeks. You may have heard or read that the body cannot lose fat this fast. This is true, but in the beginning you will be losing a lot of internal waste along with body fat. You now know that this is important for health reasons and that it also increases the efficiency of your body, making losing the remaining excess body fat faster and easier.

Set Mini-Goals

After you have set your goals, you then need to break them down into mini-goals. What is a mini-goal? A mini-goal is something so easily achievable that you cannot fail. It is like the old joke, "How do you eat an elephant?" "One bite at a time." Likewise, how do you accomplish your goals? By completing one mini-goal at a time. A mini-goal can be to make a minor change in your diet. Your first one may be to drink water before your meals and not during or after. Continue with this change and after a week, make a second small change such as eating a healthful breakfast or using only fruit for morning snacks. Another mini-goal could be to eat one less dessert a week. As you progress you can eliminate dessert twice a week, then three times and continue on to eliminate it as many times as you choose. Gradually completing more mini-goals helps you develop new health habits and progress toward completing your goals.

What if you crave chocolate and your goal is to not eat it anymore. Cleansing your body can eliminate your physical addiction, but as your body is cleansing, you will crave chocolate. To rid yourself of the physical addiction you must oppose this craving. A mini-goal would be to not eat any chocolate for one hour. Chances are you can easily resist it for at least that long. After an hour has passed, set a new mini-goal to not eat any chocolate for one hour. As each hour ends, reset your mini-goal to resist chocolate for one hour. If you cannot stop yourself from eating chocolate for an hour, make it 15 minutes or even less. Your mini-goals must be so easy that you *always* succeed, because success begets success. Each time you complete a mini-goal, it makes you feel more self-confident and capable of success. Of course, not having chocolate around the house will be extremely helpful.

The mini-goal method has helped many people stop smoking, resist junk food, and eliminate other unwanted habits. It has also helped many to create new positive habits. For example, another mini-goal can be to go to the gym and do one set of one exercise and then go home. If that is all you do, you have successfully completed your mini-goal. What often happens, however, is that once you are at the gym and have completed the first set, you then feel like continuing. You have broken the inertia of a body at rest and created some momentum. These powers are now working for you to keep your body in motion. The hardest part about doing almost anything is to break the inertia and get started. Even though mini-goals are small and easy to do, they are extremely powerful because they get you moving so the incredible powers you have at your disposal can start working for you instead of against you. Once you get started on a project or workout, it is often harder to stop than to continue. You get on a roll.

It is usually difficult for people who have never exercised to think of going to a gym or health club and completing an hour-long workout. It can feel overwhelming and keep inertia working against them. It can also be embarrassing if they are self-conscious about how they look. You will most certainly draw some stares if you are obese, but realize that most of the people there will respect and admire you for striving to improve your health and appearance. And, that respect will grow as they see you losing fat and training correctly. Some will congratulate you and others may even ask you how you are making such fast progress. You may make some new friends who lead healthy and active lifestyles. As I have said before, birds of a feather flock together. Associate with those you want to be like—those who are healthy in body, mind and spirit.

You can start doing strength training at home, but it would be limited and you could easily get discouraged due to lack of progress. For some people, it would work for a while, but unless you know how to do it correctly, you will not make much progress. You may do well training at home if you have a motivated training partner and some good equipment but most people do not have either. Do not be afraid to go to a gym because you think everyone there will look great. It is not like the television ads you may have seen with all the young, lean people in them. The majority of people (young and old) found in most gyms and health clubs do not have very good bodies, because they lack the knowledge of how to gain muscle or lose fat. A good gym or health club can be highly motivating, will usually have the equipment you need, and you may find someone to work out with who has similar goals. With the right knowledge, you can then help each other physically and emotionally to accomplish your individual goals.

To use our previous example, your initial mini-goal on your first trip to the gym may be to do one set of one exercise. Make it something easily achievable and do not criticize yourself if it is all you do. You were successful and that is what counts. After you accomplish your first mini-goal, your next one could be to go to the gym and do two sets of the same exercise or one set of two different exercises. Your third mini-goal could be to do two sets of the first exercise and one set of a new one. It may take a week or two to progress that far and it doesn't matter if it does. The point is that you are growing in confidence and ability. Knowing how to train correctly also increases your confidence and creates fast physical results, which builds your confidence even more. Chapter fifteen contains basic information about correct training.

Progress at your own pace. It is perfectly fine to take baby steps. The secret is to keep taking them. It is better to progress slowly but surely than to go "gung ho" for a short time and end up burning yourself out and quitting. The tortoise won the race because it kept plodding along at a slow but steady pace. Do not compare yourself to someone who may go to the gym the first time and work out for an hour. Look only at your own previous accomplishments and praise yourself for doing more than you have done in the past. Keep your focus on this key idea—you are making positive changes that, one by one, will gradually build and generate more power to help you. Each change helping and supporting the other makes you stronger and more able to accomplish new and larger mini-goals.

What if your goal is to lose 200 pounds of excess fat? WOW! That seems like an impossible task, doesn't it? But, what about completing a mini-goal of losing one pound of excess fat? That probably sounds quite easy. The truth is, you do not have to lose 200 pounds. All you have to do is complete your mini-goal and repeat the process two hundred times. See how easy it is? What's great is that each lost pound builds your confidence, and as you exercise, cleanse your body, and improve your thinking and eating habits, each part of your program makes the others more effective. As this positive cycle builds momentum, each excess pound will disappear faster and easier.

How do you think this book was completed? Correct—one mini-goal at a time. Use the power of mini-goals to help you achieve all of your goals.

fourteen

Lifelong Change

S ome weight-loss programs use tricks and gimmicks in an attempt to help you lose, but your mind is not fooled so success is usually short-lived. Gimmicks are unnecessary if you know the truth, however, certain psychological tools can recruit the incredible power of your subconscious mind to help you. Few people can consciously overcome their causes for being fat, because the causes are in their much stronger subconscious. Therefore, it must be dealt with there. The subconscious can be likened to a bulldozer and the conscious mind to a human body. Like learning to use your body to control and direct the power of the bulldozer, the key is to learn to use the conscious mind to control and direct the power of the subconscious. Because few people have learned to love themselves 100 percent unconditionally, the following techniques can be used to help accomplish your goals.

Visualization

Visualization can express what you want to your subconscious, but to use it successfully you must first understand how it works. Your subconscious strives to create what it believes you want but it is only positive. If you frequently use the expression that things are a "pain in the neck," it will eventually create a pain in your neck. I have noticed this with some of my patients. If you complain, your subconscious will oblige you and create more problems for you. Stop complaining and watch your life improve dramatically. Give thanks for all the blessings you already have and your subconscious will create more blessings for you. What you focus your attention on is what it will create. When you experience feelings of appreciation for yourself, others and everything in your life, you send out positive vibrations that attract more things to appreciate. Make a list of the major things you are thankful for and read it (out loud preferably) just before going to sleep every night. Feel appreciation for what you have and for anything special you enjoyed that day.

The subconscious believes that everything is directed toward it. For example, if someone cuts you off while driving and you say, "You stupid jerk," your subconscious thinks you are talking to it. You are programming yourself to feel and act like a stupid jerk. How you think, feel and talk about others will boomerang and come back to you. It will whack you in the head if it is negative, but if it is positive, you will attract more good things or become a better person. Projecting feelings of love and appreciation toward others will attract being loved and appreciated to you, and can help you learn to love yourself. It is really not difficult to do, because even the worst person in the world can be appreciated as a good example of how not to act. It may help you to project positive feelings toward others if you realize that, given the chance to get to know them, you would like many of them and some would become close friends. After all, your friends were strangers until you got to know them.

Because your subconscious is positive, you cannot use it as a deterrent. An example of this is when fat people, who want to reduce, put a picture of an extremely obese person on the refrigerator door. They mistakenly believe that the picture will deter them from overeating. What they are doing is programming their subconscious to create the fat image. The plan will usually backfire and create more fat instead of less. Everything you program into your subconscious must be what you want, not want you don't want. If you are living your life as your true spiritual self, it (you) will constantly use your subconscious power to create everything in life you need to be happy. Unfortunately, few of us live as our true selves most of the time so we counteract what it is striving to do. Luckily, we can learn to stop creating negative vibrations that block our needs from coming.

You must be particularly careful what you ask your subconscious for, because you will get it, but it may not be in the form you consciously want. Your worldly programmed conscious mind may think you need a particular thing to be happy. Your subconscious can create it for you, but it will rarely satisfy you and it frequently backfires, creating stress and unhappiness instead of the joy you anticipated. Having material possessions is your right, but if your worldly programmed ego is the source of wanting them, you will often feel unworthy to receive them. You may sabotage your life and lose them or create another way (e.g., illness or excess fat) not to enjoy them. This happens because your programmed ego does not know what makes the "real you" happy. You will have everything you need to be happy if your true self is creating your life, because it knows *exactly* what you need and can create it down to the smallest detail. The only thing capable of limiting it is your judgmental ego making you feel unworthy to enjoy all the love, satisfaction, joy, material things and opportunities your true self is attracting. The ultimate secret is to love yourself unconditionally as you are right now.

Visualization can be used three primary ways to help you accomplish your fat-losing goal. The first way is simple and takes only enough time to put a picture together. It requires finding a photograph of your body when it was as lean as you would like it to be again. It should be one where you were in a swimsuit so you can see most of your body. If you have one, make five to ten copies. Otherwise, find a picture of someone wearing underwear or a swimsuit who is lean and looks close to your height and frame size. Next, get a picture of your face, approximately the same size as the face on the picture you have found. Cut out and paste your face on this body. Make it as natural looking as possible and then make some photocopies. Some computer programs can create realistic pictures. Put the copies of this picture where you will see it as often as possible.

Here is the experience of a man who used the picture method. He was only twenty-three years old but had been fighting to lose excess fat almost his entire life. After using this method for two weeks he had lost nine pounds, even though he had made no other changes in his life. He put photocopies of the picture he had made where he would see one almost all the time. He put one next to his bed, on his bathroom mirror, on his desk at work, on his refrigerator, by his kitchen table, and even on a bookmarker he was using. He was bombarding his subconscious with the visual image of what he wanted. Even though he still had a subconscious cause for being fat, this tremendous amount of input into his subconscious was stronger than his cause so he lost weight—just by looking at a picture. But you must do more than look. You have to *feel* physically and emotionally what it will be like when your body looks like the picture. This is the secret to visualization and explains why it fails for some people.

It is easier to accomplish your fat-loss goal if the cause is eliminated, but even if the cause remains, tremendous results can be obtained using the power of your subconscious. The subconscious controls all the inner workings of your body (including fat burning) much like a fantastic computer. If you have a strong subconscious cause, you can fight against it consciously your entire life and never win, because the subconscious never sleeps and has far more power and control. The picture method is a way to use the power of your subconscious to work for you. You can use this method and guided visualization, described next, to get your fat-loss program started or to increase your progress. As you lose fat you will feel better about yourself and be more able to determine, face and eliminate your causes.

Guided visualization is another way to direct the power of your subconscious. It takes more time than the picture method but can be extremely effective if done properly. It works because your mind cannot differentiate between an "actual" experience and one that is imagined in vivid detail. To help pass the time and maintain sanity, some prisoners of war visualized playing golf on their favorite courses. When they were finally released, they returned home and played the best golf of their lives, because they had completed years of successful practice.

Start your visualization session lying face up on a bed with your eyes closed. Contract the muscles of your feet and then relax them. Do the same for your calves, thighs, buttocks and other muscles of your body. Even do your face muscles. Take slow, shallow breaths. When you feel relaxed, start to visualize in your mind's eye your new attitudes and lifestyle. See yourself waking up in the morning feeling energetic and positive. Visualize looking in the mirror at your lean, shapely body and give yourself a big smile. Picture showering your body, grooming it, shaving or applying makeup and getting ready to go to work or face the world. Visualize your entire day with as many details as possible. See yourself in recreational activities and imagine yourself going to the gym before or after work. Do not just see yourself working out; feel the energy, the strength, the vitality and sense of being alive that you get from exercising intensely. Envision your more attractive body in flattering workout clothes and see yourself making friends with others who exercise, eat well and work to stay in good shape physically and emotionally. Picture yourself shopping for new clothes and trying on the latest styles. Make sure they all fit well and look great. Do not forget to visualize eating properly at home and ordering healthful and nutritious meals in restaurants. Experience how good these natural, wholesome foods taste, and feel satisfied after eating. Feel in control knowing you have just given your body the nutrition it needs to be lean, strong and healthy.

Especially visualize the things most important to you. For example, if being fat has possibly prevented you from finding someone to share your life with, see yourself going to dances, socializing in other ways you enjoy, and meeting new people. See others being attracted not just to your nice-looking body, but to you as a person, with your newfound self-image, confidence and healthy lifestyle. If wearing stylish new clothes or participating in a particular athletic activity is important to you, picture yourself wearing those clothes or doing that activity. Remember that you must feel what it will be like, not just think about it. Our power to create comes from the feelings generated by our thoughts, not the thoughts themselves. This is the key, so feel, feel, feel. But feel only what you do want, not what you don't want. Many of the prisoners of war mentioned previously improved their golf games dramatically because they pictured only success. They never envisioned the golf ball going into the rough, sand trap or water hazard.

Another way to use guided visualization is to see what you want moving toward you. See what you want in the distance and then imagine it moving closer and closer until it is a part of you. For example, if you are a woman, see a woman in the distance going into a gym and exercising. Envision her being knowledgeable about exercise, looking great and enjoying how strong and good she feels. Gradually see this picture getting closer until you can see that the woman is you. You could imagine your fat body walking away until it cannot be seen and then your new lean body coming into view and walking toward you.

Another visualization that may work well for you is to see yourself shedding your excess fat like a snake shedding its skin, like someone taking off layers of clothing or like actors removing padding and makeup that was used to make them look fat. Use your list of reasons to be lean for other ideas on what to visualize.

If moving away from things motivates you, first see what you want to move away from close up, like it usually seems, and then visualize it moving away from you until it is completely gone. If overeating is a problem for you, see yourself shoveling food into your mouth non-stop and then see this picture moving farther and farther away until it finally disappears. Use your list of things you want to avoid for ideas.

Visualization can help eliminate your cause for being fat even if you are guessing at the cause. If the cause is eating numerous sweets and desserts, you can visualize yourself enjoying eating wholesome foods and not being tempted in the least by sweets or other desserts. If you drink alcohol because you are shy, see yourself being friendly and conversing with others without using alcohol. This is easy if you love yourself and others. Whatever your cause, you can visualize having overcome it. This may be enough to eliminate it. You can use visualization to help develop your healthier lifestyle. Make each session seem as real as possible and always experience enjoyable and desirable feelings.

Guided visualization can be done as often as you like and at any time, but the best time is just before going to sleep at night. Once you are living your dream, you can stop visualizing or use it to achieve new goals. Do your best to create the desires of your heart (your true self) for these are the only ones you will be happy with once you get them. If you visualize what your worldly programmed ego wants, you will still feel unfulfilled after you get them.

You can use visualization to help you eliminate your false programming of not being good enough or other negative feelings. Think of this false programming as memory files in a computer. See yourself transferring them to the recycle bin or trash can and then feel the sense of freedom and power when you delete them forever. Know that you have just gotten rid of hidden files that have been working behind the scenes to attract problems and unhappiness into your life.

See What You're Gaining, Not What You're Losing

If you think about it, losing excess fat is about gaining, not losing. Therefore, an excellent way to stay motivated or overcome discouragement is to look at the positive things you have gained and accomplished each day. You can do this by making two lists. One is a daily list including things like: completed 30 minutes of strength training, did an hour of fat burning on a stationary bicycle, ate fruit all day, wore pants that have not fit for five years, did not eat dessert, weighed two pounds less than yesterday, helped a friend move, and saw a beautiful sunset. Write down the loving and productive things you did, along with any measurable progress. This list is unnecessary if you are highly motivated and making good progress, but it is a good idea for everyone to do it for a few weeks. This list is especially important if you have not yet eliminated your reason for being fat. It can help you to break the inertia and start losing some fat. Making some initial progress often helps people to see and get rid of their causes more easily. Some people may lose 50 pounds before they finally discover their emotional causes. Make your daily list in the evening and read it just before going to sleep. Envision similar accomplishments the next day and how you will feel as you are doing them. Continue making a daily list as long as it is helpful.

Everyone should make another list consisting of permanent changes that have been made or experienced. It should include new health habits and what you have gained from your healthier lifestyle. List things like: take a multivitamin and mineral supplement daily, complete a strength-training program three times a week, drink water at correct times, eat more slowly and chew thoroughly, enjoy a nutritious breakfast, have dinner before 6:30 p.m., and other healthy activities. Also include such things as: have increased energy, feel more motivated to pursue creative activities, look more attractive, and enjoy increased respect from self and others. Read this list every night before bed and rejoice as you watch it grow.

Having more self-respect is an especially important benefit. Initially it can come simply from having finally taken the first step on the road to changing yourself and accomplishing the goal of permanent fat loss. You may look in the mirror on the first day and see your body as fat as ever, but you will have more self-respect and a better self-image. Look into one of your eyes and see the real you looking out. You may have previously focused on your fat body and then punished and condemned yourself. Doing this just feeds your negative cycles and worldly programming. From now on focus primarily on the spirit living inside the body. That is who you really are. Congratulate yourself for each day's accomplishments and thank yourself for the love you gave yourself that day.

Other benefits you may experience from improving your appearance and self-image are advancement in your company or a new and better job. You may start your own business or expand one you already have. You may become more active socially because you feel better about yourself and are less afraid to meet people and make new friends. You should be more capable of doing physical activities such as heavier exercise, sports and other recreational activities you enjoy or would like to learn. And don't forget about your improved sex life. You should gain more respect for your body and this could influence you to treat it better. Remember that it is a priceless gift you can take care of or destroy. The choice is yours.

More time is a valuable benefit you can enjoy from getting lean. You can stop searching for a new diet or magic pill to free you from the bondage of excess fat. Many fat people waste more time doing this than lean people spend exercising. Most of us are always wishing we had more of it, so take advantage of your newly found time—spend it wisely. Think about the time you will now have for positive activities. Time is life and the only thing any of us have. Every moment is precious and should be enjoyed. Happy moments add up to happy minutes that add up to happy hours, then days, weeks, months, years and ultimately a happy life.

You will not only have more time but increased energy and enthusiasm to accomplish more with *all* your time. Perhaps you have always wanted to write a book, start a part-time business or learn to play a musical instrument. Your body will be a stronger, more efficient vehicle to help you accomplish your goals and get more enjoyment from life. Being leaner greatly increases your chances of living more healthy and productive years. How many wealthy people would give up all they have for a few more healthy years of life? Most of them, I would guess. It is unfortunate that few of them do what it takes to acquire those years when they have the chance.

Revealing your body is like expressing your true spiritual nature. You do not have to develop your spirit, you just have to eliminate your false programming so your true self can be expressed accurately. You already have a lean body, it is just hidden under excess fat. All you have to do is uncover it. Nature created it for you to use and that is what you must do to keep it strong and healthy. You also have to fuel it with the whole foods Nature created for it. With proper exercise, you can develop a stronger and shapelier body that will be uncovered as the fat melts away.

Do not look at what you are losing. Stay focused on the positive. Think about the fresh breath you are gaining instead of the bad breath you are losing. Do not think about losing fat. See the process as uncovering and gaining the lean body underneath. Say, "My body fat level is down to 27 percent," or "My body weight is down to 150," instead of "I lost 15 pounds." Rejoice when you have to take in your clothes or buy smaller sizes, but do not buy many new clothes until you are close to your ideal weight and shape. Give your old baggy clothes to charity, because you will never need them. If you cannot let go of them, you still have a psychological cause you need to eliminate.

Do not be afraid of losing relationships with fat friends or relatives. See yourself as a good example for them. You may lose some people from your life if the main thing you had in common with them was excess fat. A few of them may choose to follow your example and uncover their own lean bodies, but do not be disappointed in them if they do not. Realize that until they are ready, nothing can make it happen. Keep in mind that if people truly care about you, their feelings toward you will not change when your body composition does. In fact, the ones worth associating with will be happy about your success. Form new, healthier relationships and move away from the ones detrimental to your happiness and well-being. Create an environment for yourself that makes getting and staying lean easy.

Keep your thoughts and feelings focused on what you want, imagine what it will feel like to be lean and healthy, and count your blessings instead of your misfortunes. As you progress, your list of what you have gained and your list of blessings will grow.

Respect Yourself

Respecting yourself in all ways can be extremely uplifting and a great self-image booster. Two ways to respect yourself (your body) come from good grooming and dressing well so you look your best. When you look good, you feel good. Keep your shoes shined brightly and you will get many compliments. Have your hair cut in the most attractive style for your face and keep it combed and styled. The right clothes and haircut can take many pounds off your appearance. This can be extremely helpful in the beginning of your program, but do not let it satisfy you and prevent you from losing your excess fat. Use it instead to help you reach your goals faster. Keep your finger and toe nails clean and trimmed. Learn and practice good grooming for your entire body. If you are a woman and you wear makeup, learn what colors are flattering for you and how to apply them so you look your best. If you are a man, keep any facial hair well trimmed and make sure it complements your facial features. Whiten your teeth if necessary and smile often to give and get the soul food that smiling provides. Do not forget that keeping your body lean and healthy is a big part of self-respect.

Have you ever seen the dramatic difference a professional makeover has on someone's appearance? You may have seen some before and after photos on television programs or at the mall portrait studio. The positive changes are sometimes almost unbelievable and they are not just physical. The physical improvements create an amazing difference in how people feel about themselves and how others respond to them. Makeover computer programs let you experiment with different looks and determine what is best for you. A physical makeover will elicit compliments from others and can greatly improve your self-image.

The beautiful actress Charlize Theron underwent an almost unbelievable transformation for the 2003 movie, *Monster*. I do not think, however, that many people would describe the character she portrayed as being physically beautiful. They gave her bad-looking teeth and an unattractive hairstyle, but she gained *only* 30 pounds of fat. Many plain-looking women would look gorgeous if they regained some lost muscle, lost 30 pounds of fat, got their teeth fixed and whitened, learned proper makeup techniques and got flattering hairstyles. Tremendous improvements can be made to someone's appearance without any cosmetic surgery, and most of the changes could be paid for with the money saved by not buying fast foods and junk foods.

If your life and environment are dirty and unorganized, chances are that your body (internally) and eating habits are the same, so respect yourself by keeping your environment clean and organized. Keeping your office, home and automobile clean and free of clutter reduces stress and makes you feel much better about yourself and your life. Respect the environment you travel through. Do not litter. Be kind to animals. Be courteous and friendly to others and respect their time by being early for work and appointments.

Whenever you do something to disrespect or harm yourself, another person, an animal or your environment, it has a negative impact on how you feel about yourself. You will feel less respectable and possibly start a cycle of negative thoughts and behaviors that could lead to depression, fat gain and harm to yourself and others. *Everything* you do has a positive or negative effect on all four aspects of your being, as does *everything* you eat and drink. You always know what you do, whether anyone else does or not, so respect yourself by associating with positive and uplifting people and doing worthwhile activities that enhance your self-worth. Improve all parts of your life by nourishing your body, mind and spirit. This will help you feel worthy of being loved, of living a longer and healthier life in a lean body, of having more money, and of living a happier and more fulfilling life.

Many Other Helpful Tools

Give yourself treats frequently—you deserve them. But give yourself valuable and rewarding treats instead of unhealthful treats like cake or ice cream. Write down all the positive treats that you will give yourself with your new lifestyle and body. Enjoy the feelings (treats) you have when you see your new body reflected in a mirror, when others compliment your appearance, when your feet, knees and back do not hurt, your clothes fit well and flatter your body, your cholesterol level goes down, your energy level goes up, and so forth. Many people want instant gratification and quite a few of them attempt to get it from eating. Sadly, most of them never feel any gratification at all or it literally lasts only for an instant. On the other hand, being lean and healthy gives lasting contentment to all parts of your being. You will feel a sense of accomplishment after exercising, satisfied after eating healthful meals and in control after resisting the temptation of foods you know are harmful to your well-being.

You will be able to buy yourself many things you want (e.g., vacations and possessions) with the money you save by not buying unhealthful foods, not going on weight-loss programs and avoiding health problems created by unhealthy eating habits. After all, the money you spend on fattening foods just goes to "waist"—or hips—or thighs. Add to your list of treats the things you can do with more money. See the benefits listed in chapter one for more ideas and include the most important ones for you. Every time you see a dessert or candy, think of all the treats you will be giving yourself if you do not eat it. Thinking about these valuable treats takes your mind off the harmful ones and gives you a new way of looking at treats—the positive and the negative ones. The list of treats you give yourself when you lose your excess fat can be long and wonderful. Add to your list as you think of more positive treats to give yourself.

A simple tool to help you avoid the temptation to overeat (go back for seconds) or eat fattening foods (like desserts) is to postpone it for five minutes. The desire will usually be gone before the five minutes is up. This is another way to use inertia to help you. You may want to spend the time thinking about why you want the food. What past, current or even imagined future event is triggering your unhealthy want? Doing this may help you discover the root cause of your excess fat. If you can determine why you want the food, you can then figure out a positive way to change your thinking and eliminate this destructive control over your behavior and your life.

Another way to short-circuit temptation is to do something you enjoy. You know—your passion—the activity you do for three hours that seems like 15 minutes. The one you get so absorbed in that the last thing you think about is eating. If you do not have at least one activity like this, you had better get busy and find one. It may be as simple as finding a good book to read. Feed your mind and soul more and your body less.

As you know, fat people tend to think and talk about food more than lean ones. Find more important things to think and talk about. Go hiking, biking, walking or just have a pleasant conversation with a lean (or soon to be lean) friend instead of baking a cake or trading cookie recipes with a fat friend. Read a health or fitness magazine instead of a baking magazine. Avoid the supermarket aisle full of candy and cookies and do not have these kinds of products in your home. Go through the produce section and look for new foods to enjoy and keep your home stocked with healthful, whole foods. A great way to eliminate the temptation to eat junk food is to eat something healthful and satisfying instead. Remember that junk food creates a junky and unhealthy body.

A good way to develop an awareness of your eating behaviors is to eat in front of a mirror so you can see yourself as others do. Be prepared, because you may not like what you see. Look into one of your eyes while eating and after you finish, write down how you were eating and what you were thinking and feeling as you ate. The purpose of this is to identify bad habits you want to change, not to judge, condemn or criticize yourself. If you start to do this, realize that your judgmental and critical behavior is another destructive habit you need to identify and eliminate. Complete this exercise as often as it takes for you to finally see the truth of how you are eating and what you need to change. Do this exercise only when you are by yourself.

Another exercise to help you understand more about your eating behaviors and feelings about food is to eat with your eyes closed. Again, do this only when you are by yourself. It is best to eat finger food or something you can eat with a spoon. After you finish, write down what you thought and felt as you were eating. This exercise helps you become more aware of the feel and taste of food, but its main purpose is to help you realize that the greatest appeal of most food is visual. This is why good chefs make the meals they prepare visually appealing. This is also why fast-food and junk-food advertisements usually have large images of what is being sold. Do not visually tempt yourself by having unhealthful foods in your house, looking at food pictures in magazines, or cruising the cookie aisle and bakery sections of the supermarket. Out of sight, out of mind is a healthy philosophy. Mute out and do not watch food commercials. I usually record television programs and my VCR automatically fast-forwards the commercials. Make sure not to watch the commercials even when fast-forwarding, because your mind can still be subliminally programmed. Be aware that advertisers also often attempt to arouse you sexually. Find positive, productive and healthy activities to do with your time instead of thinking about food. Spend your time in environments and doing activities where you can learn, create, have fun and get the nourishment you need the most—mind and soul food.

You already know that most people who overeat generally eat too fast. Because they often feel guilty about eating, they attempt to get it over with quickly. But eating fast reduces the enjoyment, because they have little time to taste anything. Then they go back for seconds or even thirds in an attempt to get some pleasure from eating. All this does is create more fat and more guilt. This lack of pleasure triggers the need in many to eat a dessert that has a strong flavor they may be able to taste. Remember that most of these people have deadened taste buds. To help break this overeating cycle and start enjoying your meals, take twice the time to eat that you normally would. Time how long you usually spend eating a typical breakfast, lunch and dinner, and then double it. Make sure the extra time is spent eating and not just talking more and eating as fast as ever. Once again, after you finish eating, write down what you thought and how you felt.

Some people advise against eating while watching television, but because many people will do it anyway I want to explain how to do it healthfully. All you have to do is put less food on your plate than you think you need. If you have excess food, you will usually be unaware of how much you are eating and momentum will keep you eating until it is all gone. A short while later, your body will let you know you ate too much. By giving yourself smaller portions, you will finish the meal and often be distracted by what you are watching so you will not think about eating more. Before you start eating, put any leftover food away so it will be difficult to run into the kitchen and load up your plate again during a commercial. If you think you need more to eat, wait for about 15 minutes. Give your body time to let you know you have had plenty already. Regular and systematic undereating is a healthy habit and the only thing proven to extend the life span of animals. It is impossible to know exactly how much to eat, but it is always better to eat less instead of more. If you are hungry in a few hours, have a healthful snack.

You sometimes hear that if you eat from a smaller plate, you will eat less and lose weight. This is true if you eat nutritious foods that provide your body's needs, but otherwise it is just a gimmick and will not work. No matter how small the plate is, if the food is lacking in nutritional value, you will keep filling it up and end up overeating.

Eating should stimulate all five senses. The sight of food is the strongest influence for most fat people and the smell of food is as important, if not more so, than taste. Try to tell the taste difference between a potato and an onion with your eyes closed and your nose plugged and you will see what I mean. Make up a few small pieces on toothpicks so you can pick one up and eat it without knowing what you have. Some people claim that smelling unhealthful foods, but not eating them, has helped them to lose excess body fat. The sense of touch is another important part of the eating experience. What is the texture of the food? Is it soft and chewy or hard and crunchy? The sound a food makes as you eat it also plays a role. Realize that the faster you eat, the less you will experience of all these sensations. Therefore, eating less food more slowly will actually increase your enjoyment of eating.

Even though many claim to be gourmets, most fat people rarely taste the food they eat. They may taste the salt and sugar on it but not the food. If salt and sugar are about the only things you ever taste, it is boring and can lead to overeating in an attempt to fulfill your taste needs. Here is something to help you understand this. Pretend you have been hired to describe and rate the taste of some of your favorite foods. Eat each food separately and rate it from zero to ten in the four basic taste sensations—sweet, sour, salty and bitter. This exercise helps you to learn to eat slowly and enjoy it. It also helps you to learn how little taste most foods have. Next, eat some of your newfound natural foods like squash, wild rice, buckwheat or rutabaga. You will probably be surprised to find their tastes rating higher than your old, unhealthful favorites—especially if you have not been eating salt for a while and your taste buds are coming back to life.

Most food processing eliminates parts of the original whole food and almost always destroys the taste. If the strong tastes of salt, sugar, fat and artificial flavors were not added, most processed foods would taste like cardboard or sawdust—not exactly the tastes that would stimulate people to eat them. Would you eat popcorn without butter or salt? I doubt it, but popcorn is one of the tastiest snacks when eaten plain. Crackers and pretzels would be completely unappealing if they were not cooked in fat and covered with salt. Even most breads are usually covered with butter, jelly, mustard, mayonnaise, ketchup or something else to give it some taste. Many processed grain snack foods are just carriers for salt and unhealthful fat. Food processing usually also eliminates the food's natural shape, smell, color, texture and sound. Everything is artificial and this leads to numerous imbalances in your body. On the other hand, natural foods supply a variety of balanced stimulation to all five of your senses. This adds greatly to the health benefits and satisfaction you get from eating. Do not settle for artificial foods when you can eat foods with real colors, real textures, real sounds when you chew them, real smells, real tastes *and* real nutrition. As I have said before, you can only enjoy *real* health if you eat *real* food.

Here are two more ways to help you change your thinking about food. Like the other exercises, do them by yourself and write down your thoughts and feelings after you finish. Sit down and look at a fattening food (or picture of it) that you are tempted to eat. Now, think of what it will do to your body. Write down if it will add fat, increase your chance of serious disease, harden your arteries, stress your pancreas, constipate you, give you indigestion, or create body odor and bad breath. Most fattening foods do all those and more. The second exercise is to write down what you could do with some foods other than eating them. For example, a donut could be used to play ring toss. Two could be giant earrings or four could be the tires for a toy truck. Look at the food and write down as many things as you can in 10 minutes. Get creative (feed your mind) and have fun (feed your soul). Creative and fun—that is what life is supposed to be, remember? Now, make a list of all the benefits you will enjoy if you do not eat the food. We have discussed a multitude of them so this should be easy. Some benefits are an improved self-image, a feeling of power and control, looking better in and out of clothes, feeling better physically and emotionally, having extra energy and getting more fun out of life. Many of the things you may not have experienced for a long time or have even forgotten about.

Some people jokingly say they are on a "see" food diet—they eat all the food they see. Unfortunately, it is not a joke for many of them. Because most of us are stimulated visually by foods, here are three ways to eliminate visual control over your behavior. One way to visually satiate yourself is to look at pictures of your favorite unhealthful foods for an hour or two. Do not, however, give into programming to eat any of them. Doing this will reduce the power that seeing these foods has over you. Another method is to sit and stare for five minutes at a food that tempts you. Do not think about answering questions, just stare at it. Use a clock or timer and after five minutes write down how you feel about the food. It is best if you do not eat the food after you finish writing but it is irrelevant if you do. Throwing it away, however, will make you feel more powerful and in control of your eating behaviors. Another satiation technique is to go to the supermarket without any means of buying anything. Walk around the bakery and candy sections and look at all the cakes, pies, cookies and other items. Stay as long as you like and then go home and write down how you felt when you were there. Break free from your slavery to unhealthful foods. These techniques usually work fast and therefore should not become subconscious programs stimulating you to eat the unhealthful foods. They are similar to eating so much chocolate in one day that you get so sick that you never want to eat it again.

Many fat people eat junk-food snacks. Do they do this because they are hungry? The answer is usually yes. You have learned that if you eat a nutritious meal, your body will not ask for food until it needs more. On the other hand, you can eat junk food all day and your body will keep asking for more, because it is starving for nutrition. Some people snack because they did not experience any satisfaction from the previous meal. Snacking is another futile attempt to get some. The Rolling Stones' song "Satisfaction" (as in "I can't get no") could be the theme song for most overeaters. Another possible reason for eating unhealthful snacks is to either create or maintain excess fat. Your emotional cause or causes for being fat stimulate this force-feeding process.

How can you prevent yourself from snacking on unbalanced and fattening foods? One way is to set a timer for five minutes whenever you get the urge for a snack. During that time, you will usually get involved doing something else and at the end of the five minutes, the desire to snack is often gone. If you still want a snack, eat something healthful. As you have learned, eating three healthful, moderately sized meals and two or three healthful snacks is a more efficient way to supply good nutrition to your body than eating two or three large meals.

Eating a snack increases some people's appetite. I believe this is caused in part because it makes them think about eating. Snacks lacking in nutritional value or containing salt or other unhealthful ingredients usually make people eat more at the next meal. Part of this reason may be caused by an emotional or physical imbalance. For some people, snacking decreases the amount they eat at the next meal. This occurs most often when a healthful, nutrient-rich snack is eaten. If you eat healthful between-meal snacks but end up eating more during your meals, look for snacks without this effect. If you cannot find any, you will be better off not eating between meals. After you have gotten lean, balanced your internal chemistry and eliminated old thinking patterns, you may be able to eat healthful snacks without overeating at the next meal.

A great way to develop healthier eating habits is to change your intent and have a positive goal. For example, instead of going out to eat and letting yourself be manipulated by food, go with the intent of eating the healthiest and most satisfying meal you can. If your goal is to enjoy a good meal and skip the dessert, it is easy to accomplish. Focus on what is truly important— the beautiful surroundings, the relaxation and the companionship of friends or loved ones. Enjoy the experience of being together and sharing life. Even if you eat alone, you can enjoy many of the same things along with some peace and solitude. Because most of the stimulation of food is visual, you can look all you want. When they bring the dessert tray, go ahead and look at everything if you so choose. You will get more out of just looking than out of eating any, and you will feel empowered and in control of yourself, your health and the shape of your body. This will give you more emotional satisfaction to go along with the physical and emotional satisfaction from the healthful meal.

We take in etheric energies when we breathe. The yogis of the East call it *prana*. Our bodies are made to use this energy. We inhale positive prana (solar energy) through the right nostril and negative prana (lunar energy) through the left nostril. We are supposed to get a balance of these energy currents but this can be disrupted when we are emotionally upset. Positive prana speeds up our metabolism and improves our digestion so we get more from what we eat. You now know the importance of this. If you have excess fat, you may want to put some cotton in your left nostril and breathe through your right one for about an hour at a time. The best time to do this is during meals and for a while afterward. This reestablishes balance between the positive and negative etheric energies. A weakened part of your body can be strengthened if you focus your thoughts on rejuvenating the area while breathing in the solar energy.

If you are thin, nervous and restless, you can reestablish balance by breathing through your left nostril for an hour a day. Breathing in lunar energy will slow your metabolism down to normal. This may be helpful for a thin person who is training properly to gain muscle mass. When yogis go on a long fast, they do not feel hungry, because they plug up their right nostrils and breathe only lunar energy. This slows down their metabolisms dramatically, thereby reducing the amount of muscle mass they would normally lose.

The following method can be helpful whether someone has a problem with overeating, making poor food choices or addiction to alcohol or drugs. It is a simple way to replace destructive habits with constructive ones. All that has to be done is to make a list of uplifting actions that can be taken instead of eating, drinking or using drugs. The list must be written (not just in your head) and have as many alternatives as possible. Whenever the urge to carry out a destructive habit occurs, do an activity on the list instead. Some examples are: listen to uplifting music and sing along or dance to it, do someone a favor, exercise, meditate, read an entertaining or inspiring book, take a walk, call a friend, watch the funniest scene from your favorite comedy movie, write in a journal or soak in a hot bath. You could write down and then give thanks (out loud) for all the good things in your life. List other soul foods and things that make you laugh, get your blood pumping and endorphins flowing, and anything else that makes you feel better about yourself and life. It is possible to make everything you do (and everything you eat and drink) improve or maintain a state of happiness and well being.

Thousands of books and audiotapes about self-improvement and personal empowerment are available. Once again, however, you must choose carefully. Some of them are like the diet books that promise you can eat whatever you want and lose your excess fat. Do not believe this. You cannot eat the same way you ate to get fat in order to get lean. It is ridiculous. People simply tell you what you want to hear to sell their products. Your life cannot change until your thoughts, feelings and behaviors change. If a book or tape promises you can change your life effortlessly without honestly looking at and changing your thinking and behavioral patterns, it is not going to help you. Some of them are filled with fancy psychological talk that may sound good but has no real truth or substance. Some of them just give you more excuses and put responsibility for your life and circumstances somewhere other than on you.

The only way to achieve lasting change is first to realize that what you are currently doing is not working. Then you have to experiment until you figure out what does work to produce the desired results. The changes you make must apply to and work in the real world, not some perfect fantasyland described in a book or tape. I once heard a story about a man who meditated in a cave in the mountains for many years. His goal was to achieve enlightenment and inner peace. When he finally felt he had attained his goal, he left the cave and went down to the village in the valley below. As he walked along the crowded street, someone accidentally stepped on his toe. The man got extremely angry and started screaming obscenities at the person. His inner peace was shattered in an instant, because he had not learned how to experience it in the world he would be sharing with others.

Life Strategies is an excellent book about permanent change. A condensed form on audiocassette is available so you can listen to it at home or in your car, but it is important to also have the book because of the exercises it contains. The author, Phillip McGraw, Ph.D., (Dr. Phil) does not beat around the bush or give you excuses. He offers real solutions to real problems we all face in the imperfect world we inhabit. If you follow his advice, you may improve your life dramatically. Remember that our own thoughts and perceptions create our own private world. You will only eliminate false thoughts and destructive behaviors, so all you will lose are the unwanted results you are currently getting—like your excess fat or drug addiction. You are not going to lose the real you when you change. On the contrary, you are going to get rid of false programming and reveal the real you inside a healthier and leaner body.

Subliminal tapes about fat loss may help you purge your mind of the false programming currently controlling your behavior. Remember that some of these may not be well designed and that even a good one should just be one of many tools you can use to change yourself and accomplish your goals.

Learning to increase your self-confidence, achieve goals, build your mind power, fill your own needs, improve your appearance, become a well-rounded person, and how to change are just some of the topics included in a self-improvement book written by me under the pseudonym T.R. Llove. It can save you from reading many books in an attempt to learn the success principles necessary to improve your life and accomplish your goals faster and easier. It was written primarily for young men so I titled it *How To Be Macho* so that they would be attracted to read a book that could help them improve their lives. The word *macho* means a strong, virile man and in my book also means a man who is successful in all areas of his life. Anyone can benefit from this book, however, because the success principles are universal. For more detailed information, visit the Web site GalahadPublishing.com.

The ultimate life-changing information can be found in the book and audiocassettes titled *Excuse Me, Your Life is Waiting* by Lynn Grabhorn. In a nutshell, she explains that your thoughts control your feelings, your feelings create certain vibrations and the vibrations attract what you think about. Like vibrations attract. Negative vibrations attract negative conditions and results, and positive vibrations attract positive conditions and results. This is a universal law that never fails. If you focus on what you do *not* want then that is exactly what you will get. The keys are to think about and *feel* only what you *do* want, experience joy in your life, focus on the positive, appreciate everything and everyone (especially yourself) and get many daily doses of soul food. I recommend this information above all other for learning to create the life you want.

Staying Lean

After you accomplish your fat-loss goal and your body is looking good, the next step is to keep it that way. As you have learned, this is what your mind was designed to create and maintain, and what your true self wants. It is the most efficient way, the healthiest way and is the least amount of work for your body. Remember that our bodies are not designed to store fat for hibernation during the winter. Being lean should be as natural and effortless as breathing. It is the way your body is meant to be and it will stay lean automatically unless a new physical cause develops or you create more fat. It is entirely up to you. Remember that you can create and maintain a lean body as easily as a fat one.

It should be easy to maintain your lean body if you have built a strong foundation by having a good reason, eliminating your causes and feeling worthy of being lean. You now also have a great deal of knowledge about balanced eating, correct exercise and your body's unique needs. You should have a better self-image and the confidence to let more of your true self (instead of your worldly programmed ego) be expressed through your mind and body. Healthy habits should have replaced most of the old unhealthy ones, and many powerful positive cycles should be working for you.

There are, however, traps you may fall into that can sabotage your success. The upcoming information should help you understand and avoid the most common pitfalls that could reverse some of your progress.

Awareness

Maintaining awareness of your body and actions is vital to staying lean. Obviously, if you start following old habits, you will get fat again. Remember that creeping obesity occurs to people with such a low degree of body awareness that they gain 15 to 20 pounds of fat before they realize anything is happening. You now know what to look out for and can occasionally check your body fat percentage to make sure it is not increasing. You can also periodically check your weight and at the first sign of a problem, find out why it is happening and deal with it. You can eliminate the cause, if a new one develops, or lose the pound of added fat before a negative cycle turns it into 20 pounds. If you have not yet eliminated the causes of why you had excess fat, you must be especially aware or you could easily fall into an old rut.

Be aware that a cause you have no experience with may develop. For example, if you were a fat single woman who now has a beautiful lean body, more men will be attracted to you. If you get married, you must realize that your husband may attempt to fatten you up if he lacks the confidence, self-esteem, and initiative to keep a great-looking lady happy and satisfied. His fear of losing you may make him subtly encourage you to get fat again. You should not have a problem unless your attractiveness to other men threatens him and he fears that he may lose you if your relationship deteriorates. If he feels secure, he will work to keep himself, you and your relationship healthy and happy.

If you are a married woman, chances are your husband will treat you differently after you lose your excess fat. More positive attention will be a treat for you, but he may show signs of jealousy if he fears losing you. He may direct his negative feelings at you or try to fatten you back up.

In times of extra stress or life-changing events, such as pregnancy, the loss of a loved one, a job or something else you value, you may fall prey to overeating or bingeing on junk food. It is normal to experience grief, depression and decreased self-worth at these times. It is easy to stop caring as much about yourself as you normally do and just think "Nothing matters so what's the use." Be aware of this possibility and understand that your digestion will not be as good, so eating less and more easily digested foods would be helpful. Also, keep in mind that exercise and good nutrition are even more important during stressful and challenging times. All parts of your body, especially your nervous system, need more vital nutrients. A stress-formula supplement of B-complex vitamins and vitamin C is helpful for restoring your life back to balance faster. Talking with supportive and understanding friends, reading uplifting books and getting as much soul food as possible is also important during these times.

Remember that your physical body and mind are merely tools your spirit has been given so it (you) can function in a physical world. It is similar to space suits or deep-sea-diving suits that allow us to function in environments we otherwise could not. The more accurately your true self is expressed through your body and mind, the less control external events have on your behavior. More thoughts, feelings and actions will come from the truth within and you will *act* based on what is, instead of *react* based on false worldly programming and the destructive habits and fears it creates.

Whenever you feel unworthy to experience love, prosperity, joy or a lean, healthy body, realize that false worldly programming is controlling you. If you are aware when this is happening, you can get in touch with the truth within you and often prevent negative behaviors. Just ask your true self what you are doing and why. It will give you the answer if you are quiet and take the time to listen. It will also direct you to what you should do.

Being mindful of your body (seeing it as it truly is) increases your awareness of other areas of your life and helps them improve or stay balanced. This prevents you from creating new causes of gaining body fat. It can also help you to help other people. Think about our marriage example. If it is obvious that your husband is making efforts to fatten you up, you will know the problem is his lack of confidence, a conditioned thought process or because he feels unworthy to be with a lean and attractive woman. Whatever the reason, you can work together to change it. If he chooses, he should be able to get what he needs to not feel threatened by your attractive body.

Do not become fanatical; just pay attention to your body composition and any changes that happen. It is easy to notice if you are starting to gain body fat. Your clothes get tighter and you see and feel it. If you check your weight every week and your body fat percentage every month or two, you should be able to easily stop potential problems long before they start. Do not worry or think about anything negative that might happen. Worry is a form of fear and the precise thing that can create new problems.

Awareness (getting in touch with your true self) is something many people strive for in the name of spiritual growth or enlightenment. It can improve all areas of your life. For example, if you are aware of a small problem starting in your relationship with your spouse, you can deal with it when it is easily solved. Small difficulties, if unnoticed or ignored, can grow into marriage-ending problems. When couples go to counselors, they often discover that what they now believe to be an unsolvable problem started out small and simply grew out of control, because neither partner was aware of what was happening. Stay alert to the possibility that a new physical or emotional cause for being fat can develop and progress.

An excellent way to develop more awareness and to experience joy in life is to learn to live in the moment. If you are not in the moment, you cannot experience the feelings that are generated from what you are doing. You are going through the motions, but not getting any joy and satisfaction from your activities. The only time you are really alive is when you are in the present moment. One of the reasons why making love is so enjoyable is that most people are in the moment for at least part of the time when they do it. When you are not living in the moment, you will probably stub your toes, bump your elbows and have other minor accidents. I believe that this is your spirit's way of attempting to wake you up and get you into the moment so you can enjoy the journey we call life and the process of learning the lessons you are here to learn. When you live in the moment, you decrease your chances of accidents and injuries and you make fewer mistakes. You also eat less and make more healthful food choices. One of my mother's favorite sayings puts it well: Yesterday's history, Tomorrow's a mystery, Today is a gift—that's why we call it the present! Be grateful for and enjoy every precious moment, because you never know how many more you will have.

Continue Your Balanced Diet

After you have uncovered your lean body, it is easy to maintain it by continuing to eat nutritious, natural foods. You will now, however, be able to eat a balance of acid- and alkaline-forming foods instead of a larger quantity of fat-burning alkaline foods. Eat a large variety of whole foods and experiment with different ones and various methods of preparing them as you add to your list of healthful favorites. If you get lax and fall into a rut, you may get bored with your meals and be tempted to eat unhealthful, fattening foods.

Always keep in mind that your daily meals should be as simple and natural as possible and provide some complete protein, but should be mostly clean-burning, easily digested energy foods that keep your body clean inside so it can function more efficiently and produce more vitality. This will maintain your lean body and prevent many health problems.

Give Your Body Regular Vacations

How would you like to work 6 to 10 hours a day, 365 days a year, for 70 or more years? That doesn't sound very healthy, does it? But that is what many people demand from their digestive systems. After a weekend of rest or a one- or two-week vacation, you usually go back to work with renewed energy and enthusiasm—if you enjoy your work. Likewise, if your digestive system gets regular rests, it has time to strengthen and rejuvenate and come back to work functioning more efficiently. I recommend giving your digestive system at least one day of rest each month and a three- to five-day vacation every spring or summer. A half to full day of rest every week along with the five-day spring vacation is even better. These rests also rejuvenate your elimination system and are good for your mind and spirit. They also save you time and money.

Giving your digestive and elimination systems time off is easy. Sunday may be the best day for you, but you can do it any day. If you ate late, excessively or both on Saturday night, just have fruit and water all day Sunday and then eat a moderate amount of food for dinner. If you have eaten well all week, on Sunday you could have a vegetable omelet or another healthful breakfast, fruit and water during the day and then a small to moderate amount of food for dinner. You may want to have some fruit and water in the morning and then crawl back into bed and cuddle with your sweetheart. If you do not have a sweetheart, take your dog for a walk. Don't have a dog? Take yourself for a walk and enjoy the wonders and beauty around you. It is all right to walk after eating fruit. Partake of some soul food and then have the omelet for brunch. Always remember how important keeping your digestive system efficient is to getting and staying lean.

Spring is the best time to do a three- to five-day cleanse, because the most cleansing fruits are in season. Nature supplies these foods to cleanse your system of the heavier foods eaten during the cold of winter. The cleaner you are inside, the fewer cleansing symptoms you will experience during your cleanse. I do not recommend cleansing longer than three days until after your body is fairly clean inside and your body weight has normalized. I do not recommend fasting with just water. Follow the cleansing recommendations in this book or another sensible cleansing program learned from another book or given to you by a healthcare professional with experience in this area.

Continue to Exercise

You must do strength training regularly to maintain your lean body mass, and to keep your body strong, your metabolism normal and your energy high. A human body is an amazing vehicle that gets more efficient with use. It will wear out someday, but it does not wear out like machines do. It has the ability to adapt and get stronger and better at whatever it is asked to do. You would most likely think someone was crazy if that person bought a beautiful new car and then let it sit and deteriorate. Sadly, that is what most people do with their bodies—they let them sit and deteriorate. Remember that if you do not use it, you will lose it. Not exercising is like not brushing your teeth and expecting them to stay white and healthy.

If you do not give your body a reason to stay strong and lean, your bones, muscles, brain and other organs will weaken, your energy and metabolism will decrease, and gaining fat will be easy. Do not forget all the other benefits of exercise such as less stress, improved sex life, a feeling of aliveness and getting more in tune with your body and its needs. Therefore, exercise must be a regular part of your new, lean lifestyle and should eventually feel as natural and necessary as sleeping and eating. It may take some time to develop an enthusiasm for strenuous exercise, just as it will take time to revitalize your taste buds and start enjoying the natural tastes of whole foods unadulterated with salt, sugar and unhealthful fats. Sooner or later you should experience joy and a sense of satisfaction from using your muscles and body as Nature intended.

Maintaining strength and lean body mass is easier than initially developing it and takes less time. This is because you will be well conditioned and rest less between sets, will have stronger nerve pathways from your brain to your muscles, will know how to do the exercises correctly and will not be pushing yourself to constantly progress. When you started, you may have been able to lift only 20 pounds in a particular exercise but can now lift 60 pounds. If you are satisfied with the level of development of the muscle being trained, continue using 60 pounds for that exercise. You never have to lift 65 pounds or more. Your workouts will then be somewhat easier, because your muscles are now strong enough to handle the amount of weight you are using. When you are just maintaining, you no longer have the motivating goal of striving to lift heavier weights, so it is important to make your exercise sessions fun and challenging in different ways. Like your nutritional program, your workouts must be varied regularly to keep them fresh and interesting. Make sure, however, to use only productive exercises and to learn how to do them correctly and safely.

I keep people's strength-building programs interesting by teaching them how to perform the two or three most productive exercises for each muscle. They may do the same exercise only once every week or ten days. Exercise can be fun, but like sex, is boring if done the same way every time. Variety keeps your body from hitting physical plateaus, reduces the chance of overstress injuries and maintains mental stimulation. You should look forward to and enjoy your exercise sessions.

You may want to keep challenging yourself by lifting heavier and heavier weights in an attempt to strengthen and build your body to its maximum potential. If this is your goal, go for it! It is a great way to stay motivated and excited. Refer to my planned book about exercise (it may be available when you read this) to learn the most efficient and fastest way to accomplish this goal. Go online to GalahadPublishing.com for information on the status of this book.

Please do not get fanatical about exercise. Some people have obsessive-compulsive behavior. It may even be one of their causes for overeating and fat gain. If obsessive-compulsive behavior is a problem for you, it must be eliminated or controlled, not simply transferred to exercising. Overexercising may be better than overeating but excessive exercise can also be harmful to your body and your life. You have learned that a healthy life has balance among the physical, mental, emotional and spiritual aspects. If one is overdone, others are neglected and an unbalanced life, with its accompanying problems, is created.

When your body is lean and shapely, the strength-training routine necessary to maintain it should take 45 to 60 minutes, two or three times a week and effective cardiovascular training requires only two or three 30-minute sessions a week. That's only 30 to 60 minutes per day, four to six days a week, a weekly total of about two-and-a-half to four-and-a-half hours. Most people waste far more time on trivial pursuits, negative activities, overeating, complaining, or because they are tired, unorganized or depressed. I have talked with many men who said they do not have time to exercise, but when asked, said they spend two to three times more time watching sports on television than I spend exercising. Just the television commercials that many people watch add up to more time. Exercising with this time (CV training can be done when watching television) is a wise way to spend it, because it gives you many benefits that are not just physical, but mental, emotional and spiritual as well. Chances are that the exercise will give you back far more time in healthy, vital years of life.

It is never too late to start exercising but, like investing money for retirement, the sooner you start the more benefits you will enjoy.

Making Faster Progress

This section is for people who want the fastest results or for those whose progress is slower than they would like it to be. I still recommend that everyone read it, because it contains information that can be helpful to anyone.

If a woman hired me to help her lose a large amount of body fat quickly (and healthfully), I would implement as many of the upcoming ideas as possible. I would first explain the program and then check to make sure that she did not have internal or structural imbalances that would slow her progress or be aggravated by exercise. Any imbalances would be dealt with either before starting or during the course of the program.

The first nutritional step would be to have her start a fruit cleanse. If her reactions were severe, the cleanse would be stopped after one day, but if she had only mild to moderate cleansing reactions, she would continue for three days. After a few light transitional meals, she would then follow a daily eating regimen of mostly alkaline-forming foods. There would not be a gradual transition from her old eating habits to healthier ones. She would eat this way for a week and then be placed on a three- to five-day apple juice cleanse. She would use natural apple juice diluted 50 percent with water and be told to sip it slowly whenever she felt hungry. She would be told to rest as much as possible and be taught that the weakness and dizziness she felt during the cleansing program is not from a lack of food, but from toxins being eliminated and energy being channeled to her organs of elimination instead of her muscles and brain. This is a vital concept to understand when following a cleansing program. After the second cleansing program she would again gradually transition back into an alkaline nutritional program. I would have her drink a glass of green vegetable juice every day, because it is highly alkaline and rich in enzymes and other nutrients necessary for the fat-burning process. The more alkaline she made her blood the faster it would burn fat to balance the pH. She would be taught the best times to eat different foods.

Along with dietary changes she would be taught how to *properly* perform strength- and muscle-building exercises. She would start with light weights to conserve energy for the cleansing process and to make it easier to learn the correct form. I would have her train six times a week with each body part being trained twice a week. In the third or fourth week, the intensity of her exercise sessions would be raised to her current strength level and then increased as fast as she could progress. Immediately after each strength-building session she would ride a stationary exercise bicycle for 40 to 60 minutes at an intensity level low enough to keep her heart rate between 110 and 120 beats per minute. If she was in a tremendous hurry to lose fat, another session of 40 to 60 minutes of fat burning would be scheduled for the evening or the morning, whichever time period was opposite of the previous session. Walking outside or on a treadmill would sometimes replace riding the exercise bike.

If my client was in an extreme hurry to get lean, her strength-building program would be split into two halves. The first half (20 to 30 minutes) would be done in the morning followed by 40 to 60 minutes of fat-burning exercise and the second half done in the afternoon with another 40 to 60 minutes of fat burning immediately after. This schedule would burn more fat, because the body starts burning stored fat sooner if the fat-burning session is done right after strength training. Because heavy exercise stimulates the release of growth hormone, splitting the strength training would increase the number of times this fat-burning hormone was released.

My client would be instructed to drink large quantities of water (at the appropriate times) to help the cleansing process and to keep the muscles well hydrated so they could function at peak efficiency and recuperate faster. If constipation became a problem during a period of rapid cleansing, she would be given an herbal laxative or, if necessary, instructed to get a colonic or take an enema to clear the blockage.

My client would take the Super Spectrim multivitamin and mineral supplement twice a day to get 24-hour coverage. She would also be tested for need and dosage of other supplements deemed necessary for her unique body to function at peak efficiency. She may be given a "fat-burning" supplement. Be aware that of the many currently available, few have any evidence of effectiveness. Many of these products contain caffeine, ephedra or other unhealthful stimulants but you may not know it by reading the ingredient list. For example, the herb guarana contains caffeine. You now know that using stimulants is not a healthy or permanent way to lose excess body fat.

I have found that some of the simpler "fat-burning" formulas containing choline, inositol, methionine, vitamin B6, betaine HCl, apple cider vinegar, lecithin, and certain herbs work fairly well when used in conjunction with an alkaline diet or healthy cleansing program. They assist the body with fat burning and internal cleansing, and none are stimulants. Three herbs I have found particularly helpful are chickweed, saffron and hyssop. My client would drink one to two glasses a day of herbal tea made from these three herbs.

I would prefer to supervise a client on a program this intense to make sure she was following it correctly. If she was doing it on her own, I would have her wear tight clothes to constantly remind her conscious and subconscious minds of her goal. She would do a visualization session just before bedtime and would have pictures of a leaner body with her face on it located where she would see one throughout the day. Most of her time would be spent focusing on what she wants.

Many people following my program have lost 15 to 25 pounds in three weeks simply by doing a few days of cleansing and eating mostly alkaline-forming foods. Some of them had not even begun to exercise. Think of what could be accomplished with the program just explained. Losses of 40 to 60 pounds in two to three months would not be out of the ordinary. Following such an intense program takes a great deal of time for exercise and rest. It would be difficult to do it and work efficiently at most occupations. Depending on your current circumstances, you may be able to use part, or all, of this example.

You can also increase your progress by forming a group with at least one friend who has read this book and wants to follow the program with you. Each of you would benefit, even if one wants to change gradually over a period of months and the other wants to dive right in to get faster results. You can help each other determine your causes for having excess fat, your reasons for losing, and what you are gaining each day. You can share meal ideas and possibly exercise together.

Do not be discouraged if you cannot find an exercise partner. Remember that you do not need anyone but yourself, because your thoughts, attitudes, actions, fat loss and all other changes in your life come from within you. External influences cannot affect you unless you attract them and give them power. Give power only to the things that bring health, joy and prosperity into your life. Just sit down and set your goals, reduce them to mini-goals and start accomplishing them. You may want to tighten your belt a notch as a constant reminder of what you are working to accomplish.

The bigger the difference between your new nutritional program and the way you were eating, the blander some of the healthful foods will initially taste. Olive oil and lemon juice on a baked potato, steamed vegetables and a salad may taste extremely bland in the beginning, but after eliminating salt and doing some internal cleansing, your mouth may water just thinking about that meal. You may want to add your favorite healthful herbs and spices, especially in the beginning. Remember that natural, wholesome foods will taste better and better as your body gets cleaner and your taste buds regain normal sensitivity.

Following the recommendations in this book should give you the leaner, stronger and more attractive body you want, along with more energy, fewer aches and pains, an improved self-image, and a happier and more satisfying life. Your goal is within your reach, because you now understand how to get there *and* how to stay there. Never forget that the only thing capable of stopping you is you. Now that you have the knowledge, progress at your own pace and develop your own course, but consistently move toward your goal—one you will find more valuable than diamonds or gold.

A human being is a part of the whole, called by us "Universe"; a part limited in time and space. He experiences himself, his thoughts and feelings as something separated from the rest—a kind of optical delusion of consciousness. This delusion is a kind of prison for us, restricting us to our personal desires and to affection for a few persons nearest us. Our task must be to free ourselves from this prison by widening our circle of compassion to embrace all living creatures and the whole of nature in its beauty. Nobody is able to achieve this completely but the striving for such achievement is, in itself, a part of the liberation and a foundation for inner security.

Albert Einstein

Gratitude is not only the greatest of virtues, but the parent of all the others.

Cicero

If you think you can do a thing or think you can't do a thing, you're right.

Henry Ford

To be what we are, and to become what we are capable of becoming, is the only end of life.

Benedict de Spinoza

The desire and pursuit of the whole is called love.

Plato

The past is gone and static.
Nothing we do can change it.
The future is before us and dynamic.
Everything we do will affect it.

Charles F. Kettering

fifteen

Strong and Shapely

Most of the talk and written material about body weight focuses on losing weight, but millions of people desperately want to gain weight. Like those who want to lose fat, they rarely define what kind of weight, but as you now know, they should strive to gain lean body mass or muscle. You have learned the many benefits of increased muscular body weight and that, once gained, it is relatively easy to maintain. Sadly, because of a lack of knowledge and an abundance of misinformation, gaining muscular body weight is often as challenging and frustrating to those who are underweight as losing fat is to those with excess. There is a good chance you will have to do both, because almost all people who are overweight with fat are underweight with muscle.

Losing body fat is easier and faster if you exercise to gain muscular body weight at the same time. Energy from stored fat can be used for your workouts and for the muscle recovery and building processes. As you have learned, every extra pound of muscle you gain increases your metabolism approximately 40 calories a day if you are moderately active. Gaining muscle helps you lose your excess body fat, makes you feel better about yourself, makes you stronger physically and emotionally, and gives you a more shapely body to uncover. More strength and muscular weight gives you greater power to do physical work or recreation and reduces mental and emotional stress. It is a vital part of a balanced life.

Exercising to build and then maintain more strength and muscle helps prevent many of the ailments that plague people as they age. Physical activities like carrying your child, skiing, playing softball or hiking all require varying degrees of skill and coordination, but your ability to do many activities well is determined largely by the strength of your muscles. If you are seventy years old but have the strength of an average twenty-year-old, you should be as capable of skiing, hiking or playing softball as you have ever been, barring injuries or other problems. And, accomplishing this at age seventy is not difficult, because the average twenty-year-old is quite weak.

Having excess body fat is like putting rocks in the back seat of your car, creating more drag and stress on the engine. Adding a more powerful engine to your car will reduce the strain on the engine because it has more power. If you should choose not to lose your excess body fat, being stronger will make it easier and less stressful to carry the weight around.

Many people have told me that they want to lose all their excess body fat and then start exercising to gain muscle. I tell them they will lose body fat much faster if they exercise to gain muscle at the same time and that when the excess fat is gone, a more shapely body will be revealed. If they get skinny, they will not look good and this often has a negative impact on someone's self-image. Then they will have to start eating more in an attempt to gain some muscular weight. This could easily cause fat gain that would stimulate even more negative feelings. It is far more efficient and their goals can be achieved much faster using stored fat for workout and muscle-building energy. Greater physical strength also helps people feel stronger mentally and emotionally, and this can be extremely helpful when developing healthier dietary habits.

Gaining muscular weight is simple if you know how to do it, but I guarantee you it is not easy. Like anything else of value it takes time and effort—but the benefits are well worth it. The effort required creates feelings that feed the soul and builds qualities such as persistence, goal attainment and consistency. The amount of time invested in efficient, correctly performed exercise is small but produces large returns. I cannot stress strongly enough the many benefits of gaining muscular body weight—*especially* for those with excess fat.

Three major steps are necessary to increase strength and lean body mass. The first and most important is to create the need. Your body is conservative with its energy, and after about age twenty-one, it will not create or maintain muscle tissue unless it has a reason. You must supply the demand. Not knowing how to do this is why most people fail in their muscle-building attempts. The second step is to supply your body with nutritious energy foods for your daily activities, to do your exercise routines and for the rebuilding process. An adequate amount (but not an excess) of complete protein is also necessary to supply certain raw materials needed for the growth process. The third step is to give your body adequate rest and enough time to complete the rebuilding process. Let's look first at what it takes to stimulate muscular growth.

Stimulating Muscular Growth

Your body maintains only the muscle strength and size necessary for your regular physical activities. For most people, this creates hardly any strength and muscle size. You have learned that this is why most of them lose muscle mass and strength as they age. The only way to stimulate your body to get stronger is to do something physically harder than you are currently doing. This is the same principle used to grow emotionally, mentally or professionally. You must push yourself to do more challenging tasks if you expect to progress in any area of your life.

Your body thrives on being used. Unlike mechanical devices that wear out with use, your body gets stronger and more efficient. It adapts to the stress of physical efforts and prepares itself to do better the next time. You will not make it far the first time you go running, because of the ache in your legs, but you will be able to go farther each time, because your body will be storing more and more glycogen (energy) in your leg muscles. If you run long distances regularly, your body will gradually reduce your body weight (fat and muscle) so the activity can be done more efficiently.

Exercising correctly for strength and muscle size stimulates your muscle fibers to enlarge and improves your coordination and mental control over your muscles. In the beginning of your training, your strength will increase dramatically, not because you are gaining new muscle but because you are learning how to better use the muscles you already have.

To make any substantial progress and to train all muscles of your body, you must join a gym or health club that has adequate strength-building equipment. Gyms are generally less expensive to join because they do not have amenities like swimming pools and saunas. Joining a health club may be worth it if you will use the extra features. Sitting in a sauna or steam room is relaxing and helps cleanse out internal toxins. This could be helpful both during and after losing your excess fat.

Stimulating muscular growth is simple. Force your muscles to work harder by lifting something heavier than you have before and increase the resistance as your muscles grow and get stronger. The weight you struggle with in your first workout will be a light warm-up after a few weeks of correct training. Many people are confused, because they have read magazine articles and books about exercise that are written by or about bodybuilders or powerlifters who use anabolic steroids and other growth- and strength-enhancing drugs. You must understand that these people can train excessively, inefficiently, or both, and still make incredible progress. Do not let this misinformation confuse you and make exercising correctly seem complicated and time-consuming.

Only one way exists to build muscle fast (without growth-enhancing drugs) and that is by regularly completing a simple, but progressively more strenuous, routine of basic exercises. The majority of my male clients have gained 10 to 15 pounds of muscle in a few months. Many have lost an equal, or greater, amount of body fat at the same time. Men have far more potential to gain muscular size than women do, because they have much higher testosterone levels. Women can get considerably stronger but most will not gain much additional muscle size. The majority of them will just build back muscle they have lost. Remember the five to seven pounds most people lose every decade? Many women will regain the nice "girlish" figure they had when they were younger. Chances are Nature gave you a relatively good body if you ate fairly well while growing up. You now know, however, that once it is fully developed it becomes your responsibility to maintain it.

Most people fail in their attempts to gain muscular weight for the same reason people fail to lose excess fat. They simply do not know how to do it. It is not because of the lack of effort many of them put into it. The problem is, they have no idea what to do or have incorrect information (most of what is available) so they put their efforts into activities that produce little, if any, results. This leads to discouragement and frequently to giving up on their goals.

To build strength and muscle you must first learn how to do it efficiently and safely. Then you should start training at a low intensity for a few weeks. This will give you time to learn correct exercise form and will condition your muscles for the heavier resistance to come. You will also be getting a rough idea of how much weight you can currently lift in each exercise. Knowing how to train so you get fast results is the key to learning to like exercise and the motivation to continue doing it. Training correctly is simple but most certainly not easy. Most people complicate their training with "fancy" routines and exercises but make it easy by lifting weights that are not heavy enough to challenge them. This produces minimal results or none at all.

It is a good idea to get a thorough physical exam prior to starting a strength-building program. Sadly, most doctors know as much about exercise as they do about nutrition—almost nothing. If possible, find a doctor who does strength training herself. Exercise is helpful for many physical ailments like diabetes, osteoporosis and most heart conditions. Almost all musculoskeletal problems can be corrected with my PMBT therapy, and some joint problems will improve if the cause is an imbalance of strength in opposing muscles or increased stress to the joint due to excess body fat. Do not do an exercise that hurts a joint, but also do not use a joint problem as an excuse not to exercise at all. People confined to wheelchairs or who have lost limbs can still exercise most of their muscles effectively if they are taught how to do it. I trained for fifteen years with a severe lower back problem and a number of other joint imbalances and have designed numerous exercise programs for people with physical limitations.

To effectively train your largest and most important muscles you must use exercises that have two joints moving at the same time. This stimulates maximum strength and muscular weight gain because you can lift the heaviest amount of weight. For example, to strengthen the shoulder muscles you must do overhead pressing movements but always lower the bar in front of your face. Never do behind-the-neck presses, because this exercise overstresses the rotator cuff muscles of the shoulders and can cause a progress-halting injury. I have successfully resolved these injuries in Mr. Universe title winners, baseball pitchers and many others, but the best thing to do is prevent them. Doing a lateral raise (a one-joint movement) with dumbbells or a machine is detrimental to building strength and size in your shoulder muscles. Likewise, the chest muscles cannot be built doing dumbbell flyes, pec deck (butterfly machine) or cable crossovers. You must use bench press exercises. Some people do dips, but I do not recommend them, because dipping bars are designed in a way that puts excessive stress on the smaller muscles in the front of the shoulders and almost none on the chest muscles. This can lead to a shoulder injury. The large middle back muscles (latissimus dorsi or lats) are built with pull-ups and pull-downs (not wide grip and not behind-the-neck) and rowing exercises with a palms down grip. The gluteal (buttock) and quadriceps (thigh) muscles are built with leg presses and full squats (done correctly), not lunges and leg extensions, which are counterproductive and stressful on the knee joints. The arms, calves, hamstrings and a few other muscles can be built with one-joint movements but are such a small part of the body's total muscle mass that training them does not stimulate much muscular weight gain.

A large number of people fail to gain muscular weight because they use many of the wrong exercises to accomplish the goal. They spend hours doing exercises that stimulate a minimal amount of strength or muscular weight gain. This has three negative effects. First, it creates the illusion they are doing something to stimulate growth. Second, it is counterproductive because it stimulates more cortisol that catabolizes (breaks down) their muscles. For people with slow metabolisms and large amounts of excess body fat, doing one-joint, leverage movements along with the heavy movements will burn a few more calories but will halt, or slow, their strength and muscular gains. Their time would be far more productive doing fat-burning exercise immediately after their *heavy* weight-training sessions. Third, excessive exercise slows down the healing process and their progress. The muscles are so depleted that they take longer to recover before they can be effectively trained again.

I have shortened many people's training programs from six, two-hour workouts a week to three, 45-minute to 60-minute workouts a week. One man went from making no progress whatsoever to adding a pound of lean body weight every week for twenty weeks. Always remember that the intensity of the exercise (not the quantity) is what makes the muscles grow larger and stronger. You could spend years working out all day and never get stronger or gain an ounce of muscle. Unfortunately, due to an abundance of misinformation, this is the most common scenario seen in gyms and health clubs. Here is an example to illustrate. My abdominal muscles are extremely strong and I have a well-defined "six pack" but I exercise them only once a week for about 10 minutes. I do not do sit-ups, leg raises or crunches. You have learned that sit-ups and leg raises are done with the hip flexor muscles and that crunches have negative effects, especially if done with added resistance. Even a beginner should not have to train their abdominal muscles more than three times a week for the same amount of time that I spend.

Some people fail in their muscle-building quests because they do upper body exercises in such a way that their arms do most of the work and the larger muscles get hardly any growth stimulation. For example, a bench press exercise should train and develop your chest muscles, but if done improperly, your triceps and the front of your shoulders do most of the work. This limits the amount of weight you can lift because these muscles are smaller and weaker than your chest muscles. It can cause an overstress injury, especially if your grip is too wide. I have treated numerous patients with rotator cuff muscle strains caused by doing this. Nothing grows when you train this way, because it overworks the arm muscles and underworks the chest, back and shoulder muscles—the ones that need stimulation if you are going to make substantial strength and muscular gains. Proper form is vital, because the arm muscles are the weak link in the larger upper body muscle exercises even when done correctly.

The biggest secret to gaining strength and muscular body weight is to train the thigh and gluteal muscles (glutes) hard. Your metabolism is stimulated, increasing the burning of body fat, and more testosterone and growth hormone is produced, causing muscular growth and fat burning. It affects your entire body and generates positive results whether your body has excess fat or is extremely thin. The appetite of thin people is naturally increased so their bodies will get the nutrients needed to grow. On the other hand, a fat body burns stored fat to help meet the energy demands for workouts and muscular growth. Fat people usually eat less than normal because of this, and also because it makes their bodies more efficient. This creates the basic-training effect that I described in chapter nine. Your thigh and glute muscles should always be the first muscles trained so they will be worked when you have maximum energy.

I have often seen people who want to gain muscular weight do no heavy exercise for their thigh and gluteal muscles. It is sometimes the main reason for their lack of progress. Exercising these muscles intensely also builds strength in your upper body muscles. Even if no other exercise is done, the thigh and gluteal muscles should be exercised hard if strength, good health and fat loss are your goals. These muscles are the source of your physical and sexual power, they support your heart and they help keep you young and active.

Many people fail in their muscular weight-gaining attempts because they do not complete the final negative repetition of each set. Let me explain. The concentric (positive) portion of an exercise occurs when you lift a weight and your muscles contract and get shorter. You normally exhale at this time. The eccentric (negative) portion of an exercise occurs when you lower the weight and your muscles lengthen. You normally inhale at this time. It is extremely common to see people struggle to do ten to twelve repetitions in an exercise and after completing the last positive repetition just drop the weight or let the lat-pulldown bar jerk their arms up. They have wasted most of their time, because the negative portion of the last repetition causes almost all of the microscopic muscle tearing that stimulates muscular growth. The previous repetitions are necessary only to fatigue the muscle enough so it will tear slightly on the last negative. Always do the negative portion of the last repetition slowly, because most of the growth inducement of the entire set is done at this time. Get the maximum benefit for your efforts. Do not throw away your progress like most people do. Lowering the weight slowly is also safer, because letting free weights or machines apply fast, jerking movements to your muscles and joints can cause injury.

Forced repetitions are the best way to increase your exercise intensity. They are done by having a workout partner help you just enough to do the positive portion of an exercise after you can no longer do any more repetitions on your own. Then you lower the weight by yourself on the negative portion. Forced repetitions are extremely beneficial but should be done only on the last two or three repetitions of your heaviest set. Because they are so intense, if you do them at all, it should be only every second or third time you train a particular muscle. I do not recommend them to anyone with less than three to six months of consistent heavy training.

Negative training is the most intense form of strength training. It requires multiple spotters and is so intense that only advanced, knowledgeable trainees should do it. It can cause injury if not done correctly.

Do not waste your time doing "drop sets" where the resistance is reduced after every few repetitions. These are ineffective, because the muscle fibers do not tear if the weight is getting lighter. Also avoid doing a different exercise for the same muscle immediately after completing another exercise. These are also ineffective, because the muscles usually have better leverage on the second exercise so they get less stress or different muscles do most of the work. Either way no muscular growth is stimulated. These and other "fancy" techniques are usually counterproductive if you are training naturally.

Most of the women I have trained or spoken with in various health clubs and gyms have been concerned about gaining muscle too quickly. This should be the least of anyone's concerns, especially women, because gaining muscle size is a slow process. You are not going to work out a few times and wake up with muscles that are larger than you want. Many women are afraid to lift heavy weights, because they believe it will cause them to "bulk up." The truth is, lifting as heavy as they can increases their strength and muscle tone faster and helps them lose body fat. They will lose inches, as their bodies get firmer and leaner. In their wildest dreams they will never get big and lean like female bodybuilders who use anabolic steroids and other growth-enhancing drugs. Even with the drugs, it still takes these women many years of heavy training.

A simple and effective way to progress is to determine how much weight you can lift for eight repetitions in each exercise. Continue to use that amount during subsequent workouts but strive to do more repetitions each time. Continue lifting the weight until you cannot lift it anymore. This is called training to failure. After you can do twelve or more repetitions in an exercise, increase the weight to an amount you can lift only seven or eight times. Use the new weight and when you can do twelve or more repetitions with it, increase the weight again. Gradually increase how much you lift until the muscle reaches the size and shape you want. To maintain the muscle at its current size, continue to train with that weight.

If you want to decrease the size of a muscle, all you have to do is train it with lighter weights. This will maintain the muscle's tone and shape, but it will get weaker and smaller, because you have reduced the need for it to maintain its strength and size. Having this degree of control over your body's size and shape is extremely uplifting for your self-image. It proves that you have the power to transform things you previously thought you could not change. Knowing that you have this power often improves other areas of your life.

After your muscles have been trained properly, they need adequate rest to repair and rebuild before being trained again. If you are a beginner, you can train each muscle three times a week, because your intensity will be low. A whole body routine of ten exercises should get you progressing nicely. After a few months, your training skill and intensity will increase and you should train each muscle only twice a week and do only half of your body (e.g., upper body or lower body) during each workout. This requires four training sessions a week and is about right for most people to build and later maintain. Three training sessions a week can also be done and the workouts just alternated. If you ever choose to push yourself extremely hard, you should train each muscle only once a week. Never train a muscle if it is still sore from a previous workout.

It is usually best to train your largest muscles first and work to the smallest. A good order for a whole body workout is quadriceps and glutes (thighs and butt), hamstrings, chest, latissimus dorsi or lats (middle back) and trapezius or traps (upper back), deltoids or delts (shoulders), biceps, triceps, abs (abdominals), lower back and calves. After thighs and glutes you could do the muscles most important to you first. For example, you can train lats before chest, triceps before biceps or lower back before abs.

The order in which you train different muscles is important even if you train different parts of your body at each session. For example, you would not want to train your triceps muscles on Monday and chest or shoulders on Tuesday or Wednesday. Remember that even when the arms are rested, they are the weak link in other upper body exercises. If your triceps are fatigued from the previous training, your weak link will be even weaker and your chest or shoulder training will suffer tremendously. In addition, the fatigued and sore triceps muscles would get overworked and possibly injured. A poorly designed program can easily lead to overstress injury to the rotator cuff muscles of the shoulders.

I do not recommend completing heavy training sessions more than four days a week, because your body's internal systems need time to recover from your strength training. Some people train hard six or seven days a week. Their logic is that they are training different muscles each time. This is true, but few people's bodies can recover sufficiently from that much training if every session is intense enough to stimulate growth. Those who use growth-enhancing drugs can do this but I highly recommend against using these dangerous substances. Training six or seven days a week can be effective if only one or two muscles are trained each day and the intensity level is cycled, but this is best left to advanced and knowledgeable trainees.

You can train long or you can train hard but you cannot do both. Strength-training sessions longer than 90 minutes are a waste of time because you get too fatigued to train efficiently. Excessively long sessions of intense exercise are often counterproductive, because they put too much stress on the body's recovery ability.

Doing counterproductive exercises, an excessive number of sets or exercises during each session, or training the same muscles too frequently can create a condition called overtraining. Excess cortisol is produced or the muscles do not get enough recovery time before they are trained again. Overtraining causes a loss of muscle size, strength and tone along with fatigue, irritability and a poor appetite. It increases the chances of a muscle strain and is a common problem among those who think that more (sets, repetitions, exercises or training sessions) is better.

You already know it is important to vary your exercise routine to make it more mentally stimulating, but because your body adapts to exercise quickly, variety helps you continue to make progress. Your gains often stop after five to six weeks if the workout stimulus is not changed. Some people like to train with the same routine for a few weeks and then switch to a new one. Others prefer to alternate two different workouts. For example, chest workout "A" can be done on Mondays and chest workout "B" on Thursdays. This is a great way to avoid plateaus and continue making progress. When I teach my patients how to train their muscles safely and effectively, I teach them the best and second best exercise for each muscle and they are told to alternate them.

Another important reason to vary your workouts regularly is to stress your muscles, tendons, ligaments and joints from slightly different angles, thereby reducing the chance of a repetitive stress injury. You may develop an overstress injury if you always do the same exercises and this can stop your progress and have other negative consequences.

The only way to make and keep your muscles strong is to lift weights that are heavy enough to challenge you, but most people never do, because they are afraid of hurting themselves. Instead of being limited by fear, they should grow with knowledge, because it is difficult to cause an injury if you train correctly. Once again, knowledge is the key to success. Unfortunately, it is difficult to find information about how to do strength training efficiently and safely. Many other people are reluctant to train intensely because they fear getting "musclebound." This fear also comes from a lack of knowledge, because building a muscle larger in diameter has no effect on its length. If you train heavy, you are bound to build some muscle (pun intended) but if done properly your flexibility should increase. I have seen many massive bodybuilders who could do the splits and had extreme flexibility in the rest of their bodies as well.

To increase flexibility during strength training you must work each muscle through its full range of motion. To do this, however, you must first learn the range of motion of each muscle. If your muscles are fully contracted and then fully stretched during each repetition, more muscle fibers are trained so more will grow and get stronger. This develops the muscles fully from origin (one end) to insertion (the other end), creating a better shape and making them more resistant to injury. Having a trainer or exercise partner help you move the weight through the last few inches of a muscle's range of motion is highly beneficial. Incomplete range of motion during strength training leads to the ends of the muscles being weaker than the belly (center) of the muscle. This makes them more susceptible to injury, because muscles get the most stress at the ends. If a muscle is strained in a trauma or repetitive activity, it will heal with scar tissue and get shorter and tighter, making you truly musclebound.

Proper strength training increases your flexibility but additional stretching will increase it even more. The best time to stretch a muscle is right after completing each set of exercise for that muscle. You get three main benefits from doing it at this time—more efficient and safer stretching because the muscle is warmed up, it helps the muscle recuperate faster for the next set of the exercise, and no additional time is used. After exercising, hanging by your hands from a chinning bar to stretch and decompress your spine is an excellent habit. Do it a few times for 20 to 30 seconds. Hanging inverted in a device that supports your upper thighs or lying on a slant board with your head at the lower end are also good habits. Inversion and slanting stretch the spinal muscles, decompress the discs between the vertebrae, and may help realign prolapsed internal organs. Slanting at about a 30-degree angle for five to ten minutes is best for older people or those with excessive body fat. Start by slanting for less time at a smaller angle. Most gyms and health clubs have adjustable slant boards and some have inversion devices. Do not hang inverted from your ankles, because this can damage your ankle or knee ligaments. Always use good sense and increase gradually whether you are walking, strength training or stretching.

Even an efficient and effective strength-training routine will produce minimal results unless you concentrate on what you are doing. Because your brain is the most important part of your strength-building program, you cannot be daydreaming, planning lunch, reading, talking or anything else during an exercise. If you are at the gym working out, you have to be "at the gym working out." Your mind must be focused on the correct performance of the exercise and feeling the muscles you are training. Concentrating on proper form also reduces the chance of injury. Most training injuries occur to people who do not know how to do exercises correctly or to those who never vary their exercise programs.

I often see people reading books or talking while doing strength-training exercises. Many of them are talking to their personal trainers who clearly know little about safe and efficient training. A trainer or workout partner should say something like "squeeze the muscle," "push," "concentrate," "focus," or "feel the muscle," with every repetition. This keeps your mind focused on the task at hand. If you train alone, you can think these things with every repetition, much like internally repeating a mantra when meditating. The bottom line is that you must feel the muscles you are training. If you do not, your training will be far less productive than it could be. You may spend years training and make little progress for all your time and effort.

To continue making progress you *must* keep records of your workouts. You will know what you did recently in a particular exercise so you can then set a mini-goal to lift the same weight more repetitions or to lift a heavier weight. This makes your workouts more challenging and fun. I see people all the time who struggle to gain muscle but never progress because they lift the same amount of weight day after day. Because it is impossible to remember what was done previously, they have no way of tracking their progress or setting new goals for subsequent workouts. I have seen tens of thousands of people working out over the years and can count on one hand the number I have seen keeping records. I have also rarely seen any personal trainers keeping records of their client's workouts.

Exercising to gain muscular weight is the same if you are thin or fat. Your diets will be different and the fat person may be doing fat-burning exercise, but the strength and muscle-building workout should be the same. Please do not let anyone convince you otherwise. Building muscle is building muscle whether it is covered with excess fat or not.

Not enough space is available here to include proper form for numerous exercises, how to arrange them, how many sets and repetitions to do and so forth. Complete instruction on training for strength and muscular weight gain will be contained in my planned exercise book. It will teach you how to avoid injuries while making the fastest possible progress. Cardiovascular training, fat burning, stretching and other valuable and necessary information will be included.

In this book I have given you most of the basic key points of effective exercise and if you apply the knowledge it can save you much time and effort. Whether you design your own exercise program or someone designs one for you, it must follow these guidelines or it will be unsafe and far less productive than it could be.

If you train hard and eat as suggested in this chapter, you should make fast progress. Consistency is paramount, along with intensity and progression in your workouts. These are the tools that will help you develop your body to its fullest natural potential or anywhere up to it you choose. You can take pride in your accomplishments knowing you have worked hard to keep your body strong, shapely and healthy.

Eating for Muscular Growth

After stimulating your muscles to grow, you have to supply them with energy and the necessary building blocks. Think about what your body needs—energy for your brain and muscles to function, energy for your workouts, digestion, elimination, other bodily functions, and energy for repair and rebuilding. As you can see, your body's primary need is for clean-burning energy foods. Fruits, vegetables, legumes and healthful fats are the best for this purpose along with a moderate amount of whole grains. This makes it easy to understand why most foods are primarily carbohydrate.

Your body also needs amino acids, the building blocks of muscular growth. Most carbohydrate foods contain incomplete protein, which lacks one or more of the essential amino acids. Nevertheless, the amino acids in carbohydrate foods can be used for repair, muscle building and other vital functions if the missing amino acids are supplied from complete protein foods or different carbohydrate foods. If your energy needs are being supplied from healthful carbohydrates and fats, then protein can be used for its primary functions instead of for energy. You already know that protein is the poorest source of energy, because it requires extensive work to digest and convert into energy.

Many years ago I ate a high-protein diet in conjunction with my strength and muscle-building workouts. As you know, the excess protein overworked my digestive system causing severe hypoglycemia. I had numerous negative reactions and it took months of fasting, cleansing and a low-protein diet to give my body the rest it needed to restore normal function. My bodybuilding progress was severely hindered, because I could not train as hard or as often during that time. This is one of many lessons I learned the hard way.

You may have read in fitness magazines and books about bodybuilding that you need large amounts of complete protein to gain muscular body weight. Do not believe it. This is the trap I fell into years ago. I have seen many people make tremendous progress eating far less complete protein than these sources say you need. It is in the best interest of people who sell protein supplements to publicize that excessive amounts are necessary. All of these supplements are processed and are often made from casein or whey protein. And, new "specially processed" products are always coming on the market to tempt you to try again. My advice is to save your money. Eating excessive amounts of protein is expensive, unhealthful and can make you fat. You may need a little more protein if you are training extremely hard, but you will get it from the extra carbohydrates you will be eating for your additional energy requirements. Because most people eat excessive amounts of complete protein, if you ate much less than you do now, you may still have more than you need.

Not much additional protein is necessary to gain muscular body weight, because your body gains muscle tissue slowly. A male has higher testosterone levels during puberty than at any other time in his life and can gain muscular weight fast if he trains correctly. Even then you would see only about a one pound increase in muscle each week. If we analyze how muscles grow, it is easy to see why hardly any extra protein is needed each day to gain a pound of muscle in a week. Skeletal muscle is approximately 70 percent water, so a pound (16 ounces) of muscle contains 11.2 ounces of water. The remaining 4.8 ounces divided by seven days is only 0.7 ounces or approximately 20 grams of complete protein a day. Even less complete protein intake than this is necessary when you consider that whole grains, legumes and vegetables contain amino acids that combine to form complete protein. Your body also reuses some of the amino acids it gets from breaking down worn out tissues. All amino acid sources contribute to an amino acid pool your body can draw from as needed. For this reason, it is unnecessary to eat a complete protein and an incomplete protein at the same time. If you get incomplete protein (from carbohydrate foods) throughout the day and some complete protein for dinner, the amino acids will be combined and used as needed.

An hour or two after a heavy workout seems to be when our bodies uptake many of the nutrients needed for rebuilding. Therefore, your post-workout meal is very important. This meal should contain about 20 to 25 grams of protein and some complex carbohydrates to replenish the glucose and glycogen used during your workout. Because you get protein from the carbohydrate foods, you need only 10 to 15 grams from complete protein foods. A good habit is to eat an apple or other fruit and take five to ten amino acid tablets immediately after your workout. This supplies energy and readily available amino acids. Then eat your post-workout meal as soon as you can. The fruit and amino acid tablets fill in the one- to two-hour gap when your meal is being digested. It has been estimated that your body can use only about 20 to 25 grams of protein at a time. This makes sense, because eating excess protein is unnecessary and will often just overtax your digestive system or be stored as fat.

Always have a bottle of water with you when you exercise and drink a little after every set or two. This has two important benefits. It keeps your muscles well hydrated so they can work at peak efficiency. If they dehydrate by even a few percent, their strength and energy is greatly reduced. Do not rely on your body's thirst mechanism, because it cannot keep up during strenuous exercise. Also, your digestive system will have enough water to make the enzymes necessary to efficiently digest your post-workout meal. Do not walk back and forth to the drinking fountain, because you will not drink enough, it wastes valuable time, and the water may not be pure.

If you have excess body fat, your hard training should naturally reduce your appetite, because your body will be burning stored fat for its additional energy needs. If you are thin, your hard training should stimulate your body to ask for, uptake and use the extra food it needs. If you supply the demand, gaining muscular body weight requires eating only slightly more of the foods your body responds to and uses best—the process is simple and natural. You should not have to force yourself to eat excessive amounts and doing it will stress your digestive system and cause fat to be gained along with the muscle.

Another widespread misconception is that thin people cannot gain muscle unless they ingest many more calories than they can get from eating whole, natural foods. Many high-calorie, weight-gaining supplements are available. Unfortunately, most of the weight people gain using these products is fat, because the majority of people who use them do not know how to train to stimulate muscular growth. It does not take many extra calories each day to gain a pound of muscle in a week, so even if you are training properly, excess calories will be stored as fat. If your training is stimulating muscle growth, your appetite should naturally increase, but if you are not gaining, gradually eat a bit more at each meal until you start gaining lean tissue. Eating more healthful fats during the day is an excellent way for thin people to get the additional calories needed to gain muscle. If you are gaining fat instead of muscle, your training program is not stimulating muscular growth and must be changed.

When I first started weight training, I read bodybuilding magazines with advertisements for various supplements. I weighed only 120 pounds so I saved my money and bought a weight-gaining powder. This was before ingredients had to be listed on the label. I naively assumed that the product contained healthful ingredients and that those selling it were interested in promoting good health. A year or two later the law was passed that required product ingredients to be listed on the label. I bought more of the product and was shocked and angry after I read the label. The ingredients in order of amount were sugar, dry milk powder and cocoa—three unhealthful ingredients that were being sold for far more than I could have bought them for at the supermarket. Needless to say, I never wasted any money on that product again.

Some products on the market contain complex carbohydrates, protein and sometimes a little fat. They usually have only a moderate number of calories. The protein source is usually either whey or casein and is not well utilized by most people. Either can cause gas and bloating, build up as internal waste or be stored as fat. Many of the complex-carbohydrate sources are unhealthful and can overload your digestive system creating similar problems. One popular product is especially bad, but is often given to hospital patients. Being used in hospitals should be your first clue that it is unhealthful. It says on the label it is scientifically formulated and recommended by doctors. Scientists who clearly know nothing about healthful nutrition formulated it and you already know that most doctors have little knowledge of healthful eating. This product claims to be good for gaining or maintaining healthy weight. The main ingredients are corn syrup, maltodextrin (corn), sugar, corn oil, cocoa powder, and sodium and calcium caseinates. You should know by now that those ingredients are bad for you physically and emotionally and do not supply any nutrients for your body to gain or maintain healthy weight.

This product is now being marketed to the general public and many similar products are also available.

There are a large number of sports and energy drinks on the market. Many of these contain unhealthful ingredients so they can cater to the distorted tastes of most people. I have yet to see one of these products that I would recommend. To add insult to injury, they are also quite expensive.

A large number of so-called health, energy, or protein bars are currently available but I have not seen any that I consider worth eating. Many of them are made from the same ingredients as the products we just discussed, they are just condensed and shaped like a candy bar. I do not recommend them, because they are processed and contain unhealthful ingredients. They are also extremely expensive. Even a bar made of ground up nuts and dates would be a poor choice, because the nuts start to go rancid as soon as the fat in them is exposed to air. Use *real* foods such as fruits, nuts or seeds as a snack when you cannot get a regular meal.

There are hundreds of products that are claimed to produce tremendous muscular growth in a short time. Do not believe it. These products generally have a picture of a huge bodybuilder who claims that using the particular product was the secret to building his amazing physique. He may have used the product a few times or many, but without the use of illegal growth-enhancing drugs he would not look anything close to the way he does. Do not fall for these false promises. Train hard and regularly on an effective program and spend your money buying a variety of real (whole and balanced) foods that will supply your body with the nutrients needed to grow with and to be strong and healthy.

If you are thin and have attempted to gain "weight" by force-feeding yourself, you may need to go on a cleansing program before your body will start gaining muscle. Yes, you may have to cleanse first to get rid of excess internal waste that is making your system inefficient. A lot of thin people are afraid to cleanse, because they fear losing weight. Banish any fear with the knowledge that you should not lose healthy tissue during your cleanse and that you will soon be gaining lean muscle if you are training to stimulate it.

If you are thin, it is helpful to gain a few pounds of body fat as you train to gain muscle, because it gives your body an energy buffer if you occasionally miss a meal or do not eat enough. Be aware, however, so you do not gain more than three or four pounds of fat. Do not worry, those few pounds can be easily eliminated after you gain the muscle you want. Check your body fat percentage occasionally so you will know if the weight you are gaining is fat or muscle. If after six weeks you have gained five pounds of muscle and four pounds of fat, reduce your food consumption until you gain only muscle.

Gaining muscular weight is a process that develops momentum over time but has daily fluctuations as you gradually gain. It is similar to losing fat but your weight increases instead of decreases. As you train hard and eat more, it may take a while before your body starts to grow. Once you get things started, however, it is easier to keep gaining, because inertia and momentum start working for you. If you are thin and skip a meal or reduce your food intake, you can slow, or stop, your momentum. It then takes more time and effort to regain it. If you have excess fat, chances are you will be eating less, but you should not skip meals. Your training must be regular and progressive and your eating consistent if you expect to make fast progress.

Muscle-Building Goals

Setting muscle-building goals should be done before starting your bodybuilding and shaping program but is included at the end of this chapter because you needed to learn certain concepts before you could set realistic goals. We all have a unique genetic potential that determines the maximum amount of muscle we can build, but it has been my experience that the average male who has never trained for it can ultimately gain 25 to 40 pounds of muscular body weight. In other words, a thin, untrained 140-pound man could realistically weigh a lean and muscular 165 to 180 pounds. A 190-pound man with quite a bit of body fat could lose 35 pounds of fat, gain 25 pounds of muscle and end up looking terrific at 180 pounds. If this same man just lost 35 pounds of fat, his body would look weak and unattractive at 155 pounds. Remember that being healthy and looking good is not just about losing "weight" or how much you weigh.

The average woman's potential to gain muscle is much less than the average man's potential, because women's bodies produce only one-fifteenth as much testosterone—the hormone primarily responsible for muscular weight gain. The small percentage of women with higher than average testosterone levels may ultimately gain 10 to 20 pounds of muscle, but this would take a few years of hard training. The majority of them would not want to gain that much so would build their bodies to the level they want and then maintain it. Most women who train intensely lose inches, keep their bones strong, maintain a normal sex drive, strengthen their muscles and improve their figures, but gain only a few pounds of muscle. This can often be accomplished in just a few months. You may not gain much muscle, but it will make a tremendous difference in how your body looks and how you feel physically and emotionally. If you currently have excess fat, you will end up weighing much less than before you began training and have a strong, shapely body you can maintain for a long time.

Before you set your strength- and muscle-building goals, sit down and assess where you are and your current physical attributes. Do you have a small, medium or large frame? How tall are you? What is your current weight and what is your body fat percentage? Some of these variations have a major impact on what you can expect to gain. To calculate your frame size, first measure your height (without shoes) in centimeters (.3937 inches). Then measure around your right wrist just above (toward your elbow) the heel of your hand. Now divide your wrist circumference (also in centimeters) into your height. For men, if the number is between 9.6 and 10.4, you have a medium frame. If it is less than 9.6, your frame is large, and if more than 10.4, your frame is small. For women, 10.1 to 11.0 is considered medium, less than 10.1 is large and more than 11.0 is a small frame.

Once you have your frame size, height, weight, body fat percentage and measurements, you are ready to start. Now you will be able to accurately monitor your progress. Do not worry about setting measurement goals. It is exciting and motivating, however, to see your measurements change. Some may not change much, but the shape and muscle-to-fat ratio should improve dramatically. If you have excess fat, all you need is a body fat percentage goal. Eat well and train hard to lower your body fat percentage and the measurements will take care of themselves. Your weight will also but you may want to have a target weight to work toward. After you have achieved your goals, there may be some areas you want to build and shape a bit more. You can set new goals at that time.

The average man starting an *effective* strength and muscle-building program can expect to gain one-half to one pound of muscle a week. After gaining 10 to 15 pounds, it may slow to a gain of one-quarter to one-half pound each week. The average woman will gain much slower and less total. If your goal is to reach your peak physical potential, you have started a never-ending quest, but most people will come close within two or three years. If you are male and all you want to do is gain 10 to 15 pounds of muscle, this can often be accomplished in a few months but then you must train to maintain it.

As you get closer to your physical potential in any athletic activity, your rate of progress will get slower. It is much easier for people who are just starting out to gain an inch on their chest and arm measurements than it is for those who have been training for a while and are closer to their physical potentials.

Another thing to consider when setting muscle-building goals is your body type. An ectomorph is thin with a fast metabolism, a mesomorph is fairly muscular with a moderate metabolism and an endomorph has a slower metabolism and tends to have higher amounts of body fat. Your body type has significant influence on how fast you gain and how much you can ultimately achieve. An ectomorph usually gains muscle more slowly than an endomorph or mesomorph, but has no trouble staying lean. If you are an endomorph, your body fat levels will need to be monitored more often so you do not gain excess fat as you gain muscle. Most endomorphs will be working toward losing body fat as they gain muscle. If you are a mesomorph, consider yourself lucky, because you can gain muscle quite fast and easily stay lean. Most of us are a combination of two of these body types but it should not be hard for you to determine your distinct type or combination.

Many thin people are afraid to eat foods containing fat but if you are primarily ectomorphic you should eat more nuts, seeds, avocados, fatty fish, healthful oils and whole grains. These good fats will supply the extra calories you need without bloating you or overloading your digestive system. Do not worry, if you eat these foods between morning and mid-afternoon they will be used for energy and not stored as body fat.

Your age influences how fast and how far you can progress. Do not feel, however, that just because you are older you cannot make dramatic improvements in your strength, body shape and composition. You have learned that a major part of aging is the loss of strength and muscle mass, and that this often leads to fat being gained subcutaneously or interlaid between the muscle fibers. Exercising to keep strength and muscle mass high and body fat low can reverse many of the effects of aging. This, along with preventing free-radical damage, keeping joints aligned and muscles flexible with PMBT treatments, and eating as you have learned, would be like finding the elusive fountain of youth. I know people who are over sixty but are stronger, healthier and look better than most people half their age. It is never too late to reap the benefits of proper exercise and wholesome, balanced nutrition.

It is important to set sensible, realistic and attainable goals. If your goals are unrealistic, you may get discouraged and quit, thereby losing out on all the amazing benefits you could enjoy. A tall, large-framed, endomorphic woman having a goal to weigh 125 pounds with 15 percent body fat would be absurd. A weight of 150 pounds with 25 percent fat would be attainable and she would look better than she would at the lower weight. There may have been a time as a young adult when your body looked good. That could be a realistic weight goal for you and the weight may even end up being more muscle and less fat than it was then.

If you are a short, ectomorphic male weighing 115 pounds, a goal of 195 pounds is never going to happen. Eat well and train hard on a productive routine and chances are you will reach your physical potential within a couple of years. Be happy with that and enjoy your life. Do not become obsessed with gaining more and make yourself unhappy in the process. If your role models are professional bodybuilders who use anabolic steroids, growth hormone, diuretics and other unhealthy drugs, you may get terribly disillusioned when you do not look like they do.

You must realize that the people who make it to the top in competitive bodybuilding have extraordinary genetic potential *and* take growth-enhancing drugs. These drugs allow them to overtrain, train with lighter weights, use numerous one joint movements and still develop huge, well-defined muscles. Without the drugs, this is physiologically impossible. Following their routines from books or magazines will cause you to overtrain, lose hard-earned muscle and possibly become discouraged and quit training. I have trained numerous people who had followed these kinds of exercise programs for years with no results. After I put them on a basic, but intense, routine they made rapid progress.

I trained for years at Gold's Gym® in Venice, California, and observed certain professional bodybuilders with much larger bodies than mine using about one-half the amount of weight I used for the same exercise. This was possible because certain drugs stimulate muscular growth with light, pumping exercises. They gain by pumping the drug into the muscles. If you train naturally, getting a pump in your muscles is detrimental and training the way they do will slow or stop your progress. I also saw huge bodybuilders lose 20 to 30 pounds of muscle in just a month or two after they stopped using the drugs. These drugs are physically harmful and often devastating emotionally when these bodybuilders see their muscles shrink rapidly and their bodies gain fat. Many of them end up looking like they have never worked out a day in their lives, because they never learned how to train without drugs.

You will never gain muscle tissue doing long marathon workouts, nor will you need or be able to use the excess calories and protein someone taking anabolic steroids or growth hormone would. I know of a professional bodybuilder who had to ingest 9,000 calories a day just to keep from losing weight during a certain cycle of steroids and growth hormone. This is not normal or natural. Therefore, do not follow the diets of the drug users either. Typically they eat brown rice and oatmeal for carbohydrates and chicken breasts, fish and egg whites for protein—all acidic foods. Fruits, vegetables and legumes are seldom eaten. Most have almost no variety in their meals and many of them eat unhealthful foods such as cake and pie when not training for a bodybuilding competition. You already know that the drugs allow body fat to be burned after the body's natural protective mechanism would have told it to stop burning fat. Because this feedback mechanism is triggered by a reduction in testosterone, anabolic steroids, which are similar to testosterone, override it. The drug user's body is unaware that body fat levels are dropping dangerously low. This is why you can never get the extreme degree of muscular definition naturally that someone using drugs can, even if you are eating better and doing much more fat-burning exercise.

Naturally training role models may be motivating for you or you could just use your own progress for inspiration. The picture method and visualization described in chapter fourteen can be used for building muscle as well as losing fat. Eat healthfully, train hard, regularly and naturally, and you can build a strong, shapely *and* healthy body that will serve you well for a long time. Enjoy the journey of life to its fullest in the most efficient and attractive vehicle you can create.

Be not afraid of life. Believe that life is worth living, and
your belief will help create the fact.

William James

Good for the body is the work of the body, and
good for the soul is the work of the soul, and
good for either is the work of the other.

Henry David Thoreau

Man's mind, once stretched by a new idea,
never regains its original dimensions.

Oliver Wendell Holmes

It is part of the cure to want to be cured.

Seneca

Most of us will do anything to be good
except change our way of living.

Anonymous

It's not what happens to us,
But what happens in us
That supremely counts.

Anonymous

EPILOGUE

All success is built on the principle of repetition. I mentioned this in the introduction but it is so important that it warrants repeating (pun intended). Winning sports teams repeat plays that win games for them, singers sing the same songs to different audiences, sales people recite the same sales pitch to different customers and lean, healthy people repeat healthful eating and exercise habits. Generally, once people learn what works for them, they simply repeat it. Whatever you do at home or work, you repeat the same successful actions. Each successful day leads to another and before long, ten successful years have gone by and eventually a successful life. Once you find the right nutritional program for you and develop some good health habits to replace the bad ones, maintaining your success requires nothing more than letting the power of habit work for you instead of against you.

Here is a saying that perfectly illustrates my point:

> I am your constant companion. I am your greatest helper or heaviest burden. I will push you onward or drag you down to failure. I am completely at your command. Half the things you do you might just as well turn over to me and I will be able to do them quickly and correctly. I am easily managed—you must merely be firm with me. Show me exactly how you want something done and after a few lessons I will do it automatically. I am the servant of all great men; and alas, of all failures as well. Those who are great, I have made great. Those who are failures, I have made failures. I am not a machine, though I work with all the precision of a machine plus the intelligence of a man. You may run me for profit or run me for ruin—it makes no difference to me. Take me, train me, be firm with me, and I will place the world at your feet. Be easy with me and I will destroy you. WHO AM I? I AM HABIT!

That saying is titled HABIT and its author is anonymous. Always keep in mind that once you bury a bad habit you do not have to visit the grave.

I am grateful to have been blessed with a brain capable of learning quite easily. Nevertheless, I had to see some of the principles in this book many times before I understood each one's true essence. I had to have one more success or failure, have the idea explained in a different way, or be given one more example before it finally became a truth I will never forget. I have done my best to simplify the principles you need and to express them in different ways to make learning them easy. If you have problems following a healthful nutritional program or are not losing fat or gaining muscle as fast as you would like to, reread the applicable section of this book and chances are you will learn why. Always remember that it is just as easy to eat and live healthfully as it is to eat and live unhealthfully.

Now a few final thoughts and reminders. The purpose of this book is to supply you with *all* the pieces of the permanent fat-loss puzzle *and* how to put them together properly so you can see and truly understand the big picture. If you think of it as a hundred-piece puzzle, I have given you the 95 pieces common to us all and numerous ideas on how to discover your five special pieces—the ones with your face on them right in the middle of the picture. Some of the concepts and beliefs are my own but are based on my more than thirty-seven years of studying nutrition, observing Nature, studying and observing human nature and on many years of nutritional and exercise experience working with my own body and numerous clients and patients. I again want to thank all the researchers, health and nutritional pioneers, spiritual teachers, philosophers, role models and others I have learned from for the lean body and healthy life I enjoy. I especially want to thank Nature for life itself, the lessons life is constantly teaching and the joy we can experience if we choose love over fear.

I do not claim to know (or that I will ever know) all the answers but I do know enough to help almost anyone accomplish the goal of permanent fat loss. You have been advised to keep learning, especially about your unique needs. Experiment and determine what is best for you and then make it a habit. Always keep your mind open to new truths, but do not let some "expert" discourage you or change your mind about something you know in your heart is true. Determine the value of new information based on the truths you have learned here. Ask yourself if Nature intended it and if it is balanced—then let your true self be your guide. The truth about UFOs may be "out there" but the truth for your health and happiness is within you. Never forget this.

Your success is important to me so please—pretty please *without* sugar on it—start again and read all the important points you have highlighted. Why? Because a *tremendous* number of concepts you did not grasp the first time will be easily understood now that you have seen the big picture. The ideas you missed the first time may be the primary keys to *your* success. You may have already started to develop a healthier lifestyle. If you have not, use visualization or the picture method explained in chapter fourteen to stimulate you to action. There are seven days in the week and none of them is named Someday. You must decide *now* that you want to be lean and healthy. Chances are that all of the knowledge you need to succeed is within you or in this book, so do not stop searching until you find your special truths. Good luck as you begin your quest. It is a wonderful journey and you have already taken some crucial steps. All you need to do is love yourself as you are, supply healthful nourishment to your body, mind and spirit, experience mostly joy in your life, enjoy each new moment and keep travelling where your heart knows you belong.

SUMMARY

Find your reason to be lean.

Discover and eliminate your causes for excess body fat.

Learn what, why, how and when to eat and drink.

Always eat when you feel hungry.

Eat a variety of whole, natural foods to supply your body's needs and leave it feeling satisfied.

Never feed your body when your mind or spirit need nourishment.

A positive and inexpensive diet is the BEST. Balanced, Efficient, Simple and Timed right.

Think about what every food and drink will do for you and your body before you ingest it and then choose good health.

Eat three moderately sized meals and one or two snacks daily.

Let your body tell you how much to eat.

Eat good food combinations.

Determine the best nutritional plan for you. Use a food diary if necessary.

Eat mostly healthful fats, fruits and whole complex carbohydrates during the day to supply your energy needs.

Eat most of your complete protein for the day at your evening meal.

Develop a number of healthful meals that you really enjoy.

Try new natural foods as you discover them.

Make and follow a one- or two-week eating schedule.

Always be prepared by having a variety of whole, natural foods available at home and when you are away.

Have a supply of foods for back-up meals.

Reverse shop at the grocery store.

Avoid the grocery store aisles with candy, soft drinks and other junk foods.

Eat organic foods and healthy meats.

Drink an adequate amount of pure water.

Drink a glass or two of water 30 to 60 minutes before eating.

Do not drink with your meals or for approximately 90 minutes after. You can drink water when eating only fruit.

Eat slowly so you will enjoy your meal more and give your body time to tell you when it has had enough.

Chew all foods well.

Eat plenty of raw foods.

Cook foods in healthful ways like steaming, baking, poaching and slow cooking.

Do not eat when you are angry or upset.

Eat foods when they are in season.

Follow my four seasons food pyramids.

If you eat late, eat less and a lighter and more easily digested meal.

Thoroughly cleanse your body if necessary.

Give your digestive system periodic rests with short cleanses.

Eat more alkaline foods if your goal is to lose excess fat.

Eat a balance of acid and alkaline foods if your goal is to maintain your current fat-to-lean ratio.

Get an adequate amount of natural, balanced light every day. Avoid unbalanced light sources as much as possible.

Learn to breathe properly so the cells of your body will get the amount of oxygen they need to be healthy.

Get an adequate amount of sleep.

Reduce or eliminate the use of alcohol, caffeine, dairy products, sugar, honey and artificial sweeteners.

Reduce or eliminate the use of salt, chocolate and cocoa, processed foods and foods containing harmful chemicals.

Do not smoke or use harmful drugs.

Choose healthful meals that are available at good restaurants.

Avoid eating desserts, especially right after a meal.

Do not eat at fast-food restaurants.

Limit "pig-out" meals to once or twice a month if you eat them at all.

Eat mostly cleansing foods the day after a pig-out meal.

Do not have unhealthful foods in your home.

Take a good multivitamin and mineral supplement every day.

Take a powerful antioxidant supplement daily.

Use other nutritional supplements as needed but get tested for need and dosage.

Do selfless service for others.

Continue learning new positive things.

See the positive side of everything and turn stumbling blocks into stepping stones.

Do positive activities that feed your mind and improve your self-image and self-confidence.

Give thanks daily for your blessings.

Eliminate as many sources of stress as possible.

Learn how to reduce any stress in your life that you cannot eliminate.

Find a way to express your creativity in positive and healthy ways.

Accept yourself 100 percent unconditionally as you are right now.

Discover and support your weak link.

Feed your children healthful foods.

Teach your children the value of eating well and exercising regularly by being a good example.

Avoid dieting and the use of unhealthful weight-loss products and drugs.

Avoid liposuction, gastric bypass and other dangerous surgeries.

Harness the six powers that make people fat to make you lean.

Follow the nutritional laws of Nature and reap the benefits.

Develop healthy thinking, eating and exercise habits.

Use the powers of inertia and momentum to help you achieve your goals.

Harness the incredible power of your subconscious mind to create your wants.

Love yourself, other people, animals, and the world around you.

Shape and strengthen your body.

Complete two to four strength-training sessions every week. Two full-body workouts or two half-body workouts and two workouts for the other half of your body.

Do fat-burning exercise after your strength-training sessions if you have time.

After you are at your best weight and body fat percentage, do one or two 30-minute cardiovascular training sessions each week if you have time.

<u>Be a lean person.</u>

Choose to be lean and healthy and it will be easy to make the choices that will create that result.

Feed your mind daily by seeing the positive side of everything, learning new things and expressing your creativity in a positive way.

Embrace and enjoy change.

Enjoy a minimum of ten minutes of three different soul-food activities daily.

Respect yourself and everything and everyone else in your life.

Associate with healthy, loving people.

Organize your life.

Pay attention to what you are eating and why.

Maintain awareness of your thought processes and keep your focus on what you do want, not what you don't want.

Buy yourself some new clothes or nice gifts with the money you save by not buying junk food or spending it on weight-loss products or medical bills caused by excess fat.

Eliminate your physical and emotional addictions to unhealthful foods and activities.

Set goals and then break them down into mini-goals that make completing them simple.

Use the picture method and visualization to help you accomplish your goals.

Develop the habits of lean people.

See what you are gaining, not what you are losing.

Eat to live, don't live to eat.

Education is not filling a bucket but
lighting a fire.
William Butler Yeats

BIBLIOGRAPHY

I acknowledge the efforts of, and thank all the people who contributed to these references but were not listed by name. I also thank all of those who contributed to the references that are not listed specifically.

Abravanel, Elliot D., M.D., and Elizabeth A. King. *Dr. Abravanel's Body Type Diet and Lifetime Nutrition Plan*. New York: Bantam Books, 1983.

Airola, Paavo, N.D., Ph.D. *Hypoglycemia: A Better Approach*. Phoenix, Arizona: Health Plus, 1977.

Atkins, Robert C., M.D. *Atkins for Life: The Complete Controlled Carb Program for Permanent Weight Loss and Good Health*. New York: St. Martin's Press, 2003.

Beers, Mark H., M.D., and Robert Berkow, M.D., editors. *The Merck Manual*. Whitehouse Station, N.J.: Merck Research Laboratories, 1999.

Bragg, Paul C., N.D., Ph.D., with Patricia Bragg, Ph.D. *Healthful Eating Without Confusion*. Desert Hot Springs, California: Health Science, 1976.

Bragg, Paul C., N.D., Ph.D., with Patricia Bragg, Ph.D. *The Miracle of Fasting*. Santa Barbara, California: Health Science, 1977.

Bruno, Frank J., Dr. *Think Yourself Thin*. New York: Harper & Row, 1972.

Cheraskin, E., M.D., D.M.D., and W. M. Ringsdorf, Jr., D.M.D., M.S., with Arline Brecher. *Psychodietetics: Food As The Key To Emotional Health*. Briarcliff Manor, New York: Stein and Day, 1974.

Christopher, John R., Dr., M.H. *Just What Is The Word Of Wisdom?* Revised ed. Provo, Utah: Dr. John R. Christopher, M.H., 1941.

Christopher, John R., M.H. *Dr. Christopher's Three Day Cleansing Program And Mucusless Diet*. Revised ed. Provo, Utah: Dr. Christopher, 1978.

Clark, Hulda Regehr, Ph.D., N.D. *The Cure For All Cancers*. San Diego, CA: ProMotion Publishing, 1993.

Clark, Hulda Regehr, Ph.D., N.D. *The Cure For All Diseases*. San Diego, CA: ProMotion Publishing, 1995.

D'Adamo, Peter J., Dr., with Catherine Whitney. *Eat Right 4 Your Type: The Individualized Diet Solution to Staying Healthy, Living Longer & Achieving Your Ideal Weight*. New York: Putnam, 1996.

Ehret, Arnold, Prof. *Prof. Arnold Ehret's Mucusless Diet Healing System*. Beaumont, California: Ehret Literature Publishing Co., 1977.

Glanze, Walter D., Managing editor. *Mosby's Medical and Nursing Dictionary*. 2nd ed. St. Louis, Missouri: C. V. Mosby Company, 1986.

Grabhorn, Lynn. *Excuse Me, Your Life Is Waiting*. San Bruno, CA: Audio Literature, 2000. (audiobook)

Gray, John, Ph.D. *What Your Mother Couldn't Tell You & Your Father Didn't Know: Advanced Relationship Skills for Better Communication and Lasting Intimacy*. New York, New York: Harper Collins Publishers Inc., 1994.

Guyton, Arthur C., M.D. *Textbook of Medical Physiology*. 7th ed. Philadelphia, PA: W.B. Saunders Company, 1986.

Kirschmann, John D., Director of Nutrition Search Inc. *Nutrition Almanac*. New York: McGraw-Hill, 1975.

Krause, Marie V., B.S., M.S., R.D., and L. Kathleen Mahan, M.S., R.D. *Food, Nutrition, and Diet Therapy*. 7th ed. Philadelphia, PA: W.B. Saunders Company, 1984.

Kroeger, Hanna, MsD, Rev. *Old Time Remedies For Modern Ailments*. Boulder, Colorado: Rev. Hanna Kroeger, MsD, 1971.

Langer, Stephen, M.D., with James F. Scheer. *Solved: The Riddle of Weight Loss*. Rochester, Vermont: Healing Arts Press, 1989.

Liddle, Verle A. and Theron C., editors. *A Thought for Today*. Volume III. Salt Lake City, UT: Liddle Enterprises, Inc.,1965.

Lindlahr, Victor H. *Eat and Reduce*. Garden City, New York: Permabooks/Doubleday & Company, 1953.

Maltz, Maxwell, M.D., F.I.C.S. *Psycho-Cybernetics*. New York: Pocket Books, Inc., 1966.

Martin, Ralph J., D.C. *The Practice of Correction of Abnormal Function: "Neurovascular Dynamics" (NVD)*. Sierra Madre, California: Ralph J. Martin, D.C., 1983.

McGraw, Phillip C., Ph.D., *Life Strategies: Doing What Works, Doing What Matters*. New York: Hyperion, 1999.

Mindell, Earl, R.Ph., Ph.D. *Earl Mindell's HERB BIBLE*. New York: Simon & Schuster/Fireside, 1992.

Ott, John N. *Health and Light*. Columbus, Ohio—Atlanta , Georgia: Ariel Press, 1973

Pitcairn, Richard H., D.V.M., Ph.D., and Susan Hubble Pitcairn. *Dr. Pitcairn's Complete Guide to Natural Health for Dogs and Cats*. Emmaus, PA: Rodale Press, 1982.

Rodale, J. I., and staff. *The Complete Book of Food and Nutrition*. Emmaus, Pennsylvania: Rodale Books, Inc., 1971.

Ryan, M. J. *Attitudes of gratitude—How to Give and Receive Joy Every Day of Your Life*. Berkeley, California: Conari Press, 1999.

Sears, Barry, Ph.D., with Bill Lawren. *The Zone: A Revolutionary Life Plan to Put Your Body in Total Balance for Permanent Weight Loss*. New York: HarperCollins, 1995.

Shelton, Herbert M. *Food Combining Made Easy*. San Antonio, Texas: Dr. Shelton's Health School, 1951.

Sifton, David W., Editor-in-Chief. *The PDR® Family Guide to Nutrition and Health™*. Montvale, N.J.: Medical Economics Company, 1995.

Snyder, Arthur W., Ph.D. *Foods That Preserve the Alkaline Reserve*. 10th ed. Los Angeles, California: Hansen's, 1962.

Valentine, Tom and Carole. *Medicine's Missing Link: Metabolic Typing and Your Personal Food Plan*. Rochester, Vermont: Thorsons Publishers, Inc., 1987.

Weil, Andrew, M.D. *Eating Well For Optimum Health: The Essential Guide to Food, Diet, and Nutrition*. New York: Alfred A. Knopf, 2000.

Numerous nutritional seminars from James M. Gerber, M.S., D.C., DABCO, DABCN and one nutritional seminar from Ernest Caldwell, D.C.

Government and specific disease-research Web sites.

A number of television health and news programs.

Thousands of articles from health newsletters, newspapers and magazines.

INDEX

A

Abravanel, Elliot D., M.D., 155
abuse, physical, verbal or sexual, 395-396
acetaldehyde, 285, 286
acetic acid, 285
acid foods, 47
acid/alkaline balance, 46-49, 205, 287
acidophilus. see Lactobacillus acidophilus
addiction(s), 287, 347, 371
  chocolate, 120
  drug, 284, 289, 346, 463, 464
  emotional, 129, 285, 347, 387-389
  food, 346
  physical, 288, 387, 388, 433, 447
  salt, 333
  sugar, 107, 333
adrenal gland dysfunction, 328
adrenaline, 100
  See also epinephrine
aflatoxin, 107, 260, 262, 265
African Americans, 124, 282, 377
African tribesman, 44, 418
aging, 297-304
ailments, mysterious, 215-216
air purifier, 73, 210, 376
Airola, Paavo, 280
albumin, 57
alcohol
  detrimental effects of, 95-98
  isopropyl, 67, 122, 259, 260, 262, 263,
   265
alcohol dehydrogenase, 285
Alcoholics Anonymous (AA), 285, 287
alcoholism, 284-290
aldehyde dehydrogenase, 285
Alexander Technique, 233
algin, 206, 208
alkaline foods, 47
allergy
  casein, 106, 345
  food, 113, 136, 167, 286, 292, 306,
   307, 331, 332, 342, 344, 345-348
aluminum, 68, 119, 142, 208, 271, 294,
  421
Alzheimer's disease, 68, 114, 127, 208,
  210, 293-295
amazake, 84, 195

American Academy of Pediatrics (AAP),
  105, 306
American Cancer Society, 261
amino acids
  essential, 56, 85, 87, 88, 486
  nonessential, 56
  pool, 487
  tablets, 148, 487
ammonia, 416
amylase
  pancreatic, 137, 306
  salivary, 137, 306
amyloid protein bundles, 295
anabolic steroids, 58, 103, 184, 308, 317,
  444, 445, 477, 481, 492, 493
anemia, 205, 305
  cow's milk and, 105
  fatigue and, 30, 332
  HCl and, 136
  iron-deficiency, 136, 211, 220, 296
  RA and, 296
  sickle cell, 210
anger, 136, 137, 138, 139
  epinephrine and, 283
  expressing, 242, 259, 265
  repressed, 242
  self-judgement and, 359
anorexia nervosa, 432
anti-aging, 298, 348
antibiotics, 165, 278, 291
  friendly bacteria and, 93
  immune system and, 93, 103
  meat and, 41, 42, 93, 184, 308
  milk and, 102, 308
antibodies, 57, 71, 104, 205, 306
antidiuretic hormone (ADH), 65
antioxidant supplements, 76, 210, 211,
  218, 219, 252, 259, 266, 304, 414
appearance, more attractive, 33-34
applied kinesiology, 386, 404
  allergy testing with, 167, 169, 347
  nutritional needs and, 169, 211-212,
   405
aromatherapy, 78
arteriosclerosis, 67, 106, 253, 254, 256
arthritic hands self-treatment video, 2, 302

F

insulin, 280, 281, 282, 283
  blood sugar and, 97, 100, 109, 110,
    277, 280, 413, 420, 428
  diabetes and, 281, 282, 440
  exercise and, 283, 420
  fat storage and, 84, 112, 148, 420
  receptors, 283
  strength training and, 223
intestinal flukes, 259, 260
iodine, 205
  sources of, 42, 118, 119, 206
  thyroid gland and, 206, 293, 324, 350
ions
  negative, 73, 242
  positive, 242, 332, 376
iron
  electrolytic, 307
  excess, 206
  foods containing, 41, 47, 88, 307
  infants and, 306
isopropyl alcohol, 67, 122, 259, 260,
  262, 263, 265

J

Jesus, 265
joint
  misalignment, 231, 232, 300, 301
  pain
    See also arthritis
    aspartame and, 114
    attention and, 363
    cause of, 226, 231, 295
    exercise and, 226, 227, 228, 302, 395,
      478
    fat loss and, 301, 401, 478
    fatigue and, 331
    food allergies and, 346
    hypoglycemia and, 278
    PMBT and, 168, 232, 233, 303, 478
    red meat and, 43, 418
    Solanaceae family and, 296
    stretching and, 232, 233
    vitamin C and, 214

K

Kelley, Dr. William D., 153

kelp, 30, 119, 120, 160, 195, 196, 206,
  208, 307
ketone bodies, 415
ketosis, 416
knowledge, 27, 405
Koplan, Jeffrey K., M.D., M.P.H., 22

L

lactalbumin, 103
lactase enzyme, 104, 269
Lactobacillus acidophilus, 105
Lactobacillus bifidus, 104
lactose intolerance, 104, 105, 347
  symptoms of, 104
laughter, benefits of, 244, 265, 375
laws
  Nature's, 20, 156, 217, 377, 429, 430,
    431, 434
  nutritional, 27, 405
laxative
  effect, 44
  herbal, 176, 472
lean, staying, **465**
lean body mass
  increasing , **476-485**
  loss of, 48, 223, 310, 320, 326, 338,
    348-350, 411
learn(ing) new things, **236**, 237, 240, 334
lecithin, 88, 253, 295, 472
legumes, **85-86**
leptin, 377
life
  longer and healthier, **31-33**, 133, 457
  unbalanced, 247, **390-395**, 470
life force, 85, 114, 123, 126, 202, 441
  definition of, 146-147
  microwave cooking and, 142
  processing and, 82, 121, 412
Life Strategies (McGraw), 464
lifestyle, lean, 343, **407-410**, 469
L-5-hydroxytryptophan (5-HTP), 329
ligand, 139, 165, 327
light
  artificial, 264, 301, 302
  blue, 75
  fluorescent, 74, 75, 293
  full-spectrum, 73-77, 214, 243, 269,
    289, 329, 375

vitamin(s) *(continued)*
  E,
    blood pressure and, 204
    blood-thinning effect of, 258
    chlorine and, 67
    iron and, 203
    low-fat diet and, 59
    magnesium and, 287
    olive oil and, 64
  fat-soluble, 59, 62, 204, 211, 428, 431
  K, 59, 204, 205
    friendly bacteria and, 67, 93, 204
    low-fat diet and, 59
  T, 295
  water-soluble, 66, 204

W

walking
  aerobic fitness and, 227, 228
  calories burned while, 426
  fat burning and, 229, 426, 471
water
  ADH and, 65
  balance, 117, 118, 205, 256, 444
  bottled spring, 67, 69
  carbonated, 65, 108
  chlorinated, 67, 93, 254
  distilled, 69, 175
  fatigue and, 64, 65, 66, 70, 98, 332
  filters, 69
  fluoridated, 67, 68, 276, 294, 308
  functions of, **64-66**
  how much, 65, 66
  muscles and, 64, 65, 271, 272, 303, 472, 487
  obesity and, 66, 117
  retention, 60, 273, 328, 336, 416, 444
  sea, 69, 119, 206
  soft, 296
  sparkling mineral, 194
  temperature, 69
  when to drink, 27, 134, 135, 174, 418, 419, 487
weakest link, your, **251-253**
weight-gaining supplements, 164, 488
weight-loss
  centers, 22, 168, 312, 423, 425, 436, 437, 439

  drugs, 22, **431**, 433, 435
  ideas, **417-427**, **431-435**
  products, 101, **427-430**
weight training. *see* exercise, strength-building
What Your Mother Couldn't Tell You & Your Father Didn't Know (Gray), 393
whey, 103, 486, 488
white willow bark, 258
wine, 102, 346, 388, 418
  allergies and, 345
  digestion and, 97, 134, 286
  obesity and, 338
"Winner's Club", 439, 440
winter
  blues, 73, 329
  foods, 43, 44, 59, 81, 83, 85, 87, 92, 192, 214, 329
  meals, **188-193**
  pyramid, **92**
Wolcott, William L., 154
work, use or action, **28**, **406**
World Health Organization (WHO), 268
writing method, the, **140**, 242

Y

yoga, 232
yogurt, 21, 90, 93, 107, 108, 226, 418
yo-yo effect, 20, 396

Z

zinc deficiency, 96, 279, 290, 296

Note: Bold listings indicate headings, subheadings and primary sections.